Wolff's
HEADACHE AND
OTHER HEAD PAIN

Erratum Slip

Wolff's Headache and Other Head Pain
SIXTH EDITION

The dosage for methysergide in the chart on page 188 is incorrect. The correct dosage is 2 mg tid-gid.

Wolff's
HEADACHE
and other head pain

Edited by

DONALD J. DALESSIO, M.D., F.A.C.P.
Senior Consultant, Division of Neurology
Scripps Clinic & Research Foundation
La Jolla, California

STEPHEN D. SILBERSTEIN, M.D., F.A.C.P.
Co-Director, Comprehensive Headache Center
at The Germantown Hospital and Medical Center
Clinical Professor of Neurology
Temple University School of Medicine
Philadelphia, Pennsylvania

Sixth Edition

New York   Oxford
OXFORD UNIVERSITY PRESS
1993

Oxford University Press

Oxford   New York   Toronto
Delhi   Bombay   Calcutta   Madras   Karachi
Kuala Lumpur   Singapore   Hong Kong   Tokyo
Nairobi   Dar es Salaam   Cape Town
Melbourne   Auckland   Madrid

and associated companies in
Berlin   Ibadan

Published by Oxford University Press, Inc.
200 Madison Avenue, New York, New York 10016

Oxford is a registered trademark of Oxford University Press

Library of Congress Cataloging-in-Publication Data

Wolff's headache and other head pain. — 6th ed. / edited by Donald J.
Dalessio and Stephen D. Silberstein.
p. cm.   Includes bibliographical references and index.
ISBN 0-19-508250-8
1. Headache.   I. Wolff, Harold G. (Harold George), 1898–
II. Dalessio, Donald J., 1931–   .   III. Silberstein, Stephen D.
IV. Wolff, Harold G. (Harold George), 1898–   .
Headache and other head pain.   V. Title: Headache and other pain.
[DNLM: 1. Headache.   WL 342 W856]
RB128.W68 1993 616.8'491—dc20
DNLM/DLC for Library of Congress   92-48683

9 8 7 6 5 4 3 2 1

Printed in the United States of America
on acid-free paper

For Jane
For Catherine, James and Kris, and Susan

To Marsha Silberstein, Milton Shy, and John Bevilacqua

Preface to the Sixth Edition

With this, the sixth edition, the life of this book spans four decades. That it is still extant, vibrant, and useful is a source of pride and gratification for its editors and authors.

Since the fifth edition, there has been an explosion of headache knowledge and information. A new international headache classification has been published and is used in this edition. We have much more information about headache epidemiology; therefore Chapter 3, "Inheritance and Epidemiology of Headache," has been completely rewritten. The serotonin theory of migraine, first formulated thirty years ago, has gained new support and emphasis with the discovery of serotonin brain receptors. The advances in this area are detailed in Chapter 4, "The Pathophysiology of Migraine." This rapidly-evolving field has spawned a new class of medications which should revolutionize headache treatment. This has been described in detail in Chapter 5, "Migraine Diagnosis and Treatment." Neuroimaging has come into its own since the previous edition, and this new information has been incorporated into Chapter 18, "Radiologic Investigation of Headache." A new chapter dealing with headache associated with abnormalities in intracranial structure or pressure (including brain tumor and post-LP headache) has been included in this edition (Chapter 19).

We have made a special effort to integrate new data with older, proven observations; still, much remains to be resolved and investigated. As Doctor Wolff observed in his preface to the first edition, here is the account as far as it has gone.

La Jolla   D.J.D.
Philadelphia   S.D.S.
April 1993

Preface to the First Edition

Since the human animal prides himself on "using his head," it is ironic and perhaps not without meaning that his head should be the source of so much discomfort. Though pain always means "something wrong," with headache it most often means "wrong direction" or "wrong pace"—a biologic reprimand rather than a threat. Thus, the vast majority of discomforts and pains of the head stem from readily reversible bodily changes, and are accompaniments of resentments and dissatisfactions. On the other hand, the headaches of brain tumor, brain abscess, fever, arteritis, meningitis, subdural and subarachnoid hemorrhage, and the pains of major neuralgias and neuritides, which call for prompt and often heroic measures, constitute only a minor portion of the total number of pains of the head. Headache may be equally intense whether its implications are malignant or benign, and though there are few instances in human experience where so much pain may mean so little in terms of tissue injury, failure to separate the ominous from the trivial may cost life or create paralyzing fear.

Some fifteen years ago, during attempts to learn about the cerebral circulation, it was noted that the major cerebral blood vessels are covered by a network of nerve fibers having to do with pain. From these elementary observations has grown a series of investigations on headache. One part of the head after the other has been explored, and thus, piece by piece, the headache picture has been put together. Happily, in the intervening years the curiosity of bold and able workers has been aroused by the problem, and the chapters that follow are mainly the results of their efforts.

Headache as a subject for investigation has fared badly through being divided among "specialists." In an effort to unify the topic, the author and his colleagues have had the temerity to transgress divisions. By thus approaching the problem from many angles and with a variety of tools, we have tried to increase the knowledge of the natural history of headaches and other head pains, and to track down some of their mechanisms, to the end that suffering may be prevented or relieved. Doubtless there is much to correct and to clarify, but here is the account as far as it has gone.

New York Hospital   H.G.W.

Acknowledgments

For the facts and formulations of this volume, we are indebted to many persons. Books are collaborative projects, and their creation is invariably the work of many hands. We especially thank our contributors, and their helpers, for sharing of time and information as we worked together toward a common goal.

Alice Green has contributed to the organization of the volume, kept the mail flowing, and helped with meeting deadlines.

James Dalessio provided invaluable help in assembling data, copyediting, and writing.

Deep appreciation to Lynne Kaiser, who knows every comma and semicolon in this book, and to Nikki Dooner, who put them there.

As always, our relationships with the editors at Oxford University Press, especially Jeffrey House, have been outstanding.

Contents

Contributors

Otto Appenzeller, M.D., Ph.D.
Professor of Neurology
University of New Mexico School of
Medicine
Albuquerque, New Mexico

Thomas J. Carlow, M.D.
Clinical Professor of Neurology and
Neuro-ophthalmology
University of New Mexico School of
Medicine
Albuquerque, New Mexico

Robert J. Coffey, M.D.
Assistant Professor of Neurosurgery
Mayo Clinic
Rochester, Minnesota

Donald J. Dalessio, M.D.
Senior Consultant in Neurology
Scripps Clinic & Research Foundation
La Jolla, California

Seymour Diamond, M.D.
Director, Diamond Headache Clinic
Adjunct Professor of Pharmacology
The Chicago Medical School
North Chicago, Illinois

Francis V. Howell, D.D.S.
Scripps Memorial Hospital
La Jolla, California

Lee Kudrow, M.D.
Director, California Medical Clinic for
Headache
Encino, California

James W. Lance, M.D.
Professor of Neurology
The Prince Henry School
Little Bay, New South Wales
Australia

John Marcelis, M.D.
Department of Medicine
Germantown Hospital and Medical
Center
Philadelphia, Pennsylvania

John Stirling Meyer, M.D.
Professor of Neurology
Baylor College of Medicine
Houston, Texas

Russell C. Packard, M.D.
Director, Headache Management and
Neurology
Pensacola, Florida

Albert L. Rhoton, Jr., M.D.
Professor of Neurosurgery
University of Florida
Gainesville, Florida

Alan H. Roberts, Ph.D.
Head, Division of Medical Psychology
Scripps Clinic & Research Foundation
La Jolla, California

Joel R. Saper, M.D.
Michigan Headache and Neurological
Institute
Ann Arbor, Michigan

Stanley G. Seat, M.D.
Division of Diagnostic Radiology
Scripps Clinic & Research Foundation
La Jolla, California

Stephen D. Silberstein, M.D.
*Co-Director, Comprehensive Headache
   Center at The Germantown Hospital
   and Medical Center*
Philadelphia, Pennsylvania

Ottar Sjaastad, M.D.
Professor of Neurology
Trondheim University Hospital
Trondheim, Norway

Donald D. Stevenson, M.D.
Chairman, Department of Medicine
Scripps Clinic & Research Foundation
La Jolla, California

W. E. Waters, M.D.
Professor of Community Medicine
*University of Southampton Faculty of
   Medicine*
Southampton, England

Gary W. Williams, M.D., Ph.D.
Head, Division of Rheumatology
Scripps Clinic & Research Foundation
La Jolla, California

Jack Zyroff, M.D.
Division of Neuroradiology
Scripps Clinic & Research Foundation
La Jolla, California

Wolff's
HEADACHE AND
OTHER HEAD PAIN

1

Diagnosis and Classification of Headache

DONALD J. DALESSIO
STEPHEN D. SILBERSTEIN

Headache has been called the most common medical complaint of civilized humans, yet severe or chronic headache is only infrequently caused by organic disease. In the United States, in 1 year, over 70% of the population have a headache, over 5% seek medical aid, and over 1% of physicians' office visits and emergency department visits are primarily for headache (Silberstein and Silberstein, 1990). For the patient headache is an illness in itself, but for the physician headache is either part of a primary headache disorder or a symptom of another illness. Whereas recurrent headaches are rarely caused by ophthalmologic problems, sinusitis, dental disorders, infection, or food allergy, they may signal the presence of catastrophic illness such as brain tumor, cerebral hemorrhage, or meningitis, and to ignore the symptom in this context is to risk the patient's life. Headache may be equally intense whether its source is benign or malignant. Many patients believe that their headache is secondary to a serious medical problem and seek not only pain relief, but also reassurance that they do not have a brain tumor. For these reasons, every physician must be knowledgeable in the diagnosis and treatment of headache.

What makes headaches hurt? What are the underlying mechanisms of headache? How can headaches best be classified? These questions are basic to an understanding of headache, and they are discussed in detail throughout this book. If the clinician appreciates how and why headache generally occurs, he or she will proceed more directly to a specific diagnosis, and a decision on therapy will follow as a natural consequence.

First, one must take the time to get a reasonable history. If the physician thinks "analgesic" as soon as the patient describes headache, nothing will be accomplished. All pain is subjective; no pain can be measured precisely. All symptoms are subjective and must be described by the patient. Many patients are not good observers of their own complaints, even when those complaints are chronic. Some individuals have difficulty verbalizing precisely what they are feeling, so the chances are that the physician will need time to probe and find out where the patient's head pain is located, what it feels like, when it occurs, how it is provoked, whether it runs in the family, and so on, before any tests are done and especially before any medication is prescribed.

Remember, then, that the diagnosis of headache often depends on patients' descriptions of their symptoms. It is helpful to discuss this dilemma directly with the patients and advise them that there are *no* precise clinical tests for many specific pain syndromes, including migraine headache, cluster headache, and the major neuralgias.

CLASSIFICATION

The taxonomy of headache has always been a problem for physicians. Since the last edition of this book, a new classification of headache has been published under the auspices of the International Headache Society (IHS). This monumental work, chaired by J. Olesen, took more than 3 years to complete and involved a steering committee and 12 subcommittees. The classification has been supported by the World Federation of Neurology Research Group on Migraine and the American Association for the Study of Headache. The new IHS classification of headache gives more precise definitions of all headache types, including the primary disorders, migraine, tension-type headache, and cluster headache, as well as secondary organic headache disorders.

Unfortunately, it has been published only once (Headache Classification Committee of the IHS, 1988) in a journal of somewhat limited circulation, and is therefore unfamiliar to many clinicians who deal with headache. Accordingly, it is reproduced in part here, as a service to the reader. An attempt has been made throughout the book to use the new classification, where it is applicable, although in some chapters the more traditional names for headache, or both old and new names, are used.

We have summarized the new classification in Table 1–1 and the rules for classification in Table 1–2. Tables 1–3, 1–4, 1–5, and 1–6, respectively, describe migraine without aura, migraine with aura, tension-type headache, and cluster headache in detail.

How should this new classification be used? In its printed form it numbers 96 pages, a formidable document. Its authors suggested that "the primary use is for research, but over the course of years it will probably influence the way we diagnose patients in our daily work." We believe that the classification represents an important step in codification of headache, and that it is already having a beneficial effect on headache studies. Although the IHS criteria are imperfect and somewhat cumbersome, they do represent an important advance in the attempt to standardize headache diagnosis. The document needs to be continually refined to make it more useful, and we have no doubt this will occur over the next decade.

In the older classification, migraine headaches were divided into two varieties, classic and common, on the basis of the presence or absence of an aura. These classifications have now been changed to reflect the presence or absence of the aura.

Table 1-1 New International Headache Society classification of headache

1. Migraine	6.3 Subarachnoid hemorrhage
1.1 Migraine without aura	6.4 Unruptured vascular malformation
1.2 Migraine with aura	6.5 Arteritis
1.3 Ophthalmoplegic migraine	6.6 Carotid or vertebral artery pain
1.4 Retinal migraine	6.7 Venous thrombosis
1.5 Childhood periodic syndromes that may be precursors to or associated with migraine	6.8 Arterial hypertension
	6.9 Headache associated with other vascular disorder
1.6 Complications of migraine	
1.7 Migrainous disorder not fulfilling above criteria	**7. Headache associated with nonvascular intracranial disorder**
	7.1 High cerebrospinal fluid pressure
2. Tension-type headache	7.2 Low cerebrospinal fluid pressure
2.1 Episodic tension-type headache	7.3 Intracranial infection
2.2 Chronic tension-type headache	7.4 Intracranial sarcoidosis and other noninfectious inflammatory diseases
2.3 Headache of the tension-type not fulfilling above criteria	7.5 Headache related to intrathecal injections
3. Cluster headache and chronic paroxysmal hemicrania	7.6 Intracranial neoplasm
	7.7 Headache associated with other intracranial disorder
3.1 Cluster headache	
3.2 Chronic paroxysmal hemicrania	**8. Headache associated with substances or their withdrawal**
3.3 Cluster headache-like disorder not fulfilling above criteria	8.1 Headache induced by acute substance use or exposure
4. Miscellaneous headaches unassociated with structural lesion	8.2 Headache induced by chronic substance use or exposure
	8.3 Headache from substance withdrawal (acute use)
4.1 Idiopathic stabbing headache	8.4 Headache from substance withdrawal (chronic use)
4.2 External compression headache	8.5 Headache associated with substances but with uncertain mechanism
4.3 Cold stimulus headache	
4.4 Benign cough headache	
4.5 Benign exertional headache	**9. Headache associated with noncephalic infection**
4.6 Headache associated with sexual activity	
5. Headache associated with head trauma	9.1 Viral infection
5.1 Acute post-traumatic headache	9.2 Bacterial infection
5.2 Chronic post-traumatic headache	9.3 Headache related to other infection
6. Headache associated with vascular disorders	
6.1 Acute ischemic cerebrovascular disorder	
6.2 Intracranial hematoma	

(continued)

Migraine without aura (Table 1–3), formerly called common migraine, is defined in terms of the duration and the quality of the attack. Note that at least five attacks fulfilling the criteria are required for diagnosis. (Trauma or organic disease as a cause, trigger, or comorbid condition, as listed in groups 5 through 11 in Table 1–1, is dealt with in Section E.)

Migraine with aura (Table 1–4), formerly classical migraine, is also precisely defined, particularly with respect to the time of onset of aura and its duration. Types of aura include (1) homonymous visual disturbance, (2) unilateral paresthesias and/or numbness, (3) unilateral weakness, and (4) aphasia or unclassifiable speech difficulty. Most common is the visual aura.

Table 1-1 New International Headache Society classification of headache (*continued*)

10. Headache associated with metabolic disorder	11.5 Nose and sinuses
10.1 Hypoxia	11.6 Teeth, jaws, and related structures
10.2 Hypercapnia	11.7 Temporomandibular joint disease
10.3 Mixed hypoxia and hypercapnia	**12. Cranial neuralgias, nerve trunk pain, and deafferentation pain**
10.4 Hypoglycemia	12.1 Persistent (in contrast to tic-like) pain of cranial nerve origin
10.5 Dialysis	12.2 Trigeminal neuralgia
10.6 Headache related to other metabolic abnormality	12.3 Glossopharyngeal neuralgia
11. Headache or facial pain associated with disorder of cranium, neck, eyes, ears, nose, sinuses, teeth, mouth, or other facial or cranial structures	12.4 Nervus intermedius neuralgia
	12.5 Superior laryngeal neuralgia
	12.6 Occipital neuralgia
	12.7 Central causes of head and facial pain other than tic douloureux
11.1 Cranial bone	12.8 Facial pain not fulfilling criteria in groups 11 or 12
11.2 Neck	
11.3 Eyes	**13. Headache not classifiable**
11.4 Ears	

Source: Headache Classification Committee of the International Headache Society (1988).

Table 1-2 General rules for classification

1. If the patient has more than one headache disorder, all should be diagnosed in the order of importance indicated by the patient.
2. To make a diagnosis, all letter headings of a set of diagnostic criteria must be fulfilled.
3. After each diagnosis, add estimated number of *headache days per year* in brackets.
4. Diagnostic criteria given at the one- or two-digit level must generally be met by the subforms, but exceptions and/or more specific criteria are listed under the subforms.
5. Patients who for the first time develop a particular form of headache in close temporal relation to onset of one of the disorders listed in groups 5–11 are coded to these groups using the fourth digit to specify type of headache. A causal relationship is not necessarily indicated, however. Preexisting migraine, tension-type headache or cluster headache aggravated in close temporal relation to one of the disorders listed in groups 5–11 are still coded as migraine, tension-type headache or cluster headache (groups 1–3). If number of headache days increase by 100% or more, the aggravating factor may be mentioned in parenthesis, but it is not coded for.
6. Code to the degree (number of digits) which suits your purpose.
7. If one headache type fits the diagnostic criteria for different categories of headache, code to the first headache category in the classification for which the criteria are fulfilled (1.7, 2.3 and 3.3 are not regarded as diagnoses if the headache also fulfills another diagnosis).
8. If a patient has a form of headache fulfilling one set of diagnostic criteria, similar episodes which do not quite satisfy the criteria also usually occur. This can be due to treatment, lack of ability to remember symptoms exactly, and other factors. Ask the patient to describe a typical untreated attack or an unsuccessfully treated attack and ascertain that there have been enough of these attacks to establish the diagnosis. Then estimate the days per year with this type of headache, adding also treated attacks and less typical attacks.
9. A major obstacle to an exact diagnosis is the reliance on patient's history to determine whether criteria are met. In less clear cases it is recommended to let the patient record attack characteristics prospectively using a headache diary before the diagnosis is made.
10. If a fourth digit is to be used in association with a diagnosis at the two-digit level, insert 0 as the third digit.

Source: Headache Classification Committee of the International Headache Society (1988).

Table 1–3 Classification of migraine without aura

1.1 Migraine without aura

Previously used terms: common migraine, hemicrania simplex

Diagnostic criteria

A. At least 5 attacks fulfilling B–D
B. Headache lasting 4 to 72 hours (untreated or unsuccessfully treated).
C. Headache has at least two of the following characteristics:
    1. Unilateral location
    2. Pulsating quality
    3. Moderate or severe intensity (inhibits or prohibits daily activities)
    4. Aggravation by walking stairs or similar routine physical activity
D. During headache at least one of the following:
    1. Nausea and/or vomiting
    2. Photophobia and phonophobia
E. At least one of the following:
    1. History, physical and neurological examinations do not suggest one of the disorders listed in groups 5–11
    2. History and/or physical and/or neurological examinations do suggest such disorder, but it is ruled out by appropriate investigations
    3. Such disorder is present, but migraine attacks do not occur for the first time in close temporal relation to the disorder

Source: Headache Classification Committee of the International Headache Society (1988).

Tension-type headache (Table 1–5) is the new term used to describe what was previously called "tension headache," "muscle contraction headache," "stress headache," and "ordinary headache." In the last edition of this book this was called muscle contraction headache. The new IHS criteria distinguish between patients with episodic tension-type headache and those with chronic tension-type headache (formerly "chronic daily headache"). The major distinguishing feature is the frequency of the headache (i.e., <15 headache days/month for episodic tension-type headache or ≥15 headache days/month for chronic tension-type headache.

Cluster headache (Table 1–6) is a nonfamilial disorder that affects men predominantly. Attacks are briefer and more frequent than migraine, strictly unilateral, and usually occur in clusters lasting weeks (episodic cluster). Attacks occurring for more than 1 year without remission or with remission lasting less than 14 days define chronic cluster.

Group 4 of the classification (Table 1–1) comprises a variety of headache disorders not associated with a structural lesion. Some, like idiopathic stabbing headache, cold stimulus headache, and benign exertional headache, may occur more frequently with the migraine syndrome or may be a part of it. The rest of the headache disorders (groups 5 through 11) are secondary to, and are considered symptomatic of, an organic disorder, although the clinical symptomology may be identical to that of one of the primary headache disorders. These are discussed in their individual chapters. The cranial neuralgias (group 12) are considered by themselves in Chapter 15.

Table 1—4   Classification of migraine with aura

1.2 Migraine with aura

Previously used terms: classic migraine, classical migraine, ophthalmic, hemiparesthetic, hemiplegic or aphasic migraine

Diagnostic criteria

A. At least 2 attacks fulfilling B

B. At least 3 of the following 4 characteristics:
   1. One or more fully reversible aura symptoms indicating focal cerebral cortical and/or brain stem dysfunction
   2. At least one aura symptom develops gradually over more than 4 minutes or 2 or more symptoms occur in succession
   3. No aura symptom lasts more than 60 minutes. If more than one aura symptom is present, accepted duration is proportionally increased
   4. Headache follows aura with a free interval of less than 60 minutes. (It may also begin before or simultaneously with the aura)

C. At least one of the following:
   1. History, physical and neurological examinations do not suggest one of the disorders listed in groups 5–11
   2. History and/or physical and/or neurological examinations do suggest such disorder, but it is ruled out by appropriate investigations
   3. Such disorder is present, but migraine attacks do not occur for the first time in close temporal relation to the disorder

1.2.1 Migraine with typical aura

Diagnostic criteria

A. Fulfills criteria for 1.2 including all four criteria under B

B. One or more aura symptoms of the following types:
   1. Homonymous visual disturbance
   2. Unilateral paresthesias and/or numbness
   3. Unilateral weakness
   4. Aphasia or unclassifiable speech difficulty

Source: Headache Classification Committee of the International Headache Society (1988).

HEADACHE DIAGNOSIS

History

Because most headache patients have normal neurologic and physical examinations, the most important tool for making a correct headache diagnosis is a detailed and relevant history (Silberstein, 1992). The most common diagnoses are tension-type headache and migraine and associated variants, including cluster headache. The headaches provoked by fever and septicemia probably rank next in frequency, and then come those due to nasal and paranasal, ear, tooth, and eye disease. The headaches of meningitis, intracranial aneurysm, brain tumor, and brain abscess, although most important and singularly dramatic, are less common.

Age at Onset

Headaches that start in childhood, in adolescence, or in the second or third decade of life are frequently migrainous. Headaches that begin later in life may have an organic etiology, such as temporal arteritis, cerebrovascular disease,

Table 1–5 Classification of tension-type headache

2.1 Episodic tension-type headache
Previously used terms: tension headache, muscle contraction headache, psychomyogenic headache, stress headache, ordinary headache, essential headache, idiopathic headache and psychogenic headache

Diagnostic criteria
A. At least 10 previous headache episodes fulfilling criteria B–D listed below. Number of days with such headache <180/year (<15/month)
B. Headache lasting from 30 minutes to 7 days
C. At least 2 of the following pain characteristics:
   1. Pressing/tightening (non-pulsating) quality
   2. Mild or moderate intensity (may inhibit, but does not prohibit activities)
   3. Bilateral location
   4. No aggravation by walking stairs or similar routine physical activity
D. Both of the following:
   1. No nausea or vomiting (anorexia may occur)
   2. Photophobia and phonophobia are absent, or one but not the other is present
E. At least one of the following:
   1. History, physical and neurological examinations do not suggest one of the disorders listed in groups 5–11

2. History and/or physical and/or neurological examinations do suggest such disorder, but it is ruled out by appropriate investigations
3. Such disorder is present, but tension-type headache does not occur for the first time in close temporal relation to the disorder

2.1.1 Episodic tension-type headache associated with disorder of pericranial muscles
Previously used terms: muscle contraction headache

Diagnostic criteria
A. Fulfills criteria for 2.1
B. At least one of the following:
   1. Increased tenderness of pericranial muscles demonstrated by manual palpation of pressure algometer
   2. Increased EMG level of pericranial muscles at rest or during physiological tests
2.1.2 Episodic tension-type headache unassociated with disorder of pericranial muscles
Previously used terms: idiopathic headache, essential headache, psychogenic headache

Diagnostic criteria
A. Fulfills criteria for 2.1
B. No increased tenderness of pericranial muscles. If studied, EMG of pericranial muscles shows normal levels of activity

(*continued*)

or tumor. Migraine often stops at menopause, but it may occasionally start at that time. Tension-type headaches can begin at any age.

Location

Is the headache bilateral or unilateral? Unilateral head pain that alternates sides suggests migraine. Strictly unilateral orbital pain of brief duration suggests cluster headache.

The headache of migraine can occur anywhere in the head and face, with the most common site being the temple. The headache usually involves either the right or the left side of the head, but may be strictly unilateral or bilateral. The headache of tooth, sinus, or eye disease usually is frontal, but the pain may

Table 1–5 Classification of tension-type headache (*continued*)

2.2 Chronic tension-type headache
Previously used terms: chronic daily headache
 	
Diagnostic criteria
A. Average headache frequency 15 days/month (180 days/year) for 6 months fulfilling criteria B–D.
B. At least 2 of the following pain characteristics:
  1. Pressing/tightening quality
  2. Mild or moderate severity (may inhibit but does not prohibit activities)
  3. Bilateral location
  4. No aggravation by walking stairs or similar routine physical activity
C. Both of the following:
  1. No vomiting
  2. No more than one of the following: nausea, photophobia or phonophobia
	D. At least one of the following:
	  1. History, physical and neurological examinations do not suggest one of the disorders listed in groups 5–11
	  2. History and/or physical and/or neurological examinations do suggest such disorder, but it is ruled out by appropriate investigations
	  3. Such disorder is present, but tension-type headache does not occur for the first time in close temporal relation to the disorder
	
	2.2.1 Chronic tension-type headache associated with disorder of pericranial muscles
	
	2.2.2 Chronic tension-type headache unassociated with disorder of pericranial muscles

Source: Headache Classification Committee of the International Headache Society (1988).

be referred to the back of the head and neck. Headaches associated with pituitary adenomas and parasellar tumors are often bitemporal.

The headaches of posterior fossa tumors, early in the development of the tumor and before the beginning of general brain displacement, are usually occipital. Headaches from supratentorial tumors, before serious brain displacement occurs, are usually frontal or vertex. If the tumor involves the dura or bone, the headache may be localized to the site of the lesion. Early in the course of the tumor or before general displacement of the brain has occurred, the headache commonly is on the side of the tumor.

Subdural hematoma may produce a headache of considerable intensity, usually localized over or near the site of the lesion, most commonly over the frontoparietal areas. The headache may be chronic, daily, but intermittent and characteristically may be continuous from the date of injury.

Although tension-type headache may be most intense in the neck, shoulders, and occiput, it can involve the frontal region. These headaches may be unilateral or bilateral.

Disease involving the dome of the diaphragm or the phrenic nerve causes pain high in the shoulder and neck. Myocardial ischemia can cause pain in the lower jaw and cervical–occipital junction.

Frequency
The frequency and pattern of headache may provide clues to the diagnosis. Cluster headache typically occurs in brief attacks, each lasting 30 to 90 minutes and recurring two to six times a day. Migraine may also occur at sporadic intervals, and thus can mimic cluster headache.

Table 1–6 Classification of cluster headache

3.1.1 Cluster headache
Diagnostic criteria
A. At least 5 attacks fulfilling B–D.
B. Severe unilateral orbital, supraorbital and/or temporal pain lasting 15 to 180 minutes untreated.
C. Headache is associated with at least one of the following signs which have to be present on the pain side:
   1. Conjunctival injection
   2. Lacrimation
   3. Nasal congestion
   4. Rhinorrhea
   5. Forehead and facial sweating
   6. Miosis
   7. Ptosis
   8. Eyelid edema
D. Frequency of attacks: from 1 every other day to 8 per day
E. At least one of the following:
   1. History, physical, and neurological examinations do not suggest one of the disorders listed in groups 5–11.
   2. History and/or physical and/or neurological examinations do suggest such disorder, but it is ruled out by appropriate investigations.
   3. Such disorder is present, but cluster headache does not occur for the first time in close temporal relation to the disorder.

3.1.2 Episodic cluster headache
Description: occurs in periods lasting 7 days to one year separated by pain free periods lasting 14 days or more.
Diagnostic criteria
A. All the letter headings of 3.1.
B. At least 2 periods of headaches (cluster periods) lasting (untreated patients) from 7 days to one year, separated by remissions of at least 14 days.

3.1.3 Chronic cluster headache
Description: attacks occur for more than one year without remission or with remissions lasting less than 14 days.
Diagnostic criteria
A. All letter headings of 3.1.
B. Absence of remission phases for one year or more with remissions lasting less than 14 days.

Source: Headache Classification Committee of the International Headache Society (1988).

Onset, Duration, Character, and Severity

The pain of cluster headache is described as deep and boring, as if a hot poker were being driven into the eye. The headaches of fever, migraine, hemangiomatous tumors, and arterial hypertension are characteristically throbbing or pulsating in quality. The headache of brain tumor and of meningitis, although occasionally pulsating, is usually of a steady, aching quality. Tension-type headache is dull, nagging, and persistent and often described as feeling as though a band were wrapped around the head.

The most intense headaches are those due to ruptured intracranial aneurysm, meningitis, fever, and migraine and those associated with malignant hypertension. Beware of the acute-onset "thunderclap" headache; it may be caused by a subarachnoid hemorrhage. Subarachnoid hemorrhage resulting from ruptured intracranial aneurysm produces a headache that is sudden in onset, reaches great intensity in a very short time, and may be associated with feelings of faintness or with unconsciousness. The onset of pain is soon followed by a stiff neck and blood in the lumbar spinal fluid. The intense headache of meningitis is accompanied by a stiff neck that prevents passive flexion of the head on the chest, although the spasm of the neck muscles associated with migraine may also inhibit neck flexion.

Headaches associated with brain tumors, brain abscesses, sinus disease, tooth disease, and eye disease are usually only moderately severe. Hemorrhage into the parenchyma of the brain may not cause headache unless the hemorrhage breaks through into the ventricular or subarachnoid spaces or produces significant brain displacement; then intense headache may result.

Course
Beware of the headache that progressively worsens; it may have an organic cause. The longer the headache has existed in its present form, the more likely it is to be benign. Cluster headache occurs in bouts that can last from 1 to 2 weeks or for as long as 4 to 5 months.

Chronologic Features
Migraine headache may be as brief as 20 or 30 minutes or may last days or, rarely, weeks. The usual headache lasts less than 24 hours. A striking singular feature of migraine is the freedom from headache between prostrating attacks. The headaches of brain tumor are intermittent and vary in intensity, but usually occur every day. Tension-type headache may persist for days, weeks, or even years.

Migraine headaches and headaches associated with hypertension frequently occur in the early morning hours, with the patient awakening with pain. Cluster headache commonly occurs after sleep onset. The headache of brain tumor may be more severe in the early part of the day, although not in the early hours of the morning, and may not have any diurnal pattern.

Migraine attacks are common during weekends, during the first portion of vacation holidays, and immediately after vacation. Attacks are commonly triggered by menstruation. Migraineurs often have their headaches on specific days of the week.

Migraine headache occurs during periods of increased conflict, tension, or stress for the individual; for example, during early fall for the schoolteacher, during rush or holiday seasons for the merchant, or during very hot or humid weather for those who feel ineffective and prostrated in such weather. Headache associated with nasal and paranasal disease is usually more common during periods when upper respiratory infections prevail, namely, the darker months of the year. Exacerbations of tic douloureux are common in the spring and fall, notably March and October. The same may be true for cluster headaches.

Prodromes and Auras
Significant prodromes, such as mood changes or changes in appetite, can occur 1 to 2 days before a migraine headache. Auras such as scintillating scotoma or paresthesias precede and define classic migraine.

Associated Signs and Symptoms
Inquire about redness or tearing of the eyes, nasal congestion, nausea, vomiting, teeth grinding, and neck stiffness or tenderness. Unilateral nasal congestion and tearing are associated with cluster headache. Nausea and vomiting are commonly associated with migraine. Teeth grinding and neck tenderness may be seen with tension-type headache.

Mucous membrane injection. Redness and swelling of the mucous membranes of the nose (with or without nosebleeds) and conjunctival injection may occur with migraine. The mucous membrane injection and engorgement may be conspicuous and give rise to headache in those with allergic sensitivities to inhalants and those in whom the nasal mucous membranes are involved during periods of major adaptive difficulties. With the exception of headache due to neoplastic invasion of paranasal structures and antral infection via the dental route, no headache associated with disease of the nasal and paranasal sinuses occurs without obvious congestion of the turbinates and nasal mucous membranes.

Gastrointestinal disturbances. Anorexia, nausea, and vomiting, although most commonly associated with migraine, may occur with any headache, and the more intense the headache the more likely these symptoms are to occur. Vomiting without nausea may occur with brain tumors, especially tumors of the posterior fossa. Nausea and vomiting with little or no headache may occur with migraine. Headache associated with sinus or eye disease is seldom associated with vomiting. Although constipation is commonly associated with migraine, diarrhea may also occur. Abdominal distention and flatulence are common in migraine and tension-type headaches but are seldom associated with other headaches.

Polyuria. Polyuria is commonly associated with migraine headache; it seldom occurs with other headaches. Tension states with headaches may be linked to urinary frequency.

Signs of depression and cognitive dysfunction. Insomnia, early-morning awakening, fatigue, anorexia, change in libido, and malaise all are signs of depression, which is frequently associated with long-standing headache. Ask about changes in behavior and thinking; check with a family member.

Mood. The wish to retire from people and responsibilities, or a dejected, depressed, irritable, or negativistic mental state bordering on prostration or stupor, is a dominant aspect of the migraine attack and may in some instances be more disturbing than the pain in the head. Apathy, listlessness, or even euphoria may be associated with brain tumor headache.

Tension-type headache may occur in a tense, irritable person, but the patient is usually willing to accept attention, massage, or medication, in contrast to the patient with a migraine headache attack, who commonly expresses the wish to be left alone. Exaltation or feelings of special well-being are rare sequels to the migraine headache attack. The suffering experienced with the headache of fever, meningitis, or ruptured aneurysm may be very great, but the mental state is that of reaction to severe pain.

Signs of neurologic dysfunction. Signs of neurologic dysfunction include weakness, paresthesia, aphasia, diplopia, visual loss, vertigo, and faintness. These signs suggest a possible space-occupying lesion or aneurysm; however, they may be part of the neurologic symptoms of migraine.

Visual disturbances. Both scintillating scotomata and visual field defects, such as unilateral or homonymous hemianopia, may occur with migraine headaches. Such visual defects may occur with brain tumor headaches when the tumor is due to a lesion of the occipital lobes or is adjacent to the visual pathways. The visual disturbances of migraine, with the exception of blurred vision and diplopia, usually precede the headache. These phenomena usually last less than 1 hour. Enlarged pupils and lacrimation may cause faulty vision during a migraine headache, but when defects in visual acuity or the fields of vision outlast the headache attack, it is likely that a cerebrovascular accident or brain tumor is the cause. Defects in color vision and colored rings about lights may occur with headache associated with glaucoma.

Vertigo and other sensory disturbances. Vertigo may be a forerunner of a migraine headache attack. Vertigo is sometimes associated with the headaches of brain tumors, although feelings of unsteadiness are more common. Fleeting vertigo occurring with sudden movement or rotation of the head often accompanies post-traumatic headache and tension-type headache.

Menière's (or labyrinthine) syndrome is occasionally associated with headache. Other sensory disturbances such as paresthesias of the hands and face may occur as a forerunner of the migraine headache. However, paresthesias that persist during the headache attack, or outlast it, are more common in patients with brain tumors or epilepsy.

Precipitating Factors
Alcohol, a newly prescribed drug, bright lights, fatigue, loss of sleep, hypoglycemia, stress, certain drugs, and food additives can provoke migraine. Migraine is often triggered by menstruation and relieved by pregnancy. Exercise or orgasm can trigger a migraine or result in the rupture of an aneurysm. Head trauma can both cause and trigger headache.

Effects of Position and Body Movement
In many instances migraine is made worse by assuming a horizontal position and is relieved by an erect position. It is often made worse by ascending stairs, by moving about rapidly, or by lifting. Sitting quietly in an upright position often proves to be most comfortable. The recumbent position may at first intensify the

headache associated with nasal and paranasal disease, but subsequently the headache subsides. A sudden change in position, usually from the sitting to the recumbent position, may intensify the headache of brain tumor. Unlike migraine headache, the headache of brain tumor is often worse when the patient is in the upright position. The head-down position aggravates most headaches, except those due to spinal drainage and occasionally those associated with brain tumor.

Straining at stool and coughing increase all but tension-type headache and that due to spinal drainage. Sharp flexion or extension of the head often reduces the intensity of post–lumbar puncture headache, whereas jugular compression increases the headache.

A major criterion that can be used in the diagnosis of cluster headache is the patient's behavior during the attack. Pacing, walking, sitting, and rocking are activities that are considered pathognomonic of this disorder. Frantic activity may occur. No other primary headache disorder is associated with such behavior.

Effect of Head Jolt

Headaches known to arise primarily from sensitization of pain-sensitive intracranial vessels (i.e., histamine headache, hypoglycemic headache, and the headaches of fever, systemic infection, "hangover," lumbar puncture, and the early postconcussive state) or inflammation of pain-sensitive intracranial arteries and veins and their adjacent structures (the headache of meningitis) are particularly sensitive to head jolting. The threshold of jolt headache during these states may be depressed 2.0 to 3.0 g or more. In patients with intracranial masses (i.e., subdural hematoma or brain tumor), the threshold of jolt headache is usually depressed and the location of the headache induced by jolting may indicate the side of the lesion. The threshold of jolt headache may be lowered during a migraine headache.

In contrast, headaches not arising from involvement of intracranial structures of the head (i.e., tension-type headache, some migraine headaches, and the headache induced by the injection of hypertonic saline into the temporal muscle) are not significantly intensified by head jolting, and the threshold to jolt headache is not lowered.

Sleep

Migraine usually does not disrupt sleep. Brain tumor, sinus disease, and tension-type headache usually do not interfere with sleep. Complaints of long periods of sleep loss because of headache may be due to coexistent anxiety or depression. The headache of meningitis usually interrupts sleep. Migraine may also occur after periods of excessively prolonged or very deep sleep. Cluster headache often occurs during rapid eye movement (REM) sleep.

Family History

Does either parent have migraine or recurrent "sick headaches?" Migraine is familial; cluster headache is not.

Multiplicity

It is not unusual for a patient to have different types of headache. The presence of pre-existing migraine does not exclude other, perhaps more ominous, headaches.

Physical Examination

The physical examination can rule out systemic causes of headache. It should include vital signs (undiagnosed hypertension, fever), funduscopy (hypertension, papilledema), and palpation of the structures in and about the face and head (local causes of headache). A neurologic examination should be conducted, but the results may be normal even in the presence of intracranial disease. Include mental status (speak to a family member about changes in behavior), cranial nerves (including pupils and eye movements), reflexes, Babinski sign, motor strength, and a careful search for any evidence of meningeal irritation, such as neck stiffness or Kernig or Brudzinski sign (Edmeads, 1988).

Tenderness

Tenderness over the aching side of the head and the nasal and paranasal sinuses, the teeth, and the ear may be conspicuous during migraine headache and for some hours thereafter. Muscles may become tender to palpation with both migraine and tension-type headache. Thus, brushing and combing the hair may be a painful experience during or after a migraine headache. With myositis and myalgia there may be tender areas in the muscles of the head and neck. Percussion of the head may cause pain over or near an underlying brain tumor or subdural hematoma.

Periostitis secondary to mastoiditis or frontal, ethmoid, or sphenoid sinus disease produces moderate to severe pain associated with focal tenderness. If the pain is sufficiently severe and continuous, it may become generalized. The tenderness or hyperalgesia associated with mastoid disease with periostitis is far greater than the hyperalgesia associated with posterior fossa brain tumor.

Tenderness at the site of a head injury is often associated with a scar and may persist for years. Tender muscles or nodules often occur in parts of the head remote from the site of injury.

Pressure on the temporal, frontal, supraorbital, postauricular, occipital, and common carotid arteries often reduces the intensity of migraine headache and headache associated with arterial hypertension. Support of the head makes any patient with headache feel more comfortable. The pain of tension-type headache may be intensified by firm manipulation of tender muscles or regions of tenderness; however, gentle massage and simple measures of physical therapy, including heat and hot packs, frequently will relieve this form of headache.

Ptosis of the eyelid may accompany the headache of brain tumor or a cerebral aneurysm of the circle of Willis, especially if there is a fixed and dilated pupil. Ptosis also occurs with ophthalmoplegic migraine, a symptom complex involving paresis of the muscles supplied by the third cranial nerve, and occasionally those supplied by the fourth and sixth cranial nerves. It usually has its onset late in the headache attack, persists for days or weeks, and may be due to edema near or about the affected cranial nerves.

Horner syndrome occurs with cluster headache. Photophobia, associated with any frontal or vertex headache, is commonly seen in patients with meningitis, migraine, nasal and paranasal disease, eye disease, brain tumor, and tension-type headache. Scleral and conjunctival injection may accompany the photophobia. If the intensity of the pain is very great, photophobia, lacrimation, and sweating of the homolateral forehead and side of the face may also occur.

When headache is associated with papilledema, it is in most instances a result of increased intracranial pressure due to an expanding intracranial mass. However, in patients with brain tumor, headache often occurs without papilledema, and papilledema without headache. In the advanced phase of hypertensive encephalopathy, headache and papilledema occur. Subarachnoid hemorrhage from a ruptured aneurysm may cause intense headache without papilledema, but it is occasionally associated with a retinal hemorrhage. Meningitis does not affect the eye grounds except possibly to induce slight suffusion, unless there is increased intracranial pressure (and papilledema). During migraine headache unilateral arterial and venous dilation in eye grounds may occur.

EMERGENCY PRESENTATION OF HEADACHE PATIENTS

Headache patients may present on an emergency basis for various reasons.

Acute Systemic Illness

The patient may have a new headache as the symptom of an acute systemic illness. Diagnosis in these cases is usually not difficult, and treatment is directed toward the underlying illness.

First or Worst Headache

The patient may have an attack of his or her "first or worst headache" (Edmeads, 1988) with or without prior history of recurrent headache, or the patient may have progressively worsening headache. This presentation may be complicated by focal neurologic signs or symptoms of intractable nausea and vomiting.

"Last Straw" Syndrome

The headache may be part of a chronic headache disorder that either has failed to respond to the usual treatment or can no longer be tolerated (the "last straw" syndrome) (Edmeads, 1988). Most patients entering the emergency department with the chief complaint of headache have a primary headache disorder or a systemic illness.

Causes for Concern

The physician should be especially concerned if the patient has any of the following symptoms (Edmeads, 1988; Silberstein, 1992):

The "first or worst" headache of the patient's life, particularly if it is of acute onset or is accompanied by other neurologic symptoms.

A headache that is subacute in onset and gets progressively worse over days or weeks.

A headache associated with fever, nausea, and vomiting that cannot be explained by a systemic illness.

A headache associated with focal neurologic findings, papilledema, changes in consciousness or cognition (such as difficulty in reading, writing, or thinking), or a stiff neck.

If a cause for concern exists, neurologic consultation, neuroimaging studies (magnetic resonance imaging or computerized tomography) or lumbar puncture may be indicated.

CONCLUSION

Most patients seeing a physician for a headache disorder have an acute exacerbation of a recurrent primary headache disorder or a headache associated with an acute febrile illness. However, all headaches should be taken seriously, and a diagnosis based on the new IHS criteria should be made, if possible prior to instituting treatment.

REFERENCES

Edmeads, J. (1988). Emergency management of headache. *Headache 28*:675–679.

Headache Classification Committee of the International Headache Society (1988). Classification and diagnostic criteria for headache disorders, cranial neuralgia, and facial pain. *Cephalalgia 8*(Suppl. 7):1–96.

Silberstein, S.D. (1992). Evaluation and emergency treatment of headache. *Headache 32*:396–407.

Silberstein, S.D. and M.M. Silberstein (1990). New concepts in the pathogenesis of migraine headache. *Pain Management 3*:297–302.

2

Pain-Sensitive Cranial Structures

ROBERT J. COFFEY
ALBERT L. RHOTON, JR.

The foundation for any study of the causes and treatments of headache is knowledge of the pain-sensitive structures and pain-conducting pathways within the cranium. Anatomic studies of postmortem human and animal material form the cornerstone on which later knowledge is built. The recent use of histochemical tracer techniques adds another dimension to the anatomic evidence regarding intracranial sensory innervation. Brain surgery performed under local anesthesia on awake patients has also contributed significant knowledge regarding the sensitivity of intracranial structures to painful stimuli. The most well known of these studies is the landmark paper of Ray and Wolff (1940), on which this chapter was based in earlier editions. Experimental stimulation during intracranial surgery on anesthetized lower animals provides corroborative, although less direct information. Finally, the examination of patients after the ablation of cranial sensory pathways by deliberate surgical interventions or destructive pathologic processes serves to correlate clinical observations with anatomic data.

This chapter reviews the anatomic, physiologic, and clinical evidence contributing to our current knowledge of the pain-sensitive intracranial structures. Pathways involved in the pains of superficial scalp origin, cranial neuralgias, cervical spondylosis, and ocular, paranasal sinus, or dental disease are discussed in separate chapters devoted to those entities. The cranial bone itself, and its endosteal venous channels, are insensitive to pain.

The following discussion first considers the anatomic and intraoperative data regarding the supratentorial pain-sensitive structures. A similar discussion of the pain-sensitive posterior fossa contents follows. The results of animal and human investigations are presented to correlate anatomic principles with clinical observations of cranial pain syndromes.

SUPRATENTORIAL DURA, DURAL SINUSES, AND MENINGEAL ARTERIES

Anatomic Data
The ophthalmic division of the trigeminal nerve (Figure 2–1) is a major source of pain-sensitive afferents for large areas of the supratentorial dura and associated venous structures (Figure 2–2). The tentorial nerve of Arnold arises as a group

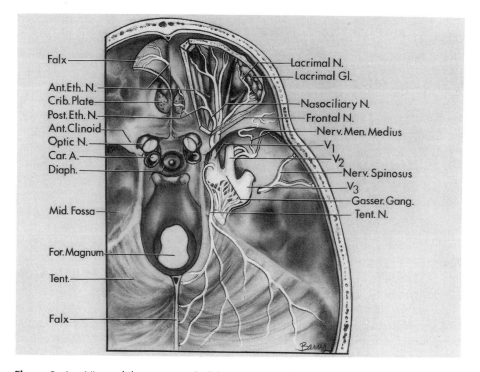

Figure 2–1. View of the anterior skull base showing the trigeminal sensory innervation of the supratentorial dura, dural sinuses, and meningeal arteries. The tentorial nerve (Tent. N.) arises from the ophthalmic division (V₁) just proximal to the superior orbital fissure. Anterior and posterior ethmoidal nerves (Ant. Eth. N., Post. Eth. N.) arise from the nasociliary branch (Nasociliary N.) of the ophthalmic division within the orbit. The nervus meningeus medius (Nerv. Men. Medius) branches from the maxillary division (V₂) proximal to the cavernous sinus. The nervus spinosus (Nerv. Spinosus) arises from the mandibular division (V₃) outside the foramen ovale and re-enters the skull through the foramen spinosum with the middle meningeal artery. Key to abbreviations: Ant. Clinoid, anterior clinoid; Car. A., carotid artery; Crib. Plate, cribriform plate; Diaph., diaphragma sellae; For. Magnum, foramen magnum; Frontal N., frontal nerve; Gasser. Gang., gasserian ganglion; Lacrimal Gl., lacrimal gland; Lacrimal N., lacrimal nerve; Mid. Fossa, middle fossa; Optic N., optic nerve; Tent., tentorium.

of branches from the superior margin of the proximal ophthalmic division within the lateral wall of the cavernous sinus just before that division enters the superior orbital fissure (Arnold, 1851). It immediately turns posteriorly within the most anterior portion of the free tentorial edge and courses close to the trochlear nerve, with which it was originally confused (Penfield and McNaughton, 1940). As the tentorium fans out in a triangular fashion, the fibers of the tentorial nerve spread out within its leaves. Here, the nerve bears no constant relation to the tentorial artery. On reaching the posterior tentorial margin at the transverse sinus, terminal branches of the tentorial nerve turn upward within the dura of the parieto-occipital convexity. The more medial branches within the tentorium

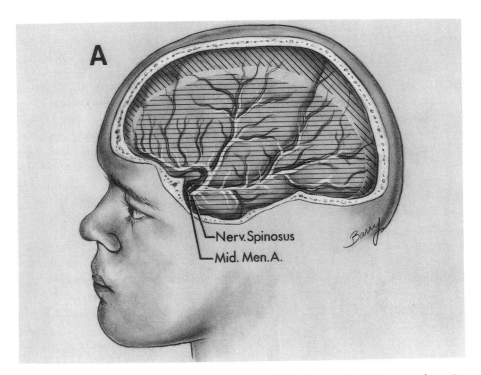

Figure 2–2. The supratentorial dural structures with their contained sinuses and meningeal arteries, shown according to their predominant sensory supply from the three divisions of the trigeminal nerve as indicated by the accompanying key. *(A)* Lateral view of the dura covering the cerebral hemisphere, showing the nervus spinosus branch of the mandibular division (Nerv. spinosus) closely following the ramifications of the middle meningeal artery (Mid. Men. A.). The narrow band of dura on either side of the superior sagittal sinus receives its innervation from the ophthalmic division through the ethmoidal and tentorial nerves (see Figures 2–1 and 2–2B and the text). *(B)* Schematic view of the tentorium (Tent.), falx, and anterior and middle fossa dural structures after removal of the convexity dura. Key to abbreviations: Crib. Plate, cribriform plate; Diaph., diaphragma sellae; Inf. Sagg. Sinus, inferior sagittal sinus; Mid. Fossa, middle fossa; Orb. Roof, orbital roof; Sphen. Ridge, sphenoid ridge; Str. sinus, straight sinus; Sup. Sagg. Sinus, superior sagittal sinus; Trans. Sinus, transverse sinus. *(C)* The dermatomal distribution of the trigeminal divisions is shown on the face. Within each dermatome is a smaller, shaded area that represents the most common site of referred pain from stimulation of dural or vascular structures innervated by each division during intracranial surgery on awake patients.

reach the straight sinus at the junction of the tentorium and falx cerebri. Here, branches turn forward to distribute themselves along the posterior two thirds of the falx for its entire width from convexity to free margin. In this fashion the tentorial nerves supply the tentorium, the superior surface of the transverse and straight sinuses, and the caudal two thirds of the falx, including the superior and inferior sagittal sinuses (Feindel et al., 1960; Kimmel, 1961b; Lance, 1982; McNaughton, 1938; McNaughton and Feindel, 1977; Netter and Mitchell, 1983;

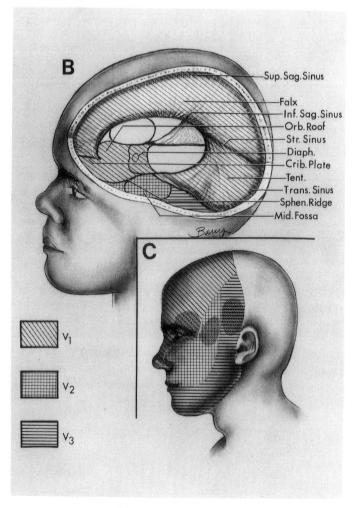

Figure 2–2.   *(Continued)*

Penfield and McNaughton, 1940). Evidence gathered during intracranial surgery on awake patients suggests that major surface tributary veins of the above-named sinuses also receive ophthalmic division innervation by means of the tentorial nerve (see below).

The dura of the diaphragma sellae is also supplied by the ophthalmic division through a small branch that arises from either the first division or its tentorial or frontal branches. According to Kimmel (1961b), this branch reaches the superior hypophyseal artery (a branch of the supraclinoid internal carotid artery), accompanies it for a short distance, and then joins the dura forming the intercavernous venous sinuses. It divides into anterior and posterior dural branches that enter the diaphragma sellae.

On entering the orbit, the ophthalmic division divides into the frontal, nasociliary, and lacrimal nerves. The nasociliary nerve traverses the common annular tendon and gives off two sensory branches: an inconstant posterior ethmoidal nerve and a more constant anterior ethmoidal nerve. Other branches of the nasociliary nerve include the infratrochlear and long ciliary nerves, as well as the sensory root of the ciliary ganglion, neither of which provides intracranial sensory innervation. The posterior and anterior ethmoidal nerves, in addition to innervating mucous membranes of the ethmoidal sinuses and nasal cavity, contribute twigs to the anterior meningeal nerves. These are formed by variable contributions from all three trigeminal divisions and provide innervation to the dura over the cribriform plate of the ethmoid bone, medial orbital roof, crista galli, and rostral one third of the falx, including the superior and inferior sagittal sinuses (Feindel et al., 1960; Kimmel, 1961b; Lance, 1982; McNaughton, 1938; McNaughton and Feindel, 1977; Netter and Mitchell, 1983; Penfield and McNaughton, 1940).

The maxillary division of the trigeminal nerve gives off a dural branch, the nervus meningeus medius of Arnold (1860), before entering the cavernous sinus. It courses laterally and anteriorly within the dura of the middle fossa floor to join the middle meningeal artery, most often the anterior branch but occasionally the main trunk or posterior branch. Closely following the artery and its branches, it supplies the dura of the anterior floor of the middle fossa along with a variable contribution from branches of the mandibular division. Branches of the nervus meningeus medius, along with the middle meningeal artery, cross the sphenoidal ridge to innervate the dural covering of the orbital roof, especially its lateral portion (Feindel et al., 1960; Kimmel, 1961b; Lance, 1982; McNaughton, 1938; McNaughton and Feindel, 1977; Netter and Mitchell, 1983; Penfield and McNaughton, 1940).

The mandibular division of the trigeminal nerve consists of a large preganglionic sensory root and the smaller motor/proprioceptive root (portio minor), which unite immediately on leaving the foramen ovale. The nerve then lies between the lateral pterygoid and tensor veli palatini muscles just anterior to the extracranial portion of the middle meningeal artery. Here, the otic ganglion is suspended from the medial surface of the nerve by its preganglionic root. The nervus spinosus of Luschka (1850) leaves the mandibular nerve posteriorly at this level to join the middle meningeal artery and re-enter the cranial cavity with that vessel through the foramen spinosum. According to Penfield and McNaughton (1940), the nervus spinosus sometimes passes directly from the third division to the artery without first leaving the skull. In all cases the nerve closely follows the middle meningeal artery and its ramifications to supply the dura over the lateral floor of the middle fossa and most of the convexity of the cranium. On reaching the vertex between the anterior and middle thirds of the superior sagittal sinus, branches of the nervus spinosus provide innervation to the "sensory watershed" region of the falx between the portions supplied by the first division through the tentorial and anterior meningeal nerves (Feindel et al., 1960; Kimmel, 1961b; McNaughton, 1938; McNaughton and Feindel, 1977; Netter and Mitchell, 1983; Penfield and McNaughton, 1940).

Cadaver dissection reveals that fibers originating in all divisions of the trigeminal nerve supply the supratentorial dura in an orderly and generally constant fashion. The first-division fibers, via the tentorial nerve, are distributed predominantly along venous structures (the major supratentorial dural sinuses), whereas the second- and third-division fibers of the nervus meningeus medius and nervus spinosus closely follow arterial structures (the middle meningeal artery and its branches).

The data gathered by investigators using the technique of retrograde axonal transport of horseradish peroxidase (HRP) in most respects confirm studies based on dissection of anatomic specimens. Steiger et al. (1982) applied HRP to various regions of supratentorial dura in the cat. When HRP was applied to the "medial aspect of the anterior cranial fossa," labeled cell bodies were found in the ophthalmic division of the trigeminal ganglion. When applied more laterally to the orbital roof dura, HRP label appeared predominantly in the maxillary division of the ganglion. Application to the tentorial dura led to labeling of first-division neurons (tentorial nerve), and HRP placed centrally along the middle fossa floor appeared in third-division neurons. Most labeled neurons in all divisions were small, supporting the notions that they subserve pain and that dural sensitivity is limited to that modality. In other recent studies, also in cats (Mayberg et al., 1984; Moskowitz, 1984), HRP applied directly to the middle meningeal artery appeared in trigeminal ganglion cells of all divisions, predominantly the ophthalmic. Likewise, tracer applied to either the anterior or posterior third of the sagittal sinus appeared in first-division neurons. Sinus ligation and falcine transection, either rostral or caudal to the HRP application site, prevented label from appearing in ganglion cells.

Despite some differences between these studies, the data are remarkably consistent with earlier morphologic investigations and support the notion that the trigeminal system is the sole source of sensory innervation to the supratentorial dura, venous sinuses, and meningeal arteries.

Stimulation Studies

Beginning with Cushing (1904), neurosurgeons have taken the opportunity to study and record the reactions of awake patients to stimulation of the various tissues during intracranial operations. Both electrical and mechanical stimulation were used commonly. The observations of most investigators are in accord with those presented by Ray and Wolff (1940) in their study (Cushing, 1909; Fay, 1931, 1937, 1939; Feindel et al., 1960; Kerr, 1961; McNaughton and Feindel, 1977; Penfield, 1935; Penfield and Norcross, 1936; Ray and Wolff, 1940; Tasker et al., 1982; Wirth and Van Buren, 1971; Wolff, 1938, 1955).

The dura over the cerebral convexity and middle fossa floor is insensitive to all modalities of stimulation, except immediately along or within a few millimeters of the meningeal arteries or dural sinuses. In contrast, the dura of the anterior fossa floor is sensitive over its entire surface. Pain arising there is referred to the ipsilateral eye and forehead. It is most intense with stimulation posteromedially at the olfactory groove. The intensity diminishes progressively as the stimulus moves anteriorly toward the frontal convexity or laterally toward the sphenoid ridge. In those regions pain sensitivity along branches of the anterior meningeal artery is maintained and referred to the forehead or back of the eye. Stimulation of the middle meningeal artery or its small branches well out onto the convexity yields pain roughly localized to the area of stimulation.

On stimulation, the superior surface of the tentorium, torcular, transverse, and straight sinuses as well as the posterior portion of the superior and inferior sagittal sinuses all refer pain to the ipsilateral forehead and eye. The anatomic basis of this phenomenon is the distribution of the tentorial nerves discussed earlier (Figure 2–3). Major surface venous tributaries of the superior sagittal, sphenoparietal, and transverse sinuses also refer pain to the cutaneous field of the ipsilateral ophthalmic division. Only one study found random pain referral phenomena, including a number of cases with bilateral or contralateral pain (Wirth and Van Buren, 1971). In general, the patterns of localized and referred pain elicited during intracranial surgery on awake patients correspond to the distribution of trigeminal fibers found in anatomic studies.

It has been the experience of most investigators that the pial surface remote from large basal vessels is insensitive to painful stimulation. However, during functional stereotactic operations on awake patients, Tasker et al. (1982) obtained painful responses to the mechanical passage of a probe or electrical stimulation through the probe in the region of the dorsal midbrain pia. The majority of these responses consisted of pain referred within the ipsilateral trigeminal ophthalmic division. Probe location was predicted from a computerized correlation of ventriculographic and stereotactic brain atlas data. Whether these responses truly represent ophthalmic division innervation of the midbrain pia or reflect incidental stimulation of the tentorium or nearby vascular structures known to have trigeminal innervation remains to be shown conclusively. The application of advanced imaging techniques, such as computerized tomography and magnetic resonance imaging, to probe localization during stereotactic surgery, may ultimately settle the question.

SUPRATENTORIAL CEREBRAL ARTERIES

Anatomic Data

The details of innervation of the vessels of the circle of Willis and their penetrating cerebral branches (Figure 2–4) have been an area of active investigation and controversy since the turn of the century (Gulland, 1898; Hassin, 1929; Huber, 1899). All modern studies have demonstrated a rich nerve plexus, of mixed sensory and vasomotor function, on the main arterial trunks at the base of the brain and their proximal pial surface branches (Lance, 1982). Despite a few reports of vascular nerves accompanying penetrating intracerebral vessels (Chorobski and Penfield, 1932; Clark, 1934; McNaughton, 1938; Penfield, 1932a; Stohr 1932), a recent electron micrographic study failed to disclose any nerve supply to those deep vessels (Dahl, 1976). The bulk of the evidence suggests that the source of afferent sensory fibers on supratentorial arterial trunks is the ophthalmic division of the trigeminal nerve.

Direct connections between the trigeminal nerve and the circle of Willis have only recently been demonstrated in primates. Ruskell and Simons (1987;

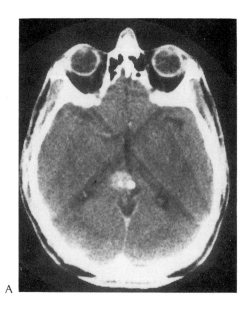

A

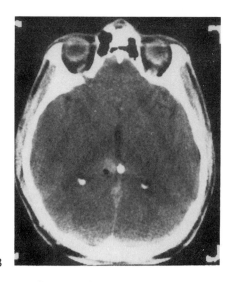

B

Figure 2–3. Trigeminal headache caused by mechanical traction on the deep venous system. (A) Contrast-enhanced computerized tomographic (CT) scan during stereotactic biopsy of a pineal region tumor (germinoma). The biopsy probe is seen in the center of the tumor; the larger midline density is calcification within the pineal gland. Manipulation of the biopsy instrument caused severe, ipsilateral ophthalmic division (V_1) pain—probably resulting from traction on tributaries of the vein of Galen and straight sinus. These structures are innervated by the tentorial nerve of Arnold, a branch of the ophthalmic division of the trigeminal nerve (V_1). (B) Postoperative CT imaging shows a small air bubble at the biopsy site within the tumor. Residual contrast enhancement was still present; no hemorrhage or other complication had occurred.

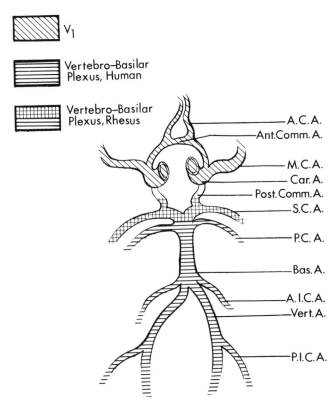

Figure 2–4. The major arterial trunks at the base of the brain are illustrated according to the source of their sensory nerve supply. The ophthalmic division of the trigeminal nerve (V₁) provides the general somatic sensory supply to the intracranial carotid (Car. A.), middle cerebral (M.C.A.), anterior cerebral (A.C.A.), anterior communicating (Ant. Comm. A.), and possibly the proximal posterior communicating (Post. Comm. A.) arteries. The vertebro-basilar plexus provides a mixed sensory–autonomic nerve supply to the vertebral (Vert. A.), basilar (Bas. A), posterior inferior cerebellar (P.I.C.A.), anterior inferior cerebellar (A.I.C.A.) and superior cerebellar (S.C.A.) arteries in the human. This plexus extends more rostrally in the rhesus monkey to supply the posterior cerebral arteries (P.C.A.) as well. The precise origin of the vertebrobasilar plexus remains an area of current research.

Simons and Ruskell, 1988) described three pathways between the trigeminal ganglion and intracranial arteries in cynomolgus monkeys (*Macaca fascicularis*). They performed detailed studies of Wallerian degeneration of nerve fibers in serial brain and cavernous sinus microscopic sections after division of the ophthalmic nerve (V₁). Observations of osmium-stained whole-mount preparations and electron microscopic studies also were performed. In *M. fascicularis*, two to six small branches of V₁ joined the sympathetic plexus on the adventitia of the internal carotid artery just proximal to its exit from the cavernous sinus. The orbitociliary nerve, a branch of V₂ in this species, also sent small branches to the carotid plexus through small nerve twigs that re-entered the cranium from the maxillary fossa through the infraorbital fissure. These investigators also reported a substantial trigeminal contribution to the sensory innervation of the upper basilar artery. A branch of the trigeminal nerve plexus within the cavernous sinus that they called the "recurrent nerve of the plexus" consistently joined the abducens nerve (VI), and traveled with it back toward the pons. Behind the cavernous sinus, the trigeminal fibers left the sixth nerve and distributed themselves along the adventitia of the basilar artery. Most branches on the basilar artery turned upward again to innervate the posterior cerebral, anterior cerebellar, and pontine perforating arteries. In accordance with earlier studies, the ophthalmic division was the principal, if not the sole source of trigeminal nerve fibers. The presence of additional, overlapping innervation from other sources more caudally along the posterior circulation (vagus, upper cervical nerves) also was confirmed indirectly in these studies.

In 1981, Mayberg et al. reported the results of applying HRP to the proximal middle cerebral artery in the cat. They found labeled cells in the ipsilateral trigeminal ganglion, predominantly the ophthalmic division, and in the ipsilateral superior cervical sympathetic ganglion. Subsequent studies employing HRP and wheat germ agglutinin (WGA) confirmed the above findings (Liu-Chen et al., 1983b; Mayberg et al., 1984; Moskowitz, 1984). The authors microscopically examined the ganglia of the trigeminal, facial, glossopharyngeal, and vagus nerves, as well as the superior cervical ganglia bilaterally. Tracer application to distal middle cerebral artery branches yielded fewer labeled cells in the trigeminal ganglion than did proximal application, suggesting a more sparse innervation distally on the vessel. Ligation and transection of the proximal middle cerebral artery prevented any retrograde transport of tracer, and no labeled cells were found. Thus, it is clear that the supratentorial vascular sensory nerves have their first-order neuron in the ophthalmic division of the trigeminal ganglion.

The second-order neuron mediating pain sensation from dural, venous, and arterial trigeminal afferents lies within the descending (spinal) trigeminal nucleus, which itself merges with the substantia gelatinosa (lamina II of Rexed) of the upper cervical cord. Projections from the spinal nucleus of the trigeminal nerve travel in the crossed and uncrossed ventral trigeminothalamic tracts (trigeminal lemniscus) to reach the ventral posteromedial thalamic nuclei, as well as the intralaminar nuclei bilaterally. General somatic afferent impulses (pain) originating in the trigeminal, vagal, and upper cervical nerves converge on the second-order neuron pool within the descending nucleus of the trigeminal nerve at the cervicomedullary junction. This may represent the anatomic basis of the pain referral phenomena seen in pathologic conditions affecting the foramen magnum region (see below) (Kerr, 1961, 1962, 1967). A recent double tracer study of trigeminal innervation of the middle cerebral artery in rats (O'Connor and van der Kooy, 1986) found that single cells within the ophthalmic division often innervated other arteries (middle meningeal) and dural structures through axonal collaterals. However, although trigeminal ganglion cells innervating the cerebral vasculature were clustered near cells innervating cutaneous fields (forehead), no collateral innervation of extra- and intracranial structures was found. This finding lends further support to the notion that central convergence, rather than peripheral axonal divergence, is the mechanism of referred pain within the trigeminal sensory system.

Stimulation Studies

The small cortical surface vessels over the convexity are insensitive to all forms of stimulation. In contrast, stimulation of the supraclinoid internal carotid artery, the proximal middle cerebral artery, and the anterior cerebral artery (pre- and postcommunicating segments) elicits pain referred to the ipsilateral eye and forehead or pterion (Figure 2–5). The large superficial middle cerebral vein and its bridging segment refer pain in the same distribution.

In summary, the trigeminal system, in addition to being the sole source of supratentorial dural and meningeal vessel sensory afferents, is also, through the ophthalmic division, the source of sensory fibers to the vessels of the anterior circulation.

INFRATENTORIAL DURA, DURAL SINUSES, AND MENINGEAL ARTERIES

Anatomic Studies

The interpretation of data from cadaver dissection studies of the posterior fossa dural nerves (Figure 2–6) has generated a controversy for over one and one-quarter centuries, which is only now being sorted out. Various investigators have implicated the facial, glossopharyngeal, vagal, spinal accessory, sympathetic, and upper three cervical nerves either alone or in various combinations as supplying painful sensation to the posterior fossa dura and associated vascular structures (Keller et al., 1985b; Kerr, 1961, 1962; Kimmel, 1961a,b; Lance, 1982; Netter and Mitchell, 1983; Pearson, 1939).

Kimmel (1961a,b) studied the posterior fossa nerves in serially sectioned human embryos. He rejected the notion of a cranial nerve source for sensory innervation of the infratentorial compartment, and advanced the theory that cells in the upper three cervical dorsal root ganglia sent fibers through the foramen magnum, hypoglossal canal, and jugular foramen in company with the respective cranial nerves. More recent studies have shown Kimmel's theory to be at least partly true. General somatic afferent fibers with cell bodies in the superior vagal ganglion form a recurrent meningeal branch that travels back through the jugular foramen. The cells of the upper two or three cervical spinal ganglia probably contribute to the recurrent meningeal branch of the vagus through interconnections at the level of the superior vagal ganglion. The superior cervical sympathetic ganglion also contributes vasomotor nerve fibers to the recurrent meningeal nerve at this level. Once inside the cranium, branches of the nerve travel superiorly and anteriorly along the walls of the sigmoid sinus to innervate dura over the petrous surface of the temporal bone. Other fibers turn posteriorly at the level of the transverse sinus to reach the falx cerebelli, occipital sinus, and dura covering the suboccipital cerebellar surface. The cen-

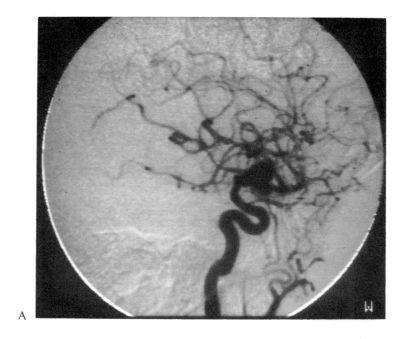

A

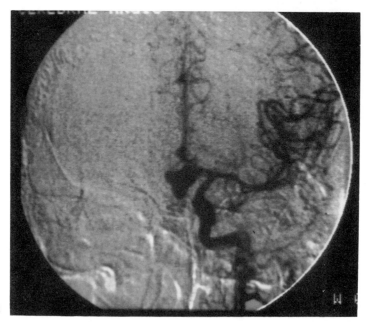

B

Figure 2–5. Headache caused by stretching and/or irritation of supratentorial vascular nerves. Cerebral angiogram, lateral view *(A)* and anteroposterior view *(B)*, showing a multilobed anterior communicating artery aneurysm that fills from the left internal carotid circulation. The patient experienced two episodes of left-sided orbitofrontal headache in the ophthalmic division (V₁) over a 10-day period before catastrophic subarachnoid hemorrhage occurred. His initial headaches were probably caused by stretching of the artery walls as the aneurysm enlarged or, alternatively, by irrigation of ophthalmic division afferents after minor aneurysmal leaks.

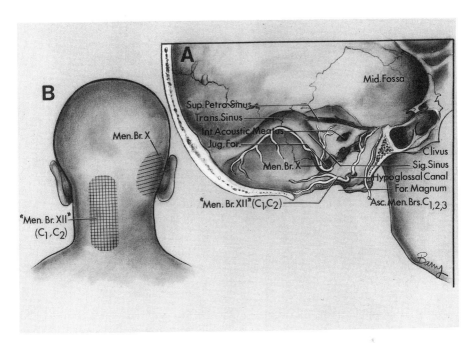

Figure 2–6. (A) The dura, dural sinuses, and meningeal arteries of the posterior fossa with their accompanying sensory nerve supply. The recurrent meningeal branch of the vagus nerve (Men. Br. X) enters the jugular foramen (Jug. For.) to innervate the dura covering the petrous surface of the temporal bone as well as the suboccipital cerebellar convexity and adjacent sinuses: sigmoid sinus (Sig. Sinus), superior petrosal sinus (Sup. Petro. Sinus), and transverse sinus (Trans. Sinus). The meningeal branch of the hypoglossal nerve (Men. Br. XII) enters the hypoglossal canal with the posterior meningeal branch of the ascending pharyngeal artery. The fibers actually arise in the upper two cervical dorsal root ganglia and provide innervation to the lateral margin of the foramen magnum (For. Magnum) and lateral posterior fossa floor. Ascending branches of meningeal rami from the upper three cervical nerves (Asc. Men. Brs. C$_{1,2,3}$) traverse the dura along the anterior craniospinal junction to supply the clivus. These reach almost to the level of the posterior clinoid processes. Key to abbreviations: Int. Acoustic Meatus, internal acoustic meatus; Mid. Fossa, middle fossa. (B) Stimulation of structures innervated by the recurrent meningeal branch of the vagus nerve elicits referred pain behind the ipsilateral ear in the distribution of the auricular (cutaneous) branch of the vagus. Sensations evoked by stimulation of the dural structures innervated by upper cervical fibers forming the meningeal branch of the hypoglossal nerve are referred to the ipsilateral occipitonuchal region within the highest cervical dermatomes. Stimulation of the ventral posterior fossa dura innervated by the ascending meningeal branches of C$_1$, C$_2$, and C$_3$ during intracranial surgery on awake patients has not been reported.

31

tral processes of vagal general somatic afferent cells synapse on second-order neurons in the ipsilateral spinal trigeminal nucleus.

Sensory fibers entering the posterior fossa through the hypoglossal canal all originate in cells of the upper two cervical spinal ganglia. They travel with the hypoglossal nerve and meningeal branch of the ascending pharyngeal artery, form a plexus within the hypoglossal canal, and emerge onto the posterior fossa floor as two branches. One extends anteriorly and laterally to innervate dura to the level of the inferior petrosal sinus. The posterior branch travels along the posterolateral margin of the foramen magnum to supply the dura of the medial posterior fossa floor.

The dura lining the anterior floor of the posterior fossa, clivus, and ventral craniospinal junction is supplied by ascending branches of meningeal rami from the upper three cervical nerves. The majority of fibers originate at the second cervical level. Anastomoses between branches from opposite sides of the body occur within the ventral dura near the midline. These branches extend rostrally almost to the level of the posterior clinoid processes (Kimmel, 1961a,b).

Studies of posterior fossa dural innervation utilizing current neuroanatomic tracer techniques have only recently been reported (Keller et al., 1985b). In the cat, application of HRP to the dura of the inferior leaf of the tentorium, the suboccipital cerebellar surface, and the clivus all led to bilateral tracer uptake in the upper three cervical dorsal root ganglia. Tracer applied to tentorial dura appears in the ophthalmic division of the trigeminal ganglion as well. Application to the suboccipital dura leads to labeling of cells in the superior vagal ganglion, presumably via the recurrent meningeal branch. A pathway to explain the appearance of HRP-labeled cells in the mandibular division of the trigeminal ganglion after application to suboccipital dura has not yet been found. HRP placed on dura covering the clivus labels cells in the superior vagal ganglion, as well as the cervical dorsal root ganglia. The finding of bilateral labeling in many cases is likely due to the intermingling of fibers from both sides of the body mentioned earlier.

Significantly, no tracer appears in the geniculate, inferior vagal (nodose), or superior or inferior glossopharyngeal ganglia. These findings are in general agreement with current concepts of posterior fossa innervation based on anatomic dissection. Interspecies variation occurs, and is especially significant in terms of the trigeminal system's contribution to the sensory innervation of posterior fossa structures.

Stimulation Studies

The patterns of referred pain elicited during the stimulation of posterior fossa dura and associated vascular channels during intracranial surgery on awake patients confirm the anatomic data presented above (Dalessio, 1980b; Kerr, 1967; Penfield and McNaughton, 1940; Pickering, 1955). As in the supratentorial compartment, the dura itself over the suboccipital cerebellar convexity is for the most part insensitive to all forms of stimulation (Ray and Wolff, 1940).

The dura covering the medial petrous surface and lateral posterior fossa floor, including the sigmoid sinus, is sensitive to stimulation, with pain referred to an area behind the ipsilateral ear. Stimulation along the lower margin of the transverse sinus and adjacent superior portion of the occipital sinus elicits pain referred to the same area. All of the previously named dural structures are innervated by the recurrent meningeal branch of the vagus nerve. The area of pain referral corresponds to the cutaneous distribution of the auricular branch of the vagus, which arises from the superior ganglion at the same level as the meningeal branch. Furthermore, intracranial section of the vagus nerve abolishes pain sensitivity in these dural structures.

The mesial posterior fossa floor surrounding the foramen magnum, the dorsal suboccipitocervical junction, and the lower portion of the occipital sinus are all sensitive to stimulation, with pain referred to the low occipital and upper cervical regions. Stimulation of branches of the posterior meningeal artery along the floor of the posterior fossa also produces low occipital–upper cervical pain. These correspond to the dural and cutaneous fields of the upper cervical roots, the pain being abolished by intradural section of the upper three cervical dorsal roots. The ventral margin of the foramen magnum, posterior fossa floor, and clivus also receive upper cervical sensory fibers, but have not been exposed and stimulated in awake patients.

Kerr found a unique role for the first cervical dorsal root, which he exposed in awake surgical patients (Kerr 1961, 1962, 1967). Electrical stimulation of C_1 intradural fibers caused frontal headache in the distribution of the ipsilateral trigeminal ophthalmic division. Central processes from pseudounipolar cells in the first cervical spinal ganglion synapse with their second-order neurons within the spinal trigeminal nuclear complex at the cervicomedullary junction. Kerr proposed central processing at this level as a mechanism to explain the phenomenon of fronto-orbital headache due to tonsillar herniation or a foramen magnum lesion compressing and irritating the first cervical root (Figure 2–7).

INFRATENTORIAL CEREBRAL ARTERIES

Anatomic Studies

Aside from revealing the presence of a perivascular nerve plexus on the surface of the vertebrobasilar vessels and their branches, studies of stained cadaver material have contributed little toward uncovering the origin of such nerves (see Figure 2–3). A sympathetic contribution via the perivertebral plexus exists, but its relevance to sensory innervation is doubtful.

Cadaver dissections have shown that the rostral extent of the vertebrobasilar nerve plexus varies among species. In the human it includes the superior cerebellar arteries, whereas in the rhesus monkey it extends onto the posterior cerebral arteries (McNaughton, 1938). Thus, data from anatomic tracer studies or physiologic experiments performed on lower animals may not accurately explain headache phenomena observed in humans. This is especially true for the posterior cerebral and posterior communicating arteries, which may represent a sensory watershed between the trigeminal and vagocervical innervation territories.

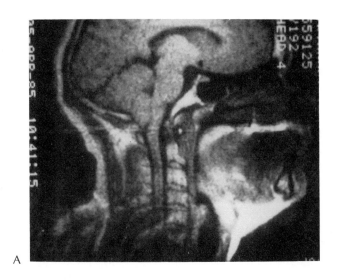

A

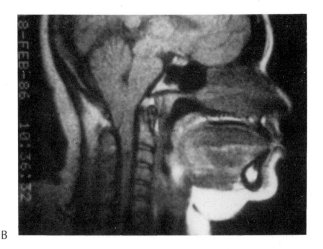

B

Figure 2–7. Fronto-orbital headache associated with tonsillar herniation. Sagittal magnetic resonance images of two patients with Chiari malformation and severe, bilateral ophthalmic division headache associated with tonsillar herniation that distorted high cervical (C_1, C_2) root fibers. Central processing of C_2 afferent impulses within the dorsal horn and descending (spinal) trigeminal nuclear complex was the mechanism proposed by Kerr (1961, 1962, 1967) to explain trigeminal pain in the setting of a foramen magnum lesion. The patient in A had no other symptoms. The patient in B had a more extensive malformation that caused an eye movement disorder and symptoms of cervical hydromyelia (cavity in spinal cord seen at and below C_3). Neither patient had hydrocephalus. Frontal headaches were relieved in both patients by decompressive surgery.

Keller and others (1985a) examined the ganglia of the trigeminal, facial, glossopharyngeal, and vagal nerves, as well as dorsal root ganglia of the upper three cervical nerves and the superior cervical, stellate, and sphenopalatine ganglia in a series of cats after application of HRP or WGA-HRP to the caudal basilar artery. They found positive label uptake in cells of the superior cervical, stellate, sphenopalatine, trigeminal, and superior vagal ganglia (although the label in the latter was considered to be spurious). Of these ganglia, only the trigeminal mediates general somatic (pain) sensation. Later investigators found contributions from the first three cervical dorsal root ganglia to the sensory innervation of the vertebrobasilar vessels in the cat and in the rat. Saito and Moskowitz (1989) analyzed the substance P content of cerebral arteries before and after cervical ganglionectomy in cats. Arbab et al. (1986) used WGA-HRP tracer studies to obtain similar data in rats. Both studies support the schema presented in Figure 2–4. The few intraoperative observations of basilar artery branch stimulation in humans also suggest a nontrigeminal source for sensory nerves to those vessels. Thus, the precise origins of and pathways for painful sensation from posterior fossa arterial structures that remained unsettled a few years ago (Lance, 1982) are now being elucidated.

Stimulation Studies

Ray and Wolff (1940) stimulated a circumferential pontine perforating branch of the basilar artery and the internal auditory artery. Both caused pain referred behind the ipsilateral ear, suggesting innervation by the vagus nerve.

Stimulation of the intradural segment of the vertebral artery or its branch, the posterior inferior cerebellar artery, causes diffuse pain referred to the occiput or to the upper cervical dermatomes. Thus, the pain referral patterns observed during the stimulation of posterior fossa structures in awake surgical patients correspond to the distribution of general somatic afferent fibers revealed by some anatomic studies, but questioned by others.

CLINICAL OBSERVATIONS

Since Cushing reported the loss of middle fossa dural sensitivity following removal of the trigeminal ganglion (Cushing, 1904), clinical observation of a large number of patients after surgical, pharmacologic, or pathologic interruption of intracranial pain pathways has contributed much to understanding the anatomic principles underlying headache mechanisms. The trigeminal and vagus nerves, along with the dorsal roots of the upper three cervical spinal nerves, are the only structures whose destruction has consistently abolished intracranial pain sensitivity in the regions outlined earlier in this chapter. Ganglionectomy, rhizotomy, chemical gangliolysis, brainstem injury, or syringomyelia with accompanying anesthesia in intracranial regions appropriate to the locale of the lesion abolish headache resulting from histamine injection, direct dural or vascular stimulation, pneumography, or migraine in the anesthetic zone (Carmichael and Woolard, 1933; Cushing, 1904; Graham and Wolff, 1937; Northfield, 1938; Pickering, 1939; Schumacher et al., 1940; Sutherland and Wolff 1938; Von Storch et al., 1940; Wolff, 1938).

Among the structures that clinical observation has shown are not of importance in the generation or conduction of intracranial pain are the facial, glossopharyngeal, and sympathetic nerves. Destruction of these nerves has no effect on dural pain sensitivity, histamine headache, or migraine. Operations have been performed specifically for the relief of headache. However, it is appropriate to mention here that procedures not based on sound anatomic principles have not withstood the test of time.

Thus, operations such as superficial temporal or middle meningeal artery ligation (Craig, 1933), cervical or periarterial sympathectomy (Dandy, 1931; Penfield, 1932b), petrosal neurectomy (Gardner et al., 1947; Kunkel and Dohn, 1974; Sachs, 1969), and therapeutic pneumography or lysis of subdural adhesions (Penfield and Norcross, 1936; Penfield and McNaughton, 1940) as treatments for headache are no longer performed. Most of Penfield's patients were relieved of their headaches only after a denervation procedure that included the ophthalmic division of the trigeminal nerve. The surgical treatment of medically intractable cluster headache (chronic migrainous neuralgia, periodic migrainous neuralgia, petrosal neuralgia) has remained a recurring theme in the neurosurgical and otorhinologic literature. Although petrosal neurectomy has been abandoned, a series of operations that included transection of the nervus intermedius or removal of the sphenopalatine ganglion has been reported recently (Cepero et al., 1987; Kunkel and Dohn, 1974; Morgenlander and Wilkins, 1990; Rowed, 1990; Wake and Hitchcock, 1987). A critical review of these more recent studies provides little support for the interruption of autonomic pathways in the treatment of headache disorders. Most series included section, coagulation, or manipulation of the trigeminal nerve. However, partial trigeminal section that did not cause dense sensory loss in the ophthalmic division (V_1) was accompanied by a high postoperative pain recurrence rate (77 to 92%) in one carefully analyzed series (Morgenlander and Wilkins, 1990). In fact, Onofrio and Campbell (1986) reported results with trigeminal rhizotomy or radiofrequency lesioning alone for cluster headache superior to those other investigators had reported for surgical procedures that involved multiple nerves. All patients who experienced a good or excellent result had dense sensory loss in V_1. The effects of trigeminal lesions on the pressor response elicited by painful stimulation of intracranial structures in anesthetized animals lend further support for the exclusive role of the fifth nerve in mediating supratentorial pain sensations (Leake et al., 1927; Levine and Wolff, 1932; Wall and Pribram, 1950).

In accordance with anatomic data, clinical observations have established a definite, albeit limited, role for the upper cervical nerve roots in the production of headache pain. So-called third occipital headache, sometimes accompanied by radiation from the suboccipital region (C_2 and C_3 dermatomes) to the vertex or forehead (V_1 distribution) has been studied by a number of investigators (Bogduk and Marsland, 1986; Edmeads, 1988; Jansen et al., 1989; Poletti and Sweet, 1990). In highly selected patients, local anesthetic blockade or surgical decompression of the involved roots has temporarily or permanently relieved pain. The central convergence of pain sensation (general somatic afferents) from cervical and trigeminal dermatomes within the spinal trigeminal nucleus and tract, as outlined above, is the most plausible explanation for these phenomena.

More recently, the effect of lesions of the trigeminal ganglion, cervical dorsal roots, and cervical sympathetic ganglia on the levels of substance P and other pain-associated peptides in the pial vessels of various species has been studied. Depletion of substance P in the anterior circle of Willis after trigeminal ganglionectomy again underscores the key role of the trigeminal system in mediating head pain from supratentorial structures. Whereas evidence regarding the source of substance P in the vertebrobasilar circulation was inconclusive a few years ago (Liu-Chen et al., 1983a,b,c; Moskowitz, 1984; Moskowitz et al., 1983; Norregaard et al., 1983), recent studies have shed considerable light on the subject (see above; see also Chapters 4 and 5).

So far the mechanisms and pathways involved in the transmission of pain due to pathologic processes within the cerebral parenchyma or ventricular system have not been addressed. The cerebral substance itself and the ventricular ependyma are insensitive to all forms of stimulation. Thus, pain associated with intracerebral lesions or hydrocephalus arises as a consequence of effects on the pain-sensitive structures discussed in the previous sections of this chapter.

Depending on the size, location, and mass effect of a particular lesion, the affected pain-sensitive structures may be located either nearby, at a distance, or both (Dalessio, 1980a). A more detailed discussion of headache and brain tumor appears in Chapter 19; however, the anatomic principles of pain sensitivity associated with intracranial mass lesions bear mentioning here. According to Ray and Wolff (1940) and Kunkle, Ray, and Wolff (1942), the mechanisms include the following: (1) traction on venous sinuses or their tributaries; (2) traction on meningeal arteries; (3) traction on the large arteries at the base of the brain; (4) direct pressure on cranial or cervical pain-sensitive nerves; (5) dilation of intracranial arteries; and (6) inflammation of any pain-sensitive structure.

Processes that affect local pain-sensitive structures reproduce the various pain patterns elicited during intraoperative stimulation studies as described above. Mass lesions that produce displacements or herniation syndromes at a distance elicit pain of a generalized or falsely localizing nature. One special instance is the phenomenon of displacement of the underlying large vessels of the circle of Willis by distention of the third ventricle in patients with hydrocephalus or tumor. This produces severe generalized headache. Another special phenomenon is the frontal headache that accompanies tonsillar herniation or a mass lesion of the foramen magnum, associated with upper cervical root traction. Central processing of afferent signals at the level of the spinal trigeminal nucleus has been discussed earlier as a possible mechanism in such cases.

In summary, all available evidence supports an orderly somatotopic representation of the supratentorial pain-sensitive meningeal and vascular structures within the trigeminal system. Pain sensation from posterior fossa structures is carried centrally by the vagus nerve, the upper three cervical nerves, and possibly the trigeminal afferents as well. The patterns of pain referral from experimental or pathologic stimulation of sensitive structures generally follow the dermatomal distribution of the structures' nerve supply. The convergence of trigeminal, vagal, and cervical afferents on second-order neurons in the spinal trigeminal nucleus and dorsal horn at the cervicomedullary junction unites pain impulses encoded from all portions of the cranium centrally. The anatomic principles outlined in this chapter form the basis for an understanding of the mechanisms and rational treatment of head pain.

REFERENCES

Arbab, M.A.R., L. Wiklund, and N.A. Svendgaard (1986). Origin and distribution of cerebral vascular innervation from superior cervical, trigeminal and spinal ganglia investigated with retrograde and anterograde WGA-HRP tracing in the rat. *Neuroscience 19:695.*

Arnold, F. (1851). *Handbuch der Anatomie des Menschen.* A. Emmerling and Herder, Freiberg, Germany.

Arnold, F. (1860). *Icones Nervorum Capitis.* J.C.B. Mohr, Heidelberg, Germany.

Bogduk, N. and A. Marsland (1986). On the concept of third occipital headache. *J. Neurol. Neurosurg. Psychiatry 49:775.*

Carmicheal, E.A. and H.H. Woollard (1933). Some observations on the fifth and seventh cranial nerves. *Brain 56:109.*

Cepero, R., R.H. Miller, and K.L. Bressler (1987). Long-term results of splenopalatine ganglionectomy for facial pain. *Am. J. Otolaryngol. 3:171.*

Chorobski, J. and W. Penfield (1932). Cerebral vasodilator nerves and their pathway from the medulla oblongata, with observations on the pial and intracerebral vascular plexus. *Arch. Neurol. Psychiatry 28:1257.*

Clark, S.L. (1934). Innervation of the choroid plexuses and the blood vessels within the central nervous system. *J. Comp. Neurol. 60:21.*

Craig, W.M. (1933). Localized headache associated with lesion of meningeal vessels. *JAMA 100:816.*

Cushing, H. (1904). The sensory distribution of the fifth cranial nerve. *Bull. Johns Hopkins Hosp. 15:213.*

Cushing, H. (1909). A note upon the faradic stimulation of the post-central gyrus in conscious patients. *Brain 32:44.*

Dahl, E. (1976). Microscopic observations on cerebral arteries. In *The Cerebral Vessel Wall* (J. Cervos-Navarro et al., eds.), pp. 15–21, 61–66. Raven Press, New York.

Dalessio, D.J. (1980a). Clinical observations on headache. In *Wolff's Headache and Other Head Pain* (D.J. Dalessio, ed.), 4th ed., Chapter 25. Oxford, New York.

Dalessio, D.J. (1980b). Pain sensitive structures within the cranium. In *Wolff's Headache and Other Head Pain* (D.J. Dalessio, ed.), 4th ed., Chapter 3. Oxford, New York.

Dandy, W.E. (1931). Treatment of hemicrania (migraine) by removal of the inferior cervical and first thoracic sympathetic ganglion. *Bull. Johns Hopkins Hosp. 48: 357.*

Edmeads, J. (1988). The cervical spine and headache. *Neurology 38:1874.*

Fay, T. (1931). Certain fundamental cerebral signs and symptoms and their response to dehydration. *Arch. Neurol. Psychiatry 26:452.*

Fay, T. (1937). Mechanism of headache. *Arch. Neurol. Psychiatry 37:471.*

Fay, T. (1939). Problems of pain reference to the extremities, their diagnosis and treatment. *Am. J. Surg. 44:*52.

Feindel, W., W. Penfield, and F. McNaughton (1960). The tentorial nerve and localization of intracranial pain in man. *Neurology 10:*555.

Gardner, W.S., A. Stowell, and R. Dutlinger (1947). Resection of the greater superficial petrosal nerve in the treatment of unilateral headache. *J. Neurosurg. 4:*105.

Graham, J.R. and H.G. Wolff (1937). Mechanism of migraine headache and action of ergotamine tartarate. *Assoc. Res. Nerv. Dis. Proc. 18:*638.

Gulland, L. (1898). The occurrence of nerves on intracranial blood vessels. *BMJ 2:*781.

Hassin, G.B. (1929). The nerve supply of the cerebral blood vessels, a histologic study. *Arch. Neurol. Psychiatry 22:*375.

Huber, C.G. (1899). Observations on the innervation of the intracranial vessels. *J. Comp. Neurol. 9:*1.

Jansen, J., A. Bardosi, J. Hildebrandt, and A. Lucke (1989). Cervicogenic, hemicranial attacks associated with vascular irritation or compression of the cervical nerve root C2. Clinical manifestations and morphological findings. *Pain 39:*203.

Keller, J.T., A. Beduk, and M.C. Saunders (1985a). Origin of fibers innervating the basilar artery of the cat. *Neurosci. Lett. 58:*263.

Keller, J.T., M.C. Saunders, A. Beduk, and J.G. Jollis (1985b). Innervation of the posterior fossa dura of the cat. *Brain Res. Bull. 14:*97.

Kerr, F.W.L. (1961). A mechanism to account for frontal headache in cases of posterior fossa tumors. *J. Neurosurg. 18:*605.

Kerr, F.W.L. (1962). Facial, vagal and glossopharyngeal nerves in the cat: Afferent connections. *Neurology 6:*264.

Kerr, F.W.L. (1967). Evidence for a peripheral etiology of trigeminal neuralgia. *J. Neurosurg. 26*(Suppl.):168.

Kimmel, D.L. (1961a). Innervation of spinal dura mater and dura mater of the posterior cranial fossa. *Neurology 11:*800.

Kimmel, D.L. (1961b). The nerves of the cranial dura mater and their significance in dural headache and referred pain. *Chicago Med. School Q. 22:*16.

Kunkel, R.S., and D.F. Dohn (1974). Surgical treatment of chronic migrainous neuralgia. *Clev. Clin. Q. 41:*189.

Kunkle, E.C., B.S. Ray, and H.G. Wolff (1942). Studies on headache: The mechanisms and significance of the headache associated with brain tumor. *Bull. N. Y. Acad. Med. 18:*400.

Lance, J. (1982). Causes of headache. In *Mechanism and Management of Headache,* 4th ed., Chapter 5. Butterworths, London.

Leake, C.D., A.S. Loevenhart, and C.W. Muehlberger (1927). Dilatation of cerebral blood vessels as a factor in headache. *JAMA 88:*1076.

Levine, M. and H.G. Wolff (1932). Cerebral circulation: Afferent impulses from the blood vessels of the pia. *Arch. Neurol. Psychiatry 28:*140.

Liu-Chen, L.Y., P.H. Han, and M.A. Moskowitz (1983a). Pia arachnoid contains substance P originating from trigeminal neurons. *Neuroscience 9:*803.

Liu-Chen, L.Y., T. Liszcak, S.A. Gillespie et al. (1983b). Substance P-containing fibers in middle cerebral arteries—origin and ultrastructure. *Neurosci. Soc. Proc. 13:*294.

Liu-Chen, L.Y., M.R. Mayberg, and M.A. Moskowitz (1983c). Immunohistochemical evidence for a substance P-containing trigeminovascular pathway to pial arteries in cats. *Brain Res. 268:*162.

Luschka, H. (1850). *Die Nerven in der harten Hirnhaut.* H. Laupp, Tubingen, Germany.

Mayberg, M., R.S. Langer, N.T. Zervas, and M.A. Moskowitz (1981). Perivascular meningeal projections from cat trigeminal ganglia: Possible pathways for vascular headaches in man. *Science 213:*228.

Mayberg, M.R., N.T. Zervas, and M.A. Moskowitz (1984). Trigeminal projections to supratentorial pial and dural blood vessels in cats demonstrated by horseradish peroxidase histochemistry. *J. Comp. Neurol. 223:*46.

McNaughton, F.L. (1938). The innervation of the intracranial blood vessels and dural sinuses. *Assoc. Res. Nerv. Dis. Proc. 18:*178.

McNaughton, F.L. and W.H. Feindel (1977). Innervation of intracranial structures: A reappraisal. In *Physiological Aspects of Clinical Neurology* (F.C. Rose, ed.), Chapter 19. Blackwell, Oxford, England.

Morgenlander, J.C. and R.H. Wilkins (1990). Surgical treatment of cluster headache. *J. Neurosurg. 72:*866.

Moskowitz, M.A. (1984). The neurobiology of vascular head pain. *Ann. Neurol. 16:*157.

Moskowitz, M.A., T.V. Norregaard, L.Y. Liu-Chen et al. (1983). VIP, CCK, and met-enkephalin in pia arachnoid and cerebral arteries after unilateral lesions of the cat trigeminal ganglia. *Neurosci. Soc. 13:*576.

Netter, F.H. and G.A.G. Mitchell (1983). Cranial nerves. In *The CIBA Collection of Medical Illustrations,* Vol. I, Part I, Sect. 5. (prepared by F.H. Netter). CIBA, West Caldwell, NJ.

Norregaard, T.V., R.C. Weatherwax, and M.A. Moskowitz (1983). The effects of lesioning the trigeminal, superior cervical sympathetic, C2 and C3 ganglia on substance-P in cat cerebral arteries. *Neurosci. Soc. Proc. 13:*455.

Northfield, D.W.C. (1938). Some observations on headache. *Brain 61:*133.

O'Connor, T.P. and D. van der Kooy (1986). Pattern of intracranial and extracranial projections of trigeminal ganglion cells. *J. Neurosci. 6:*2200.

Onofrio, B.M. and J.K. Campbell (1986). Surgical treatment of chronic cluster headache. *Mayo Clin. Proc. 61:*537.

Pearson, A.A. (1939). The hypoglossal nerve in human embryos. *J. Comp. Neurol. 71:* 21.

Penfield, W. (1932a). Intracerebral vascular nerves. *Arch. Neurol. Psychiatry 27:*30.

Penfield, W. (1932b). Operative treatment of migraine and observations on the mechanism of vascular pain. *Trans. Am. Acad. Ophthalmol. 37:*50.

Penfield, W. (1935). A contribution to the mechanism of intracranial pain. *Assoc. Res. Nerv. Dis. Proc. 15:*399.

Penfield, W. and F. McNaughton (1940). Dural headache and innervation of the dura mater. *Arch. Neurol. Psychiatry 44:*43.

Penfield, W. and N.C. Norcross (1936). Subdural traction and posttraumatic headache, study of pathology and therapeusis. *Arch. Neurol. Psychiatry 36:*75.

Pickering, G.W. (1939). Experimental observations on headache. *BMJ 1:*4087.

Pickering, G.W. (1955). Experimental observations on headache. *Int. Arch. Allergy 7:* 1955.

Poletti, C.E. and W.H. Sweet (1990). Entrapment of the C2 root and ganglion by the atlanto-epistrophic ligament: Clinical syndrome and surgical anatomy. *Neurosurgery 27:*288.

Ray, B.S. and H.G. Wolff (1940). Experimental studies on headache pain-sensitive structures of the head and their significance in headache. *Arch. Surg. 41:*813.

Rowed, D.W. (1990). Chronic cluster headache managed by nervus intermedius section. *Headache 30:*401.

Ruskell, G.L. and T. Simons (1987). Trigeminal nerve pathways to the cerebral arteries in monkeys. *J. Anat. 155:*23.

Sachs, E. Jr. (1969). Further observations on surgery of the nervus intermedius. *Headache 9:*159.

Saito, K. and M.A. Moskowitz (1989). Contributions from the upper cervical dorsal roots and trigeminal ganglia to the feline circle of Willis. *Stroke 20:*524.

Schumacher, G.A., B.S. Ray, and H.G. Wolff (1940). Experimental studies on headache. Further analysis of histamine headache and its pain pathways. *Arch. Neurol. Psychiatry 44:*701.

Simons, T. and G.L. Ruskell (1988). Distribution and termination of trigeminal nerves to the cerebral arteries in monkeys. *J. Anat. 159:*57.

Steiger, H.J., J.M. Tew Jr., and J.J. Keller (1982). The sensory representation of the dura mater in the trigeminal ganglion of the cat. *Neurosci. Lett. 31:*231.

Stohr, P.J. (1932). Nerves of the blood vessels, heart, meninges, digestive tract and urinary bladder. In *Cytology and Cellular Pathology of the Nervous System,* Vol. 1, Sect. 8 (W. Penfield, ed.), p. 383. Hoeber, New York.

Sutherland, A.M. and H.G. Wolff (1938). Experimental studies on headache. Observations on the mechanism of headache in migraine, hypertension and fever therapy. *Trans. Am. Neurol. Assoc. 64:*103.

Tasker, R.R., L. Organ, and P.A. Hawrylyshyn (1982). Pial responses. In *The Thalamus and Midbrain of Man,* Chapter 12. Charles C Thomas, Springfield, IL.

Von Storch, J.J.C., L. Secunda, and C.M. Krinsky (1940). Production and localization of headache with subarachnoid and ventricular air. *Arch. Neurol. Psychiatry 43:* 326.

Wake, M. and E. Hitchcock (1987). A review of treatment modalities for periodic migrainous neuralgia. *Pain 31:*345.

Wall, P.D. and K.H. Pribram (1950). Trigeminal neurotomy and blood pressure response from stimulation of lateral cerebral cortex of *Macaca mulatta. J. Neurophysiol. 13:*409.

Wirth, F.P., Jr. and J.M. Van Buren (1971). Referral of pain from dural stimulation in man. *J. Neurosurg. 34:*630.

Wolff, H.G. (1938). Headache and cranial arteries. *Trans. Assoc. Am. Physicians 53:* 193.

Wolff, H.G. (1955). Headache mechanisms. *Int. Arch. Allergy 7:*210.

3

Inheritance and Epidemiology of Headache

W.E. WATERS
STEPHEN D. SILBERSTEIN
DONALD J. DALESSIO

Headache, one of the most common medical symptoms, is a common reason for consulting a doctor. Despite this, it was not until the second half of the 20th century that its inheritance and epidemiology received any detailed study. Many clinicians have made systematic observations based on their experience with patients. Conclusions from clinic-based reports, even those comprising a large consecutive series of patients, may not be confirmed by rigorous study of a defined population, since individuals who consult a medical practitioner are often different from those who do not. Those who go to a doctor with headache may have more severe pain, more prolonged symptoms, or more frequent attacks than those who do not seek medical attention, and they are likely to differ in other respects, such as intelligence and social class, as well (see below). These findings make any review of the inheritance and epidemiology of headache difficult, because many reports in the medical literature are based on selected series of patients and many sufferers of headache and migraine do not seek medical attention.

The other difficulty in reviewing the inheritance and epidemiology of headache is the problem of definitions. For most headache disorders there are no anatomic, biochemical, or physiologic markers that are useful for diagnosis in epidemiologic research. Diagnosis rests on the symptoms patients report, and these may be distorted or forgotten, particularly if mild or temporally remote. Even the presence or absence of headache may not always be easy to determine in epidemiologic surveys because some headaches may not be reported either on direct questioning by doctors or on questionnaires. Population-based studies may provide data that are difficult to assess because of widely different response rates in different subgroups (i.e., those who cooperate as opposed to those who do not). Epidemiologic studies have used different definitions and different methods, which may make direct comparisons inappropriate. These and other epidemiologic problems have been considered in detail (Linet and Stewart, 1984; Waters, 1986). This chapter emphasizes findings based on representative populations using defined methods, which are noted because this information will determine how confident one can be about the accuracy and comparability of results.

Defining types of headache in a way suitable for epidemiologic study is perhaps even a greater problem than providing a definition of headache. "Definitions" such as those given by the World Federation of Neurology (1970), which include some of the characteristic features of the condition, are more in the nature of descriptions and are not precise enough for use in epidemiologic studies. Indeed, epidemiologic studies have questioned whether migraine is a separate entity, distinct from other headaches, or simply part of a spectrum of headache of varying degrees of severity (Waters, 1973; Ziegler, 1976).

Previous migraine definitions stressed the three features of migraine: unilateral headache, the presence of a warning, and nausea and vomiting. Some stressed the paroxysmal nature of the pain and a positive family history. None of these criteria were subjected to careful analysis.

Waters (1970, 1986) found little cross-correlation between the three key features of migraine, suggesting that these symptoms do not form an important syndrome. In terms of headache severity, he found that the three key symptoms occurred together more frequently as headache severity increased. The distribution of headache severity spans a continuum from mild attacks that usually do not have unilateral distribution, warning, or nausea to severe headaches that frequently are accompanied by the key features of migraine.

Using the results of a telephone interview survey of 10,109 individuals ages 12 to 29 years in Washington County, Maryland, Celentano et al. (1990) analyzed the frequency, pain, and duration of recent (within 4 weeks) headache attacks. They found that, when migraine and tension-type headache symptoms occurred at the same time, the resultant headaches were moderate in intensity. Symptoms usually associated with migraine (nausea, aura, photophobia) were infrequent but resulted in severe headaches.

Although in the past definitions of migraine and other types of headache were sometimes acknowledged to pose problems, the situation was aggravated by those who still believed that they could clinically diagnose almost all sufferers. This was evidenced by an epidemiologic study of general practitioners, many of whom could not diagnose their own migraine headache (Waters, 1972). It is now accepted that earlier definitions were unsatisfactory. The new "Classification and Diagnostic Criteria for Headache Disorders, Cranial Neuralgias, and Facial Pain" (Headache Classification Committee of the International Headache Society, 1988) accepts that operational diagnostic criteria must be introduced, although this process may be tedious and irritating. Otherwise, if previously available criteria are used, they do not "characterize that patient precisely, but are almost synonymous with stating that the patient has . . . [been diagnosed] according to the opinion of the investigator." This is certainly a difficult problem for epidemiologic studies, which seek to determine the prevalence of various types of headache. The classification of the International Headache Society (IHS) appears to be a great improvement over previous attempts. Its criteria have been criticized as being confusing and, sometimes, arbitrary and dogmatic; however, detailed published evidence of its robustness are now becoming available (Rasmussen et al., 1991). New epidemiologic studies based on these definitions have already appeared and are beginning to clarify the field.

INHERITANCE

Many headache investigators acknowledge, and some stress, that migraine is familial. It is not clear whether familial aggregation occurs as a result of genetic or nongenetic mechanisms. Because families tend to share the same living conditions, headache that runs in families may be environmentally or genetically determined. Many reports in the literature are surprisingly vague and nonspecific; although they may mention a "positive family history," they do not define "positive" or "family." The World Federation of Neurology (1970) included the familial history of migraine in its definition of the condition, as do some authors. They then looked for the familial factor in migraine. However, familial aggregation cannot be studied when family history is part of the definition; it is essential that family history be excluded from headache definitions and case identification, because this practice selects for familial cases. Although many headache and migraine sufferers report similar problems in other members of their families, migraine is a highly prevalent condition. The critical point is whether migraine is more prevalent in the relatives of those with migraine than it is in the relatives of those without migraine. Few studies have even attempted to address this point.

The literature is almost unanimous in stating that migraine is inherited, but there is no consensus on the type of inheritance. Dominant inheritance (Allan, 1928), dominant inheritance with greater penetration in females (Barolin, 1970), recessive inheritance with incomplete penetrance (Goodell et al., 1954), and multifactorial inheritance related to several genes (Dalsgaard-Nielsen and Ulrich, 1973) have all been proposed. McKusick (1988) noted that "familial aggregation of migraine is undoubted," but few have ever attempted to test this in a scientific manner.

Epidemiologic Evidence

In a study using random samples of subjects with no headache, subjects with headache, and subjects with migraine, all selected from a population-based study, first-degree relatives of all the groups living in a defined area were visited at home by a trained interviewer and questioned about headaches that occurred in the previous year (Waters, 1971). The response rate was over 99% of the 524 first-degree relatives: a prevalence of migraine (strictly defined) of 10% was found in the relatives of the probands with migraine, compared with a prevalence of only 5 or 6% in the relatives of the other groups. These differences are less than expected from the literature and were in fact not statistically significant. However, the findings came from interviews of first-degree relatives of migraineurs and suitable controls, all identified from a community study.

Other controlled studies have shown a positive family history among patients with migraine ranging from 34 to 71% (Ash-Upmark, 1953; Bille, 1962; Childs and Sweetnam, 1961; Couch et al., 1986; Ely, 1930; Lennox, 1941). These studies indicate that migraineurs have about a sixfold greater family history of migraine compared to controls. The probands in all of these studies were clinic based. Headache reports from patients are often inaccurate (Dalsgaard-Nielsen et al., 1970); thus, studies of family pedigree based on secondhand histories may be unreliable and may introduce bias. The method of ascertainment can alter dramatically the estimate of familial aggregation. Nonblind assessment based on clinical samples may elevate the degree of familial aggregation, and the "family history method"—as opposed to direct interview—may lead to a two- to threefold underestimation of disease prevalence in relatives (Merikangas, 1990). Waters' low rates may be based on bias in clinic-based samples. They may also be based on a severity effect comparable with a polygenetic model. Persons with more severe cases may go to the clinic and may have greater genetic loading, and such cases may be more heritable.

Few investigators of headache have attempted to separate bias (a systematic type of error, tending to occur in one particular direction) from random error (which generally matters rather less in epidemiologic studies). Some rare forms of headache, such as hemiplegic migraine, are so uncommon that they cannot readily be studied by population surveys. When a number of cases of a rare condition are found in the same family, it is unlikely to be due to chance. An environmental cause should be considered, especially if the inheritance does not seem to correspond with any known genetic pattern.

Twin Studies

Comparison of the disease prevalence in monozygotic (MZ) and dizygotic (DZ) twins allows genetic analysis. These studies have "built-in" controls (Lucas, 1977). Members of a twin pair are concordant when they are affected similarly and discordant when only one is affected. For a condition under genetic control, the twin study method predicts that MZ twins will be more concordant than DZ twins. Many twin studies on migraine have been based on small numbers of cases and others have lacked detailed information on zygosity. Table 3–1 provides the details of the three most important studies of headache in twins.

These studies provide some evidence of inheritance for both migraine and severe headache, but are less convincing than might have been suspected from the results of the numerous uncontrolled clinical studies. In fact, the evidence is weaker than that in Table 3–1. Because migraine is more common in women than in men, one would expect some degree of concordance in the data. When Lucas (1977) analyzed the DZ twins of the same sex, the concordance rate was similar to that in MZ twins. Care was taken in these twin studies to reduce errors, but the possibility of bias still exists. Lucas (1977) concluded that there is "a much lower genetic factor in migraine than previously thought." In addition, MZ twins have more in common than DZ twins. They are more likely to be treated similarly based on their similar appearance.

Table 3–1   Details of three studies of inheritance of headache in twins

Country	Sample	Findings	Reference
Denmark	Danish twin study—1,900 unselected twins	Migraine found in only 84 subjects (2.2%). There were 6 concordant pairs of monozygotic twins among 18 with migraine in at least one, and 3 concordant pairs of dizygotic twins among 57 with migraine in at least one.	Harvald and Hauge (1956)
United States	Wide advertisements yielded 106 twins	Of 41 pairs of monozygotic twins, 11 had at least one individual and 2 had both affected by severe headaches. Of 65 pairs of dizygotic twins, 16 had at least one individual and 2 had both affected by severe headaches.	Ziegler et al., (1975)
England	1,300 twins on London Institute of Psychiatry's twin register	Concordance rates for migraine were 26% in monozygotic twins and 13% in dizygotic twins.	Lucas (1977)

PREVALENCE OF HEADACHE AND MIGRAINE

Adults

One of the main tasks of epidemiology is to measure how common various diseases are in the general population. One useful measure is the *period preva-lence,* defined as the proportion of a particular population that has a particular condition during a defined period of time. Many studies have used the year immediately preceding the survey, and data obtained by questionnaires sent to a representative sample of a defined population, to determine period preva-lence. Data from a survey in the United Kingdom on all headaches are presented in Table 3–2. In all age groups, headache is more common in women than in men. Prevalence in both sexes declines with age. Rasmussen et al. (1991) found a total lifetime prevalence of headache of 99% in women and 93% in men (see below).

Prior to the IHS criteria, there were no agreed-on definitions of migraine

Table 3–2   Prevalence of headache in the previous year (percentages)

	Age groups (years)			
	21–34	35–54	55–74	75 and over
Men	74.0	69.0	53.3	21.7
Women	92.3	82.6	66.2	55.2

Source: Pontypridd survey (Waters, 1986).

Table 3–3 Prevalence of migraine (based on clinical validation of a questionnaire) in the previous year (percentages)

	Age groups (years)			
	21–34	35–54	55–74	75 and over
Men	16.8	16.4	12.6	4.9
Women	30.1	26.0	16.6	10.3

Source: Pontypridd survey (Waters and O'Connor, 1975).

for epidemiologic studies. Some of the characteristic features of migraine are surprisingly common in those with headache in the general population. For example, of all women with a headache in the previous year, 48% had a unilateral distribution of the pain, 48% had nausea with the headache, and 28% had a warning that the attack was coming. This is consistent with the suggestion that migraine and tension-type headache may differ only in severity and have overlapping symptoms (Waters, 1986). Because migraine is a clinical diagnosis, a comparison between a neurologist's clinical diagnosis and the data obtained from questionnaires is an appropriate method of determining migraine prevalence (Waters and O'Connor, 1975). This (Table 3–3) gives a much higher migraine prevalence than most previous studies. Migraine prevalence in other studies has varied greatly, from less than 1% to more than a quarter of the total population (Waters, 1986). This variation may be due to both the variety of migraine definitions and the use of clinic-based or doctor-based studies. Nearly half the patients clinically diagnosed as having migraine in the clinical validation of the questionnaire had never consulted a doctor for their headaches, and only 23% had done so in the previous year (Waters and O'Connor, 1971). Clinic- or physician-based studies will therefore considerably underestimate the true prevalence of migraine. Whatever the view of the actual prevalence in Table 3–3—and this depends on the definitions and diagnosis—the table does present data in different age groups in men and women separately, and all these figures were obtained in a similar way. With this "internal consistency," it is evident that migraine, like all headache, is more prevalent in women than in men and that its prevalence declines with age in both sexes. Studies have now been conducted in many different locations, such as in a Mediterranean culture (D'Alessandro et al., 1988) and in a Bangkok slum (Phanthumchinda and Sithi-Amorn, 1989). The absolute prevalence rates in these studies are dependent on how one diagnoses migraine.

Linet et al. (1989) examined headache prevalence among adolescents and young adults using cross-sectional data from the Washington County, Maryland, telephone interview survey. They attempted to evaluate a subject's most recent headache and the associated symptoms. More than 57% of men and 76% of women experienced their most recent headache in the 4 weeks before the interview. A lifetime history of one or more headaches was reported by 90.8% of men and 95.8% of women. The 4-week migraine prevalence was 3.0% in men and 7.4% in women. Absence from school or work was reported in 1.2 to 4.5% of subjects. Only 14.6% of men and 28.0% of women had consulted a physician for headache. This study suggests that headache clinic– and office practice–based studies focus on a small fraction of all headache sufferers. The lower incidence of migraine in the study is due to the 4-week restriction (as opposed to 3-month or 1-year periods) and the tighter diagnostic criteria used.

The prevalence of chronic migraine headache in the United States has been reported to have increased 60% in the 1980s, from 25.8:1,000 to 41:1,000 persons (MMWR, 1991), according to answers given by a representative sample of the population when periodically asked, on a checklist, if they had a "migraine headache." No definitions were given to the sample because no criteria were used. This finding could result from improved recognition and reporting of "migraine," without an increase in prevalence, or it could represent a true increase in migraine prevalence.

The new headache classification (Headache Classification Committee of the IHS, 1988) has now been used in epidemiologic studies, but it does pose some additional problems in considering an appropriate length of time for a period prevalence. The diagnostic criteria for migraine without aura (formerly called common migraine) require at least five attacks, and those for migraine with aura (formerly called classic migraine) require only two attacks. These arbitrary definitions will therefore result in the ratio of these two types of migraine being dependent on the duration of the period chosen for the measurement of prevalence.

Rasmussen et al. (1991) presented the first prevalence study of specific headache types using the operational diagnostic criteria of the IHS. One thousand 25- to 64-year-old men and women from part of Copenhagen County were randomly selected and were invited to have a general health examination. The participation rate was 76%. The difference in headache prevalence in nonparticipants was not quantitatively important. The authors found lifetime prevalences of any kind of headache, migraine, and tension-type headache were 93%, 8%, and 69%, respectively, in men and 99%, 25%, and 88%, respectively, in women. Prevalence of migraine in the previous year had been 6% in men and 15% in women, and the corresponding prevalence of tension-type headache 63% and 86%. The point prevalence ("Do you have a headache today?") was 11% in men and 22% in women. In this study there was no significant difference in migraine prevalence rates according to age.

Stewart et al. (1992) utilized a modified version of the new IHS definition for migraine in a 1989 study of 15,000 households selected to be representative of the U.S. population. A designated member of each household was asked if there was a member with "severe headache." Each household member between the ages of 12 and 80 with "severe headache" then completed a questionnaire. Stewart et al.'s criteria differed from those of the IHS in that the lifetime number of previous migraine attacks and the headache duration were not considered. (The overwhelming majority of cases met these criteria anyway.) Subjects with severe daily headaches were not considered to have migraine. In 17.6% of women and 5.7% of men, one or more migraine headaches occurred per year. Migraine prevalence varied by age and was highest in both men and women between the ages of 25 and 55 years, peaking near age 40 and decreasing

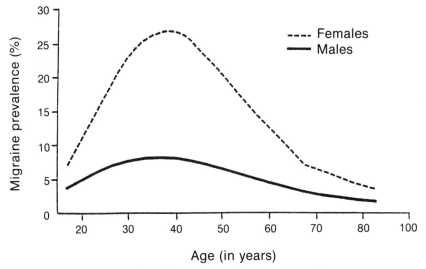

Figure 3–1. Migraine prevalence by age. Prevalence increased from 12 to 38 years of age in both females and males; peak was considerably higher among females. (Reproduced with permission from Stewart, W. F., R. B. Lipton, D. D. Celentano, and M. L. Reed (1992). Prevalence of migraine headache in the United States. *JAMA* 267:64–69.)

in both groups after this age (Figure 3–1). Prevalence was 60% higher in low-income groups compared to high-income groups. Prevalence was lower in higher income groups (Figure 3–2).

Migraine prevalence in this study may be lower than in other studies because analysis was done only of subjects with "severe headache." Subjects with moderate headache, or aura without headache, would have been excluded. The higher prevalence of migraine in lower economic groups is contrary to the belief that migraine is a disease of the higher socioeconomic groups. People from high-income groups were much more likely to report a medical diagnosis of migraine. At least in the United States, it appears that migraine is a disease of higher income people in the doctor's office, but not in the community. People from higher income households are more likely to consult physicians and therefore be disproportionally included in clinic-based studies (Lipton et al., 1992).

The higher prevalence of migraine in the lower socioeconomic groups may reflect a downward socioeconomic drift; may be a side effect of poor diet, stress, or poor medical care; or may represent poorer subjects categorizing their headaches as more "severe." This study, unlike that of Rasmussen et al., found a decrease in migraine prevalence with age. Table 3–4, adopted from Rasmussen, shows the headache prevalence in prior studies, many of which did not use the IHS criteria and many of which were physician or clinic based. In addition, results from several recent studies are added.

Much of the above discussion focuses on prevalence, the proportion of the population with disease in a definite period of time. Incidence, on the other hand, refers to the number of *new cases* that arise in a defined population over

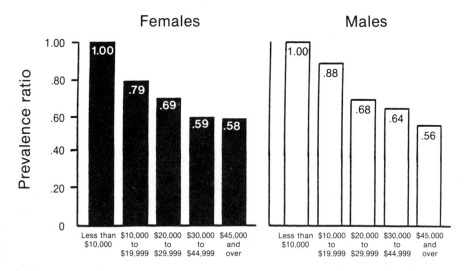

Household income

Figure 3–2. Prevalence ratio of migraine by income. Ratio decreased with increasing income. Ratio adjusted for age and race, which may alter relationship. (Reproduced with permission from Stewart, W. F., R. B. Lipton, D. D. Celentano, and M. L. Reed (1992). Prevalence of migraine headache in the United States. *JAMA 267*:64–69.)

a defined period of time. Stewart et al. (1991) estimated migraine incidence using cross-sectional rather than longitudinal data which came from the telephone interview survey in Washington County, Maryland. Subjects report both headache symptoms and the age of onset of their symptoms. This study was performed prior to the publication of the new IHS criteria. Definition of migraine without aura required one of the following headache accompaniments: (1) nausea or vomiting with unilateral head or eye pain; (2) photophobia and throbbing pain with nausea or vomiting and unilateral head or eye pain. Migraine with aura subjects, in addition, had to report two visual prodrome symptoms beginning no more than 1 hour before the headache. The study used reported age of symptom onset and then corrected for "telescoping" to estimate age incidence. (Telescoping refers to the phenomenon of reporting events in the past at a time closer to the present; it is a ubiquitous source of error in research based on recall.)

The estimate of age-specific and sex-specific incidence rates for the onset of migraine with and without aura was based on the 392 men and 1,018 women identified as migraineurs. Of these, 27% of the men and 28% of the women had migraine with aura. For men, the age-specific incidence of migraine with aura peaked 3 to 5 years earlier than migraine without aura. The peak incidence of migraine with aura, at or about 5 years of age, was 6.6:1,000 person-years. The peak incidence for migraine without aura was 10:1,000 person-years at between 10 and 11 years of age. New cases of migraine were uncommon in men in their 20s. In women, the onset of migraine began at a later age. The highest incidence of migraine with aura occurred between ages 12 and 13 (14.1:1,000 person-years), and migraine without aura peaked between ages 14 and 17 (18.9:1,000 person-years). New-onset migraine was relatively common among women in their late 20s.

Children

Headaches are prevalent in children: Bille (1962) found that the headache prevalence among 8,993 schoolchildren in Uppsala, Sweden, increased from 39% at age 6 to over 70% by age 15. Waters (1986) found that 85% of boys and 95% of girls between the ages of 13 and 15 had had a headache in the previous year. The symptoms that are characteristic of migraine are also common in children, as assessed by self-administered questionnaires, but there has been no satisfactory clinical validation of such questions in children. Other symptoms, such as abdominal pain, are commonly present in children with migraine. Diagnostic criteria are particularly difficult in this age group (Hockaday, 1988). Pioneering studies of childhood migraine were conducted in Sweden by Bille (1962, 1990). Using a restrictive definition of migraine that has not been followed in all subsequent studies, Bille showed that migraine prevalence was similar in boys and girls (mean 3.9%) aged 7 to 10 but higher in girls after puberty. Bille used Vahlquist's (1955) criteria, which included paroxysmal headache separated by pain-free intervals and two or more of the following: nausea, scotomata, unilateral pain, and positive family history.

Cluster Headache

Most cluster headache studies report on the "relative frequency" of cluster headache compared to migraine and find a ratio between 1:5.6 and 1:47.1. Selection may produce considerable bias in these ratios. One study of cluster prevalence in 10,000 18-year-old men being considered for national service in Sweden, consisting of a questionnaire followed by clinical examination, showed a 0.09% prevalence (Ekbom et al., 1978). Cluster headache is rare in children (Bille, 1990).

CHARACTERISTICS OF SUBJECTS WITH HEADACHE AND MIGRAINE

Authors of earlier clinical studies have been impressed with various characteristics that have been described as being more or less frequent in subjects with headache and migraine. Such associations should, however, be based on epidemiologic surveys and not simply on patients attending a doctor, because of selection bias. Physician- and clinic-based studies had given the clinical impression that migraine sufferers were more intelligent and of a higher social class. Using school classes as a "measure" of intelligence, Bille (1962) found that this was not the case in schoolchildren. In adults, epidemiologic studies using intelligence testing and occupation as a measure of intelligence and social class found no evidence of higher social class or intelligence being associated with migraine (Waters, 1971). In fact, Stewart et al. (1992) found that migraine preva-

Table 3–4 Some prevalence studies of different forms of headache in America and Western Europe

Study, country	Sample source	Respondents (N)	Age	Time-period prevalence	Headache %M	Headache %F	Headache %Both	Migraine %M	Migraine %F	Migraine %Both	Tension-type headache %M	Tension-type headache %F	Tension-type headache %Both
D'Alessandro et al., (1988), Italy	General population	1,154	>7	Prev. 1 yr	35.3	46.2		9.3	18.0	16.1			
Crisp et al. (1977), UK	General population	727	Adults	Lifetime / Prev. 2 yr	68.9	93.7		9.8 / 8.9	25.7 / 19.5		28.8	34.5	
Dalsgaard-Nielsen and Ulrich (1973), Denmark	Doctors	461	25–85	Lifetime				14	22	16			
Duckro et al. (1989), USA	Nonclinic, telephone sampled	500	>21	Lifetime / Past 3 mo				(very severe headache) 11.2 / 8.8	20.4 / 15.2	15.8 / 12.0			
Hollnagel and Nørrelund (1980), Denmark	General population	1,052	40	?	69	85	77	8	18	13			
Linet et al. (1989), USA	General population	10,169	12–29	Lifetime / 4 weeks	90.8 / 57	95.3 / 76							
Markush et al. (1975), USA	Women serving as control group for cerebrovascular disease	451	15–44	Prev. 1 yr		76.5		3.0	7.4 / 23.5				

Reference	Population	No.	Age	Prevalence									
Nikiforow (1981), Finland	General population	200	>15	Lifetime	69	83	91	11	35	24.5	37	42	40
				Prev. 1 yr			77						
Philips (1977), UK	General practice	597	16–60	Prev. 6 mo		74	89		10	21		65	68
Rasmussen et al. (1991), Denmark	General population	740	25–64	Lifetime	93	99	96	8	25	16	69	88	78
				Prev. 1 yr	11	22	16	6	15	10	63	86	74
				Point				0	0	0	9	16	12
Schnarch and Hunter (1980), USA	Shopping center	1,293	Adults	Prev. 1 yr			7.3						
Stewart et al. (1992), USA	General population	20,468	12–80	Year				5.7	17.6				
Waters and O'Connor (1971), UK	General population (women)	2,933	20–64	Prev. 1 yr		78.7			19			61	
Waters (1972), UK	General practitioners	882	35–54	Prev. 1 yr				14	26				
Waters (1974, 1975), UK	General population	1,718	>21	Prev. 1 yr	63.5	78.4		14.9	23.2		43		
Ziegler et al. (1977), USA	Church congregations	1,809	>15	Lifetime	82.6	84.2		40.9 (disabling headache)	50.2		41.7 (mild headache)	34.0	

Source: Rasmussen et al. (1991), with some additions.

lence was increased in lower socioeconomic groups. Among those with migraine, individuals who had seen a doctor were more likely to be of a higher social class and to be, on the average, more intelligent. This was evidence of *selection*—those who sought medical attention were biased toward higher social class and intelligence than other migraine sufferers who did not consult a doctor.

A number of hypotheses about possible causal factors, such as visual acuity, ocular muscle imbalance, and blood pressure, have been similarly tested in representative groups of subjects selected from the general population with no headache, headache, and migraine. Little convincing evidence was found that these are actually associated with migraine (Waters, 1986), except that a higher proportion of the migraineurs had hyperphoria with near vision. In conducting such studies, it is important to make the assessments blindly, with the observer being unaware of the subject's diagnosis to reduce the danger of bias. Defects of visual acuity, ocular muscle imbalance, and blood pressure are unlikely to be etiologic factors, or even statistical associations, in headache or migraine. Epidemiologic studies cannot show that the headache (or migraine) may not be related to these conditions in individual cases; they can only show that these conditions are as common in the general population as in those persons with migraine, those with headache, and those with neither. Because these conditions may vary with age or sex, all comparisons between the headache, migraine, and no-headache groups must be standardized for age and sex.

Some studies have looked at personality and headache. Migraine, episodic tension-type, and chronic tension-type headache cases selected from a community sample were studied by Philips (1976, 1977). These groups were indistinguishable from each other on any of the four personality dimensions measured by the personality questionnaire, but differences were found in those taking certain treatments. Using a random sample of civil servants with migraine, nonmigrainous headaches, and no headache, Henryk-Gutt and Rees (1973) obtained details of personal, medical, and family histories by interview. This study gave evidence that migraine was associated with increased N scores on the Eysenck Personality Inventory, increased anxiety and somatization scores on the Minnesota Multiphasic Personality Inventory (women only), and increased hostility scores on the Buss Scale. These differences were statistically significant, but in the initial study only 54% of questionnaires were returned completed correctly, which may have introduced bias, because the response rate varied between 31 and 77% (Henryk-Gutt and Rees, 1973).

A study in schoolchildren in Holland failed to find many of the recorded differences between those with migraine, headache, and no headache, but it did find that migraine and tension headache sufferers were characterized by the following personality traits: achievement motivation, rigidity, fear of failure, and low impulsiveness (Passchier, 1985). This may be a function of the pain they experience or the result of bias. Köhler and Kosanic (1992) studied 69 migraineurs age and sex matched to 69 controls, and found no difference between the groups in ambition, orderliness, and rigidity.

In a population study of 162 adults who participated in the Washington County, Maryland, telephone interview survey, Brandt et al. (1990) found a higher prevalence of psychological symptoms of anxiety and depression in migraine sufferers independent of headache frequency. In a prospective study of 27- to 28-year-olds in Zurich, Switzerland, Merikangas et al. (1990) found an association between migraine and anxiety that manifested itself 3 to 4 years before the appearance of migraine. In this age group, depression alone (without anxiety) was more common in nonmigraineurs. These two studies suggest that the migraine syndrome may have different manifestations at different times in the life cycle. Anxiety may appear in early childhood, followed by migraine and then depression. The duration of the disease may be more important than the frequency of the attacks in determining the presence of associated psychological conditions.

Stewart et al. (1989), analyzing results of the telephone interview survey in Washington County, Maryland, found that individuals with panic disorder or panic syndrome reported more frequent occurrence of headaches during the preceding week. They also reported longer and more frequent migraine headaches than did individuals without a history of panic attack. Males with a panic disorder were seven times more likely to report migraine than those without this condition. Could this be a result of a higher incidence of somatization or hypochondriacal behavior among those with migraine or panic attack, could they both be caused by an underlying condition, or could they cause each other? Which of these choices is correct is not clear at this time.

Breslau and Davis (1992) examined prospectively the risk for major depression and panic disorder in persons with a prior history of migraine. Nine hundred ninety-five young adults ages 21 to 30, recruited from a large health maintenance organization in Detroit, Michigan, were interviewed in 1989 and reinterviewed in 1990. At baseline, 12.9% of the sample met the IHS criteria for lifetime migraine prevalence. A history of migraine at baseline increased fourfold the risk for major depression after 14 months. A history of anxiety disorder had a major modifying effect on this risk. Subjects without migraine or anxiety have a 2.5% rate of major depression. Subjects with anxiety alone or migraine without anxiety had a 5.8% rate, and subjects with both migraine and anxiety had a 21.9% rate of major depression. Subjects with migraine were 12 times more likely to develop panic disorder than subjects without a history of migraine. The rate of development of major depression or panic disorder in patients with past migraine (15.4%) was slightly higher than in persons with active migraine (13%), suggesting that these disorders are *not* a reaction to current migraine attack. This again suggests that these disorders share a common pathophysiology. Persons with migraine with aura have an increased lifetime prevalence of suicide attempts and suicidal ideation. The authors will attempt to give precise estimates of the risk in further prospective studies.

CONCLUSION

Epidemiologic studies have failed to confirm many of the clinical hypotheses about the causes of headache and migraine. We still know remarkably little about why some individuals suffer from these symptoms and others do not. The genetic element is very much less in population studies and in twin studies and has been over-emphasized in the clinical literature. Most of the positive findings from recent research are related to "trigger" factors that determine the timing of the attack in those who are susceptible (Waters, 1990). Thus migraine sufferers may relate their attacks to missing a meal, or to the beginning of menstruation (Silberstein and Merriam, 1991). Such factors are related to the onset of the attack, but many other individuals can miss meals or have menstrual periods without ever suffering from headache or migraine.

Large population-based studies in the United States and Denmark have shed light on many epidemiologic issues. The lifetime headache prevalence is over 90% in men and 95% in women, most of whom have never seen a physician for headache, especially in the United States. Lifetime migraine prevalence is 29% in women and 8% in men in Copenhagen, whereas 4-week prevalence is 7.4% in women and 3.0% in men. The prevalence of migraine may be increasing in the United States, but this is uncertain.

Anxiety and depression are frequently associated with migraine. Subjects with panic disorders have more frequent headaches and migraine. Patients with a history of migraine (and anxiety) have an increased risk of developing major depression. Migraineurs are at increased risk of developing a panic disorder. The genetics of migraine are uncertain and need further study using systematic interviews of all first degree relatives of migraine cases and controls. The frequency, severity, and underdiagnosis of migraine and the associated disability attest to the importance of this disorder.

REFERENCES

Allan, W. (1928). The inheritance of migraine. *Arch. Intern. Med. 42*:590–599.

Ash-Upmark, E. (1953). Inverted nipples and migraine. *Acta Med. Scand. 167*:191–197.

Barolin, G.S. (1970). Migraine families and their EEGs. In *Background to Migraine: Third Migraine Symposium*, pp. 28–36. Heinemann, London.

Bille, B. (1962). Migraine in school children. *Acta Paediatr. Scand. 51*(Suppl. 136): 1–151.

Bille, B. (1990). The development of pediatric headache research. *Headache Q. 1*:39–42.

Brandt, J., D. Celentano, W. Stewart et al. (1990). Personality and emotional disorder in a community sample of migraine headache sufferers. *Am. J. Psychiatry 147*: 303–308.

Breslau, N. and G.C. Davis (1992). Migraine, major depression and panic disorder: A prospective epidemiologic study of young adults. *Cephalalgia 12*:85–90.

Celentano, D.D., W.F. Stewart, and M.S. Linet (1990). The relationship of headache symptoms with severity and duration of attacks. *J. Clin. Epidemiol. 43*:983–994.

Childs, A.J. and M.T. Sweetnam (1961). A study of 104 cases of migraine. *Br. J. Indust. Med. 18*:234–236.

Couch, J.R., C. Bearss, and S. Verhulst (1986). Importance of maternal heredity in the etiology of migraine. *Neurology 36*(Suppl.):99.

Crisp, A.H., R.S. Kalucy, B. McGuinness et al. (1977). Some clinical, social and psychological characteristics of migraine subjects in the general population. *Postgrad. Med. J. 53*:691–697.

D'Alessandro, R., G. Benassi, P.L. Lenzi et al. (1988). Epidemiology of headache in the Republic of San Marino. *J. Neurol. Neurosurg. Psychiatry 51*:21–27.

Dalsgaard-Nielsen, T., H. Engberg-Pedersen, and H.E. Holm (1970). Clinical and statistical investigations of the epidemiology of migraine; an investigation of the onset age and its relation to sex, adrenarche, menarche and the menstrual cycle in migraine patients, and of the menarche age, sex, distribution and frequency of migraine. *Dan. Med. Bull. 17*:138–148.

Dalsgaard-Nielsen, T. and M.D. Ulrich (1973). Prevalence and heredity of migraine and migrainoid headaches among 461 Danish doctors. *Headache 12*:168–172.

Duckro, P.N., R.C. Tait, and R.B. Margolis (1989). Prevalence of very severe headache in a large US metropolitan area. *Cephalalgia 9*:199–205.

Ekbom, K., B. Ahlborg, and R. Schele (1978). Prevalence of migraine and cluster headache in Swedish men of 18. *Headache 18*:9–19.

Ely, F.A. (1930). The migraine-epilepsy syndrome. *Arch. Neurol. Psychiatry 24*:943.

Goodell, H., R. Lewontin, and H.G. Wolff (1954). Familial occurrence of migraine headache. *Arch. Neurol. Psychiatry 72*:325–334.

Harvald, B. and M. Hauge (1956). A catamnestic investigation of Danish twins. *Dan. Med. Bull. 3*:150–158.

Headache Classification Committee of the International Headache Society (1988). Classification and diagnostic criteria for headache disorders, cranial neuralgias, and facial pain. *Cephalalgia 8*(Suppl. 7):1–96.

Henryk-Gutt, R. and W.L. Rees (1973). Psychological aspects of migraine. *J. Psychosom. Med. 17*:141–153.

Hockaday, J.M. (1988). Definitions, clinical features, and diagnosis of childhood migraine. In *Migraine in Children* (J.M. Hockaday, ed.), pp. 5–24. Butterworth, London.

Hollnagel, H. and N. Nørrelund (1980). Headache among 40-year-olds in Glostrup. *Ugeskr. Laeger 142*:3071–3077.

Köhler, T. and S. Kosanic (1992). Are persons with migraine characterized by a high degree of ambition, orderliness, and rigidity? *Pain 48*:321–323.

Lennox, W.G. (1941). *Science and Seizures: New Light on Epilepsy and Migraine.* Harper, New York.

Linet, M.S. and W.F. Stewart (1984). Migraine headache: Epidemiologic perspectives. *Epidemiol. Rev. 6*:107–139.

Linet, M.S., W.F. Stewart, D.D. Celentano et al. (1989). An epidemiologic study of headache among adolescents and young adults. *JAMA 261*:2211–2216.

Lipton, R.B., W. Stewart, D.D. Celentano, and A.I. Reed (1992). Undiagnosed migraine: A comparison of symptom-based and self-reported physician diagnosis. *Arch. Intern. Med. 156*:1–6.

Lucas, R.N. (1977). Migraine in twins. *J. Psychosom. Res. 21*:147–156.

Markush, R.E., R.K. Herbert, A. Heyman, and W.M. O'Fallon (1975). Epidemiological study of migraine symptoms in young women. *Neurology 25*:430–435.

McKusick, V.A. (1988). *Mendelian Inheritance in Man,* 8th ed. Johns Hopkins University Press, Baltimore.

Merikangas, K.R. (1990). Genetic epidemiology of migraine. In *Migraine: A Spectrum of Ideas* (M. Sandler and G. Collins, eds.), pp. 40–50. Oxford University Press, New York.

Merikangas, K.R., J. Angst, and H. Isler (1990). Migraine and psychopathology. Results of the Zurich cohort study of young adults. *Arch. Gen. Psychiatry 47*:849–853.

MMWR (1991). Prevalence of chronic migraine headaches—United States, 1980–1989. *MMWR 40*:331–338.

Nikiforow, R. (1981). Headache in a random sample of 200 persons: A clinical study of a population in northern Finland. *Cephalalgia 1:*99–107.

Passchier, J. (1985). *Headache and Stress.* VU Uitgeverij, Amsterdam.

Phanthumchinda, K. and C. Sithi-Amorn (1989). Prevalence and clinical features of migraine: A community survey in Bangkok, Thailand. *Headache 29:*594–597.

Philips, C. (1976). Headache and personality. *J. Psychosom. Res. 20:*535–542.

Philips, C. (1977). Headache in general practice. *Headache 16:*322–329.

Rasmussen, B.K., R. Jensen, M. Schroll, and J. Olesen (1991). Epidemiology of headache in a general population—a prevalence study. *J. Clin. Epidemiol. 44:* 1147–1157.

Schnarch, D.M. and J.E. Hunter (1980). Migraine incidence in clinical vs nonclinical populations. *Psychosomatics 21:*314–325.

Silberstein, S.D. and G.R. Merriam (1991). Estrogens, progestins, and headache. *Neurology 41:*786–793.

Stewart, W.F., M.S. Linet, and D.D. Celentano (1989). Migraine headaches and panic attacks. *Psychosom. Med. 51:*559–569.

Stewart, W.F., M.S. Linet, D.D. Celentano et al. (1991). Age and sex-specific incidence rates of migraine with and without visual aura. *Am. J. Epidemiol. 34:*1111–1120.

Stewart, W.F., R.B. Lipton, D.D. Celentano, and M.L. Reed (1992). Prevalence of migraine headache in the United States. *JAMA 267:*64–69.

Vahlquist, B.C. (1955). Migraine in children. *Int. Arch. Allergy Appl. Immunol. 7:* 348–355.

Waters, W.E. (1970). Community studies of the prevalence of headache. *Headache 9:* 178–186.

Waters, W.E. (1971). Migraine: Intelligence, social class, and familial prevalence. *BMJ 2:*77–81.

Waters, W.E. (1972). Headache and migraine in general practitioners. In *The Migraine Headache and Dixarit,* pp. 31–44. Boehringer Ingelheim, Bracknell, England.

Waters, W.E. (1973). The epidemiological enigma of migraine. *Int. J. Epidemiol. 2:* 189–194.

Waters, W.E. (1974). *The Epidemiology of Migraine.* Boehringer Ingelheim, Bracknell, England.

Waters, W.E. (1975). Epidemiological data relevant to prognosis in migraine in adults. *Dan. Med. Bull. 22:*89–91.

Waters, W.E. (1986). *Headache* (Series in Clinical Epidemiology). PSG Publishing Co., Inc., Littleton, MA.

Waters, W.E. (1990). The epidemiology of migraine: Where are we now? *Headache Q. 1:*43–44.

Waters, W.E. and P.J. O'Connor (1971). Epidemiology of headache and migraine in women. *J. Neurol. Neurosurg. Psychiatry 34:*148–153.

Waters, W.E. and P.J. O'Connor (1975). Prevalence of migraine. *J. Neurol. Neurosurg. Psychiatry 38:*613–616.

World Federation of Neurology (1970). Definition of migraine. In *Background to Migraine: Third Migraine Symposium,* pp. 181–182. Heinemann, London.

Ziegler, D.K. (1976). Epidemiology and genetics of migraine. In *Pathogenesis and Treatment of Headache,* pp. 19–29. Spectrum, New York.

Ziegler, D.K., R.S. Hassanein, and J.R. Couch (1977). Characteristics of life headache histories in a nonclinic population. *Neurology 27:*265–269.

Ziegler, D.K., R.S. Hassanein, D. Harris, and R. Stewart (1975). Headache in a nonclinic twin population. *Headache 14:*213–218.

4

The Pathophysiology of Migraine

JAMES W. LANCE

In *Dr. Willis' Practice of Physicke,* published in 1684, 9 years after the death of Thomas Willis, headache is ascribed to increased blood flow to the head, which "distends the vessels, greatly blows up the membranes, and pulls the nervous fibres one from another, and so brings to them painful corrugations or wrinklings" (Knapp, 1963). Vascular distention as the primary cause of headache was questioned by Liveing (1873), who subtitled his classic monograph *A Contribution to the Pathology of Nerve-Storms.* Gowers (1893) wrote: "We must not ascribe too much significance to throbbing, or to the increase in the pain by the causes of vascular distension; these may be due merely to the oversensitiveness of the central structures."

Although the studies of Wolff and his colleagues concentrated on the reactions of extracranial vessels during migraine, Wolff (1963) left open the possibility that vascular changes were secondary to a central neural discharge:

> According to the neurogenic concept of vascular headache of the migraine type, any noxious factor within the brain that threatens survival of the cerebrum may induce cerebral vasodilatation. If this be sufficiently great, the arteries on the outside of the head dilate. With the liberation of chemical factors such as proteases and polypeptides, edema and a lowering of the pain threshold are engendered. Tenderness and headache ensue. . . . It is conceivable that the initial event within the head is vasoconstriction, resulting in ischemia. (p. 385)

Whether the symptoms of migraine are determined by changes in the cerebral, meningeal, and extracranial circulations and humoral agents that react with them or the primary event is a neural discharge remains controversial to the present day. These hypotheses are not mutually exclusive and may well prove to be complementary. Certain groups of symptoms can be recognized within the conceptual framework of migraine that may recur in a specific phase of each attack, may be present in some episodes but not in others, and probably employ diverse neurovascular mechanisms.

SYMPTOM COMPLEXES IN MIGRAINE

Any attempt to explain the pathophysiology of migraine must account for the following components of the attack.

> *Premonitory symptoms:* Mood changes (commonly a sense of elation associated with hyperactivity), increased appetite (particularly for sweet foods), and excessive yawning may precede migraine by as long as 24 hours on at least some occasions in about one third of migrainous patients (Blau, 1980; Drummond and Lance, 1984). These symptoms are presumably of hypothalamic origin.

> *Focal neurologic symptoms:* These may arise from the cerebral cortex, brainstem, or cerebellum and may anticipate the onset of headache, as in the aura of classic migraine, or may appear during the headache phase. In either case, the neurologic symptoms may progress as a "slow march" (e.g., spreading fortification spectra or paresthesias that indicate sequential involvement of areas of cerebral cortex), or as a patchy impairment of neurologic function that suggests a diffuse but unevenly distributed process affecting cortical function.

> *Headache:* Headache is unilateral in two thirds of patients and commonly starts as a dull ache at the occipitonuchal junction, or in one temple, which then spreads over that side of the head or the whole head or may remain localized as a "bar of pain" extending from the eye to the occiput. The pain is usually constant and unremitting but assumes a pulsatile or throbbing quality when severe. It may consistently affect the same side of the head or may move from side to side, even in the one migrainous episode. Pain may radiate down the neck to the shoulder or, in some cases, to the arm and even the leg on the same side of the body, suggesting that the spinothalamic tract has collaborated with trigeminal pathways in the production of pain.

> *Prominent scalp vessels:* The frontal branches of the superficial temporal artery become distended in about one third of patients, venous engorgement may be seen, and heat loss increases from the affected area, while pressure over the prominent vessels eases the headache to some extent (Drummond and Lance, 1983). Most patients appear pale and "dark under the eyes" as the headache worsens, although exceptional patients flush before or during the attack.

> *Sensory hyperacuity:* Light may be perceived as dazzling or may provoke pain, sounds may appear unnaturally loud, and smells may be more intense during (or even before) the headache phase. Sensitivity of the scalp to touch and muscular hyperalgesia may develop during, and outlast, the headache phase.

> *Gastrointestinal symptoms:* Nausea sometimes precedes the onset of headache but commonly evolves as the attack progresses and may culminate in vomiting. Diarrhea afflicts about 20% of patients (Lance and Anthony, 1966).

ORIGIN OF MIGRAINE HEADACHE

Pain Pathways

Brain substance is insensitive to pain. The studies of Ray and Wolff (1940) showed that pain may be referred to the frontotemporal area from the dura, the intracranial segment of the internal carotid artery, the proximal few centimeters of the anterior and middle cerebral arteries, a portion of the cerebral veins and venous sinuses, the middle meningeal artery, and the superficial temporal artery. Afferent nerves from these blood vessels have their cell bodies in the part of the Gasserian ganglion corresponding to the ophthalmic division of the trigeminal nerve (Moskowitz, 1984). Stimulation of structures in the posterior fossa causes pain in the occipital region and upper neck (Ray and Wolff, 1940), whereas stimulation of the upper three cervical posterior roots refers pain to the vertex as well as the back of the head and neck. Kerr (1961a) reported that stimulation of the first cervical root in humans consistently caused frontal and orbital pain. He also demonstrated that afferent fibers from the first and second cervical roots converged with fibers in the spinal tract of the trigeminal nerve on second-order neurons in the posterior horn of the spinal cord (Kerr, 1961b). This convergence provides a pathway for referral of pain from the neck to the front of the head and vice versa.

Stimulation of the superior sagittal sinus and middle meningeal artery in the cat activates cells in the trigeminal nucleus caudalis (Davis and Dostrovsky, 1986; Lambert et al., 1979; Strassman et al., 1986) and in the dorsolateral quadrant of the second cervical segment of the spinal cord (Lambert et al., 1991; Zagami et al., 1987). Increased metabolic activity in these areas can then be demonstrated by autoradiography following the intravenous injection of 2-deoxyglucose (Goadsby and Zagami, 1991). Afferents from these vessels project to the ventroposteromedial nucleus and the medial nucleus of the posterior complex (Davis and Dostrovsky, 1988; Zagami and Lambert, 1990) (Figure 4–1). Some of these afferent fibers travel to the thalamus by way of the upper cervical spinal cord (Angus-Leppan et al., 1989).

Source of Pain
Graham and Wolff (1938) observed that the severity of migraine headache lessened after the injection of ergotamine tartrate as the amplitude of temporal artery pulsation declined. This, together with the old observation that compression of the common carotid or temporal arteries often alleviated the pain, suggested that arterial distention was an important factor in producing migraine headache. From studies of more than 5,000 records of temporal artery pulsations in 75 patients, Tunis and Wolff (1953) selected 10 migrainous patients for special analysis. They found that temporal artery pulse amplitudes became more variable and larger for up to 3 days before the onset of headache and that the mean amplitude during headache was greater than in headache-free periods. Blau and Dexter (1981) assessed the contribution of extracranial arteries to migraine headache by inflating a sphygmomanometer cuff around the patient's head. Of 47 patients, only 21 experienced relief from headache after inflation

of the pericranial cuff, whereas the majority complained that their headaches were aggravated by coughing, jolting, or holding their breath, indicating an intracranial component to head pain. Drummond and Lance (1983) compared the pulse amplitude of the superficial temporal artery and its main frontotemporal branch with the intensity of pain felt in the temple while the ipsilateral common carotid and temporal arteries were compressed alternately. Of 62 patients, selected only by the presence of a unilateral migrainous headache, the pain appeared to be of extracranial vascular origin in about one third, was of mainly intracranial (or meningeal) vascular origin in one third, and had no detectable vascular component in the remaining one third. In the subgroup with increased arterial pulsation in the frontotemporal region, thermography demonstrated increased heat loss from this area, and temporal artery compression eased the headache.

Headache does not depend on increased cerebral perfusion, because migraine without aura (common migraine) is not usually associated with alteration of cerebral blood flow (Olesen et al., 1981b) and the headache of migraine with aura (classic migraine) usually starts while blood flow is still reduced (Lauritzen et al., 1983a; Olesen et al., 1990). Kobari et al. (1989) found that local cerebral blood flow was increased during migraine headaches but this increase was not related to the side on which the headache was experienced. Migrainous headache may be relieved by ergotamine (Norris et al., 1975) or codeine (Sakai and Meyer, 1978), although cerebral perfusion remains increased. In any event, vascular dilatation by itself would not cause headache. In periarterial fluid sampled during migraine headache, Chapman et al. (1960) found a polypeptide similar to the polypeptide found in blister fluid that they named "neurokinin." This bradykininlike substance was postulated to set up a sterile inflammatory response in the vessel, which thus became pain sensitive. Serotonin may also be implicated because it is known to be released from platelets during migraine headache (Anthony et al., 1967) and potentiates the pain-producing effect of bradykinin when injected into a human arm vein (Sicuteri, 1967). Friberg et al. (1991) estimated by transcranial Doppler sonography that flow in the territory supplied by that artery was unaltered; they deduced that the lower velocity was caused by dilation of the middle cerebral artery. Following the intravenous infusion of 2 mg of the 5-hydroxytryptamine (5-HT) agonist sumatriptan, the headache was relieved within 30 minutes while the velocity of flow in the middle cerebral artery returned to normal.

Pain from tender muscles may add a nonvascular component to migraine headache. Excessive contraction of the temporal, masseter, and neck muscles is common in migrainous patients (Lous and Olesen, 1982), more so than in patients with "tension-type headache," and becomes evident just before the headache reaches its maximum (Bakke et al., 1982). Tfelt-Hansen et al. (1981) found that infiltration of tender muscle areas with local anesthetic or normal saline relieved migraine headache within 70 minutes in 28 of 48 patients. Serotonin and bradykinin potentiated the pain-producing effects of one another when injected into the temporal muscle of normal volunteers but did not evoke headache (Jensen et al., 1985). The sites of muscle contraction in migraine correlate with the spatial distribution of pain and tenderness, suggesting that it is a secondary phenomenon but one that nonetheless contributes to headache.

In summary, the headache of migraine is not necessarily associated with dilatation of extracranial arteries or increased cerebral perfusion, although it is aggravated by vascular pulsation. It appears to be of intracranial origin at least as often as extracranial origin, and it may be related to increased sensitivity of vessels or perivascular structures. Whether or not central trigeminal pathways are also hyperexcitable, and whether or not their spontaneous discharge may initiate migraine headache, are discussed below.

Endogenous Pain Control Pathways

Interneurons control pain perception using enkephalins and possibly γ-aminobutyric acid as their transmitter substances to gate the inflow from peripheral pain pathways by presynaptic and probably postsynaptic inhibition in the dorsal horn of the spinal cord (Basbaum and Fields, 1978, 1984). These inhibitory interneurons are modulated by monoaminergic pathways descending from the brainstem, which also have a direct effect on dorsal horn cells. The serotonergic pathway passes downward from the periaqueductal gray matter of the midbrain to the nucleus raphe magnus in the midline and also to lateral medullary nuclei (Duggan, 1982) to regulate the discharge of neurons in trigeminal and spinal pain pathways. A complementary noradrenergic tract originates from the locus ceruleus in the upper pons and descends in the dorsolateral funiculus of the spinal cord. There is evidence that the electrophoretic administration of serotonin and noradrenaline near the bodies of dorsal horn cells reduces their rate of discharge (Duggan, 1982), but the precise manner in which monoaminergic pathways are effective in pain control is unknown. It appears likely that depletion of monoamines could open the pain control gates and lead to the perception of aching in the head and neck, as postulated by Sicuteri (1976).

Even in periods of freedom from migraine, migrainous subjects carry with them susceptibility to head pain. Raskin and Knittle (1976) found that cold drinks or ice cream evoked headache in 93% of migrainous patients compared with only 31% of control subjects. One third of patients with "ice-cream headache" state that this pain involves precisely the same part of the head as their habitual migraine headache (Drummond and Lance, 1984). Moreover, 42% of migrainous patients are prone to sudden jabs of pain in the head ("ice-pick pains"), compared with 3% of nonheadache controls (Raskin and Schwartz, 1980). Drummond and Lance (1984) found that ice-pick pains coincided with the site of the customary headache in 40% of patients. The trigeminal pathways may thus become activated spontaneously in paroxysms lasting a fraction of a second (ice-pick pains) or may be activated reflexly for seconds or minutes by sudden cooling of the pharynx (ice-cream headache). This indicates a persisting disinhibition of trigeminal pathways in migrainous patients, suggesting that the trigeminal system could also discharge excessively for hours or days to provide a neural origin for migraine headache.

VASCULAR CHANGES

Vascular Reactivity between Headaches

Pulsation of the superficial temporal artery in migrainous patients does not differ from that of normal controls at rest, nor does it differ on changing posture from sitting to standing, but it does increase more during exercise on the side habitually affected by migraine headache (Drummond and Lance, 1981). A similar increase was noted in migrainous patients during a stressful mental arithmetic test (Drummond, 1982) or when subjects viewed slides of fatal traffic accidents (Pratt, 1985). However, Goudswaard et al. (1985) found that, during the sustained stress of a student examination, temporal pulse amplitude did not increase in migrainous patients as much as it did in control subjects. Physiologic reactions in a target organ participating in the production of symptoms is known as "symptom specificity" and could indicate that some neurovascular reflexes are hyperactive in migrainous patients even between attacks.

Reactivity of intracranial vessels is also asymmetric in the resting state. The vasodilator response to carbon dioxide is greater in migrainous patients than in normal subjects, more so on the side affected most recently by headache (Sakai and Meyer, 1979). Moreover, blockade of α-adrenergic receptors or stimulation of β receptors was shown to increase cerebral blood flow more on the side of headache or the side recently affected by headache (Yamamoto and Meyer, 1980). Conversely, α receptor stimulation diminished cerebral perfusion more on the affected side. Yamamoto and Meyer explained these findings by sympathetic denervation hypersensitivity.

Observations on Cerebral Blood Flow and Cortical Spreading Depression

Migraine with Aura (Classic Migraine)
Since the introduction of radioactive xenon measurement techniques, cerebral blood flow has been shown to diminish by about 20% during the aura phase of classic migraine (Table 4–1). Studies undertaken in Copenhagen to measure the

Table 4–1 Cerebral and extracranial blood flow in migraine

Reference	No. of patients	Reduction during prodrome (%)	Increase during headache (%)	Increase after headache (%)
O'Brien (1971)	18	23	8	
Skinhøj (1973)	10	50	0–90	
Simard and Paulson (1973)	1	50	—	
Hachinski et al. (1978)	5	0–40	0–30	20
Henry et al. (1978)	12	—	0–40	
Sakai and Meyer (1978)	43	20 (general) 35 (focal)	35 (i.c.) 50 (e.c.)	20
Olesen et al. (1981a)	8	20 (general) 36 (focal)	—	
Andersen et al. (1988)	12	—	—	20
Kobari et al. (1989)	12	—	25–35	

Key to abbreviations: i.c., intracranial circulation; e.c., extracranial circulation.

regional cerebral blood flow (rCBF) from one hemisphere by 254 detectors after intracarotid injection of ^{133}Xe (which precipitates migraine with aura in some patients) have given a more precise picture of the sequence of events. In some patients with migrainous aura (Olesen et al., 1981a) or hemiplegic migraine (Friberg et al., 1987), patchy areas of increased blood flow were seen before the cerebral blood flow diminished. Diminution of the flow started in the occipital region and extended forward as a "spreading oligemia" (Olesen et al., 1981a). The wave of oligemia progressed over the cortex at 2.2 mm/minute irrespective of arterial territories, stopping short at the central and lateral sulci, although the frontal lobes also became oligemic independently in some patients (Lauritzen et al., 1983a). Spreading oligemia typically began before the patient noticed local neurologic symptoms, reached the sensorimotor area only after the appropriate symptoms had started, and outlasted these symptoms. Oligemia lasted several hours and was followed by delayed hyperemia (Andersen et al., 1988). The headache usually started while cerebral blood flow was still diminished. From these studies, the authors concluded that cortical oligemia was a reflection of the cortical spreading depression (CSD) of Lãeo (1944) that is responsible for the slow march of fortification spectra and other neurologic symptoms previously calculated to traverse the cortex at about 3 mm/minute.

Lauritzen and his colleagues (1982) showed that induced spreading depression in the rat was accompanied by a transient hyperemia for some 3 minutes followed by a 20 to 25% depression of cerebral blood flow for 60 minutes or more. Comparable changes have been found in the gyrencephalic cortex of the cat (Piper and Duckworth, 1989). CSD has been described in the human hippocampus and caudate nucleus during stereotactic surgery by Sramka et al. (1977–78). Because this is the only description in humans, the frequency and importance of CSD as a pathophysiologic entity is unknown. There have been no studies that have provided direct evidence of the phenomenon in human neocortex. Gloor (1986) reported in a letter that he had not observed electroencephalographic (EEG) changes consistent with CSD during human neurosurgery. Barkley et al. (1990), using magnetoencephalography, have demonstrated large-amplitude waves, long-duration decrements in EEG amplitude, and large-amplitude DC shifts in migraine patients during headache (14 migraine with aura, 3 migraine without aura). The latter two changes are similar to those seen during CSD in animals and suggest that these findings may represent evidence of CSD in humans.

Cerebrovascular reactivity is altered in the low flow areas observed during the aura. Olesen et al. (1981a) demonstrated reduced increase in cortical flow accompanying cortical activation. Three groups using ^{133}Xe clearance have found that reactivity to hypercapnia is impaired during the aura of migraine (Lauritzen et al., 1983b; Sakai and Meyer, 1979; Simard and Paulson, 1973). Sakai and Meyer considered that autoregulation was impaired, whereas Lauritzen et al. found that it was not disturbed. Because loss of carbon dioxide reactivity and reduced cortical blood flow during functional activation with preservation of autoregulation are characteristics of CSD (Lauritzen, 1984; Piper and Duckworth, 1989), their convincing demonstration during the migrainous aura would help to define a pathophysiologic role for CSD in humans.

rCBF has been studied by single-photon emission computerized tomography during spontaneous attacks of migraine after the inhalation of [133]Xe (Lauritzen and Olesen, 1984). Of 11 patients examined during attacks of classic migraine in the headache phase, areas of cortical hypoperfusion were found on the appropriate side in 8, posteriorly in 7, and anteriorly in 1. The mean decrease in rCBF was 17 ± 7% (rCBF 41 to 66 ml/100 g/minute), which persisted for about 4 to 6 hours. Three patients did not exhibit any flow changes when studied 30 minutes to 3 hours after the onset of the attack. In no patient was rCBF increased, although patients were examined during severe headache.

Re-evaluation of cerebral blood flow studies to allow for the influence of scattered radiation on the recording from areas of low flow during the aura has shown that flow dropped to 16 to 23 ml/100 g/minute, below the critical level for cortical function, in the most underperfused areas in the majority of patients (Skyhøj-Olsen et al., 1984). This degree of ischemia is sufficient to explain transient and possibly persistent neurologic deficits.

Migraine without Aura (Common Migraine)

The findings of studies of cerebral blood flow in migraine without aura have not been consistent (see Table 4–1). Olesen et al. (1981b) and Lauritzen and Olesen (1984) were unable to demonstrate any change, whereas increased cortical perfusion was reported by Sakai and Meyer (1978) and Kobari et al. (1989), with the latter study also showing increases in the thalamus and basal ganglia. Kobari et al. found that flow was augmented by 25 to 35% during headache, whether it was preceded by an aura or not, but that the changes were not related to the side of the headache. Géraud et al. (1989) described areas of hypoperfusion (clinically silent oligemic areas) as well as regions of hyperperfusion coexisting in patients with common migraine.

Conclusion

It therefore appears that the focal neurologic symptoms of classic migraine, whether arising as an aura or developing during the headache phase, are accompanied by diminished cortical perfusion of the appropriate part of the opposite cerebral hemisphere. On some occasions a wave of hypoperfusion may advance slowly over the cortex in association with a slow march of visual or other neurologic symptoms, whereas on other occasions it presumably persists as a local or diffuse cortical oligemia responsible for static symptoms. It is not possible to deduce with certainty from current techniques whether constriction of the cortical microcirculation precedes or follows diminution in cortical neuronal activity. However, Adams et al. (1989) found that stimulation of the locus ceruleus at frequencies that reduced cerebral blood flow in the cat had no consistent effect on the resting discharge of neurons in the visual cortex, suggesting that an important action of this brainstem projection was constriction of the microcirculation.

It is clear that the presence or absence of headache does not depend on cortical blood flow but that dilatation of the middle cerebral artery, and possibly other intracranial arteries may contribute to the perception of pain.

Observations on Extracranial Blood Flow

Extracranial blood flow generally increases during migraine headache (Sakai and Meyer, 1978), but no change in blood flow could be demonstrated in the temporal muscles (Jensen and Olesen, 1985) or in the subcutaneous tissue of the temple on the side affected by headache (Jensen, 1987). The frontal branches of the superficial temporal artery increase in amplitude during migraine headache in one third of patients (Drummond and Lance, 1983). In this subgroup, increase in heat loss from this area can be demonstrated by thermography, and compression of the temporal artery eases the pain. Iversen et al. (1990) have shown that the lumen of the temporal artery is wider on the painful side during unilateral headache, compared with relative constriction of other arteries.

Mitochondrial Abnormalities

In recent years, mitochondrial defects have been found in association with multisystem disorders, and syndromes such as "myoclonic epilepsy with ragged red fibers" and "mitochondrial myopathy, encephalopathy, lactic acidosis, and strokelike episodes" (MELAS) have been identified. Dvorkin et al. (1987) described nine patients who suffered from intractable epilepsy, severe migraine headaches (with prominent visual symptoms in seven), and occipital infarction or other cerebral lesions. Muscle biopsy disclosed ragged red fibers in two of four patients, suggesting that the disorder was related to the MELAS syndrome. The authors commented that perusal of the literature showed that migraine headaches or, in younger patients, episodic vomiting attacks were common in MELAS, which appears to be transmitted by nonmendelian maternal inheritance.

Montagna et al. (1988) investigated nine patients with migraine, five of whom had suffered a migrainous stroke, for defects of mitochondrial energy metabolism. Abnormalities of respiratory chain enzymes were detected in all patients, blood levels of lactate on exertion were elevated, and ragged red fibers were found on muscle biopsy in one case. It is thus probable that the vascular changes caused by mitochondrial disease ("mitochondrial microangiopathy") may be responsible for some cases of migrainous stroke.

BLOOD PLATELETS, VASOACTIVE AGENTS, AND BIOCHEMICAL CHANGES

Blood Platelets

Platelet dense bodies, the storage organelles for serotonin, are increased in migrainous patients between attacks (D'Andrea et al., 1989c). Do platelets aggregate more easily in migrainous patients, particularly during a headache? Kalendovsky and Austin (1975) demonstrated that platelets from migrainous patients aggregated more readily than controls, a difference most marked in those patients with complicated migraine, of whom four of seven also showed increased coagulability of the blood. Hyperaggregability of blood platelets in migrainous patients was confirmed by Couch and Hassanein (1977) and Deshmukh and Meyer (1977), who found that platelet aggregation increased during the prodromal phase but diminished during headache. Kruglak et al. (1984), however, could find no significant difference between the platelets of migrainous patients and those of controls in headache-free periods and only a small *increase* in aggregability during headache, which was of statistical but questionable clinical significance. Hanin et al. (1985) could not demonstrate any variation from normal controls of platelets from blood taken during the migraine attack or in headache-free periods.

How can this conflicting evidence be reconciled? Perhaps platelet aggregation takes place in subgroups of migrainous patients or is demonstrable only by certain techniques. Certainly the changes are not so constant as to influence views on the pathogenesis of migraine, although they may be a factor in migrainous infarction.

Irrespective of the degree of platelet aggregation, there is evidence for a platelet release reaction in migraine, as judged by the increase in β-thromboglobulin, a measure of total platelet activation, during headache (Gawel et al., 1979). This has relevance to the changes in plasma serotonin levels in migraine (discussed below). The content of monoamine oxidase B (MAO-B), which assists the metabolism of phenylethylamine (not serotonin), has been reported to be low in the platelets of migrainous patients, but Glover et al. (1981) found that this was true only for male patients. With the possible exception of MAO content, blood platelets in migrainous patients seems to be remarkably normal, and their role in migraine is probably limited to aggregation in some instances and the release of serotonin (Fozard, 1982).

Serotonin (5-Hydroxytryptamine)

Platelet serotonin content increases before migraine attacks and falls during the headache phase in most migraine patients (Anthony et al., 1967, 1969). This applies only to migraine without aura, but free 5-HT is released into the plasma during headache whether the headache is preceded by an aura or not (Ferrari et al., 1989b). Anthony et al. first reported that a serotonin-releasing factor was present in the blood during migraine headache, an observation since confirmed by Dvilansky et al. (1976) and Mück-Šeler et al. (1979) but not by Ferrari et al. (1987). The agent concerned is of less than 50,000 molecular weight (Anthony and Lance, 1975) and has not been identified, although adrenaline, noradrenaline, free fatty acids, and immune complexes are possible contenders. The main metabolite of serotonin, 5-hydroxyindoleacetic acid, is excreted in excess in the urine of some patients during migraine attacks (Curran et al., 1965; Sicuteri et al., 1961). The intramuscular injection of reserpine lowers plasma serotonin and evokes a typical headache in those susceptible to migraine, which is relieved by the intravenous injection of serotonin (Anthony et al., 1967; Kimball et al., 1960). Normal subjects experience only a dull, nonspecific headache after reserpine.

Free serotonin, after release from platelets, could possibly exert vasomotor effects before it is absorbed to vessel walls or metabolized because it is a potent constrictor of extracranial arteries in monkeys (Spira et al., 1976) and in humans

(Carroll et al., 1974; Lance et al., 1967). The isolated human basilar artery constricts more readily in response to serotonin than to noradrenaline (Carroll et al., 1974), but the infusion of serotonin into the monkey vertebral artery does not produce any significant change (Lambert et al., 1984a), presumably because of autoregulation in the intact circulation. It seems unlikely that the amount of serotonin released from platelets during migraine headache would be sufficient to cause any vascular constriction, at least in the anesthetized monkey (Spira et al., 1976), but it may possibly combine with bradykinin or other peptides to render the arterial wall sensitive to painful dilation.

Changes in plasma serotonin may be an index of changes of serotonergic transmission within the central nervous system. Serotonin is implicated in at least three important pathways of potential application to migraine: (1) a direct projection from the dorsal raphe nucleus to the cerebral cortex, (2) an indirect projection to cranial vessels via the parasympathetic component of the facial nerve, and (3) the inhibitory system descending from the nucleus raphe magnus that operates the enkephalinergic pain control system.

Serotonin Receptors

Four main groups of 5-HT receptors have been classified by ligand-binding studies (Humphrey and Feniuk, 1987). 5-HT$_1$ receptors are plentiful in layers 1 and 2 of the cortex, the posterior hypothalamus, central gray matter, raphe nuclei, and substantia gelatinosa (Pazos et al., 1987a), the two latter areas being concerned, respectively, with the endogenous pain control system and the entry portal for pain impulses into the spinal cord. 5-HT$_2$ receptors are present in the subcortical gray matter, cerebral cortex (layers 3 and 5), brainstem, and spinal cord (Pazos et al., 1987b). 5-HT$_3$ receptors are distributed mainly in the lower brainstem and substantia gelatinosa (Waeber et al., 1989). 5-HT$_4$ receptors have been recently described (Dumuis et al., 1991). The central action of 5-HT$_1$ receptors is mainly inhibitory, whereas the action of 5-HT$_2$ receptors is mainly excitatory.

Receptors on cerebral arteries are mostly 5-HT$_1$–like and those on temporal arteries are predominantly 5-HT$_2$. The meningeal arteries contain both types of receptor (Edvinsson and Jansen, 1989). 5-HT$_3$ receptors are present on afferent neurons in the cranial vessels and presumably play some part in mediating vascular pain, although 5-HT$_3$ antagonists have not proven to be successful in relief of migraine.

The 5-HT$_1$ agonist sumatriptan (previously designated GR43175) has proven to be effective in relieving established migraine attacks (Dahlof et al., 1989; Ferrari et al., 1989a) and is known to constrict isolated human basilar artery by acting on 5-HT$_1$ receptors (Parsons & Whalley, 1989). Since sumatriptan penetrates the blood–brain barrier poorly (Sleight et al., 1990), it is likely that its beneficial effect depends on constriction of cranial vessels or the prevention of a sterile inflammatory reaction in perivascular tissues.

Ergotamine and sumatriptan block the extravasation of plasma protein from dural vessels induced by trigeminal ganglion stimulation in the rat (Buzzi and Moskowitz, 1989). Because both drugs also blocked extravasation produced by capsaicin (which releases substance P from nerve terminals) but not the effect of substance P itself, it may be deduced that they act at a prejunctional site on the nerve terminal.

The part played by 5-HT$_2$ receptors in migraine remains uncertain. Prophylactic agents such as methysergide and pizotifen, which are mainly 5-HT$_2$ antagonists, also have some 5-HT$_1$ agonist activity, and the selective 5-HT$_2$ antagonist ICI 169,369 was found to be of doubtful efficacy in a small open pilot trial (Davies and Steiner, 1990).

Catecholamines

Whereas studies of serotonin levels in migraine have been reasonably consistent between laboratories, estimates of noradrenaline have varied widely. In headache-free periods, the level of noradrenaline was found to be elevated in platelets (D'Andrea et al. 1989b) and in plasma (Schoenen et al., 1985), although Gotoh et al. (1984) had reported low values. Plasma levels of noradrenaline have been reported as increased before (Hsu et al., 1978) and during (Anthony, 1981) migraine headache, whereas Fog-Møller et al. (1978) found a progressive decline during headache, reaching significance 1 to 2 hours before headache reached its peak.

The final enzyme in the synthesis of noradrenaline is dopamine β-hydroxylase (DBH), serum levels of which reflect the amount of sympathetic activity. Serum DBH levels in migrainous patients without headache are almost double those of patients with tension-type headache and normal controls (Gotoh et al., 1976) and were shown to increase in 19 out of 20 patients at some stage during migraine headache. The high level of DBH in migraine has been confirmed by Anthony (1981). One of the main catabolites of catecholamines, vanillylmandelic acid, also known as p-hydroxy-m-methoxymandelic acid, is excreted in excessive amounts by some, but not all, patients at the time of migraine headache (Curran et al., 1965; Curzon et al., 1969; Sicuteri et al., 1962). It thus appears that noradrenergic activity increases before, and in the initial stages of, migraine headache. Published studies agree that the adrenaline level does not alter.

Noradrenaline is contained in neurons of the locus ceruleus, which projects diffusely to the cerebral cortex and also plays a part in the endogenous pain control system. Stimulation of the locus ceruleus causes release of noradrenaline from the adrenal medulla (Goadsby, 1985). Peripheral actions of noradrenaline include vasoconstriction mediated by α receptors and vasodilation mediated by β receptors. Noradrenaline also releases free fatty acids, which may in turn release serotonin from platelets (see Figure 4–4 below).

Dopamine concentration in platelet-rich plasma increases after migraine headache has been established for an hour or so (Eadie and Tyrer, 1985). Migrainous patients are more susceptible to the emetic effect of apomorphine and the hypotensive effect of bromocriptine, both of which are dopamine agonists (Fanciullacci et al., 1980; Sicuteri, 1977). Dopamine may thus mediate some of the symptoms of migraine, such as nausea and vomiting.

Histamine

Whole-blood histamine is significantly increased after migraine headache (Anthony and Lance, 1971). Receptors responsible for the vasodilator effect of histamine are of the H$_2$ variety in the external carotid circulation of monkeys

(Lord et al., 1981) and humans (Glover et al., 1973) and mainly of the H_2 type in the internal carotid circulation of monkeys (Lord et al., 1981). For these reasons, the H_2 blocking agent cimetidine has been subjected to controlled trials for the prevention of migraine but has not proven to be effective when administered alone or in combination with a H_1 blocking agent (Anthony et al., 1978). This does not exclude the possibility that histamine is released from mast cells in perivascular tissues.

The injection of histamine or the histamine-liberating substance 48/80 into the external carotid artery is said to cause pain (Sicuteri, 1967); thus, liberated histamine may contribute to the vascular component of migraine. However, the infusion of histamine into the internal carotid artery at a rate of 10 to 50 μg/minute does not increase rCBF or cause headache in migrainous subjects (Krabbe and Olesen, 1980). It must be concluded that histamine is of little, if any, importance in the genesis of migraine.

Tyramine and Phenylethylamine

Tyramine is formed from the amino acid tyrosine by decarboxylation, and phenylethylamine is derived from phenylalanine by a similar process. Both substances are present in normal foods—tyramine in old cheeses and gamy meat and phenylethylamine in chocolate. Both have been implicated in "dietary migraine." The controversial literature was reviewed by Kohlenberg (1982), who analyzed the methodology of conflicting studies and concluded cautiously that "the tyramine hypothesis appears to have some validity." Further careful studies are required before these dietary factors can be considered important in the pathophysiology of migraine.

Excitatory Amino Acids

D'Andrea et al. (1989a) reported that the platelet content of glutamate and aspartate was increased during headache-free periods in patients subject to migraine with aura, when compared with normal controls and migrainous patients without aura. The glutamate level rose further during headache. Ferrari et al. (1990) measured these amino acids in plasma and found the level to be elevated in migrainous patients between attacks, more so in those patients whose migraine was accompanied by an aura, and to increase further during headache. If a similar defect were shown to exist in the cortex, it could render neurons and glial cells more susceptible to spreading depression.

Peptides

The discovery that peptides are present in cerebral neurons, autonomic fibers, and afferent pathways has drawn attention to their possible relevance to migraine.

Vasoactive Peptides

The peptide story goes back to the report of Chapman et al. (1960) of a bradykininlike substance, termed "neurokinin," in the perivascular tissue of the temple during migraine headache. Bradykinin is a nonapeptide with a vasodilator and hypotensive action that is released by kallikrein from kininogen, an α-globulin. Plasma kininogen is diminished at the end of a migraine attack (Sicuteri et al., 1963; Sjaastad, 1970), and the blood level of a bradykinin-releasing enzyme is increased. Kinins are also increased in venous blood (Sjaastad, 1970). Sicuteri (1967) has shown that the pain-producing effect of bradykinin injected into a hand vein is potentiated by serotonin. However, the intravenous infusion of bradykinin in humans (Fox et al., 1961) or the intradermal injection of bradykinin into the temporal area (Elkind et al., 1964) does not cause headache.

Nerve fibers containing substance P, calcitonin gene-related peptide (CGRP), vasoactive intestinal polypeptide (VIP), and neuropeptide Y have been identified in the walls of human cerebral arteries obtained at operation (Edvinsson et al., 1987). Neuropeptide Y exerts a direct constrictor action but the other peptides are vasodilators, with CGRP being the most potent. After ablation of the trigeminal ganglion in the cat, the cerebrovascular content of substance P was found to be depleted (Moskowitz, 1984). Following thermocoagulation of the trigeminal ganglion in human patients, the levels of substance P and CGRP in the external jugular blood rose sharply at the same time as the cutaneous distribution of the affected divisions flushed (Goadsby et al., 1988). De Marinis et al. (1984) noted that the facial flushing response to the intravenous injection of histamine was diminished on the side of a previous trigeminal ganglion thermocoagulation, suggesting that the neural content of vasodilator peptides had been depleted. The observations in human subjects are supported by the laboratory studies of Zagami et al. (1990), who reported that levels of CGRP and VIP rose in the external jugular vein of the cat after the superior sagittal sinus was stimulated. The possible relevance of this to migraine became apparent when Goadsby et al. (1990) demonstrated that the level of CGRP (but not substance P or VIP) rose in external jugular blood on the side of migraine headache, suggesting that this peptide may mediate the peripheral dilatation that is often apparent at this time.

In contrast, in cats the vasodilator peptide associated with the parasympathetic projection through the facial nerve appears to be VIP. This efferent pathway leaves the facial nerve as the greater superficial petrosal nerve, which makes synaptic contact with cells adjacent to the carotid siphon (the carotid ganglion) before continuing as the vidian nerve to the sphenopalatine ganglion. Fibers loop back from this ganglion to the carotid siphon (Walters et al., 1986) as well as emerging to innervate peripheral blood vessels (Figure 4–2). The carotid ganglion comprises 100 to 150 neurons, some containing substance P, CGRP, and neuropeptide A, whereas others contain VIP (Hardebo et al., 1989). The axons from these cells have been shown in the rat to innervate the internal carotid artery and the proximal parts of its branches. Stimulation of the trigeminal nerve or ganglion in cats causes vasodilation in the extracranial circulation by two means (Lambert et al., 1984b). The first is mediated by a reflex employing the greater superficial petrosal nerve as its efferent pathway and releasing VIP as the vasodilator agent (Goadsby and Macdonald, 1985). The second, which persists after section of the trigeminal root, is probably caused by antidromic activation of trigeminal fibers, releasing CGRP and substance P as described above. Stimulation of the trigeminal nerve (Goadsby and Duckworth,

1987) and the facial nerve in the cat causes regional increases in cortical blood flow that, in the latter case, was found to be associated with a fourfold increase in the local release of VIP (Goadsby and Shelley, 1990). It thus appears probable that the release of vasodilator peptides (summarized in Figure 4–1) plays a part in the vascular phenomena of migraine, whereas there is no evidence as yet that vasoconstrictor peptides have any relevance.

Opioid Peptides

Endogenous opioids have been implicated as inhibitory neurotransmitters liberated from interneurons in the central regulation of pain pathways. They comprise β-endorphin, enkephalins, and dynorphins. There have been conflicting reports on plasma β-endorphin levels in migraine. Bach et al. (1985) studied 17 patients without and 11 patients with aura and could not demonstrate any significant change between attacks and headache-free periods. Nappi et al. (1985) found that the β-endorphin content of cerebrospinal fluid (CSF) was low during headache-free periods of patients subject to migraine without aura. Anselmi et al. (1980) reported that CSF enkephalins were significantly lowered during migraine headache when compared with samples taken in headache-free periods and those from normal controls. Plasma methionine–metenkephalin levels are higher in migrainous patients than in normal controls and increase further during headache (Ferrari et al., 1987; Mosnaim et al., 1986). The extent to which these changes in blood and CSF reflect central opioid function remains uncertain. It is interesting that the intramuscular injection of 0.8 mg naloxone shortened the migrainous aura in most patients but, when the aura followed its usual course, the ensuing headache was of normal severity (Sicuteri et al., 1983).

Prostaglandins

Prostaglandins (PGs) are long-chain unsaturated fatty acids derived from arachidonic acid with potent constrictor and dilator effects. During migraine headache, plasma levels of PGE_1 do not alter (Anthony, 1976) but the level of PGE_2-like substances has been shown to fall significantly, by 41%, in contrast with its elevation found in cluster headache (Nattero et al., 1984).

The intravenous infusion of PGE_1 into normal subjects has been reported to evoke headache indistinguishable from migraine (Carlson et al., 1968), but the intravenous administration of prostacyclin in migrainous patients caused only a dull headache unlike the subjects' spontaneous attacks (Peatfield et al., 1981b). Nonsteroidal anti-inflammatory agents with prostaglandin antagonist activity are used in the treatment of migraine and presumably help to reduce the sterile inflammatory reaction that is thought to take place around dilated blood vessels.

Free Fatty Acids

The blood level of free fatty acids increases in fasting patients who subsequently develop headache (Hockaday et al., 1971) and is significantly elevated during migraine headache (Anthony, 1976, 1978). Anthony postulated that free fatty

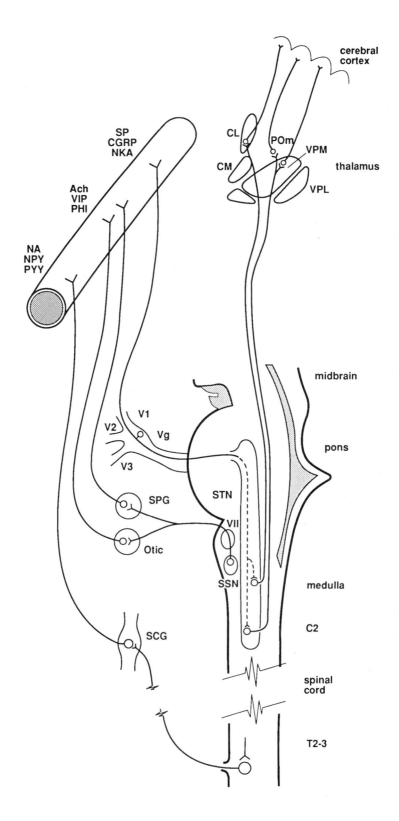

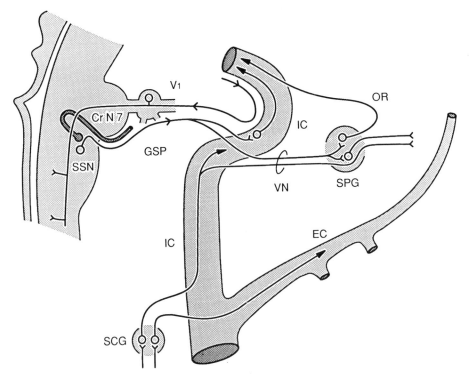

Figure 4–2. Autonomic control of the cranial circulation. Parasympathetic fibers arise in the superior salivatory nucleus (SSN) and accompany the facial nerve (CrN7) before branching off as the greater superficial petrosal (GSP) nerve to synapse on cells in the wall of the internal carotid (IC) artery while other fibers pass on with sympathetic fibers in the Vidian nerve (VN) to the sphenopalatine ganglion (SPG). Post-ganglionic neurons innervate branches of the external carotid (EC) artery as well as looping back to the internal carotid artery, via orbital rami (OR). Sympathetic fibers from the superior cervical ganglion (SCG) form a plexus in the walls of both internal and external carotid arteries. Afferent fibers from the internal carotid circulation traverse the first division of the trigeminal nerve (V_1). (From Lance, J.W. (1993). *The Mechanism and Management of Headache*, 5th ed., By permission of Butterworth-Heinemann, London.)

←

Figure 4–1. Central pain pathways and neurotransmitters associated with afferent and efferent pathways in the trigeminovascular system. Vascular afferent fibers have their cell bodies in the Gasserian ganglion (Vg), and descend in the spinal tract of the trigeminal nerve (STN) before synapsing in nucleus caudalis and the second cervical (C2) segment of the spinal cord. The second order neurons project to the ventroposteromedial (VPM), the intralaminar or centrolateral (CL) nuclei of the thalamus and the medial nucleus of the posterior complex (POm). The centromedial (CM) and ventroposterolateral (VPL) nuclei are also marked on the diagram.

Abbreviations for transmitters are as follows: (a) Trigeminovascular system; Substance P (SP); Calcitonin gene-related peptide (CGRP); Neurokinin A (NKA). (b) Parasympathetic fibers arising in the superior salivatory nucleus (SSN) that emerge in the seventh cranial nerve (VII) and traverse the sphenopalatine ganglion (SPG) and otic ganglion. Acetylcholine (ACh); Vasoactive intestinal polypeptide (VIP); Peptide histidine isoleucine (PHI); (c) Sympathetic fibers originating in the superior cervical ganglion (SCG). Norepinephrine (noradrenaline, NA); Neuropeptide Y (NPY); Peptide YY (PYY). (From Goadsby, P.J., A.S. Zagami, and G.A. Lambert (1991). *Headache 31:* 365–371, by permission of the editor.)

acids might be responsible for the release of serotonin from blood platelets in migraine.

Glucose

Missing a meal may precipitate migraine, presumably because of hypoglycemia (Blau and Cumings, 1966). Migrainous patients have a poor hyperglycemic response to glucagon, suggesting impaired mobilization of liver glycogen (de Silva et al., 1974).

Electrolytes

The measurement of brain phosphates by magnetic resonance imaging after the intravenous injection of ^{31}P has enabled the indirect assay of magnesium content by examining the chemical shift properties of the ^{31}P resonance signals. By using this noninvasive technique, Welch et al. (1989) found that magnesium ion concentration was lower during migraine headache. This preliminary result suggests a basis for cerebral hyperexcitability that could render the brain susceptible to spreading depression.

Sodium and fluid are retained before and during migraine headache (Campbell et al., 1951), but this is probably a secondary phenomenon because the use of diuretics does not prevent attacks (Schottstaedt & Wolff, 1955).

Hormones

Premenstrual migraine recurs each month when plasma estradiol and progesterone levels fall and may be deferred by maintaining an artificially high level of estradiol (Somerville, 1972). Nattero et al. (1979) reported high plasma levels of both hormones in migrainous patients on the 26th day of the menstrual cycle, unlike Somerville, who found that hormone levels did not differ from those of normal subjects.

Eleven female migrainous patients given the "triple test" (thyrotropin-releasing hormone, luteinizing hormone–releasing hormone, insulin) showed a significantly greater increase in the secretion of prolactin, but not other hormones, than controls (Awaki et al., 1989). This could be explained by diminished dopaminergic or increased serotonergic transmission.

Mean values of cortisol were not found to be significantly higher in migrainous patients (Ziegler et al., 1979), but the circadian rhythm of its secretion was disturbed.

Immune Complexes

Lord and Duckworth (1977) found breakdown products of the third complement component (C_3) in the plasma of three headache-free patients, each of whom developed a migraine attack within 24 hours, whereas none of the 28 patients without detectable breakdown products had a headache within this period. Immune complexes were present significantly more often at the onset of headache in those patients without than in those with aura (Lord and Duckworth, 1978). Jerzmanowski and Klimek (1983) found that the mean value for the C_3 fraction in 54 migrainous patients between attacks was lower than that of 70 control subjects. Other investigations (Behan et al., 1981; Moore et al., 1980) have not found any difference in complement components or immune complexes between the migrainous and the control groups. The possible precipitation of migraine by immune reactions remains an open question.

NEURAL CHANGES IN MIGRAINE

Cortical Events

Lashley (1941) plotted the expansion of his own visual scotoma in migraine and calculated that the visual cortex was being compromised by some process advancing at about 3 mm each minute, a rate corresponding to that of "spreading depression" as described in the cortex of experimental animals by Leão (1944). Studies of rCBF during the aura indicate that a wave of oligemia sweeps over the cortex slowly at a similar velocity of 2 to 5 mm/minute (Lauritzen et al., 1982). Positron emission tomography has shown that the rate of glucose metabolism in the cerebral cortex diminishes in the early stages of migraine attacks induced by the injection of reserpine (Sachs et al., 1985). Vasoconstriction may be the primary event because rCBF can be reduced to a critical level in classic migraine (Skyhøj-Olsen et al., 1984).

The contingent negative variation (CNV) is a slow negative potential recorded over the scalp preceding motor activity in a reaction-time task. It is a readiness potential that is thought to be mediated by a central catecholaminergic pathway. The amplitude of the CNV is significantly higher in migraineurs receiving no prophylactic therapy than in patients with tension headache and normal controls, but returns toward normal values when the patients are treated with β blockers (Maertens de Noordhout et al., 1985). This increase in CNV, and also in the amplitude of visual evoked potentials recorded in migrainous patients (Gawel et al., 1983), suggests an increased central excitatory state in the cortex itself or in the nonspecific and specific afferent projections to the cortex. Indirect support is given to this view by the finding of Fanciullacci et al. (1974) that migrainous patients are unduly susceptible to hallucinogenic drugs.

Hypothalamus

Premonitory symptoms, such as elation, hunger, thirst, and drowsiness, preceding migraine headache by up to 24 hours, suggest a hypothalamic disturbance (Herberg, 1975). The hypothalamopituitary axis appears to be normal in migrainous patients when assessed by conventional tests (Rao and Pearce, 1971). Prolactin secretion is inhibited by tuberoinfundibular neurons using dopamine as a transmitter and is increased by serotonin, probably through a prolactin-releasing factor. A levodopa loading test was found to reduce the prolactin level during attacks of common migraine but to increase it when migraine headache was accompanied by neurologic symptoms and signs (Vardi et al., 1981). This suggests that some factor antagonistic to dopamine, such as serotonin, overcame the inhibitory effect of dopamine in classic migraine. The periodicity of migraine is probably determined by an "internal clock," such as the suprachiasmatic nucleus, that may activate the hypothalamus well in advance of other structures mediating the migraine attack, but proof of this is lacking.

Autonomic Nervous System

Appenzeller et al. (1963) reported that the dilator response of forearm vessels to heat was impaired in migrainous patients, but this was not confirmed by French et al. (1967) or Hockaday et al. (1967). Downey and Frewin (1972) found that resting blood flow in the hand was higher in migrainous patients than in controls and that the reduction in flow in response to a cold stimulus was less.

The pupillary diameter of migrainous patients had been studied by Fanciullacci (1979), who found that oral fenfluramine, which has sympathomimetic properties, induced less mydriasis in migraineurs than in normal controls. Eye drops of 5% guanethidine, a drug that depletes stores of noradrenaline, provoked a greater and more prolonged miosis in migraineurs than in controls, whereas the instillation of 1% phenylephrine, which causes only a slight dilation of the normal pupil, produced mydriasis in migrainous patients. Fanciullacci concluded that noradrenaline stores in the iris were depleted and that the receptors were hypersensitive in migraine; curiously, however, he observed no difference between sides in unilateral migraine, although Drummond (1987) found consistent pupillary changes on the side of habitual headache. Denervation hypersensitivity of the iris was confirmed by Gotoh et al. (1984), who also demonstrated a decrease in blood pressure overshoot in the Valsalva maneuver and a tendency toward orthostatic hypotension in migrainous patients compared with controls. Sweating of the dorsum of the hand in response to local intradermal injection of 0.05 ml of 1% pilocarpine was found to be diminished in migrainous patients (Hamada et al., 1985), suggesting a sympathetic deficit without denervation hypersensitivity.

Pupillary changes may develop at an early age in migrainous patients. Battistella et al. (1989) described supersensitivity of the pupils to phenylephrine in 18 children age 16 years or less who were subject to migraine with aura. The same response was apparent in all adult patients with migraine without aura. Drummond (1990) confirmed his earlier results in 80 patients with unilateral migraine and found that pupillary supersensitivity on the side affected by headache correlated with increased heat loss from the ipsilateral forehead and orbit during headache, suggesting that an ocular sympathetic deficit may contribute to the localized vasodilation observed. The most likely mechanism, as has been suggested for the partial Horner syndrome of cluster headache, is that connections of the greater superficial petrosal nerve with the carotid ganglion (Figure 4–1) release vasodilator peptides (Figure 4–2) in the wall of the internal carotid artery, thus producing edema of the arterial wall that compromises the periarterial sympathetic plexus.

Brainstem Control of the Cranial Circulation

The discovery of intrinsic noradrenergic and serotonergic pathways from the brainstem to the cerebral cortex may prove to be of relevance to the neurologic symptoms and vascular changes of migraine.

Locus Ceruleus

The locus ceruleus is located near the wall of the fourth ventricle in the upper pons and is the largest collection of noradrenaline-containing neurons in the brain. It receives afferent fibers from the insular and visual cortex, amygdala, hypothalamus, brainstem reticular formation, raphe, vestibular nucleus, and tractus solitarius—all areas related to internal and external sensory stimuli or to the affective state. It projects to the cerebral cortex mainly through a dorsal bundle of fibers passing through the septum, turning backward through the cingulum, and sending lateral projections to all areas of the neocortex. In the squirrel monkey, noradrenergic fibers are distributed particularly to layers III, V, and VI of the visual cortex, in contrast with serotonergic fibers from the raphe nuclei, which terminate in layer IV (Morrison et al., 1982). The locus ceruleus also projects to the hypothalamus, thalamus, medial and lateral geniculate nuclei, facial nerve nucleus, and spinal nucleus of the trigeminal nerve and spinal cord, predominantly ipsilaterally. The upstream projection seems to be related to the state of awareness, with a subpopulation of locus ceruleus neurons that switch off just prior to and during the rapid eye movement (REM) phase of sleep (Foote et al., 1983). Maximal activity in the locus ceruleus neurons occurs at times of arousal and vigilance. Their effect on target organs is, in general, to reduce spontaneous activity and enhance the activity evoked by sensory systems. The downstream projection from the locus ceruleus is, at least in part, related to pain control mechanisms.

Hartman et al. (1980) found that electrical or chemical stimulation of locus ceruleus neurons bilaterally in the monkey decreased cerebral blood flow and increased vascular permeability without associated changes in blood pressure or pulse rate. De la Torre et al. (1977), using the hydrogen washout technique, showed that unilateral stimulation of the locus ceruleus at 1.5/second reduced rCBF. Goadsby et al. (1982) confirmed that cerebral vascular resistance increased—that is, blood flow fell—by about 20% with low-frequency stimulation of monkey locus ceruleus. In contrast, external carotid resistance diminished—that is, blood flow increased—as the frequency of locus ceruleus stimulation increased. The extracranial vasodilator effect was later shown to be mediated by the greater superficial petrosal branch of the facial nerve. These changes, which were predominantly ipsilateral, bear a striking resemblance to the vascular changes accompanying classic migraine.

Raphe Nuclei

Serotonin-containing neurons from the midbrain raphe project rostrally in the medial forebrain bundle and are distributed to the hypothalamus and dorsal thalamus and diffusely to the cerebral cortex (Moore et al., 1978). In the visual cortex of the monkey, serotonergic nerve terminals are distributed chiefly to spiny stellate cells of layer IV, the layer that receives incoming geniculocalcarine fibers (Morrison et al., 1982). The nucleus raphe dorsalis and medianus send an ascending serotonergic pathway that innervates blood vessels of the cerebral microcirculation in the rat cortex (Reinhard et al., 1979). A serotonergic innervation has also been demonstrated on intrinsic brainstem vessels of monkeys and rats (di Carlo, 1977), on rabbit vertebral arteries (Griffith et al., 1982), and on the vertebrobasilar system of cats (di Carlo, 1981), the latter originating from the nucleus raphe pallidus and obscurus in the brainstem.

Stimulation of the nucleus raphe dorsalis increases cerebral blood flow in the monkey. It dilates both internal and external carotid circulations, through connections with the facial (greater superficial petrosal) nerve (Goadsby et al., 1985a,b). The extracranial vasodilation is comparable with the reflex effects of locus ceruleus stimulation. The ascending projections of the midbrain raphe nuclei have been implicated in the control of sleep behavior and neuroendocrine regulation, as have noradrenergic pathways. It appears that catecholaminergic and serotonergic projections from the brainstem exert an influence on both neuronal discharge and vascular supply to the cerebral cortex, although whether these pathways are complementary or at times antagonistic (analogous to sympathetic and parasympathetic autonomic nervous systems) remains to be determined.

The Trigeminovascular Reflex

Thermocoagulation of the Gasserian ganglion for tic douloureux, a procedure that would be very painful if the patient were not anesthetized, produces a facial flush in the distribution of the division or divisions coagulated (Drummond et al., 1983). Lambert et al. (1984b) showed that electrical stimulation of the Gasserian ganglion diminished carotid resistance and increased blood flow and facial temperature in cats by a reflex pathway traversing the trigeminal root as its afferent limb and the greater superficial petrosal branch of the facial nerve as its efferent limb. A minor component of the response, particularly that elicited from the third division, persisted after section of the trigeminal root, almost certainly caused by the liberation of vasoactive peptides from antidromic activation of trigeminal nerve terminals of a vasoactive agent such as substance P (Moskowitz, 1984). The main reflex vasodilator response to stimulation of the locus ceruleus, raphe nuclei, or trigeminal nerve is mediated by the sphenopalatine and otic ganglia and employs VIP as its neurovascular transmitter (Goadsby and Macdonald, 1985).

A pathway has thus been established that can account for extracranial vascular dilatation accompanying a primary pain-producing excitation of trigeminal pathways, a mechanism that may prove relevant to the vascular changes of migraine. A suitable name for this phenomenon might be the trigeminovascular reflex (Figure 4–3).

Synthesis

Migraine is a neurovascular reaction in response to sudden changes in the internal or external environment. Each individual has a hereditary "migrainous threshold," with the degree of susceptibility depending on the balance between

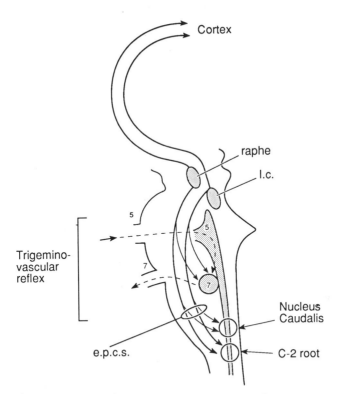

Figure 4–3. The trigeminovascular reflex. Stimulation of the trigeminal nerve increases blood flow in both intra- and extracranial circulations by its connections with the parasympathetic outflow illustrated in Figure 4–2. Stimulation of the nucleus raphe dorsalis and locus ceruleus (l.c.), the latter with stimulation only at high frequencies, produce vasodilatation through the same pathway. Both raphe and l.c. project diffusely to the cerebral cortex where low frequency l.c. stimulation reduces cerebral blood flow. Nucleus raphe magnus and l.c. also play a part in the endogenous pain control system (e.p.c.s.) modulating the transmission of pain impulses in nucleus caudalis and the upper cervical spinal cord (C_2 root).

excitation and inhibition at various levels of the nervous system. Such a balance may be influenced by magnesium deficiency, excitatory amino acids, monoamines, opioids, and other factors outlined earlier in this chapter. Neural and vascular elements both contribute to headache.

Vascular constriction and dilatation take place at different stages of the migraine attack, leading to a suggestion that migraine may be allied to Raynaud phenomenon and variant angina, but the reaction of the digital arteries to cold is normal (Corbin and Martyn, 1985). The injection of contrast media into the carotid or vertebral arteries can initiate phenomena resembling the aura and headache of migraine, and the intake of vasodilator drugs can cause headache in migrainous subjects. The release of 5-HT from platelets at the onset of migraine was thought to induce constriction of small vessels and to sensitize larger arteries to distention so that later dilatation caused pain, but animal studies have shown that the amount of 5-HT liberated could not cause a significant change in cerebral or extracranial blood flow (Spira et al., 1976). The 5-HT receptors in migrainous arteries do not differ from those of normal controls (Skarby et al., 1982), so there is no evidence for specific sensitivity to the action of 5-HT. Nevertheless, the facts remain that the injection of reserpine induces migraine as it lowers platelet 5-HT and that the intravenous infusion of 5-HT relieves spontaneous and induced migraine headache. The 5-HT_1–like agonist sumatriptan has proven effective in relieving migraine, presumably by some peripheral action because it does not pass readily through the blood–brain barrier.

Vasodilatation is unlikely to cause pain unless it is accompanied by sensitization of the vessel wall or a sterile inflammatory reaction in the perivascular tissues. Moskowitz and his colleagues have shown that the intravenous injection of capsaicin or stimulation of the trigeminal nerve for 5 minutes induces plasma extravasation from dural vessels in rats, an effect blocked by ergotamine, dihydroergotamine, and methysergide (Saito et al., 1988). The reaction to capsaicin, which releases substance P, was blocked in guinea pigs by sumatriptan, although the reaction to substance P itself was unaffected, suggesting that sumatriptan acts at a prejunctional site (Buzzi and Moskowitz, 1989). Moskowitz (1984) suggested that his experimental findings showed how the trigeminal nerve, or the central nervous system via the trigeminal nerve, could provoke unilateral vascular changes and that the antidromic release of vasodilator peptides from the nerve could induce the sterile inflammatory reaction responsible for headache. Moskowitz thought that spreading depression of the cortex during the aura phase of migraine might depolarize trigeminal nerve fibers surrounding the pial arteries and thus initiate the headache phase of migraine. If this were the case, headache would always develop on the side of the head responsible for the cerebral symptoms (e.g., a left visual field aura would be followed by a right-sided headache). Most authors agree that the headache appears as often as not on the inappropriate side (Peatfield et al., 1981a).

Olesen et al. (1990) have also sought to link the phenomena underlying the aura phase with the development of headache. They found that the majority of patients studied did have their headache on the side relevant to the production of the aura but, even so, 3 of their 38 patients experienced their unilateral headache on the "wrong" side. Of 19 patients with bilateral headache, aura symptoms were bilateral in 6 and unilateral in 13. Of 10 patients with bilateral aura, 6 developed bilateral and 4 unilateral headache. The correlation between the cortical process responsible for the aura (probably allied to or identical with spreading depression) and the ensuing headache is therefore close but not absolute. There is no evidence that ischemia alone is sufficient to cause headache, and we must account for the greater number of patients who experience migraine headache without aura or the converse, aura without headache.

About one quarter of all patients have experienced premonitory symptoms of elation, a craving for sweet foods, or excessive yawning, suggesting that the migrainous process starts in the hypothalamus. Other patients are subject to headaches at regular intervals, irrespective of any external circumstances, indicating that the process is regulated by some biologic clock. Others may respond to stress, relaxation after stress, or excessive afferent stimuli, such as glare, noise, or strong perfumes. At times, the relationship is so close that it suggests a reflex cortical response. For example, exposure to flickering light may induce a visual aura within minutes.

Wherever the process starts in the brain, it is likely that activation of brainstem nuclei follows. Welch et al. (1988) postulated that the orbitofrontal and limbic cortices trigger the intrinsic noradrenergic system through the locus ceruleus. In our laboratory, we have demonstrated in cats and monkeys that stimulation of the locus ceruleus at low frequencies can reduce cerebral blood flow by about 20% and, at higher frequencies, can increase extracranial blood flow by the same amount (Goadsby and Lance, 1988). These vascular changes closely resemble those seen in migraine (Lance et al., 1983). We have also demonstrated that stimulation of the serotonergic nucleus raphe dorsalis and the trigeminal system will increase both intracranial and extracranial blood flow by a reflex pathway employing the greater superficial petrosal nerve as its efferent limb and releasing VIP as the vasodilator agent (Figures 4–3 and 4–4). This provides a mechanism for brainstem activity to produce secondary vascular changes and ties together the above theories. Feedback from cerebral, dural, or extracranial vessels via the trigeminal nerve could intensify these changes, leading to a vicious circle intensifying pain. Vomiting is most likely caused by the action of dopamine or 5-HT on the area postrema of the medulla (Cahen, 1974).

The other factor that must be considered in the pathogenesis of migraine is the endogenous pain control pathway. There is presumably some partial or segmental defect in this pathway in migrainous patients because spontaneous jabs of pain (ice-pick pains) and the reflex response to ingestion of cold foods or drinks (ice-cream headache) are felt in the area habitually affected by migraine headache in about one third of patients. Migraine headache may thus represent a more prolonged discharge of a partially disinhibited group of neurons when subjected to the cerebral and brainstem influences described above. It is interesting to note in this context that 15 of 175 patients in whom electrodes had been inserted into the periaqueductal gray matter for the relief of intractable pain developed migrainelike headaches (Raskin et al., 1987). It thus appears that the endogenous pain control system can be switched off as well as on by such electrode placements. The locus ceruleus and raphe nuclei are part of this pathway, and their descending projections modulate the transmission of painful impulses in the trigeminal system (Figures 4–3 and 4–4).

Excessive activity of monoaminergic pathways could account for the vascular changes of migraine, including those accompanying the aura, and a subsequent phase of monoamine depletion could accentuate a pre-existing deficiency in the pain gateway, whether a particular attack originates centrally or is triggered by vascular or other afferent input. The locus ceruleus exerts an inhibitory effect on the contralateral nucleus (Buda et al., 1975), which could account for migraine headache being predominantly unilateral.

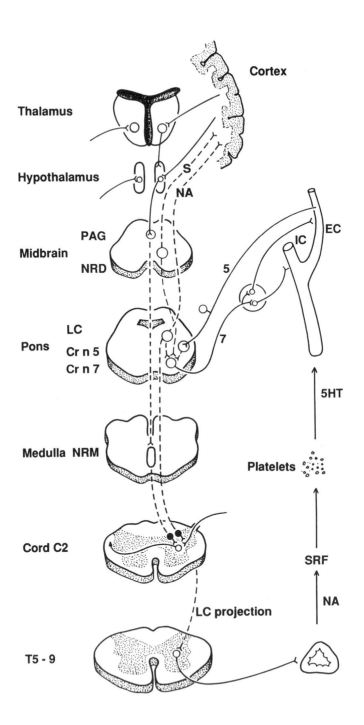

Cortex

Thalamus

Hypothalamus

S

NA

PAG

Midbrain

NRD

5

IC

EC

LC

Pons

Cr n 5

Cr n 7

7

5HT

Medulla NRM

Platelets

Cord C2

SRF

LC projection

NA

T5 - 9

CONCLUSIONS

Migraine has been presented as an unstable trigeminovascular reflex with a segmental defect in the pain control pathway, thus permitting excessive discharge of part of the spinal nucleus of the trigeminal nerve and its thalamic connections in response to excessive afferent input or corticobulbar drive. The end result is interaction between brainstem and cranial blood vessels, with the afferent impulses from the latter intensifying pain perception through the trigeminovascular reflex. Diffuse projections from the locus ceruleus to the cerebral cortex could initiate cortical oligemia and possibly spreading depression. Activity in this system could account for the migrainous aura that may occur quite independently of the headache, although one commonly follows the other. The headache phase may be interrupted by therapy aimed at either the central or peripheral end of the trigeminovascular reflex. Although many aspects remain unexplained, this hypothesis fits the observations made in patients with migraine as well as the experimental findings in laboratory animals. It also provides a rationale for medication directed toward the central nervous system as well as the peripheral end organ, the cranial blood vessel.

←——

Figure 4–4.   The neurovascular hypothesis for migraine. Brainstem mechanisms are triggered by descending pathways from the cerebral cortex (in response to emotion or stress), from the thalamus (in response to excessive afferent stimulation, light, noise, or smells), or from the hypothalamus (in response to changes in the internal environment or "internal clocks"). Nucleus raphe dorsalis (NRD) and locus ceruleus (LC) project diffusely to the cerebral cortex, employing serotonin (S) and norepinephrine (noradrenaline, NA), respectively, as transmitter agents. LC causes constriction of the ipsilateral cortical microcirculation through this direct pathway. Stimulation of NRD, LC, or the trigeminal nerve (5) induces dilatation of the extracranial circulation (EC), by connections with the parasympathetic component of the facial nerve (7) (the greater superficial petrosal nerve) and the sphenopalatine and otic ganglia, and releases vasoactive intestinal peptide as a peripheral transmitter agent ("the trigeminovascular reflex"). NRD causes dilatation in the internal carotid circulation (IC) through the same indirect pathway. Stimulation of the LC area causes release of NA from the adrenal gland by its connection with the intermediolateral cell column of the thoracic cord (LC projection). NA, or a serotonin (5-HT) releasing factor (SRF) liberated by NA, causes a platelet release reaction. Free serotonin released from platelets increases the sensitivity of vascular receptors, thus augmenting the afferent inflow through the trigeminal nerve (5). The spinal tract of the trigeminal nerve (not illustrated) descends to the second cervical segment of the spinal cord (C2) where it converges with fibers from the second cervical root onto second order neurons in the pain pathway. Transmission at this synapse is regulated by inhibitory neurons (black circles) which, in turn, are modulated by the endogenous pain-control pathway descending from the periaqueductal gray matter (PAG) through nucleus raphe magnus (NRM), and from LC. Activity in brainstem monoaminergic pathways is thus able to replicate the vascular changes of migraine as well as to regulate the perception of pain arising from cranial vessels. (Reproduced from Lance, J.W., G.A. Lambert, P.J. Goadsby, and A.S. Zagami (1990). Contribution of experimental studies to understanding the pathophysiology of migraine. In *Migraine: A spectrum of ideas* (M. Sandler and G. Collins, eds.), p. 30. Oxford University Press, Oxford, by permission of the editors.)

REFERENCES

Adams, R.W., G.A. Lambert, and J.W. Lance (1989). Stimulation of brainstem nuclei in the cat: Effect on neuronal activity in the primary visual cortex of relevance to cerebral blood flow and migraine. *Cephalalgia* 9:107–118.

Andersen, A.R., L. Friberg, T. Skyhøj Olsen, and J. Olesen (1988). Delayed hyperemia following hypoperfusion in classic migraine. Single photon emission computed tomographic demonstration. *Arch. Neurol.* 45:154–159.

Angus-Leppan, H., G.A. Lambert, P. Boers et al. (1989). The cervical spinal cord is a relay centre for the central nervous system processing of input from the cranial vasculature. *Cephalalgia* 9(Suppl. 10):137–138.

Anselmi, B., E. Baldi, F. Casacci, and S. Salmon (1980). Endogenous opioids in cerebrospinal fluid and blood in idiopathic headache sufferers. *Headache* 20:294–299.

Anthony, M. (1976). Plasma free fatty acids and prostaglandin E in migraine and stress. *Headache* 16:58–63.

Anthony, M. (1978). Role of individual free fatty acids in migraine. *Res. Clin. Stud. Headache* 6:110–116.

Anthony, M. (1981). Biochemical indices of sympathetic activity in migraine. *Cephalalgia* 1:83–89.

Anthony, M., H. Hinterberger, and J.W. Lance (1967). Plasma serotonin in migraine and stress. *Arch. Neurol.* 16:544–552.

Anthony, M., H. Hinterberger, and J.W. Lance (1969). The possible relationship of serotonin to the migraine syndrome. *Res. Clin. Stud. Headache* 2:29–59.

Anthony, M. and J.W. Lance (1971). Histamine and serotonin in cluster headache. *Arch. Neurol.* 25:225–231.

Anthony, M. and J.W. Lance (1975). The role of serotonin in migraine. In *Modern Topics in Migraine* (J. Pearce, ed.), p. 107–123. Heinemann, London.

Anthony, M., G.D.A. Lord, and J.W. Lance (1978). Controlled trials of cimetidine in migraine and cluster headache. *Headache* 18:261–264.

Appenzeller, A., K. Davison, and J. Marshall (1963). Reflex abnormalities in the hands of migrainous subjects. *J. Neurol. Neurosurg. Psychiatry* 26:447–450.

Awaki, E., T. Takeshima, K. Mikamo et al. (1989). A neuroendocrinological study in female migraineurs: Prolactin and thyroid stimulating hormone responses. *Cephalalgia* 9(Suppl. 10):53–54.

Bach, F.W., K. Kensen, N. Blegvad et al. (1985). Beta-endorphin and ACTH in plasma during attack in common and classic migraine. *Cephalalgia* 5:177–182.

Bakke, M., P. Tfelt-Hansen, J. Olesen, and E. Møller (1982). Action of some pericranial muscles during provoked attacks of common migraine. *Pain* 14:121–135.

Barkley, G.L., N. Tepley, S. Nagel-Leiby et al. (1990). Magnetoencephalographic studies of migraine. *Headache* 30:428–434.

Basbaum, A.I. and H.L. Fields (1978). Endogenous pain control mechanisms: Review and hypothesis. *Ann. Neurol.* 4:451–462.

Basbaum, A.I. and H.L. Fields (1984). Endogenous pain control systems: Brainstem spinal pathways and endorphin circuitry. *Annu. Rev. Neurosci.* 7:309–338.

Battistella, P.A., R. Ruffilli, and F. Zacchello (1989). Pupillary adrenergic sensitivity and idiopathic headache in pediatric patients. *Headache* 29:163–166.

Behan, W.M.H., P.O. Behan, and W.F. Durward (1981). Complement studies in migraine. *Headache* 21:55–57.

Blau, J.N. (1980). Migraine prodromes separated from the aura: Complete migraine. *BMJ* 21:658–660.

Blau, J.N. and J.N. Cumings (1966). Method of precipitating and preventing some migraine attacks. *BMJ 2:*1242–1243.

Blau, J.N. and S.L. Dexter (1981). The site of pain origin during migraine attacks. *Cephalalgia 1:*143–147.

Buda, M., B. Roussel, B. Renaud, and J-F. Pujol (1975). Increase in tyrosine hydroxylase activity in the locus coeruleus of the rat brain after contralateral lesioning. *Brain Res. 93:*564–569.

Buzzi, M.G. and M.A. Moskowitz (1989). GR43175, a 5-HT-like agonist, blocks neurogenic plasma protein extravasation in dura mater. *Cephalalgia 9*(Suppl. 10): 27–28.

Cahen, R.L. (1974). Emetic effect of biogenic amines. *Res. Clin. Stud. Headache 3:* 227–244.

Campbell, D.A., K.M. Hay, and E.M. Tonks (1951). An investigation of salt and water balance in migraine. *BMJ 2:*1424–1429.

Carlson, L.A., L.-G. Ekelund, and L. Orö (1968). Clinical and metabolic effects of different doses of prostaglandin E in man. *Acta Med. Scand. 183:*423–430.

Carroll, P.R., P.W. Ebeling, and W.E. Glover (1974). The responses of the human temporal and rabbit ear artery to 5-hydroxytryptamine and some of its antagonists. *Aust. J. Exp. Biol. Med. Sci. 52:*813–823.

Chapman, L.F., A.O. Ramos, H. Goodell et al. (1960). A humoral agent implicated in vascular headache of the migrainous type. *Arch. Neurol. 3:*223–229.

Corbin, D. and C. Martyn (1985). Migraine is not a manifestation of a generalized vasospastic disorder. *Cephalalgia 5*(Suppl. 3):458–459.

Couch, J.R. and R.S. Hassanein (1977). Platelet aggregability in migraine. *Neurology 27:*843–848.

Curran, D.A., H. Hinterberger, and J.W. Lance (1965). Total plasma serotonins 5-hydroxyindoleacetic acid and *p*-hydroxy-*m*-methoxymandelic acid excretion in normal and migrainous subjects. *Brain 88:*997–1010.

Curzon, G., M. Barrie, and M.I.P. Wilkinson (1969). Relationships between headache and amine changes after administration of reserpine to migrainous patients. *J. Neurol. Neurosurg. Psychiatry 32:*555–561.

Dahlof, C., P. Winter, and S. Ludlow (1989). Oral GR43175, a 5-HT1-like agonist, for treatment of the acute migraine attack. *Cephalalgia 9*(Suppl. 10):351–352.

D'Andrea, G., A.R. Cananzi, R. Joseph et al. (1989a). Platelet excitatory aminoacids in migraine. *Cephalalgia 9*(Suppl. 10):105–106.

D'Andrea, G., K.M.A. Welch, S. Nagel-Leiby et al. (1989b). Platelet catecholamines in migraine. *Cephalalgia 9:*3–5.

D'Andrea, G.K., K.M.A. Welch, J.M. Riddle et al. (1989c). Platelet serotonin metabolism and ultrastructure in migraine. *Arch. Neurol. 46:*1187–1189.

Davies, P.T.G. and T.J. Steiner (1990). Serotonin S2 receptors and migraine: A study with the selective antagonist ICI 169,369. *Headache 30:*340–343.

Davis, K.D. and J.O. Dostrovsky (1986). Activation of trigeminal brainstem nociceptive neurons by dural artery stimulation. *Pain 25:*395–401.

Davis, K.D. and J.O. Dostrovsky (1988). Responses of feline thalamic neurons activated by stimulation of the middle meningeal artery and sagittal sinus. *Brain Res. 454:* 89–100.

De la Torre, J.C., J.W. Surgeon, and R.H. Walker (1977). Effects of locus coeruleus stimulation on cerebral blood flow in selected brain regions. *Acta Neurol. Scand. Suppl. 64:*104–105.

De Marinis, M., N. Martucci, F.M. Gagliardi et al. (1984). Trigeminal control of craniofacial vasomotor response: 1. Histamine test in patients with unilateral gasserian ganglion lesions. *Cephalalgia 4:*243–251.

Deshmukh, S.V. and J.S. Meyer (1977). Cyclic changes in platelet dynamics and the pathogenesis and prophylaxis of migraine. *Headache 17:*101–108.

De Silva, K.L., M.A. Ron, and J. Pearce (1974). Blood sugar response to glucagon in migraine. *J. Neurol. Neurosurg. Psychiatry 37:*105–107.

Di Carlo, V. (1977). Histochemical evidence for a serotonergic innervation of the microcirculation in the brainstem. In *Neurogenic Control of the Brain Circulation* (C. Owman and L. Edvinsson, eds.), pp. 55–58. Pergamon Press, Oxford, England.

Di Carlo, V. (1981). Serotoninergic innervation of extrinsic brainstem blood vessels. *Neurology (NY) 31*(2):104.

Downey, J.A. and D.B. Frewin (1972). Vascular responses in the hands of patients suffering from migraine. *J. Neurol. Neurosurg. Psychiatry 35:*258–263.

Drummond, P.D. (1982). Extracranial and cardiovascular reactivity in migrainous subjects. *J. Psychosom. Res. 26:*317–331.

Drummond, P.D. (1987). Pupil diameter in migraine and tension headache. *J. Neurol. Neurosurg. Psychiatry 50:*228–231.

Drummond, P.D. (1990). Disturbances in ocular sympathetic function and facial blood flow in unilateral migraine headache. *J. Neurol. Neurosurg. Psychiatry 53:* 121–125.

Drummond, P.D., A. Gonski, and J.W. Lance (1983). Facial flushing after thermocoagulation of the gasserian ganglion. *J. Neurol. Neurosurg. Psychiatry 46:*611–616.

Drummond, P.D. and J.W. Lance (1981). Extracranial vascular reactivity in migraine and tension headache. *Cephalalgia 1:*149–155.

Drummond, P.D. and J.W. Lance (1983). Extracranial vascular changes and the source of pain in migraine headache. *Ann. Neurol. 13:*32–37.

Drummond, P.D. and J.W. Lance (1984). Neurovascular disturbances in headache patients. *Clin. Exp. Neurol. 20:*93–99.

Duggan, A.W. (1982). Brainstem control of the responses of spinal neurones to painful skin stimuli. *TINS 5:*127–130.

Dumuis, A., M. Sebben, E. Monferini, M. Nicola, M. Turconi, H. Ladinsky, and J. Bockaert (1991). Azabicycloalkyl benzimidazolone derivatives as a novel class of potent agonists at the 5-HT$_4$ receptor positively coupled to adenylate cyclase in brain. In *Pharmacology*. Springer-Verlag, Berlin.

Dvilansky, A., S. Rishpon, I. Nathan et al. (1976). Release of platelet 5-hydroxytryptamine by plasma taken from patients during and between migraine attacks. *Pain 2:*315–318.

Dvorkin, G.S., F. Andermann, S. Carpenter et al. (1987). Classical migraine, intractable epilepsy and multiple strokes: A syndrome related to mitochondrial encephalomyopathy. In *Migraine and Epilepsy* (F. Anderman and E. Lugaresi, eds.), pp. 203–232. Butterworth, London.

Eadie, M.J. and J.H. Tyrer (1985). *The Biochemistry of Migraine*, p. 65. MTP Press, Lancaster, England.

Edvinsson, L., R. Edman, I. Jansen et al. (1987). Peptide-containing nerve fibers in human cerebral arteries: Immunochemistry, radioimmunoassay, and in vitro pharmacology. *Ann. Neurol. 21:*431–437.

Edvinsson, L. and I. Jansen (1989). Characterization of 5-HT receptors mediating contraction of human cerebral, meningeal and temporal arteries: Target for GR43175 in acute treatment of migraine? *Cephalalgia 9*(Suppl. 10):39–40.

Elkind, A.H., A.P. Friedman, and J. Grossman (1964). Cutaneous blood flow in vascular headache of the migrainous type. *Neurology (Minneap.) 14:*24–30.

Fanciullacci, M. (1979). Iris adrenergic impairment in idiopathic headache. *Headache 19:*8–13.

Fanciullacci, M., G. Franchi, and F. Sicuteri (1974). Hypersensitivity to lysergic acid diethylamide (LSD-25) and psilocybin in essential headache. *Experentia 30:* 1441–1442.

Fanciullacci, M., S. Michelacci, C. Curradi, and F. Sicuteri (1980). Hyperresponsiveness of migraine patients to the hypotensive action of bromocriptine. *Headache 20:*99–102.

Ferrari, M.D., E.M. Bayliss, S. Ludlow, and A.J. Pilgrim (1989a). Subcutaneous GR43175 in the treatment of acute migraine: An international European study. *Cephalalgia 9*(Suppl. 10):348.

Ferrari, M.D., M. Frolich, J. Odink et al. (1987). Methionine-enkephalin and serotonin in migraine and tension headache. In *Current Problems in Neurology, Vol. 4, Advances in Headache Research* (F. Clifford Rose, ed.), pp. 227–234. John Libbey, London.

Ferrari, M.D., J. Odink, K.D. Bos et al. (1990). Neuroexcitatory plasma amino acids are elevated in migraine. *Neurology 40:*1582–1586.

Ferrari, M.D., J. Odink, C. Tapparelli et al. (1989b). Serotonin metabolism in migraine. *Neurology 39:*1239–1242.

Fog-Møller, F., I.K. Genefke, and B. Bryndum (1978). Changes in concentration of catecholamines in blood during spontaneous migraine attacks and reserpine-induced attacks. In *Current Concepts in Migraine Research* (R. Greene, ed.), pp. 115–119. Raven Press, New York.

Foote, S.L., F.E. Bloom, and G. Aston-Jones (1983). Nucleus locus ceruleus: New evidence of anatomical and physiological specificity. *Physiol. Rev. 63:*844–914.

Fox, R.H., R. Goldsmith, D.J. Kidd, and G.P. Lewis (1961). Bradykinin as a vasodilator in man. *J. Physiol. (Lond.) 157:*589–602.

Fozard, J.R. (1982). Serotonin, migraine and platelets. In *Progress in Pharmacology* (P.A. Van Zwieten and E. Schonbaum, eds.), pp. 135–146. Gustav Fischer Verlag, Stuttgart.

French, E.B., B.W. Lassers, and M.G. Desai (1967). Reflex vasomotor responses in the hands of migrainous subjects. *J. Neurol. Neurosurg. Psychiatry 30:*276–278.

Friberg, L., J. Olesen, H.K. Iversen, and R. Sperling (1991). Migraine pain associated with middle cerebral artery dilatation: Reversal by sumatriptan. *Lancet 338:* 13–17.

Friberg, L., T.S. Olsen, P.E. Roland, and N.A. Lassen (1987). Focal ischaemia caused by instability of cerebrovascular tone during attacks of hemiplegic migraine. A regional cerebral blood flow study. *Brain 110:*917–934.

Gawel, M., M. Burkitt, and F. Clifford Rose (1979). The platelet release reaction during migraine attacks. *Headache 19:*323–327.

Gawel, M., J.F. Connolly, and F. Clifford Rose (1983). Migraine patients exhibit abnormalities in the visual evoked potential. *Headache 23:*49–52.

Géraud, G., M. Bessou, N. Fabre et al. (1989). Heterogeneous cerebral blood flow during spontaneous attacks of migraine with and without aura: A 99m Tc-HMPAO SPECT study. *Cephalalgia 9*(Suppl. 10):31–32.

Gloor, P. (1986). Migraine and regional cerebral blood flow. *Trends Neurosci. 2:*21.

Glover, V., R. Peatfield, R. Zammit-Pace et al. (1981). Platelet monoamine oxidase activity and headache. *J. Neurol. Neurosurg. Psychiatry 44:*786–790.

Glover, W.E., P.R. Carroll, and N. Latt (1973). Histamine receptors in human temporal and rabbit ear arteries. In *International Symposium on Histamine H2 Receptor Antagonists,* pp. 169–174. Smith Kline and French, Welwyn Garden City, NJ.

Goadsby, P.J. (1985). Brainstem activation of the adrenal medulla in the cat. *Brain Res. 327:*241–249.

Goadsby, P.J. and J.W. Duckworth (1987). The effect of stimulation of the trigeminal ganglion on regional cerebral blood flow in the cat. *Am. J. Physiol. 253:* R270–R274.

Goadsby, P.J., L. Edvinsson, and R. Ekman (1988). Release of vasoactive peptides in the extracerebral circulation of man and the cat during activation of the trigemino-vascular system. *Ann. Neurol. 23:*193–196.

Goadsby, P.J., L. Edvinsson, and R. Ekman (1990). Vasoactive peptide release in the extracerebral circulation of humans during migraine headache. *Ann. Neurol. 28:* 183–187.

Goadsby, P.J., G.A. Lambert, and J.W. Lance (1982). Differential effects on the internal and external carotid circulation of the monkey evoked by locus coeruleus stimulation. *Brain Res. 249:*247–254.

Goadsby, P.J. and J.W. Lance (1988). Brain stem effects of intra- and extracerebral circulations. Relations to migraine and cluster headache. In *Basic Mechanisms of Headache* (J. Olesen and L. Edvinsson, eds.) pp. 413–427. Elsevier, Amsterdam.

Goadsby, P.J. and G.J. Macdonald (1985). Extracranial vasodilatation mediated by intestinal polypeptide (VIP). *Brain Res. 329:*285–288.

Goadsby, P.J., R.D. Piper, G.A. Lambert, and J.W. Lance (1985a). The effect of activation of the nucleus raphe dorsalis (DRN) on carotid blood flow. I The monkey. *Am. J. Physiol. 248:*257–262.

Goadsby, P.J., R.D. Piper, G.A. Lambert, and J.W. Lance (1985b). The effect of activation of the nucleus raphe dorsalis (DRN) on carotid blood flow. II The cat. *Am. J. Physiol. 248:*263–269.

Goadsby, P.J. and S. Shelley (1990). High-frequency stimulation of the facial nerve results in local cortical release of vasoactive intestinal polypeptide in the anesthetised cat. *Neurosci. Lett. 112:*282–289.

Goadsby, P.J. and A.S. Zagami (1991). Stimulation of the superior sagittal sinsus increases metabolic activity and blood flow in certain regions of the brainstem and upper cervical spinal cord of the cat. *Brain 114:*1001–1011.

Gotoh, F., T. Kanda, F. Sakai et al. (1976). Serum dopamine B-hydroxylase in migraine. *Arch. Neurol. 33:*656–657.

Gotoh, F., S. Komatsumoto, N. Araki, and S. Gomi (1984). Noradrenergic nervous activity in migraine. *Arch. Neurol. 41:*951–955.

Goudswaard, P., J. Passchier, and A. van Boxtel (1985). Physiological reactions of migraine patients on real-life stress. *Cephalalgia 5*(Suppl. 3):30–31.

Gowers, W. (1893). *Diseases of the Nervous System,* Vol. 2, pp. 836–866. P. Blakiston, Philadelphia.

Graham, J.R. and H.G. Wolff (1938). Mechanism of migraine headache and action of ergotamine tartrate. *Arch. Neurol. Psychiatry 39:*737–763.

Griffith, S.G., J. Lincoln, and G. Burnstock (1982). Serotonin as a neurotransmitter in cerebral arteries. *Brain Res. 247:*388–392.

Hachinski, V.C., J.W. Norris, P.W. Cooper, and J.G. Edmeads (1978). Migraine and the cerebral circulation. In *Current Concepts in Migraine Research* (R. Greene, ed.), pp. 11–15. Raven Press, New York.

Hamada, J., F. Gotoh, Y. Ishikawa et al. (1985). Autonomic nervous function in migraine—quantitative determination of perspiration and retinal vasomotor activity. *Cephalalgia 5*(Suppl. 3):460–461.

Hanin, B., M.-G. Bousser, J. Olesen et al. (1985). Platelet aggregation study in migraine patients between and during attacks. *Cephalalgia 5*(Suppl. 3):398–399.

Hardebo, J.E., N. Suzuki, and R. Ekman (1989). Morphological and functional substrates for neurogenic inflammation in the human internal carotid artery. Implications for cluster headache. *Cephalalgia 9*(Suppl. 10):17–18.

Hartman, B.K., L.W. Swanson, M.E. Raichle et al. (1980). Central adrenergic regulation of cerebral microvascular permeability and blood flow, anatomic and physiologic evidence. *Adv. Exp. Med. Biol. 131*:113–126.

Henry, P.Y., J. Vernhiet, J.M. Orgogozo, and J.M. Caille (1978). Cerebral blood flow in migraine and cluster headache. *Res. Clin. Stud. Headache 6*:81–88.

Herberg, L.J. (1975). The hypothalamus and aminergic pathways in migraine. In *Modern Topics in Migraine* (J. Pearce, ed.), pp. 85–95. Heinemann, London.

Hockaday, J.M., A.L. Macmillan, and C.W.M. Whitty (1967). Vasomotor reflex response in idiopathic and hormone-dependent migraine. *Lancet 1*:1023–1028.

Hockaday, J.M., D.H. Williamson, and C.W.M. Whitty (1971). Blood glucose levels and fatty acid metabolism in migraine related to fasting. *Lancet 1*:1153–1156.

Hsu, L.K.G., A.H. Crisp, R.S. Kalucy et al. (1978). Nocturnal plasma levels of catecholamines, tryptophan, glucose and free fatty acids and the sleeping electroencephalograms of subjects experiencing early morning migraine. In *Current Concepts in Migraine Research* (R. Greene, ed.), pp. 121–130. Raven Press, New York.

Humphrey, P.P.A. and W. Feniuk (1987). Pharmacological characterization of functional neuronal receptors for 5-hydroxytryptamine. In *Neuronal Messengers in Vascular Function* (A. Nobin, C. Owman, and B. Arneklo-Nobin, eds.). pp. 3–19. Elsevier, Amsterdam.

Iversen, H.K., T.H. Nielsen, J. Olesen et al. (1990). Arterial responses during migraine headache. *Lancet 336*:837–839.

Jensen, K. (1987). Subcutaneous blood flow in the temporal region of migraine patients. *Acta Neurol. Scand. 75*:310–318.

Jensen, K. and J. Olesen (1985). Temporal muscle blood flow in common migraine. *Acta Neurol. Scand. 72*:561–570.

Jensen, J., U. Pedersen-Bjergaard, C. Tuxen et al. (1985). Nociception and pressure-pain threshold in the temporal muscle following local injection of bradykinin and serotonin. *Cephalalgia 5*(Suppl. 3):24–25.

Jerzmanowski, A. and A. Klimek (1983). Immunoglobulins and complement in migraine. *Cephalalgia 3*:119–123.

Kalendovsky, Z. and J.H. Austin (1975). Complicated migraine: Its association with increased platelet aggregability and abnormal plasma coagulation factors. *Headache 15*:18–35.

Kerr, F.W.L. (1961a). A mechanism to account for frontal headache in case of posterior fossa tumours. *J. Neurosurg. 18*:605–609.

Kerr, F.W.L. (1961b). Trigeminal and cervical volleys. *Arch. Neurol. 5*:171–178.

Kimball, R.W., A.P. Friedman, and E. Vallejo (1960). Effect of serotonin in migraine patients. *Neurology (Minneap.) 10*:107–111.

Knapp, R.D. Jr. (1963). Reports from the past 2. *Headache 3*:112–122.

Kobari, M., J.S. Meyer, M. Ichijo et al. (1989). Hyperperfusion of cerebral cortex, thalamus and basal ganglia during spontaneously occurring migraine headaches. *Headache 29*:282–289.

Kohlenberg, R.J. (1982). Tyramine sensitivity in dietary migraine: A critical review. *Headache 22*:30–34.

Krabbe, A.A. and J. Olesen (1980). Headache provocation by continuous intravenous infusion of histamine. Clinical results and receptor mechanisms. *Pain 8*:253–259.

Kruglak, L., I. Nathan, A.D. Korczyn et al. (1984). Platelet aggregability, disaggregability and serotonin uptake in migraine. *Cephalalgia 4*:221–225.

Lambert, G.A., N. Bogduk, J.W. Duckworth, and J.W. Lance (1979). Trigeminal correlates of craniovascular sensation. *Proc. Aust. Physiol. Pharmacol. Soc. 10*:231P.

Lambert, G.A., J.W. Duckworth, N. Bogduk, and J.W. Lance (1984a). Low pharmacological responsiveness of the vertebro-basilar circulation in *Macaca nemestrina* monkeys. *Eur. J. Pharmacol. 102:*451–458.

Lambert, G.A., N. Bogduk, P.J. Goadsby et al. (1984b). Decreased carotid arterial resistance in cats in response to trigeminal stimulation. *J. Neurosurg. 61:*307–315.

Lambert, G.A., A.S. Zagami, N. Bogduk et al. (1991). Cervical spinal cord neurones receiving sensory input from the cranial vasculature. *Cephalalgia 11:*75–85.

Lance, J.W. and M. Anthony (1966). Some clinical aspects of migraine: A prospective survey of 500 patients. *Arch. Neurol. 15:*356–361.

Lance, J.W., M. Anthony, and A. Gonski (1967). Serotonin, the carotid body and cranial vessels in migraine. *Arch. Neurol. 16:*553–558.

Lance, J.W., G.A. Lambert, P.J. Goadsby, and J.W. Duckworth (1983). Brain stem influences on the cephalic circulation: Experimental data from cat and monkey of relevance to the mechanism of migraine. *Headache 23:*257–265.

Lashley, K.S. (1941). Patterns of cerebral integration indicated by the scotomas of migraine. *Arch. Neurol. Psychiatry 46:*331–339.

Lauritzen, M. (1984). Long-lasting reduction of cortical blood flow of the brain after spreading depression with preserved autoregulation and impaired CO_2 response. *J. Cereb. Blood Flow Metab. 4:*546–554.

Lauritzen, M., M.B. Jørgensen, N.H. Diemer et al. (1982). Persistent oligemia of rat cerebral cortex in the wake of spreading depression. *Ann. Neurol. 12:*469–474.

Lauritzen, M. and J. Olesen (1984). Regional cerebral blood flow during migraine by Xenon-133 inhalation and emission tomography. *Brain 107:*447–461.

Lauritzen, M., T. Skyhøj Olesen, N.A. Lassen, and O.B. Paulson (1983a). Changes in regional cerebral blood flow during the course of classical migraine attacks. *Ann. Neurol. 13:*633–641.

Lauritzen, M., T. Skyhøj Olsen, N.A. Lassen, and O.B. Paulson (1983b). Regulation of regional cerebral blood flow during and between migraine attacks. *Ann. Neurol. 14:*569–572.

Leão, A.A.P. (1944). Spreading depression of activity in the cerebral cortex. *J. Neurophysiol. 7:*359–390.

Liveing, E. (1873). *On Megrim, Sick-Headache, and Some Allied Disorders: A Contribution to the Pathology of Nerve-Storms.* J. and A. Churchill, London.

Lord, G.D.A. and J.W. Duckworth (1977). Immunoglobulin and complement studies in migraine. *Headache 17:*163–168.

Lord, G.D.A. and J.W. Duckworth (1978). Complement and immune complex studies in migraine. *Headache 18:*255–260.

Lord, G.D.A., E.J. Mylecharane, J.W. Duckworth, and J.W. Lance (1981). Effects of histamine H1- and H2-receptor antagonists in the cranial circulation of the monkey. *Clin. Exp. Pharmacol. Physiol. 8:*89–100.

Lous, I. and J. Olsen (1982). Evaluation of pericranial tenderness and oral function in patients with common migraine, muscle contraction headache and 'combination headache.' *Pain 12:*385–393.

Maertens de Noordhout, A., M. Timsit-Berthier, and J. Schoenen (1985). Contingent negative variation (CNV) in migraineurs before and during prophylactic treatment with beta-blockers. *Cephalalgia 5*(Suppl. 3):34–35.

Montagna, P., T. Sacquegna, P. Martinelli et al. (1988). Mitochondrial abnormalities in migraine. Preliminary findings. *Headache 28:*477–480.

Moore, R.Y., A.E. Halaris, and B.A. Jones (1978). Serotonin neurons of the midbrain raphe: Ascending projections. *J. Comp. Neurol. 180:*417–437.

Moore, T.L., R.E. Ryan Jr., D.A. Pohl et al. (1980). Immunoglobulin, complement and immune complex levels during a migraine attack. *Headache 20:*9–12.

Morrison, J.H., S.L. Foote, M.E. Molliver et al. (1982). Noradrenergic and serotonergic fibers innervate complementary layers in monkey primary cortex: An immunohistochemical study. *Proc. Natl. Acad. Sci U.S.A. 79:*2401–2405.

Moskowitz, M.A. (1984). The neurobiology of vascular head pain. *Ann. Neurol. 16:* 157–168.

Mosnaim, A.D., J. Chevesich, M.E. Wolf et al. (1986). Plasma methionine enkephalin. Increased levels during a migraine episode. *Headache 26:*278–281.

Mück-Sěler, D., Ž. Deanović, and M. Dupelj (1979). Platelet serotonin (5-HT) and 5-HT releasing factor in plasma of migrainous patients. *Headache 19:*14–17.

Nappi, G., F. Facchinetti, E. Martignoni et al. (1985). Plasma and CSF endorphin levels in primary and symptomatic headaches. *Headache 25:*141–144.

Nattero, G., D. Bisbocci, and F. Ceresa (1979). Sex hormones, prolactin levels, osmolarity and electrolyte patterns in menstrual migraine—relationship with fluid retention. *Headache 19:*25–30.

Nattero, G., J.S. Franzone, L. Savi, and R. Cirillo (1984). Serum prostaglandin-like substances in cluster headache and common migraine. In *Progress in Migraine Research 2* (F. Clifford Rose, ed.), pp. 199–204. Pitman, London.

Norris, J.W., V.C. Hachinski, and P.W. Cooper (1975). Changes in cerebral blood flow during a migraine attack. *BMJ 3:*676–677.

O'Brien, M.D. (1971). Cerebral blood changes in migraine. *Headache 10:*139–143.

Olesen, J., L. Friberg, T. Skyhøj Olsen et al. (1990). Timing and topography of cerebral flow, aura and headache during migraine attacks. *Ann. Neurol. 28:*791–798.

Olesen, J., B. Larsen, and M. Lauritzen (1981a). Focal hyperemia followed by spreading oligemia and impaired activation of rCBF in classical migraine. *Ann. Neurol. 9:* 344–352.

Olesen, J., P. Tfelt-Hansen, L. Henricksen, and B. Larsen (1981b). The common migraine attack may not be initiated by cerebral ischaemia. *Lancet 2:*438–440.

Parsons, A.A. and E.T. Whalley (1989). Characterization of the 5-hydroxytryptamine receptor which mediates contraction of the human isolated basilar artery. *Cephalalgia 9*(Suppl. 9):47–51.

Pazos, A., A. Probst, and J.M. Palacios (1987a). Serotonin receptors in the human brain—III, Autoradiographic mapping of serotonin-1 receptors. *Neuroscience 21:* 97–122.

Pazos, A., A. Probst, and J.M. Palacios (1987b). Serotonin receptors in the human brain—IV. Autoradiographic mapping of serotonin-2 receptors. *Neuroscience 21:* 123–139.

Peatfield, R.C., M.J. Gawel, and F. Clifford Rose (1981a). Asymmetry of the aura and pain in migraine. *J. Neurol. Neurosurg. Psychiatry 44:*846–848.

Peatfield, R.C., M.J. Gawel, and F. Clifford Rose (1981b). The effect of infused prostacyclin in migraine and cluster headache. *Headache 21:*190–195.

Piper, R.D. and J.W. Duckworth (1989). Changes in cerebral blood flow associated with the spreading depression of Leão in the cat. *Cephalalgia 9*(Suppl. 10):298–299.

Pratt, J.M. (1985). Stress-induced superficial temporal artery flow differences between migraine and muscle-contraction headache groups. *Cephalalgia 5*(Suppl. 3):488.

Rao, N.S. and J. Pearce (1971). Hypothalamic-pituitary-adrenal axis studies in migraine with special reference to insulin sensitivity. *Brain 94:*289–298.

Raskin, N.H., Y. Hosobuchi, and S. Lamb (1987). Headache may arise from perturbation of the brain. *Headache 27:*416–420.

Raskin, N.H. and S.C. Knittle (1976). Ice cream headache and orthostatic symptoms in patients with migraine headache. *Headache 16:*222–225.

Raskin, N.H. and R.K. Schwartz (1980). Ice-pick-like pain. *Neurology 30:*203–205.

Ray, B.S. and H.G. Wolff (1940). Experimental studies on headache. Pain sensitive structures of the head and their significance in headache. *Arch. Surg. 41:*813–856.

Reinhard, J.F., Jr., J.E. Liebmann, A.J. Schlosberg, and M.A. Moskowitz (1979). Serotonin neurons project to small blood vessels in the brain. *Science 206:*85–87.

Sachs, H., J. Russell, D. Christmas, and A. Wolf (1985). Positron emission tomographic studies on induced migraine. *Cephalalgia 5*(Suppl. 3):456–457.

Saito, K., S. Markowitz, and M.A. Moskowitz (1988). Ergot alkaloids block neurogenic extravasation in dura mater. Proposed action in vascular headaches. *Ann. Neurol. 24:*732–737.

Sakai, F. and J.S. Meyer (1978). Regional cerebral hemodynamics during migraine and cluster headache measured by the 133Xe inhalation method. *Headache 18:* 122–132.

Sakai, F. and J.S. Meyer (1979). Abnormal cerebrovascular reactivity in patients with migraine and cluster headache. *Headache 19:*257–260.

Schoenen, J., A. Maertens de Noordhout, and P.J. Delwaide (1985). Plasma catecholamines in headache patients: Clinical correlations. *Cephalalgia 5*(Suppl. 3):28–29.

Schottstaedt, W.W. and H.G. Wolff (1955). Variations in fluid and electrolyte excretion in association with vascular headache of the migraine type. *Arch. Neurol. Psychiatry 73:*158–164.

Sicuteri, F. (1967). Vasoneuroactive substances and their implication in vascular pain. *Res. Clin. Stud. Headache 1:*6–45.

Sicuteri, F. (1976). Migraine, a central biochemical dysnociception. *Headache 16:* 145–159.

Sicuteri, F. (1977). Dopamine, the second putative protagonist in headache. *Headache 17:*129–131.

Sicuteri, F., M. Boccuni, M. Fanciullacci, and G. Gatto (1983). Naloxone effectiveness on spontaneous and induced perceptive disorders in migraine. *Headache 23:* 179–183.

Sicuteri, F., M. Fanciullacci, and B. Anselmi (1963). Bradykinin release and inactivation in man. *Int. Arch. Allergy 22:*77–84.

Sicuteri, F., G. Franchi, S. Michelacci, and S. Salmon (1962). Aumento della escrezione urinaria dell'acido vanilmandelico, catabolita delle catecolamine durante l'accesso emicranico. *Settim. Med. 50:*13–16.

Sicuteri, F., A. Testi, and B. Anselmi (1961). Biochemical investigations in headache: Increase in hydroxyindoleacetic acid excretion during migraine attacks. *Int. Arch. Allergy 19:*55–58.

Simard, D. and O.B. Paulson (1973). Cerebral vasomotor paralysis during migraine attack. *Arch. Neurol. 29:*207–209.

Sjaastad, O. (1970). Kinin- and histamine-investigations in vascular headache. In *Kliniske Aspekter i Migraeneforskningen,* pp. 61–69. Nordlundes Bogtrykkeri, Copenhagen.

Skarby, T., P. Tfelt-Hansen, F. Gjerris et al. (1982). Characterization of 5-hydroxytryptamine receptors in human temporal arteries: Comparison between migraine sufferers and non-sufferers. *Ann. Neurol. 12:*272–277.

Skinhøj, E. (1973). Hemodynamic studies within the brain during migraine. *Arch. Neurol. 29:*95–98.

Skyhøj Olsen, T., M. Lauritzen, and N.A. Lassen (1984). Focal ischemia during migraine attacks in patients with classical and complicated migraine. *Acta Neurol. Scand. Suppl. 98:*258–259.

Sleight, A.J., A. Cervenka, and S.K. Peroutka (1990). In vivo effects of sumatriptan (GR43175) on extracellular levels of 5-HT in the guinea pig. *Neuropharmacology 29:*511–513.

Somerville, B.W. (1972). The role of oestradiol withdrawal in the etiology of menstrual migraine. *Neurology (Minneap.) 22:*355–365.

Spira, P.J., E.J. Mylecharane, and J.W. Lance (1976). The effect of humoral agents and antimigraine drugs on the cranial circulation of the monkey. *Res. Clin. Stud. Headache 4:*37–75.

Sramka, M., G. Brozek, J. Bures, and P. Nadvornik (1977–78). Functional ablation by spreading depression: Possible use in human stereotactic neurosurgery. *Appl. Neurophysiol. 40:*48–61.

Strassman, A., P. Mason, M. Moskowitz, and R. Macievicz (1986). Response of brainstem trigeminal neurons to electrical stimulation of the dura. *Brain Res. 379:* 242–250.

Tfelt-Hansen, P., I. Lous, and J. Olesen (1981). Prevalence and significance of muscle tenderness during common migraine attacks. *Headache 21:*49–54.

Tunis, M.M. and H.G. Wolff (1953). Long term observations of the reactivity of the cranial arteries in subjects with vascular headache of the migraine type. *Arch. Neurol. Psychiatry 70:*551–557.

Vardi, J., S. Flechter, D. Ayalon et al. (1981). L-dopa effect on prolactin plasma levels in complicated and common migrainous patients. *Headache 21:*14–20.

Waeber, C., D. Hoyer, and J.M. Palacios (1989). 5-hydroxytryptamine3 receptors in the human brain: Autoradiographic visualization using (3H) ICS 205-930. *Neuroscience 31:*393–400.

Walters, D.W., S.A. Gillespie, and M. Moskowitz (1986). Cerebrovascular projections from the sphenopalatine and otic ganglia to the middle cerebral artery of the cat. *Stroke 17:*488–494.

Welch, K.M.A., S. Nagel-Leiby, and G. D'Andrea (1988). The biological and behavioral basis of migraine. In *Basic Mechanisms of Headache* (J. Olesen and L. Edvinsson, eds.), pp. 447–456. Elsevier, Amsterdam.

Welch, K.M.A., N.M. Ramadan, H. Halvorson et al. (1989). Low brain magnesium in migraine. *Cephalalgia 9*(Suppl. 10):51–52.

Wolff, H.G. (1963). *Headache and Other Head Pain.* Oxford University Press, New York.

Yamamoto, M., and J.S. Meyer (1980). Hemicranial disorder of vasomotor adrenoceptors in migraine and cluster headache. *Headache 20:*321–335.

Zagami, A.S., P.J. Goadsby, and L. Edvinsson (1990). Stimulation of the superior sagittal sinus in the cat causes release of vasoactive peptides. *Neuropeptides 16:*69–75.

Zagami, A.S. and G.A. Lambert (1990). Stimulation of cranial vessels excites nociceptive neurones in several thalamic nuclei of the cat. *Exp. Brain Res. 81:*552–566.

Zagami, A.S., G.A. Lambert, and J.W. Lance (1987). Studies in the cat on the pathway for vascular head pain. *Cephalalgia 7*(Suppl. 6):7–9.

Ziegler, D.K., R.S. Hassanein, A. Kodanez, and J.C. Meek (1979). Circadian rhythms of plasma cortisol in migraine. *J. Neurol. Neurosurg. Psychiatry 42:*741–748.

5

Migraine: Diagnosis and Treatment

STEPHEN D. SILBERSTEIN
JOEL R. SAPER

Migraine, an episodic headache disorder often accompanied by neurologic, gastrointestinal, and psychological changes, occurs in at least 19% of women, 10% of men, and 4% of children. The term "migraine" is derived from the Greek word *hemicrania,* introduced by Galen in approximately 200 A.D. (McHenry, 1969).

Most migraine descriptions stress what Waters (1986) refers to as the three features of migraine: the unilateral distribution of the headache, the presence of a warning (often visual), and nausea or vomiting. The Ad Hoc Committee on Classification of Headache (Friedman et al., 1962) described vascular headache of migraine type as:

> Recurrent attacks of headache, widely varied in intensity, frequency, and duration. The attacks are commonly unilateral in onset; are usually associated with anorexia and sometimes with nausea and vomiting; in some are preceded by, or associated with, conspicuous sensory, motor, and mood disturbances; and are often familial. (p. 14)

The new international classification of headache attempts to impart greater precision to the definition of migraine. Migraine headaches were formerly divided into two varieties: classic and common (Silberstein, 1984). Now common migraine is called "migraine without aura" (1.1) and classic migraine is called "migraine with aura" (1.2), the aura being the complex of focal neurologic symptoms that initiates or accompanies an attack. (Headache Classification Committee of the International Headache Society, 1988). At most only 30% of migraine headaches are "classic" (Ziegler and Hassanein, 1990). The same patient may have headache without aura, headache with aura, and aura without headache. To establish a diagnosis of migraine under the International Headache Society (IHS) classification, certain attributes must be present and organic disease must be excluded.

Migraine without aura (1.1) is the new IHS term for common migraine. To establish a diagnosis, five attacks are needed, each lasting 4 to 72 hours and having two of the following four characteristics: unilateral location, pulsating quality, moderate to severe intensity, and aggravation by routine physical activity. In addition, the attacks must have at least one of the following: nausea and/or vomiting and/or photophobia and phonophobia.

To make a diagnosis of *migraine with aura* (1.2), the new term for classic migraine, at least two attacks with any three of four features are required: one or more fully reversible aura symptoms; aura developing over more than 4 minutes; aura lasting less than 60 minutes; and headache following aura with a free interval of less than 60 minutes.

Migraine with aura is subdivided into migraine with typical aura (1.2.1) (homonymous visual disturbance, unilateral numbness or weakness, or aphasia); migraine with prolonged aura (1.2.2) (aura lasting more than 60 minutes); familial hemiplegic migraine (1.2.3); basilar migraine (1.2.4); migraine aura without headache (1.2.5); and migraine with acute-onset aura (1.2.6). Other varieties of migraine include ophthalmoplegic (1.3), retinal (1.4), and childhood periodic syndromes (1.5).

Complications of migraine (1.6) include status migrainosus (1.6.1) (an attack of headache or aura lasting more than 72 hours) and migrainous infarction (1.6.2) (a neurologic defect not reversible in 7 days).

Some have suggested that, whereas the old ad hoc criteria were not sufficiently specific, the new IHS criteria are too complex and cumbersome (Rapoport, 1992; Solomon and Lipton, 1991). Solomon and Lipton (1991) have proposed a simple set of criteria for diagnosing migraine without aura requiring the presence of any two of four symptoms (unilateral headache, pulsating quality, nausea, and photophobia and phonophobia). A similar headache must have occurred in the past and organic disease must be excluded. These criteria are sensitive and specific in differentiating migraine without aura from chronic daily headache. They were not tested against episodic tension-type headache, which is the most difficult type of headache to differentiate from migraine and which some believe may be related to migraine (Zeigler, 1985). In particular, these criteria did not include aggravation of pain by routine physical activity, which Iverson et al. (1990) found extremely useful in separating migraine from tension-type headache. Iverson's group thought that the intensity of pain helped separate migraine (moderate to severe pain) from tension-type (mild to moderate pain) headache. Their criteria were both sensitive and specific, but they believe that the criteria could be improved with regard to quantifying the accompanying symptoms.

CLINICAL FEATURES OF MIGRAINE (TABLE 5–1)

Most patients develop migraine in the first three decades of life; some develop it in the fourth, and even the fifth decade.

Blau (1980) has divided the migraine attack into five phases: the prodrome, which occurs hours or days before the headache; the aura, which immediately precedes the headache; the headache itself; the headache termination; and the postdrome phase. Migraine without aura consists of the headache, its termina-

Table 5–1   Characteristics of migraine

	Adult series		Juvenile series	
	Oleson (1978)	Selby & Lance (1960)	Congdon & Forsyth (1979)	Barlow (1984)
Number of patients	750	500	300	300
Family history		55%	88%	89.7%
Headache				
Throbbing quality	47%			66%
Hemicranial distribution	56%	67%	31%	22%
Nausea and/or vomiting	86%	87%	94%	62%
Photophobia/phonophobia	49%	82%		*a*
Aura				
Visual (teichopsia, scotomata)	20%	36%	16%	5%
Numbness (face, hands)		33%	2%	0.5%

a Common.

tion, and the postdrome. Migraine with aura consists of the aura, the headache, its termination, and the postdrome. Both may have associated prodromes.

Prodrome

Premonitory phenomena can occur hours to days before the headache and consist of mental, neurologic, or general (constitutional, autonomic) symptoms. Mental symptoms include depression, euphoria, irritability, restlessness, mental slowness, hyperactivity, fatigue, and drowsiness. Neurologic phenomena include photophobia, phonophobia, and hyperosmia, among others. General prodromal symptoms include a stiff neck, a cold feeling, sluggishness, increased thirst, increased urination, anorexia, diarrhea, constipation, fluid retention, and food cravings.

Two types of migraine prodromes are described: nonevolutive, which precede the attack by up to 48 hours; and evolutive, which start approximately 6 hours before the attack, gradually increasing in intensity and culminating in the attack. A dopaminergic mechanism has been suggested (Amery et al., 1986a,b). The presence of a prodrome is common—Blau (1980) found it in 28 of 50 migraineurs, and Isler (1986) found it in 65 of 100 migraineurs with equal frequency in migraine with or without aura.

Aura

The migraine aura is a complex of focal neurologic symptoms that precedes or accompanies an attack. Most aura symptoms develop over 5 to 20 minutes and usually last less than 60 minutes (Headache Classification Committee of the IHS, 1988). The aura can be characterized by visual, sensory, or motor phenomena, and may also involve language or brainstem disturbances.

Headache usually occurs within 60 minutes of the end of the aura if it occurs at all. The IHS criteria are used to distinguish the aura of migraine from a focal seizure or transient ischemic attack (TIA) (Peatfield, 1987). The headache may begin before or simultaneously with the aura, or the aura may occur alone. If the aura is prolonged, it may meet the criteria for what formerly was called complicated or hemiplegic migraine. Patients can have more than one type of aura with a progression from one symptom to another. Most patients with a sensory aura also have a visual aura (Zeigler and Hassanein, 1990).

Visual aura is the most common of the neurologic events and often has a hemianoptic distribution. The aura may consist of photopsia (the sensation of unformed flashes of light before the eyes) or scotoma (partial loss of sight) (Hachinski et al., 1973; Hupp et al., 1985; Lance and Anthony, 1966; Wilkinson, 1986).

The most characteristic visual aura, almost diagnostic of migraine, is the fortification spectrum or *teichopsia* (Greek; "town wall" and "vision") (Selby and Lance, 1960; Wilkinson, 1986). Ten percent of Selby and Lance's (1960) patients reported teichopsia. The patient may first notice a geometric unformed scotoma, usually, but not always, beginning near the point of fixation, that spreads outward or migrates across the visual field with a scintillating edge of often zigzag, flashing, or occasionally colored phenomena.

Visual distortions and hallucinations, speculated to represent Lewis Carroll's descriptions in *Alice in Wonderland,* can occur. These attacks occur more commonly in children, are usually followed by a headache, and are characterized by (Hosking, 1988; Sacks, 1985):

1. Complex disorder of visual perception (metamorphopsia, micropsia, macropsia, zoom or mosaic vision)
2. Complex difficulties in the perception and use of the body (apraxia and agnosia)
3. Speech and language disturbances
4. States of double or multiple consciousness associated with déjà vu or jamais vu
5. Elaborate dreamy, nightmarish, trancelike, or delirious states

Sensory phenomena (Jensen et al., 1986; Friedman et al., 1962) are characterized by paresthesias that frequently begin in the hand, migrate anatomically to the elbow, arm, and neck and then often to the tongue and lips (cheiro-oral migraine).

Motor disturbance and aphasia. A transient focal fatigue or true monoparesis or hemiparesis may be part of the aura of migraine (Jensen et al., 1986; Selby and Lance, 1960). Difficulty speaking or understanding language can occasionally occur.

Migraine aura without headache. Periodic neurologic dysfunction, which may be part of the migraine aura, can occur in isolation without the headache (Whitty, 1967). These phenomena (scintillating scotoma; recurrent sensory, motor, and mental phenomena) can only be accepted as migraine after full investigation and prolonged follow-up. Headache occurring in association with the symptoms of aura will help confirm the diagnosis (Silberstein, 1990). Ziegler and Hassanein (1990) reported that 44% of their patients who had headache with aura had aura without headache at some time.

Levy (1988) looked at the incidence of transient (<24 hours) neurologic loss among neurologists at Cornell. Thirty-two percent (25 of 80) had transient central nervous system (CNS) dysfunction, most commonly (15 of 25) visual (field cuts, obscurations, scotomata). Ten of 35 had nonvisual symptoms (hemiparesis, clumsiness, paresthesias, dysarthria). Migraine was reported in 29% (23 of 80). Forty-four percent reporting transient CNS dysfunction (11 of 25) had migraine, whereas 22% (12 of 50) of the nonreporters had migraine. Follow-up for up to 5 years showed that none developed any residual deficit or chronic neurologic disorder, suggesting that these are benign migrainous accompaniments.

Fisher (1980) described late-life migrainous accompaniments, which are transient neurologic phenomena frequently not associated with headache. He has reported on 188 patients over the age of 40; 60% were men and 57% had a history of recurrent headache. They developed an attack or attacks of episodic neurologic dysfunction with variable recurrence (1 attack, 27%; 2 to 10 attacks, 45%; >10 attacks, 28%). The attacks lasted from 1 minute to 72 hours. Fisher considered scintillating scotoma to be diagnostic of migraine even when it occurred in isolation, whereas other episodic neurologic symptoms (paresthesias, aphasia, and sensory and motor symptoms) needed more careful evaluation.

Fisher (1986) believed that transient migrainous accompaniments—scintillating scotomas, numbness, aphasia, dysarthria, and motor weakness—may occur for the first time after the age of 45 and be easily confused with TIAs of cerebrovascular origin. Diagnosis in all but the most classic cases is still by exclusion.

Headache (Table 5–1)

The headache of migraine can occur at any time of the day or night, but occurs most frequently on arising in the morning (Selby and Lance, 1960). The onset is usually gradual; the pain peaks and then subsides, and usually lasts between 4 and 72 hours in adults and 2 and 48 hours in children (Headache Classification Committee of the IHS, 1988). The headache is bilateral in 40% and unilateral in 60% of cases; it consistently occurs on the same side in 20% of patients (Selby and Lance, 1960). Migraineurs with alternating headache do not develop more consistent lateralization of headache with time (Whitty and Hockaday, 1968).

The head pain varies greatly in intensity, ranging from annoying to incapacitating. The pain is usually constant, and often described as tight or bandlike (50%) but, particularly when severe, it will assume a throbbing quality (50%) (Selby and Lance, 1960). During an attack, pain may move from one part of the head to another, and may radiate down the neck into the shoulder. The pain is commonly aggravated by physical activity or simple head movement. Patients prefer to lie down in a dark quiet room. Scalp tenderness occurs in two thirds of patients during or after the headache. This tenderness may involve the head and neck, and prevent the patient from lying on the affected side (Drummond, 1987).

Many migraineurs will have interictal headaches that do not meet the criteria for migraine (Olesen, 1978). These headaches will usually be shorter and less severe and meet the criteria of episodic tension-type headache. Some patients note that their headache begins as a tension-type headache and builds into a "migraine" (Drummond and Lance, 1984; Olesen, 1978). Other patients may have chronic tension-type or chronic daily headache with superimposed bouts of migraine (combination headache) (Graham, 1968; Mathew et al., 1982, 1987; Saper, 1983).

Patients with migraine may also have short-lived jabs of pain, lasting for seconds, occurring between more characteristic migraine attacks. The pain is described as an "icepick," "needle," "nail," "jabs and jolts," or "pinprick" headache, and occurs in about 40% of migraineurs (Raskin and Schwartz, 1980).

Associated Phenomena

The debilitation of migraine may arise more from the accompanying symptoms than from the headache itself. Characteristically the attacks of pain are accompanied by a variety of other symptoms.

Gastrointestinal (Table 5–1)
Anorexia is common, and food craving can occur; nausea is typical; and vomiting is frequent (Olesen, 1978; Selby and Lance, 1960). The associated gastroparesis contributes to gastrointestinal distress and poor absorption of oral medication (Boyle et al., 1990; Saper, 1983; Volans, 1978). Diarrhea occurs in 16% of patients (Selby and Lance, 1960).

Neuropsychological Accompaniments
Many patients will have signs of sensory hyperexcitability manifested by photophobia, phonophobia, and osmophobia, and seek a dark, quiet room (Drummond, 1986; Selby and Lance, 1960). Some will have lightheadedness and vertigo (Kuritzky et al., 1981). The symptoms of the prodrome, such as exhilaration, agitation, fatigue, lethargy, disorientation, hypomania, anger, rage, or depression, can continue into the headache. Constitutional, mood, and mental changes are almost universal.

Other Symptoms
Fluid retention can occur hours to days before the headache. Frank edema can occur just before the attack, and polyuria occurs during and after the headache, with resolution of the fluid retention (Dalessio, 1980). Patients (10 to 20%) may have nasal stuffiness during a migraine attack, followed in some by profuse nasal secretion as the attack terminates (Raskin, 1988).

Postdrome
Following the headache, the patient may feel tired, washed out, irritable, and listless or have impaired concentration. Muscle weakness and aching, and anorexia or food cravings can occur (Blau, 1982).

MIGRAINE VARIANTS

Basilar Migraine

Basilar migraine was originally called "basilar artery migraine" (Headache Classification Committee of the IHS, 1988) or "Bickerstaff's migraine" (Bickerstaff, 1987). Initially, Bickerstaff thought this was mainly a disorder of adolescent girls, but it affects all age groups and both sexes, with the usual migraine female predominance.

The aura generally lasts less than 1 hour and is usually followed by a headache. The visual aura frequently begins with a hemianoptic field disturbance, but can rapidly involve both visual fields, leading at times to temporary blindness. The visual aura is usually followed by ataxia, dysarthria, vertigo, tinnitus, bilateral paresthesia, nausea or vomiting, and change in level of consciousness and cognition, which, when marked, defines confusional migraine.

Confusional Migraine

Confusional migraine (Headache Classification Committee of the IHS, 1988; Hosking, 1988) occurs more commonly in boys than girls, with an incidence of about 5%. Clinical features include a typical aura, a headache (which may be insignificant), and confusion, which may precede or follow the headache. The confusion is characterized by inattention, distractibility, and difficulty maintaining speech and other motor activities. The electroencephalogram (EEG) may be abnormal during the attack. Agitation, memory disturbances, obscene utterances, and violent behavior are not uncommon. Single attacks are most common, and multiple attacks rare. Both may be triggered by mild head trauma. If the level of consciousness is more profoundly disturbed, *migraine stupor* lasting 2 to 5 days can occur.

The differential diagnosis includes drug ingestion, metabolic encephalopathies (Reye syndrome, hypoglycemia), viral encephalitis, the postictal state, and acute psychosis.

Ophthalmoplegic Migraine

Ophthalmoplegic migraine presents with acute attacks of third nerve palsy associated with a dilated pupil. Rarely the fourth and sixth cranial nerves are involved. The unilateral eye pain is migrainous in quality. The duration of ophthalmoplegia is variable, from hours to months.

The differential diagnosis includes berry aneurysm and chronic sinusitis with a mucocele. However, most cases of ophthalmoplegic migraine fit the criteria for the Tolosa-Hunt syndrome of painful ophthalmoplegia (Hansen et al., 1990): steady, gnawing, boring, eye pain; involvement of nerves of the cavernous sinus; symptoms lasting days or weeks; spontaneous remission, with recurrent attacks occurring after months or years; computerized tomography or magnetic resonance imaging scans demonstrating confinement to the cavernous sinus; and steroid responsiveness.

Hemiplegic Migraine

The Headache Classification Committee of the IHS (1988) has subdivided hemiplegic migraine into sporadic and familial forms, both of which typically begin in childhood and cease with adulthood. Whitty (1986) and Bradshaw and Parsons (1965) believe that this separation is not justified and that both may be part of the same syndrome. Forty-seven percent of Bradshaw and Parsons' (1965) patients had a family history of migraine; 18% had a family history of hemiplegic migraine. The age of onset of hemiplegic migraine may be earlier than that of common migraine, and the attacks themselves are frequently precipitated by minor head injury. Changes in consciousness ranging from confusion to coma are a feature, especially in childhood, and occurred in 23% of Bradshaw and Parsons' series (1965).

The hemiplegia may be part of the aura and last less than 1 hour (migraine with typical aura). However, the headache may precede the hemiparesis or be absent. The onset of the hemiparesis may be abrupt, last for days or weeks, and simulate a stroke (Whitty, 1986). All of Bradshaw and Parsons' (1965) patients had associated paresthesias; 88% had visual auras and 44% had speech disturbances. Weakness lasted less than 1 hour in 58% of patients; however, it lasted 1 to 3 hours in 14%, 3 to 24 hours in 12%, and between 1 day and 1 week in 16% of patients.

The headache can be generalized (29%), contralateral (47%), or ipsilateral (22%) to the hemiparesis. Before assessment, 17% of Bradshaw and Parsons' (1965) patients had had a single neurologic episode, 37% had had between two and six episodes, and the remainder had had more than seven attacks. The longer lasting episodes were associated with more profound weakness and tended to be less frequent in their recurrence.

The prevalence of hemiplegic migraine is uncertain and varies from 4 to 30% (Selby and Lance, 1960; Whitty, 1986). The differential diagnosis of hemiplegic migraine includes focal seizures, stroke, homocystinuria, and MELAS syndrome (mitochondrial myopathy, encephalopathy, lactic acidosis, and strokelike episodes) (Hosking, 1988).

Alternating Hemiplegia of Childhood

Alternating hemiplegia of childhood is a rare disease that begins in infancy and is characterized by sudden, repeated attacks of hemiplegia involving each side alternately, lasting hours to days, and associated with dystonic features. During an attack, the child is acutely uncomfortable and has signs of autonomic disturbance. This is a progressive disorder with onset before 18 months, producing a fixed motor deficit, retardation, and dyskinesias. Fifty percent of patients with alternating hemiplegia have a family history of migraine. In contrast to alternating hemiplegia, hemiplegic migraine is not a progressive disorder and is not associated with dystonia or retardation. Flunarizine in a double-blind controlled study has been shown to be effective in alternating hemiplegia (Casaer, 1989).

MIGRAINE IN CHILDREN

Children frequently have migraine or tension-type headache. Bille (1962) studied the occurrence of headache in 8,993 school children in Uppsala and found that headache prevalence increased from 39% at age 6 to over 70% by age 15. Migraine prevalence (probably underestimated by overstrict criteria), equal in boys and girls, was 3.9%. Goldstein and Chen (1982) reviewed a number of reports of migraine prevalence in children and adults. Migraine prevalence was equal in boys and girls prior to puberty. After puberty, the expected female predominance was observed.

Specific definitions of migraine (Barlow, 1984), as well as the IHS criteria, may be useful for epidemiologic studies but are not as valuable for the diagnosis of the individual child. Bille (1962) required a periodic headache plus two of the following associated symptoms: visual aura, nausea, vomiting, one-sided pain, or familial occurrence. His criteria do not take into account severity, photophobia, sonophobia, and exacerbation by movement, nor exclusion of symptomatic causes, and overrepresent migraine with aura. Hockaday (1988a) has proposed that recurrent paroxysmal headache in childhood should be accepted as migraine provided there is a return to full normal health between attacks and that other causes of headache have been excluded. The details of the distribution and quality of the headache are not always easily obtainable in children and may not be helpful to the diagnosis (Hockaday, 1988a).

Most children's migraine series (Barlow, 1984; Congdon and Forsythe, 1979; Hockaday, 1988a), have shown migraine without aura to be more common than migraine with aura. However, other authors have reported a higher prevalence of migraine with aura (Bille, 1962; Zammarano et al., 1989). Some authors (Hockaday, 1988a; Manzone et al., 1989) comment on the attack being briefer (less than an hour) and more frequent than in adults; others found the attack to last all day in patients seeking medical attention (Symon and Russell, 1989). The migraine headache is usually bilateral in younger children and unilateral in older children (Table 5–1).

Associated Symptoms

All authors agree on the prominence of vegetative symptoms in children's migraine attacks. The most common are the gastrointestinal complaints of nausea and vomiting, occurring in up to 90% of attacks (Barlow, 1984; Congdon and Forsythe, 1979; Sillanpaa, 1983). Nausea may become less frequent in older children. Comparing Barlow's (1984) and Congdon and Forsythe's (1979) series to Selby and Lance's (1960) and Oleson's (1978) series, the incidence of nausea and vomiting is as high in adults as in children (Table 5–1). Other symptoms include diarrhea, increased micturition, sweating, thirst, edema, and lacrimation.

Visual aura is one of several criteria generally used to define migraine. Despite this, there is significant variability in its incidence. Bille (1962), who used the presence of aura as part of his definition, found visual aura in 50% of his cases, Hockaday (1988a) in 9%, and Barlow (1984) in 5%. Wendorff (1989) and Sillanpaa (1983) independently reported on the increased incidence of visual aura in older children.

Differences in Children with Migraine

Migraineurs do not differ from their peers in socioeconomic status or intelligence. The reported tendency (Bille, 1962) to be more serious, tidy, and vulnerable to frustration and anxiety and less self-confident may be a function of the pain they experience (Hockaday, 1988a).

Prognosis

Many children, followed prospectively in open or double-blind drug studies, show a progressive reduction in headache in both the treated and control groups (up to 50%). Several investigators (Congdon and Forsythe, 1979; Hockaday, 1988a) have reported significant long-term migraine remissions. Bille (1989) followed a cohort of children with severe migraine for up to 37 years. As young adults, 62% were migraine free for more than 2 years, but after 30 years only 40% continued to be migraine free. This suggests that migraine is a lifelong disorder.

Childhood Migraine Equivalents

The periodic syndrome, abdominal migraine, and cyclic vomiting are not included under the IHS criteria for migraine (1.5), despite the view that they may be "migraine equivalents."

Periodic Syndrome
The periodic syndrome of Wyllie and Schlesinger (1933) is a combination of one or more of the following symptoms:

1. Cyclic vomiting or repeated bilious attacks
2. Recurrent vague abdominal pain
3. Recurrent headaches
4. Dizzy spells
5. Periodic attacks of fever
6. Periodic attacks of limb and joint pains or stiffness (prevalence alone may be 4.5% "growing pains")

This syndrome most likely includes many cases of juvenile migraine, particularly when headache is present (Barlow, 1984).

Cyclic Vomiting
A common reason for recurrent episodic vomiting may be migraine. Many children and adults with migraine will have a history of cyclic vomiting (40%), and children with cyclic vomiting will frequently develop migraine. A single episode is indistinguishable from an acute gastrointestinal illness. Many patients have been reported to have associated pallor and photophobia (Barlow, 1984; Hockaday, 1988b).

Abdominal Migraine

Paroxysmal abdominal pain occurs in 10% of school-age children. Associated symptoms include pallor (38%), headache (23%), and vomiting (22%) (Hockaday, 1988b). Some studies have shown a relationship of paroxysmal abdominal pain to migraine (Salmon, 1983), but other long-term studies are not as certain. The differential diagnosis includes celiac disease, appendicitis, and temporal lobe seizures. Sorge et al. (1989) found that in 52% of 42 children there was an organic cause of recurrent abdominal pain; lactose intolerance was the most common cause of this syndrome (8 of 22), followed by oxyuriasis (7 of 21). Forty-three percent of the patients had migraine (18 patients). Eleven migraine patients had a functional cause of their abdominal pain (61%), whereas seven (39%) had an organic cause.

Benign Torticollis in Infancy

Benign torticollis in infancy consists of recurrent attacks of head tilt occurring during the first year of life and persisting a few months to several years. There is no specific precipitating factor; attacks occur predominantly in the morning and last hours to a day. Associated symptoms may include irritability, drowsiness, pallor, redness, and signs of dysequilibrium (Deonna, 1988).

Benign Paroxysmal Vertigo of Childhood

Benign paroxysmal vertigo of childhood is characterized by multiple, brief, sporadic episodes of true vertigo occurring in otherwise healthy children. The children stop all activities, appear frightened and refuse to move or stand, and may have nausea and vomiting. This also may be a migraine equivalent of childhood or adolescence. The IHS criteria require a normal neurologic examination and a normal EEG, because recurrent vertigo can be a symptom of epilepsy (tornado epilepsy) (Deonna, 1988).

RELATIONSHIP BETWEEN MIGRAINE AND EPILEPSY

There is no clear epidemiologic evidence that migraine and epilepsy are linked. There is no evidence that frequent, long-lasting, severe, or complicated migraine leads to epilepsy. It is not uncommon for alteration and loss of consciousness to occur during a migraine attack (Deonna, 1988; Hockaday and Newton, 1988).

Many of the abnormal EEGs reported in childhood migraine are now believed to be normal variants (posterior slowing, 14 + 6 phantom spike and wave, psychomotor variant, small sharp spikes). Some EEGs become abnormal at the site of the aura interictally. During an attack of migraine with aura, a slow wave focus can develop (Andermann, 1987).

Some epileptic subjects experience headache as part of their typical attack and at other times may have only headache. Brevity of attack is not a distinguishing feature for a seizure. Visceral symptoms may be seen in both. Continuous EEG monitoring may be required to make the diagnosis.

Ehrenberg (1991) studied the relationship between migraine and epilepsy in the adult seizure clinic at the Tufts New England Medical Center. Twenty percent of 395 patients (79) had migraine, and, of these, 3% (13) had their epileptic seizures during or immediately after a migraine aura. In two patients, the entire sequence from migraine aura through a partial seizure and culminating in a generalized tonic-clonic seizure was recorded. Better seizure control was obtained with "antimigraine" medication in four patients.

TREATMENT OF MIGRAINE

Principles of Care and General Approach

Effective headache treatment depends on making an accurate diagnosis, ruling out alternate etiologies, ordering appropriate studies, and addressing the psychological impact of the headache. Patients with recurrent headache often believe that their complaints have not been taken seriously. They are often worried that they have a life-threatening condition such as a brain tumor or an aneurysm. Just as they want headache relief, patients want to know what is wrong with them (Packard, 1979) and to be assured that the physician is committed to relieving their distress.

Once a diagnosis of migraine has been made, it is important to reassure the patient and relieve the anxiety that frequently plagues headache sufferers. Patients are relieved to find out that their headache is neither secondary to an organic disorder nor merely psychogenic. It is good practice to educate the patient about his or her disorder with a detailed description of suspected mechanisms of headache and common precipitating factors. Contributing psychological factors should be pursued.

Once the proper relationship between the physician and the patient (and family) is established, the factors that contribute to the pain and to its relief should be addressed (Saper, 1989). Current theory on pathogenesis suggests that central or peripheral mechanisms are incited by internal or external stimuli. Effective control, therefore, requires reduction or modification of activating factors and of central or peripheral instability, and educational intervention to redirect the patient's activities.

A headache calendar can be a useful tool in accurately establishing the actual frequency, intensity, and duration of headache and the presence of associated symptoms such as aura or nausea and vomiting. Provoking factors, such as menses, missed meals, or too little sleep, can be identified. Once a treatment program has been prescribed, the calendar can be used to show the effectiveness of both symptomatic and preventive treatment (Dalessio, 1987).

Wilkinson (1988b) has suggested that headache treatment consists of: (1) prevention of attacks by avoidance of triggers; (2) the use of nonpharmacologic treatments such as relaxation, biofeedback, and acupuncture; (3) the treatment of the acute attack; and (4) long-term prophylactic therapy. To this we strongly advise adding periodic reassessment and reconsideration of the treatment plan.

Avoidance of Provoking/Activating Factors (Triggers)

Migraine patients are afflicted by a disorder that renders them physiologically and perhaps psychologically hyperresponsive to a variety of internal and external stimuli, including hormonal changes, dietary factors, environmental changes, sensory stimuli, and stress (Saper, 1983; Silberstein and Silberstein, 1990). Too much or too little sleep, missed or delayed meals, menstruation, alcohol, certain foods and food additives, light glare, and odors have all been reported to provoke or activate migraine in susceptible individuals. Provoking factors do not always trigger an attack of migraine; this may reflect chronobiologic changes in sensitivity to provocation.

Migraine is frequently provoked by environmental, psychological, and neuroendocrine perturbations. The prodromes of migraine (chocolate craving, anxiety, exhilaration, or depression) can be mistaken for migraine triggers.

Van den Bergh et al. (1987) collected information on provoking factors in 217 migraineurs. Most patients (85%) were spontaneously aware of one or more factors. The main reported activating factors were specific foods (44.7%), menstruation (49%), alcoholic beverages (51.0%), and stress (48.8%).

Diet

A good deal of controversy exists about the role food allergy plays in migraine. The most common cause of what patients commonly call "food allergy" is food aversion—a psychological response to the food itself (Bix et al., 1984).

Most food reactions are chemically mediated—for example, lactose intolerance (Bayless et al., 1975); nitrites ("hot dog headache") (Raskin, 1981); monosodium glutamate, which is believed to be responsible for the "Chinese restaurant syndrome" (Schaumberg et al., 1969); and perhaps aspartame (Koehler and Glaros, 1988; Schiffman et al., 1987), red wine (Littlewood et al., 1988), and alcohol (Raskin, 1981). Chocolate is probably not a migraine-provoking factor (Moffett et al., 1974).

The use of elimination diets and clinical ecology is controversial (Egger et al., 1983; Ferguson, 1990; Jewett et al., 1990; MacDonald et al., 1989). It is our belief that most patients with headache do not require severely restricted diets, but they should avoid foods or additives that they believe might have a provocative effect on their headaches. Migraineurs should avoid alcohol, particularly red wine, large amounts of monosodium glutamate, and perhaps cured meats (nitrites). They should not skip meals or overindulge in sugar. The value of avoiding strong cheeses, pickled herring, chicken liver, and chocolate is unproven. Patients with a lactase deficiency should use supplemental lactase (Lactaid). Elimination diets may be necessary in selected instances (Raskin, 1988).

Sleep

Too much or too little sleep can provoke migraine, as can shift work or jet lag. Patients with migraine need proper sleep hygiene. They should maintain a regular bedtime and avoid sleeping in on weekends.

Hormonal Factors and Migraine

Menstrual migraine. Migraine attacks are linked to the period of menses in 60% of women, and exclusively to this period (true menstrual migraine) in 14% (Epstein et al., 1975). An attack can occur before, during, or after menstruation, or at the time of ovulation. Premenstrually it may be accompanied by other features of premenstrual syndrome, including mood changes, backache, breast tenderness and swelling, and nausea (American Psychiatric Association, 1987). During menstruation migraine is often associated with dysmenorrhea. Menstrual migraine is frequently refractory to treatment that otherwise benefits typical attacks. The mechanism is uncertain but most likely involves estrogen withdrawal, which may trigger migraine attacks in susceptible women. Somerville (1975) reported that the headache of menstrual migraine occurred during or after the simultaneous fall of estrogens and progesterone, and that giving estrogens premenstrually delayed the onset of migraine but not menstruation. In contrast, progesterone administration delayed menstruation but did not prevent the migraine attack. Somerville concluded that estrogen withdrawal may trigger migraine attacks in susceptible women. Estrogen-withdrawal migraine requires several days of exposure to high levels of estrogen (Silberstein and Merriam, 1991).

Migraine and pregnancy. Migraine may worsen in the first trimester of pregnancy but significantly improve during later pregnancy. Twenty-five percent of women have no change. Women with a history of menstrual migraine typically have an improvement of all their migraine types with pregnancy, perhaps as a result of sustained high estrogen levels (Lance and Anthony, 1966; Ratinahirana et al., 1990; Somerville, 1972a).

Migraine and menopause. In general, migraine prevalence decreases with advancing age (Goldstein and Chen, 1982). Menopause may bring regression, worsening, or no change in migraine. Estrogen replacement therapy can exacerbate migraine or prevent natural improvement (Raskin, 1988; Saper, 1983; Silberstein and Merriam, 1991). There is no evidence that hysterectomy or oophorectomy is an effective or reasonable treatment of migraine at any age (Alvarez, 1940).

Migraine and oral contraceptives. The oral contraceptives most commonly used in the United States contain combinations of estrogen and progestin taken 21 days each month. Controversy persists as to whether the use of oral contraceptives in migraineurs imposes a greater than expected risk of stroke (Bickerstaff, 1975). However, the Collaborative Group for the Study of Stroke in Young Women (1975) did not confirm reports of a greater risk of stroke in migraine patients using oral contraceptives, but suggested that migraine, itself, may be a risk factor for stroke. The neurologic risk associated with the use of oral contraceptives in migraine patients, particularly those with migraine with aura, remains uncertain.

Oral contraceptives can induce, change, or alleviate headache. They can provoke the first migraine attack, most often in women with a family history of migraine. Existing migraine may exacerbate, and headaches may predictably occur on the days off the contraceptive. The headache pattern may become more severe and/or frequent and may be associated with neurologic symptoms. Refractoriness to standard treatment is often noted. Generally, data from neurologic or migraine clinics show an increased incidence, severity, and refractoriness of migraine in oral contraceptive users. Studies from contraceptive clinics and general practitioners are more favorable.

Four double-blind, placebo-controlled studies (Cullberg, 1972; Goldzieher et al., 1971; Nilsson and Solvell, 1967; Silbergeld et al., 1971) revealed no difference in headache incidence between patients taking oral contraceptives and those taking placebo. Both groups had a decreasing incidence of headache with continued duration of observation. In most women the headache pattern does not change, and some may actually experience improvement in headache (Silberstein and Merriam, 1991).

Oral contraceptives may generate new headache or aggravate or ameliorate pre-existing headache. Women with cardiovascular or cerebrovascular risk factors or moderate to severe neurologic events in migraine, especially those who smoke, should avoid the use of oral contraceptives.

Other Provoking Phenomena

Environmental factors, including weather or temperature change, light glare, pungent odors, and high altitude, are cited as provoking migraine headache in susceptible individuals (Van den Bergh et al., 1987). Head and neck pain of another cause may also provoke migraine. Physical exertion from exercise or sexual activity can incite headache (Blau, 1987). Stress and anxiety, particularly the poststress letdown phase, and head trauma can precipitate a migraine headache (Blau, 1987; Lance, 1982; Raskin, 1988; Saper, 1983; Speed, 1989; Van den Bergh et al., 1987).

Nonpharmacologic Treatment

General measures for migraineurs might include regular exercise, good health practices, regular mealtimes, adequate sleep, and maintaining accustomed patterns of activity (Saper, 1983). There appears to be growing evidence that chronobiologic phenomena play an important role in the provocation or the actual pathogenesis of migraine. Migraine patients appear less capable of adjusting to changes in expected external stimuli, such as mealtimes, awakening and retiring times, or even stress excitation. Patients should attempt "chronobiologic regulation"—that is, regularity in their daily activities of living. Meals should be at approximately the same time every day, and retiring and awakening times, particularly the latter, should be about the same. In every way possible, the weekends should approximate the rest of the week, including the time of breakfast and the amount of food taken early in the morning.

The nonpharmacologic techniques of relaxation training, biofeedback, hypnosis, and formal psychotherapy may be useful in selected patients, and are discussed in detail in Chapter 21. With an acute attack, the patient should avoid uncomfortable sensory stimuli. If possible, he or she should retire to a dark, quiet room. Ice packs or heat may be useful adjuncts. Lance (1988) has described a new device incorporating a cooling compartment that encircles the head and a separate warming compartment that is applied to the vertex. The device (Migra-lief) reduced the severity of the migraine headache in 15 of 20 patients.

Because migraine is a recurrent disorder, periodic follow-up medical management is required. A typical pattern of continuing care would be a follow-up visit at 1 month, at 6 weeks, and every 2 to 3 months thereafter. At each visit the effects and side effects of medications should be reviewed and the headache calendar examined. Routine blood work, blood levels of medication, and drug screens can be obtained if necessary (Dalessio, 1987).

Pharmacotherapy

General Considerations

The physician must choose between two general approaches to pharmacologic treatment: symptomatic (reversal, abortive) and preventive (prophylactic) treatment. Concurrent approaches are required in most patients with recurring and severe headache. Symptomatic treatment attempts to abort, reduce, or actually reverse a headache once it has begun, whereas preventive therapy is administered in an attempt to prevent the headache or reduce the frequency and severity of anticipated attacks.

Most authorities believe that symptomatic treatment is appropriate for most acute attacks and should be employed a maximum of 2 to 3 days per week. Preventive therapy should be considered when attacks occur more frequently than three to four times a month. However, a global statement cannot be made and each case must be considered individually. For example, a treatment that emphasizes the preventive approach might be utilized for a patient with infrequent attacks in whom symptomatic treatment is unsuccessful, contraindicated, or likely to be used excessively. Alternately, patients with infrequent attacks (not exceeding 2 to 3 days/week, however) in whom the preventive medication might be contraindicated or in whom compliance is a serious problem might be better served with a program emphasizing the symptomatic approach (Mathew, 1990a). Before starting a woman on any medication, it is important to ascertain that she is not pregnant and is utilizing an effective means of birth control.

Neuropharmacology of Migraine Treatment

Serotonin, or 5-hydroxytryptamine (5-HT), is found widely distributed throughout the body, with major concentrations in the gastrointestinal tract (90%), the platelets (8%), and the brain. Sicuteri et al. (1961) originally observed that there is an increase in the urinary concentration of the serotonin metabolite 5-hydroxyindoleacetic acid during a migraine attack; however, others have not been able to replicate this finding (Ferrari and Odink, 1989).

A direct relationship between serotonin and migraine is suggested by the observation that headache can be precipitated by reserpine (a serotonin releasor and depletor), relieved by serotonin, and blocked by pretreatment with methysergide (a 5-HT_{1C} and 5-HT_2 receptor antagonist) (Fozard and Gray, 1989;

Lance, 1990). Unstable serotonergic transmission in the myenteric plexus could account for the gastrointestinal symptoms of migraine.

There are at least four classes of 5-HT receptors: $5\text{-}HT_1$, $5\text{-}HT_2$, $5\text{-}HT_3$, and $5\text{-}HT_4$ (Dumuis et al., 1991); all have been identified in the brain. The $5\text{-}HT_1$ and $5\text{-}HT_2$ receptors are modulated by estrogens, perhaps accounting for hormone-induced headache (Silberstein and Merriam, 1991). Aging results in a decrease in serotonin receptors and an improvement in migraine. The $5\text{-}HT_1$ receptor is inhibitory and the $5\text{-}HT_2$ and $5\text{-}HT_3$ receptors excitatory. Stimulation of the $5\text{-}HT_3$ receptor, which is present in the area postrema and substantia gelatinosa, produces nausea, vomiting, and activation of autonomic reflexes (Peroutka, 1990a,b).

In humans there are at least four $5\text{-}HT_1$ receptor subtypes: $5\text{-}HT_{1A}$, $5\text{-}HT_{1B}$, $5\text{-}HT_{1C}$, and $5\text{-}HT_{1D}$. The search to characterize serotonin receptors in the vasculature led to the identification of the $5\text{-}HT_1$–like receptor (Humphrey et al., 1990). Some believe that the $5\text{-}HT_1$–like receptor is identical to the $5\text{-}HT_{1D}$ receptor (Peroutka, 1990a,b); others believe it is an entirely new receptor type (Saxena and Ferrari, 1989). The $5\text{-}HT_{1D}$ receptor is a widespread autoreceptor that modulates neurotransmitter release within the nervous system. Receptor activation inhibits release of 5-HT, norepinephrine, acetylcholine, and substance P.

Stimulation of the $5\text{-}HT_2$ receptor results in neuronal depolarization in the CNS. In other organs it produces vasoconstriction, bronchoconstriction, gastrointestinal smooth muscle contraction, and platelet aggregation.

It is currently believed that most specific antimigraine symptomatic drugs interact with the $5\text{-}HT_1$ receptor, although it is uncertain whether this is their mode of therapeutic action (Raskin, 1988) (Table 5–2). Sumatriptan (GR43175)

Table 5–2 Antimigraine drug potencies at $5\text{-}HT_{1D}$ receptor subtypes

	Receptor affinity (K_i, nmol/liter)
Acute	
Sumatriptan	17
Dihydroergotamine	19
Prophylactic	
Methysergide	120
Pizotifen	>1,000
Alprenolol	>1,000
Amitriptyline	>1,000
Cyproheptadine	>1,000
Nifedipine	>1,000
Pindolol	>1,000
Propranolol	>1,000
Verapamil	>1,000
Timolol	>1,000
Atenolol	>1,000
Diltiazem	>1,000

Reproduced with permission from Peroutka, S.J. (1991). Developments in 5-hydroxytryptamine receptor pharmacology in migraine. *Neurol. Clin.* 8:829–838.

(Humphrey et al., 1990; Peroutka, 1990a,b), a serotonin analogue used in the acute treatment of migraine, has been found to be a specific agonist at the 5-HT_{1A}, 5-HT_{1B}, and 5-HT_{1D} receptors, with no significant binding activity at the 5-HT_2, 5-HT_3, adrenergic, dopaminergic, or muscarinic receptor sites.

Dihydroergotamine (DHE) (Callaham and Raskin, 1986), an ergot derivative, is effective in the treatment of acute migraine. Peroutka (1990a,b) has shown that DHE and sumatriptan strongly bind to the 5-HT_{1A}, 5-HT_{1B}, and 5-HT_{1D} receptors. DHE also binds to the 5-HT_{1C}, 5-HT_2, α_1- and α_2-noradrenergic, and dopaminergic receptors. The acute antimigraine action of both drugs is related to their high affinity and agonism for the 5-HT_1 receptor. However, the location of the 5-HT_1 receptor responsible for their acute antimigraine effectiveness is still uncertain.

Sumatriptan and DHE close cerebral arteriovenous shunts in cats and dogs. Heyck has proposed that migraine is due to the opening of these shunts in humans, but there are no strong supporting data for this theory (Spierings, 1984).

Recently, Moskowitz and colleagues have demonstrated that the antimigraine drugs ergotamine (Saito et al., 1988) and sumatriptan (Buzzi and Moskowitz, 1990) (a 5-HT_1 receptor agonist) acutely block the development of neurogenically induced inflammation in the rat dura mater. These drugs work by blocking neurotransmission in small unmyelinated C fibers. Methysergide works in this model only after chronic administration; this is consistent with its clinical usefulness as a prophylactic antimigraine drug (Moskowitz, 1990). The nonsteroidal anti-inflammatory drugs also block the development of neurogenic inflammation; the mechanism of this action is less certain. DHE and sumatriptan may also help in modulation of the central serotonergic pain system.

Raskin (1988) and Peroutka (1990a,b) believe that most of the prophylactic antimigraine drugs interact with the 5-HT_2 receptor (Table 5–3). The prophylactic 5-HT drugs methysergide, pizotofen, and cyproheptadine bind avidly and are antagonistic to the 5-HT_2 receptor, which is concentrated in the frontal cortex. Methysergide also shows modest binding to the 5-HT_1 receptor, where it may be an agonist (Peroutka, 1990a,b). The tricyclic antidepressants block 5-HT reuptake, may block the 5-HT_2 receptor, and may down-regulate the 5-HT_2 receptor (Peroutka, 1990a,b). Recently Brewerton et al. (1988) found that m-chlorophenylpiperazine, a major metabolite of the antidepressant trazodone and a selective 5-HT_{1B} and 5-HT_{1C} agonist, could induce migraine headache in humans. It is likely that this effect is mediated at 5-HT_{1C} receptors in humans (Fozard and Gray, 1989).

Methysergide, cyproheptadine, and pizotofen are, in addition to being 5-HT_2 receptor antagonists, 5-HT_{1C} receptor antagonists. Many have considered their migraine prophylactic effectiveness to be a function of 5-HT_2 receptor antagonism (Peroutka, 1990a,b). The fact that ketanserin, a more selective 5-HT_2 than 5-HT_{1C} receptor antagonist, is not an effective migraine preventative casts doubt on the unifying 5-HT_2 mechanism in migraine prophylaxis and suggests that the 5-HT_{1C} receptor may be of central importance (Fozard and Gray, 1989). Since Peroutka (1990a,b) believes that the 5-HT_{1C} receptor is part of the 5-HT_2 "family," this argument may be in part semantic.

Table 5–3 Antimigraine drug potencies at 5-HT$_2$ receptor subtypes

	Receptor affinity (K_i, nmol/liter)
Acute	
Dihydroergotamine	78
Sumatriptan	>1,000
Prophylactic	
Cyproheptadine	2.2
Pizotifen	3.6
Methysergide	5.7
Amitriptyline	23
Verapamil	140
Nifedipine	320
Diltiazem	>1,000
Propranolol	>1,000
Alprenolol	>1,000
Pindolol	>1,000
Timolol	>1,000
Atenolol	>1,000

Reproduced with permission from Peroutka, S.J. (1991). Developments in 5-hydroxytryptamine receptor pharmacology in migraine. *Neurol. Clin. 8*:829–838.

Although speculative, it can be said that drugs that *stimulate* the inhibitory 5-HT$_1$ receptor seem to produce acute headache relief, whereas drugs that *antagonize* the excitatory 5-HT$_2$ (or 5-HT$_{1C}$) receptor or down-regulate it are effective prophylactic agents.

Treatment of the Prodrome

Premonitory symptoms, such as elation, hunger, thirst, and drowsiness, which precede the headache by as much as 24 hours, suggest a hypothalamic disturbance, perhaps mediated by dopamine and serotonin. The periodicity of migraine and the flow of symptoms from prodrome to aura to headache may be regulated by the hypothalamic arcuate nucleus (see Chapter 4).

In a double-blind, placebo-controlled trial, Waelkens et al. (1986) found that 30 mg of domperidone (an antidopaminergic drug that may not pass the blood–brain barrier), taken at the earliest appearance of the premonitory symptoms, prevented 66% of headache attacks. For maximum efficacy, the drug must be taken at the first appearance of the nonevolutive premonitory symptoms (those that do not merge into the headache and that occur at least 6 hours before the attack). Taking the medication for evolutive prodromal symptoms (occurring within 6 hours of the attack) was not as effective. Spierings (1989) has found that metoclopramide may be as effective as domperidone.

Treatment of the Aura

In migraine with aura, a wave of oligemia spreads forward from the occipital area, precedes the aura, and persists into the headache phase (Oleson and Edvinsson, 1988). The rate of progression of oligemia is the same as the rate of the spreading electrical depression measured by Leāo (1944), who electrically stimulated exposed rabbit cortices and monitored the induced changes in electrical activity, which spread over the cortex at a rate of 2 to 3 mm/minute. Recent squid magnetoencephalogram studies suggest the existence of spreading depression in humans with migraine (Simkins et al., 1989), implying that spreading depression may be the mechanism that produces the aura (see Chapter 4) (Blau, 1984; Pearce, 1984; Raskin, 1990a; Welch et al., 1990).

Wolff (Dalessio, 1980) found that the inhalation of 10% carbon dioxide in air for 5 minutes was temporarily effective in decreasing the visual aura of migraine. The inhalation of 10% carbon dioxide with 90% oxygen was always effective in abolishing the aura of migraine and preventing the development of the expected headache. When headache was present, the effect of 10% carbon dioxide with 90% oxygen was unpredictable. Alvarez (1934) found that the inhalation of 100% oxygen for 15 to 120 minutes produced relief in 42% of his patients. The earlier the treatment, the better the result. Alvarez's patients had a more unpredictable result compared to Wolff's and required longer treatment.

Wolff concluded that the migraine aura was caused by a primary vasoconstriction that could be overridden by the administration of the potent vasodilator arterial carbon dioxide. However, experimental studies on cortical spreading depression (CSD) offer another explanation. Hypercapnic hyperoxia inhibits the propagation of CSD. Thus the effects of hypercapnia on the migraine aura may be mediated by inhibition of CSD (Lauritzen, 1986).

Wolff found that the inhalation of small amounts of amyl nitrite could temporarily reverse the preheadache scotoma in some subjects. The inhalation of larger amounts of amyl nitrite produced generalized vasodilation, hypotension, and an enlargement of the scotoma.

Kupersmith et al. (1979) found that the inhalation of isoproterenol (using a medihaler) at the onset of the aura could abort the neurologic or visual deficit of migraine with aura and basilar migraine. In some cases the resulting headache was unaffected; in others it became more severe with the use of isoproterenol.

In a 15-year-old girl with migraine with prolonged aura, Goldner and Levitt (1987) found that the administration of 10 mg of sublingual nifedipine was effective within 10 to 15 minutes in reversing the focal neurologic symptoms (including aphasia and a mild right hemianopia). Miller and Santoro (1985) reported similar results in patients with migraine and lupus. The actual value of treatment for the aura is uncertain, as is the mechanism that causes the aura.

Treatment of the Acute Migraine Headache

Patients with moderate to severe periodic attacks not amenable to nonpharmacologic treatment should be instructed to use abortive medication for the acute headache attack. Symptomatic medication is appropriate even in patients who are using preventive medication. To prevent escalation of the headache, treatment should begin as early as possible. Often the headache begins with pain of mild to moderate severity and is described as tension type. As the headache increases in severity, it frequently is described as migrainelike. Thus the treatment of migraine and episodic tension-type headache overlap, unless there is a preceding aura (Silberstein, 1984).

At the first sign of headache or neck pain, patients should remove themselves from situations of sensory overstimulation. If possible, they should rest in a dark quiet room, apply an ice pack, and use the symptomatic medication. Symptomatic headache medications include analgesics, antiemetics, anxiolytics, nonsteroidal anti-inflammatory drugs (NSAIDs), ergots, steroids, major tranquilizers, narcotics, and, more recently, selective 5-HT$_1$ agonists. The physician should have a treatment strategy utilizing one or more of these medications in headaches of different severity (Silberstein, 1991).

Overuse of Headache Medications

Patients with frequent headaches are prone to overuse both analgesics and ergotamine. This excessive use can be characterized by the regular daily intake of analgesics; the regular use (more often than four times a week) of combination analgesics containing barbiturates or sedatives; or the regular use (more often than twice a week) of ergotamine tartrate (Anderson, 1988; Diamond and Dalessio, 1982; Mathew, 1990b; Saper, 1983, 1987b, 1989, 1990a; Saper and Jones, 1986; Wilkinson, 1988a).

Medication overuse by headache-prone patients produces chronic refractory headache, with growing dependence on and addiction to symptomatic medication (Saper, 1983, 1986). Withdrawal (abstinence) symptoms following discontinuation of symptomatic medication (including increased headache) and refractoriness to prophylactic medications are common (Mathew, 1990b; Saper, 1983, 1986). Kudrow (1982) has reported that prophylactic amitriptyline is not effective if daily analgesics are continued. In the majority of patients, stopping the symptomatic medication will result in headache improvement after a period of increased headache (analgesic washout period) (Baumgartner et al., 1989; Rapoport et al., 1989; Saper, 1986). In addition to the induction of chronic refractory headache, each class of medication has unique side effects: ergotism, analgesic nephropathy, gastrointestinal problems (including dyspepsia and ulcers), and anemia.

Raskin (1986) and Silberstein (1990) have shown that detoxification can be enhanced by using repetitive intravenous DHE to control the headaches and promote return to intermittent migraine.

Drug-Related Headache

During the Second International Workshop on Drug-Related Headache at the University of Tübingen in 1986, the participating experts agreed on the following characteristics of drug-related headache (Wilkinson, 1988):

1. More than 20 headache days per month
2. Daily headache duration exceeding 10 hours
3. Intake of analgesic or migraine drugs on more than 20 days/month
4. Regular intake of analgesics and/or ergotamine preparations in combination with barbiturates, codeine, caffeine, antihistamines, or tranquilizers
5. Increase in the severity and frequency of headaches after discontinuation of drug intake (rebound headache)
6. The nature of the underlying headache (e.g., migraine, tension head-

ache, cluster headache, post-traumatic headache, or cervicogenic headache) is not related to the syndrome.

Transformed/evolutive migraine. Overuse of analgesics and/or ergotamines by patients with tension-type headache or intermittent migraine can lead to the development of chronic daily headache. Kudrow (1982), Saper (1983, 1986, 1987b), Mathew et al. (1987), Isler (1982), and Rapoport and Weeks (1988) have all written extensively on the concept of transformed or evolutive migraine. Saper (1983) reported that 80% of his patients with transformed migraine had onset of migraine by age 26 and transformation to chronic daily headache by age 41. These patients were typically women, frequently clinically depressed. Periodically, these chronic daily headache sufferers had superimposed acute migraine headaches.

"Chronic daily headache" is a term that has been widely employed to describe the phenomenon of head pain on a daily or almost-daily basis. Unfortunately, the term is a wastebasket for any type of headache that may occur in this pattern. In this chapter, we are referring to that subset of daily chronic headache patients who have experienced a transformational migraine, in which periodic, occasional migraine has transformed or evolved to a more frequent pattern, usually daily, with periodic, superimposed migrainous attacks. A better term for this phenomenon might be "pernicious migraine" or "progressive migraine," thereby suggesting a progressive evolution from the periodic pattern, but at the same time distinguishing it from all other daily chronic headache origins, which might include a long list of physiologic and psychological entities.

Preventing drug-related headache. Specific limits on the use of abortive medications are necessary in order to prevent the development of both analgesic and ergotamine overuse. Wilkinson (1988a), Saper (1986), Mathew et al. (1987), and Scholz et al. (1988) have compared ergotamine intake in patients with and without chronic daily headache. In the groups without chronic daily headache, the maximum ergotamine intake was 24 mg/month. However, one patient with chronic daily headache consumed only 7 mg of ergotamine per month. The frequency of days of ergotamine use (treatment days, events) is as important as, if not more important than, the total monthly dose (Saper, 1983, 1986). Rebound can develop in patients taking as little as 0.5 to 1 mg of ergotamine 3 times a week.

Scholz et al. (1988) studied the consumption of simple analgesics, comparing patients with and without rebound headache. Patients with rebound headache consumed between 1,200 and 1,500 mg of analgesics a day. Increased caffeine, but not codeine, consumption was correlated with the development of chronic daily headache. Barbiturate consumption was significantly higher (60 to 500 mg/day; mean 160 mg/day) in patients with chronic daily headache than in those without chronic daily headache (mean <60 mg/day).

Fisher (1988) attempted to refute the concept of analgesic rebound headache by denying its existence in patients using analgesics for arthritis. His criticism highlights the point that rebound headaches only occur in headache-prone patients. There is significant individual sensitivity to the effects of drug overuse, and not all patients will develop drug-induced headache.

Dose limits for the use of preventive medications should be set below the dose that might produce chronic daily headache. The actual limit of symptomatic drug use and its duration beyond which rebound occurs is unknown. For practical purposes, we provide general and arbitrary guidelines that we employ based on our experience. We believe it is just as important to limit the number of treatment days the drug is used per month (events) as the maximum amount of drug used per month, to maintain a drug-free interval between the days of drug use.

Another strategy to limit overuse is to use different classes of medications. Polypharmacy can be either detrimental or beneficial in this regard. Its benefit may be enhanced by alternating the use of symptomatic medications with similar mechanism of action in an attempt to provide drug-free days. Use of the same symptomatic medication, such as analgesics or ergotamine derivatives, should be avoided. In cluster headache and menstrual migraine syndromes, some relaxation of these restrictions is appropriate. The rebound phenomenon has not been clearly identified in cluster headache patients, who might suffer from a condition imposing a different level of vulnerability to the rebound phenomenon.

SYMPTOMATIC TREATMENT

Nonprescription Medications

The symptomatic treatment of headache begins with the use of analgesics. Most people find relief for their headache by using a simple analgesic such as aspirin (Murray, 1964) or acetaminophen, either alone or in combination with caffeine. Caffeine, which is present in many over-the-counter (OTC) preparations, has been shown not only to potentiate the analgesic action of these drugs but also to be an analgesic itself (Ward et al., 1991). Ibuprofen, in various OTC preparations, is a NSAID that is effective in the symptomatic relief of headache (see below).

In a placebo-controlled, double-blind study in patients with either tension or tension–vascular headache, Peters et al. (1983) found both aspirin and acetaminophen superior to placebo. The danger of Reye syndrome makes acetaminophen preferable to aspirin in children younger than 15 (Silberstein, 1990). Acetaminophen is preferable to aspirin or the other NSAIDs in patients with gastritis or bleeding disorder.

The dose of aspirin or acetaminophen should be limited to 1,000 mg per individual attack, with a maximum of 4,000 mg/day. We recommend no more than 3 usage days per week unless there is some overriding medical reason. For side effects of the simple analgesics, see the *Physicians' Desk Reference for Nonprescription Drugs* (Barnhart, 1991b).

Prescription Analgesics

If the patient does not respond to the simple analgesics, a combination of aspirin or acetaminophen with butalbital may be prescribed. These combinations may have the following advantages:

1. Combining two analgesics with different mechanisms of action can enhance analgesia (Beaver, 1984; McQuay et al., 1989).
2. Caffeine not only enhances the analgesia of aspirin and acetaminophen (140%) (Beaver, 1984) and ibuprofen (240%) (Forbes et al., 1991), but is itself analgesic (Ward et al., 1991).
3. Lower doses of different drugs reduce side effects.
4. The use of barbiturates or benzodiazepam can alleviate anxiety. Any value of the barbiturate may be via a central effect: sedation or pain modulation (Saper, 1990a).
5. Analgesic combination drugs also offer product convenience (Beaver, 1984).

However, some physicians believe that these combinations are more likely to lead to overuse and dependence, and may not offer additional pain control sufficient to justify their use.

Commonly used combinations include aspirin or acetaminophen plus butalbital, a short-acting barbiturate effective in reducing anxiety (Silberstein, 1984). These combinations, available with caffeine (Fiorinal, Fioricet, Esgic) or without caffeine (Phrenilin), may be prescribed. For an individual attack, patients should take one or two tablets or capsules immediately, with a maximum of six per attack. The most frequent adverse reactions are drowsiness and dizziness.

The combination of acetaminophen, isometheptine (a sympathomimetic), and dichlorphenazone (a chloral hydrate derivative) (Midrin) has been shown to be safe and effective in headache treatment (Ryan, 1974; Yuill et al., 1972). The initial dose of Midrin is two capsules, with a maximum of five capsules per attack. Midrin is contraindicated in patients with glaucoma, renal failure, significant hypertension, or heart or liver disease, and in patients using monoamine oxidase (MAO) inhibitors. Adverse reactions include transient dizziness and skin rash.

If a stronger analgesic is required, use a combination of aspirin, caffeine, butalbital, and codeine (Fiorinal with codeine) or acetaminophen with codeine, or acetaminophen, butalbital, and codeine (Phrenilin with codeine). For an individual attack, patients should take one to two capsules immediately, with a maximum of six per attack. Although Scholz et al. (1988) found that codeine use did not correlate to the development of chronic daily headache, prudence calls for a smaller monthly use of combination analgesics with codeine.

In general, we recommend no more than 2 to 3 usage-days per week, with strict monthly limits of these agents to prevent overuse. Monthly limits should be established below maximal allowable usage, although individual consideration on a patient-by-patient basis is appropriate.

More potent narcotic analgesics such as propoxephene, oxycodone, hydrocodone, meperidine, morphine, and hydromorphone are available alone or in

Table 5–4 Oral doses of narcotics equivalent to 10 mg parenteral morphine

Drug	Oral dose (mg)	Oral-to-parenteral dose ratio	Parenteral dose (mg)
Morphine			
Single dose	60	6:1	10
Repeated dose	30	3:1	10
Hydromorphone (Dilaudid)	7.5	5:1	1.5
Meperidine (Demerol)	300	4:1	75
Codeine	200	1.5:1	130

Reproduced with permission from Foley, K.M. (1985). The treatment of cancer pain. *N. Engl. J. Med. 313*:84–95.

combination with simple analgesics. Because of the danger of narcotic addiction, their use should be limited, but they are not contraindicated. Saper (1990b) has suggested that narcotic analgesics may be considered for patients with infrequent, moderate to severe forms of migraine that do not respond to standard, non-narcotic measures. This is particularly true in patients who have not over-used medication or violated treatment recommendations. These medications should be avoided or used cautiously and restrictively in patients who have demonstrated addictive tendencies or have a family history of addictive disease. Setting strict limits and offering small amounts of medication seems a prudent way to provide relatively safe medication, in a manner that avoids the risk of excessive use, to patients otherwise resistant to treatment (Portenoy, 1990). Meperidine, for example, may be useful in the pregnant patient, and occasional use of narcotics in the patient who cannot tolerate or does not respond to ergot derivatives and other symptomatic medications is considered appropriate.

Dosages of narcotics should be adjusted to account for the difference in bioavailability between the oral, parenteral, and rectal routes of administration (Table 5–4). Narcotics should be limited to one or two doses per week. Although admittedly controversial, some pain authorities have argued that the liberal use of narcotics in intractable headache (e.g., intractable menstrual migraine) or special circumstances (e.g., elderly patients in whom the otherwise standard treatment of ergotamine is contraindicated) is justifiable.

Nonsteroidal Anti-inflammatory Drugs

At least five different types of NSAIDs (Pradalier et al., 1988) can be used for headache treatment. These include the salicylates, propionic acid, aryl and heterocyclic acids, meclophenamates, and piroxicam. Ibuprofen is now available as an OTC medication in a 200-mg dosage (Table 5–5) (Insel, 1990).

The major mechanism of action of NSAIDs is the inhibition of the enzyme cyclo-oxygenase, preventing the synthesis of prostaglandins (Campbell, 1990). In addition, some NSAIDs (ketoprofen, indomethacin, diclofenac) decrease the synthesis of leukotrienes by inhibiting 5-lipo-oxygenase (Brooks and Day, 1991; Campbell, 1990). One NSAID (meclofenamate) may be a direct prostaglandin receptor antagonist. In addition, NSAIDs interfere with a variety of membrane-associated processes, including the activity of NADPH oxidase in neutrophils and phospholipase C in macrophages (Brooks and Day, 1991).

Table 5-5   Nonsteroidal anti-inflammatory drugs

Salicylates	Aryl and heterocyclic acids
Diflunisal (Dolobid)	Tolmetin (Tolectin)
Propionic acids	Indomethacin (Indocin)
Ibuprofen (Motrin, Advil)	Diclofenac (Voltaren)
Naproxen (Naprosyn)	Sulindac (Clinoril)
Naproxen sodium (Anaprox)	Meclofenamate (Meclomen)
Fenoproxen (Nalfon)	Piroxican (Feldene)
Ketoprofen (Orudis)	

NSAIDs can be used symptomatically or preventively and should be considered for the treatment of menstrual migraine, exertional migraine, benign orgasmic cephalgia, hemicrania continua, and ice pick headache (Raskin, 1988). In order to be effective, NSAIDs must be given in adequate doses. If one NSAID is ineffective, another should be tried.

Side effects seen with all the NSAIDs include gastrointestinal upset, peptic ulcers and bleeding, abdominal pain, constipation, diarrhea, nausea, occasional paradoxical headache, lightheadedness, dizziness, somnolence, tinnitus, and fluid retention. The more lipid-soluble NSAIDs penetrate the CNS more effectively and may have greater central effects (Brooks and Day, 1991). All NSAIDs are associated with an increased risk for peptic ulcer disease, the risk increasing with the dosage of the NSAID (Griffin et al., 1991), and aggravation of existing gastrointestinal inflammatory disease. Contraindications to NSAIDs include active ulcer disease, gastritis, kidney disease, and bleeding disorders.

The NSAIDs most commonly used for headache relief are listed in Table 5-5. The dose should be limited to the maximum for each drug. In some cases it can be repeated in 1 to 2 hours (naproxen, ibuprofen) as long as the maximal dose is not exceeded. Indomethacin (Indocin) is available as a 50-mg rectal suppository, which is useful in patients with severe nausea and vomiting. Ketorolac (Toradol) is the first NSAID that can be given parenterally (available as 15-, 30-, and 60-mg Cartrix for intramuscular (IM) injection). Klapper and Stanton (1991) found that ketorolac (60 mg IM) was less effective than DHE and metoclopramide given intravenously (IV) in the treatment of acute migraine headache.

Patients using NSAIDs should be monitored for gastrointestinal blood loss, renal dysfunction, worsening of hypertension, and aggravation of colitis. Their use should be limited to one week of continuous daily use perimenstrually or three times per week when used regularly. It is not known if NSAIDs can produce rebound headache, but some authors have implicated these drugs (Henry et al., 1985).

Combination Therapy

The City of London Migraine Clinic (Wilkinson, 1988b) and the Copenhagen Acute Headache Clinic (Olesen et al., 1979) (both outpatient clinics) use the combination of acetaminophen or aspirin, metoclopramide, and diazepam in the acute treatment of headache. This regimen combines an analgesic, an antiemetic, and an anxiolytic. The London and Copenhagen programs each begin with a screening history and physical examination. The patients are then given 10 mg metoclopramide IM, 1 g aspirin or 1 g acetaminophen, followed by 5 mg diazepam (Insel, 1990). Ninety percent of the patients in the Copenhagen program had migraine; 67% left the clinic free of all symptoms and 25% left with a mild headache. The mean length of stay was 4 hours, the median 5.9 hours (range, minutes to several days). There was no correlation between initial pain severity and pain relief, but it took longer to cure patients who had more severe headaches. Ergotamine or piperazine was used for treatment failure. Both Wilkinson (1988b) and the Copenhagen group (Olesen et al., 1979) stressed that the combination of sleep, an antinauseant, a simple analgesic, and (in one third of patients) ergotamine tartrate provided relief within 3 to 4 hours for most patients who were well enough to get to the clinic.

Use of Ergotamine and Dihydroergotamine

Barring contraindications, ergotamine is the treatment of choice for moderate to severe migraine (Zeigler, 1987) if analgesics do not provide headache relief or produce significant side effects. Ergotamine tartrate, originally derived from a rye fungus (*Claviceps purpurea*), is an ergopeptide that consists of a natural D-lysergic acid linked to a tricyclic peptide moiety by a peptide bond.

Ergotamine has α-adrenergic and serotonergic agonist activity and vasoconstricting actions, stimulating arterial smooth muscle through serotonin receptors. It also constricts venous capacitance vessels. Both ergotamine and DHE are agonists at the serotonin 5-HT_{1A}, 5-HT_{1B}, and 5-HT_{1D} receptors, which have been implicated in the genesis and treatment of migraine (Peroutka, 1990a,b). DHE is a derivative of ergotamine that has been reduced at the 9–10 double bond on the D-lysergic acid moiety.

DHE differs from ergotamine (Berde and Stuermer, 1978). Although both DHE and ergotamine inhibit the reuptake of noradrenaline at sympathetic nerve endings, DHE is a weaker arterial vasoconstrictor but almost as potent a venoconstrictor as ergotamine, constricting venous capacitance vessels while having a negligible effect on resistance vessels. DHE is a more potent α-adrenergic blocker than ergotamine and inhibits the baroreceptor circulatory reflex. In both animals and humans, DHE is much less emetic and has less effect on the uterus than ergotamine. It is very difficult to induce experimental gangrene in the rat's tail with high doses of DHE.

Neither drug has an effect on cerebral hemisphere blood flow (Andersen et al., 1987; Hachinski et al., 1978), suggesting that their effect in migraine is independent of any cerebrovascular vasoconstrictor properties. Moskowitz (1990) has shown that DHE and ergotamine block the development of neurovascular inflammation in the trigeminal vascular system by inhibiting transmission in small unmyelinated C fibers. This may be a mechanism of amplification of headache pain and may account for the secondary blood vessel changes occasionally seen in migraine.

Goadsby and Gundlach (1991) have recently shown that radiolabeled DHE, injected intravenously in the cat, passes through the blood–brain barrier and labels nuclei in the brainstem and spinal cord that are intimately involved in pain transmission and modulation. Lance (1986) has, in addition, shown that one of these nuclei—the caudal trigeminal nucleus—was activated by stimulation of the sagittal sinus, and that this activity was transmitted to the thalamus. Both ergotamine and DHE, in clinically active doses, suppressed this activation (Lambert et al., 1986).

These data strongly suggest that the ergot alkaloids, ergotamine and DHE, exert their antimigraine effect by a receptor-mediated neural pathway both in the CNS and in the trigeminal nerve.

Dosage Forms and Bioavailability

Clinically, ergotamine tartrate is available as a sublingual preparation (Ergostat), and, in combination with caffeine, as an oral tablet (Cafergot, Wigraine) and a suppository (Cafergot, Wigraine). Caffeine has been shown to enhance the oral absorption of ergotamine (Schmidt and Fanchamps, 1974) and recently to have an analgesic effect on its own (Ward et al., 1991). Ergotamine, in combination with a barbiturate and a belladonna alkaloid, is no longer commercially available.

The bioavailability of ergotamine is highly dependent on the route of administration. Ergotamine given by suppository to normal volunteers produced blood levels 20- to 30-fold higher than the same dose given orally (Figure 5–1) (Sanders et al., 1986). The oral absorption of ergotamine is erratic, which has extremely important clinical implications.

Ergotamine Dosing Strategies

Some headache authorities recommend predetermining the subnauseating dose of ergotamine prior to its initial use, at a time when the patient is headache free (Raskin, 1988). This will avoid overdosing and increased headache and nausea, and underdosing and lack of efficacy. Using 1-mg ergotamine tablets (Cafergot or Wigraine), the patient takes one, then two, then four, and finally six tablets at different times, titrating upward until nausea develops (Silberstein, 1991). Alternatively, one, two, and three sublingual 2-mg tablets of ergotamine (Ergostat) can be used.

Since the rectal route of administration produces higher blood levels than the oral form, the patient should start with one fourth of a suppository, then one third, then one half, and finally a full suppository at different times to predetermine the subnauseating dose. At the time of the acute headache attack, the predetermined subnauseating dose (usually one third to one half of a suppository) should be taken (Silberstein, 1991).

Ergotamine tartrate. For individual attacks, patients can take up to six (1-mg) tablets, two suppositories, or six inhalations. Monthly limits are 8 events, 24 (1-mg) tablets, 12 suppositories, or 24 inhalations. In certain circumstances, a liberalization of these limits may be appropriate (e.g., cluster headache, intractable menstrual migraine).

If a patient cannot tolerate the use of ergotamine because of nausea, he or she can be pretreated with metoclopramide (Volans, 1978), prochlorperazine

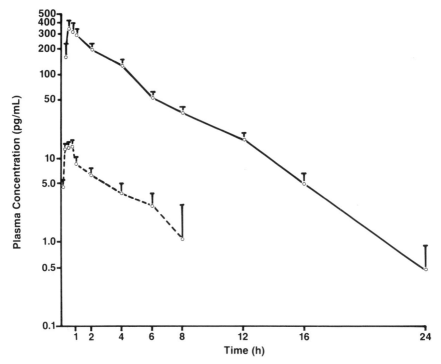

Figure 5–1.   Mean plasma concentrations following single 2-mg oral (----) and rectal (——) doses of ergotamine in healthy volunteers (mean ± SEM). (Adapted from Sanders et al. [1986].)

(Kanto et al., 1981), phenergan (Silberstein, 1991), or a mixture of a barbiturate and a belladonna alkaloid. Oral metoclopramide might also enhance oral absorption of ergotamine. If patients cannot tolerate or obtain no relief from ergotamine, they should be instructed in the use of DHE.

DHE Dosing
DHE (Raskin, 1988) is currently available only in 1 mg/ml ampules, which can be administered IM, subcutaneously (SC), or IV. A nasal spray preparation has been formulated and is awaiting FDA approval. Bioavailability and blood levels are highest with IV injection (Kanto et al., 1981) and most erratic with SC injection (Schran and Tse, 1985). Patients can be taught to self-administer IM DHE.

   A trial to determine the subnauseating dose of DHE can be done at a time when the patient is headache free (Raskin, 1988). The patient should take up 1 mg of DHE in a 3-ml syringe with a 1-inch 22-gauge needle. The patient first injects 0.25 mg (0.25 ml) IM, then additional 0.25-mg increments every 15 minutes until a maximum of 1.0 mg has been injected or nausea has developed. The incidence of nausea is much lower with IM than with IV injection and lower still than seen with oral or rectal ergotamine tartrate (Raskin, 1988; Tillgren, 1947).

Dosage for individual attacks should be limited to 1 mg IM or IV (maximum of 3 mg/day). Monthly limits are 18 ampules or 12 events. DHE, unlike ergotamine, may not produce rebound headache, but this remains uncertain. We recommend limiting its use to prevent overuse of IM injections and the development of refractoriness. Exceptions include cluster headache, menstrual migraine, and use during detoxification.

DHE may produce nausea in some patients. Pretreatment with metoclopramide, promethazine, or a combination of atropine and a barbiturate, or perhaps ondansetron, might counter this side effect and treat the nausea associated with the migraine as well.

Contraindications to the use of ergotamine tartrate or DHE include renal or hepatic failure; pregnancy; coronary, cerebral, and peripheral vascular disease; hypertension; and sepsis.

DHE nasal spray. DHE, applied as a nasal spray, is rapidly absorbed, with peak plasma concentrations occurring within 45 minutes. The bioavailability is 40% of the same dose given intramuscularly. A large multicenter double-blind, placebo-controlled study found that, in 82% of patients, DHE nasal spray (1.0 mg) either completely controlled or partially improved headache within 90 to 120 minutes. The side effects of nasal DHE are mild and transient and include nasal stuffiness, nausea, and rarely vomiting (Lataste, 1989).

Adjunctive Treatment

The associated symptoms of migraine, such as nausea and vomiting, can be as disabling as the headache pain itself. Gastric stasis and delayed gastric emptying associated with migraine can decrease the effectiveness of oral medication (Boyle et al., 1990; Tfelt-Hansen et al., 1980; Volans, 1978). In addition, the medications used to treat migraine can produce nausea, as can migraine itself. Therefore, antiemetics, such as metoclopramide (Reglan), available in tablets, syrup, and injectable form (dose 10 to 20 mg), can be extremely useful in the treatment of migraine. In addition, metoclopramide decreases the gastric atony and enhances the absorption of coadministered medications (Albibi and McCallum, 1983). Promethazine (Phenergan), available in tablet, liquid, suppository, and injectable forms (dose 25 to 50 mg), is also useful for the control of nausea and vomiting but, unlike metoclopramide, does not enhance gastric emptying (Silberstein, 1990). Some patients find promethazine more tolerable than metoclopramide because it has fewer extrapyramidal side effects.

Hydroxyzine (dose 50 to 100 mg orally, 75 mg IM) may be useful in controlling both nausea and headache. Perphenazine (dose 2 to 4 mg orally, 5 mg IM), chlorpromazine (dose 25 to 50 mg orally, 25 to 100 mg per rectum), and prochlorperazine (dose 10 mg IM or per rectum) may be similarly useful, and are discussed in more detail later (see "Treatment of Severe Persistent [Pernicious] Migraine").

Recently ondansetron (Zofran), a new selective 5-HT$_3$ receptor antagonist that has no antidopaminergic activity and no effect on gastrointestinal motility, has become available for IV infusion (dose 0.15 mg/kg diluted in 50 ml of 5% dextrose or normal saline solution).

Preventive Medications Used for Symptomatic Headache Treatment

β-Adrenergic Blockers in Acute Treatment of Migraine

Featherstone (1983b) and Tokola and Hokkanan (1978) have suggested that propranolol (40 to 80 mg) can abort an acute attack of migraine with or without aura. However, Fuller and Guiloff (1990) could not demonstrate propranolol's effectiveness in a placebo-controlled, double-blind study. This could be a result of a large placebo effect in the open studies or a failure to study a subset of migraineurs who might respond to propranolol.

Calcium Antagonists in Acute Treatment of Migraine

Intravenous verapamil (10 mg) and sublingual nimodipine (40 mg) have not been effective in treating acute attacks of migraine (Andersson and Vinge, 1990). Nifedipine may be used for the treatment of the aura of migraine but is ineffective in treating the headache (Scholz and Hoffert, 1987). Some recent studies suggest that IV (Pfaffenrath et al., 1990; Soyka et al., 1989) or sublingual (Takeshima et al., 1988) flunarizine is effective in the acute treatment of migraine, perhaps in part because of its dopaminergic blocking effect.

New Abortive Treatment

Sumatriptan, a selective 5-HT$_1$ agonist, is effective in placebo-controlled, double-blind studies when given orally (Patten, 1991) or SC (Ensink, 1991). Oral sumatriptan (200 mg) was 75% effective in decreasing headache to mild or no pain within 2 hours. Side effects, which occurred in 48% of the patients, included nausea or vomiting. In one study, SC sumatriptan (6 mg) was 73% effective in decreasing headache to mild or no pain (Ensink, 1991). Side effects, which occurred in 62% of the patients, were usually mild and transient and included warmth, heaviness, and tingling.

Cady et al. (1991), in a placebo-controlled, double-blind study of 1,104 patients, found sumatriptan (6 mg SC) was more effective than placebo in reducing moderate or severe headache to mild or no pain (70 versus 22%) and in completely relieving pain (49 versus 9%) after 1 hour. No additional benefit of a second injection of sumatriptan, given at 1 hour, was noted.

Sumatriptan (Imitrex) is now available in the United States in a 6 mg SC dosage form using an autoinjector. SC sumatriptan is well tolerated, effective and indicated for the acute treatment of migraine with or without aura. It is not indicated for use in hemiplegic or basilar migraine. Recurrent headache requiring a second dose of the drug occurs in up to 38% of patients (The Subcutaneous Sumatriptan International Study Group, 1991). Contraindications include ischemic heart disease (angina, myocardial infarction, silent myocardial infarction, signs or symptoms of ischemic heart disease), Prinzmetal angina, uncontrolled hypertension, and hypersensitivity to sumatriptan. Sumatriptan should not be used intravenously because of the risk of coronary vasospasm. Consideration should be given to giving the first dose in the physician's office if coronary artery disease is suspected.

The dose of sumatriptan is 6 mg SC. This can be repeated once in 24 hours, with an hour between doses. Sumatriptan should not be taken within 24 hours of ergotamine preparations.

We do not know if using sumatriptan more than 2 days a week poses a risk of rebound headache.

TREATMENT OF SEVERE, PERSISTENT (PERNICIOUS) MIGRAINE

Intermittent, self-limited migraine can evolve into a daily headache pattern, sometimes reaching an intensity that requires aggressive parenteral intervention. The term "status migrainosis" has been informally applied to a state of intractable, debilitating pain, and often arises from a setting in which the patient has become dependent on one or more symptomatic medications, usually analgesics or ergotamine tartrate (Edmeads 1988, Raskin 1990c; Saper, 1986, 1987b, 1990a). Recently, status migrainosis has been classified as an entity by the IHS.

The symptoms of this condition, which might be termed "pernicious migraine," include the progressive intensification of severe, debilitating pain, accompanied by the usual characteristics of acute migraine (nausea, vomiting, light sensitivity, etc.) and by increasing prostration. Dehydration, electrolyte alterations, autonomic disturbances, and emotional despair are generally present (Edmeads, 1988). The so-called rebound headache is characterized by the regular, dependable, and predictable development of a headache within hours of the waning therapeutic effect of the last dose of medication. The phenomenon is self-perpetuating and occurs insidiously in patients with pre-existent, intermittent migraine (Saper 1986, 1987b).

Many patients have a history of progressively increasing use of symptomatic medications. Although one can argue that the overuse of symptomatic medication is the result, not the cause, of the progressive form of headache, it is the prevailing belief of most authorities that the overuse of ergotamine tartrate and/or centrally acting analgesic is of primary importance in the pathogenesis of this refractory state. It is generally believed that a state of refractoriness to symptomatic medications and the progression to this pernicious form of migraine can occur even with the use of simple analgesics such as aspirin or acetaminophen at a seemingly innocuous level of 1,200 to 1,500 mg/day (Raskin 1990c; Scholz et al., 1988).

The mechanism by which this phenomenon can occur is uncertain. A central effect on adrenergic mechanisms thought to be related to headache was noted in a study of 200 patients with ergotamine dependency (Saper, 1986). More recently, Fields (1991) has noticed an increased firing of the so-called on-cells (the pain-facilitating neurons) during the period of narcotic withdrawal. Together with the recognition that headache, backache, and abdominal pain are common features of narcotic withdrawal (Jaffe, 1985) and the finding in animals that implanted opiates result in reduced production of endogenous opiatelike substances (Prezewlocki et al., 1979), Fields' observation offers a possible explanation of those circumstances that may contribute to rebound.

General Approach

The patient with acute, pernicious migraine may require hospital admission, particularly if the symptoms are accompanied by dependency on medication. The medication protocols listed below are acceptable and effective in the emergency room setting, but the presence of drug dependency and "rebound" will frequently render any temporary improvement short lived, with the presentation repeated soon thereafter.

The principles of treatment for patients with refractory, severe migraine include: (1) fluid and electrolyte replacement, (2) drug detoxification, (3) intravenous pharmacotherapy to control pain, and (4) concurrent implementation of migraine prophylaxis.

Hospitalization

The concept of hospitalizing headache patients is not without controversy. Nonetheless, since the development and initial description of the first inpatient unit specifically directed at the treatment of intractable headaches in 1979 (Van Meter and Saper, 1981), specialty hospital services in particular, and hospital care in general, have provided a critical therapeutic benefit to patients with severe treatment-resistant headache. The primary orientation of a specialty hospital program is the administration of aggressive, acute medical headache management in a setting that can address coexistent and contributing disturbances. These include toxic medication reactions, dependency syndromes, and the behavioral and psychological features that often accompany this clinical syndrome, such as the fear of headache (cephalgiaphobia), which promotes excessive, obsessive use of symptomatic treatments (Saper, 1990a; Silberstein et al., 1990).

A prospective outcome evaluation has demonstrated long-term benefits in patients with intractable headache (Lake et al., 1990). This study reported that a 64% reduction in the mean number of days of severe or incapacitating headache was sustained, with a corresponding increase in the mean number of headache-free days. Dysfunctional days dropped by 70% and clinical depression by 69%. A mean percentage of subjective improvement of 70% was noted, with 87% of patients reporting at least a 50% reduction in headache. Silberstein and Silberstein (1992) have reported similar long-term benefit. Most patients (87%) detoxified from analgesic or ergotamine overuse as part of an inpatient program continued to do well when re-evaluated at 2-year follow-up after hospitalization.

Criteria developed jointly with the Michigan Blue Cross and Blue Shield for the admission of patients with intractable, primary head pain include:

1. Severe, intractable pain accompanied by dependence on analgesic or ergotamine medication.
2. Severe, intractable headache accompanied by dehydration or requiring parenteral therapy for pain interruption.
3. Severe, intractable headache in the presence of significant neurologic, medical, or psychiatric illnesses, sufficient to require acute medical management not available or inappropriate on an outpatient basis.

These criteria presume that, when possible, aggressive, good faith outpatient efforts have preceded the admission and failed to achieve adequate treatment success.

Hospital Protocols

Detoxification Guidelines

The following protocol is employed by one of the authors (J.R.S.):

1. Fluid replacement. Experience demonstrates that a large number of patients are clinically or subclinically dehydrated as a result of prolonged nausea and vomiting, a presumed increase in insensible fluid loss from protracted pain, and increased diuresis accompanying severe migraine and/or excessive ingestion of caffeine, often present in analgesic and ergot preparations. Twenty-four to 48 hours of fluid and electrolyte replacement have, by personal observation (J.R.S.), enhanced treatment efficacy and the withdrawal and detoxification process.
2. Ergotamine tartrate can be discontinued abruptly if DHE is administered. Otherwise, a tapering regimen over 2 to 3 days is recommended.
3. Analgesics not containing opiates can be stopped abruptly, although abdominal cramping, muscle aches, and malaise are frequently noted when high dosage has been sustained for a prolonged period.
4. Combined analgesics containing barbiturate should be discontinued gradually. Rapid discontinuation can be achieved by giving 30 to 60 mg of phenobarbital three times a day for several days and then tapering.
5. Narcotic withdrawal must be carried out slowly. Side effects can be reduced by giving clonidine hydrochloride and/or phenobarbital or a benzodiazepine derivative (Bakris et al., 1982; Gold et al., 1980).

Treatment of Pain and Nausea Both in the Emergency Room and during Hospitalization

Intravenous DHE. Callaham and Raskin (1986) have shown that the combination of 5 mg prochlorperazine IV followed by IV DHE is a safe and effective means of terminating a migraine attack. Belgrade et al. (1989) have shown that the combination of IV metoclopramide and IV DHE is more effective in treating an acute migraine attack than is IM meperidine. More recently, Raskin (1990b) has advocated mixing 10 mg (2 ml) of prochlorperazine and 1 mg (1 ml) of DHE in a syringe and injecting 2 ml of the mixture IV. If the headache is not relieved in 15 to 30 minutes, the remainder of the dose can be injected.

Repetitive intravenous DHE. Intravenous DHE has become the mainstay of the acute symptomatic treatment for intractable headache (Edmeads, 1988; Raskin, 1986; Silberstein et al., 1990). Raskin (1986) found that repetitive IV DHE was effective in eliminating intractable headache in 89% of patients within 48 hours. Intravenous diazepam was only partially effective in eliminating such headaches (13% within 3 to 6 days). Silberstein et al. (1990) also found that repetitive IV DHE was effective in eliminating prolonged migraine, cluster headache, and chronic daily headaches with or without rebound. It is argued that intravenous DHE has a sustained therapeutic effect, but it is uncertain whether this observation is directly related to the effects of the DHE (Raskin, 1986; Silberstein et al., 1990) or the active metabolite 8-OH-DHE (Aellig, 1984; Muller-Schweinitzer,

1984), the termination of drug "rebound" (Diener et al., 1988; Saper, 1986), or the removal of the patient from a stressful environment (Silberstein et al., 1990).

Patients treated with DHE should have a heparin lock inserted for administration of medication. The patients are pretreated with metoclopramide (Reglan 10 mg IV), which is continued as needed before each infusion of DHE. DHE is initially administered at a test dose of 0.5 mg (0.25 in younger children) given via IV push over 3 to 5 minutes. If the headache persists, another 0.5 mg of DHE is given and 1.0 mg of DHE is administered every 8 hours (Figure 5–2). If the patient is controlled on 0.5 mg of DHE, the dose is continued every 8 hours. If nausea persists, the next dose of DHE can be reduced to 0.25 mg. DHE is tapered and discontinued if the patient is headache free or fails to respond to the medication.

Neuroleptic therapy. Controlled studies have shown that intravenous chlorpromazine (Bell et al., 1990; Lane and Ross, 1985; Lane et al., 1989) and prochlorperazine (Callaham and Raskin, 1986; Jones et al., 1989) are effective in controlling intractable headache. Chlorpromazine (0.1 mg/kg repeated up to three times) was more effective than the combination of meperidine and dimenhydrinate. Callaham and Raskin (1986) found that 5 mg prochlorperazine IV was

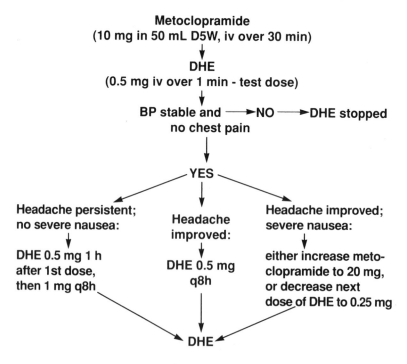

Figure 5–2. Protocol for the use of repeated intravenous DHE.

effective in treating emergency room patients. Jones et al. (1989) found that 10 mg prochlorperazine IV was more effective than placebo in treating emergency room patients. Although neuroleptics are locally irritating when given IV, they are more effective than when given by suppository or IM.

Neuroleptics may be used as an adjunct treatment for nausea or as primary therapy. Neuroleptics can be administered orally, rectally, IM, or IV. The patient must be monitored carefully for hypotension and sedation. Orthostatic hypotension can be avoided by maintaining the patient supine for several hours following neuroleptics.

Chlorpromazine (Thorazine) can be administered IV (10 to 25 mg three to four times per day) diluted in 20 to 30 ml of saline by rapid drip or "slow push" over several minutes. Chlorpromazine can also be administered IM or rectally.

Prochlorperazine (Compazine) can be administered intravenously 7.5 to 15 mg over 5 to 10 minutes via a saline drip or "slow push" (Callaham and Raskin, 1986; Jones et al., 1989).

Perphenazine (Trilafon; 5 mg IM), haloperidol (Haldol; 5 mg IM), and thiothixene (Navane; 5 mg IM) can also be used as primary or adjunct treatment for intractable migraine (Silberstein et al., 1990). Metoclopramide (10 mg IV or IM) can be used as an antiemetic.

Corticosteroids. Studies have suggested that corticosteroids are effective in the treatment of headache (Gallagher, 1986; Klapper and Stanton, 1991; Levine et al., 1987). One study demonstrates that dexamethasone given intravenously at a dose of 6 mg following pretreatment with intravenously administered metoclopramide is effective in the treatment of acute migraine headache (Klapper and Stanton, 1991). Another suggests that the addition of dexamethasone to a narcotic regimen provides added relief (Gallagher, 1986). Clinical experience also supports the view that oral steroids can assist in terminating an otherwise refractory migraine (Saper, 1989; Silberstein et al., 1990). High-dose intravenous steroids, alone or in conjunction with neuroleptics or DHE, can terminate a refractory headache cycle (Saper, 1990b; Silberstein et al., 1990).

Hydrocortisone can be given IV in the following manner: 100 mg via a saline "drip" over 10 minutes every 6 hours for 24 hours; every 8 hours for 24 hours; every 12 hours for 24 hours; and then a final dose.

Dexamethasone (Decadron) can be administered IV or IM, starting at a dose of 8 to 20 mg/day in divided doses, rapidly tapering over 2 to 3 days.

Parenteral narcotics and benzodiazepines. Raskin (1990c) suggested that morphine (4 mg) can be given by slow IV "push" during the first 24 hours of acute head pain. Diazepam (5 to 10 mg) given orally or parenterally with appropriate precautions has been used by some to help terminate an attack by inducing sleep (Wilkinson, 1988b; Zeigler, 1987).

Implementation of a Preventive Program

Most patients requiring this level of acute intervention will benefit from the simultaneous implementation of a preventive treatment program. On discharge, acute attacks of migraine subsequent to the termination of the intractable attack can be treated with standard symptomatic interventions, although avoidance of the previously overused agents is recommended in order to avoid recidivism and a recurrence of dependency.

Treating Emotional Problems or Substance Overuse

Although most authorities reject the belief that psychological factors represent the primary mechanism leading to the intractable state of severe headache, there is little doubt that behavioral disturbances, including cephalgiaphobia (fear of the next headache), depression, and acute emotional upset, contribute to the complexity of the syndrome and to its treatment. A behavioral therapeutic orientation and a problem-solving approach to these problems is recommended. It is not advisable to suggest to the patient that he or she experiences headaches "as a result" of these factors, because there is little evidence to suggest that this is true. The psychological disturbances noted in this population of patients may well be the consequence of a neuropsychiatric accompaniment to the migraine phenomenon, not its cause.

Patients with treatment-resistant headache who resort to excessive medication usage for pain control or to maintain functional status should not be stereotyped as, or confused with, those with a primary substance-abuse disorder. However, all patients overusing medication require education and counseling in proper medication usage. Some require more intensive formal programs.

Maintenance Therapy

Most patients with intractable (pernicious) migraine will require maintenance intervention and continuing care after acute treatment is completed. Ongoing and regularly scheduled medical visits, appropriate adjustment of medication, careful attention to the amount of symptomatic medication used, and general supportive and educational measures are all necessary. Recurring episodes of intractable migraine can occur despite otherwise appropriate treatment and may be an expected component of the pernicious form of migraine.

GENERAL PRINCIPLES OF PREVENTIVE THERAPY AND TREATMENT

Use of preventive medication should be considered when attacks occur at least three to four times a month; when symptomatic medications are contraindicated, overused, or ineffective; or when special circumstances exist (i.e., a headache attack is so disruptive that prevention is necessary). If preventive medication is indicated, it is best to start with a low dose, slowly increasing it and administering a full trial of 2 to 6 months. To obtain maximal benefit of preventive medication, the patient should not be taking interfering medications (such as vasodilators, estrogens, or oral contraceptives) or overusing analgesics or ergot derivatives. Migraine headache may improve with time independent of treatment; if the headaches are well controlled, consider a drug holiday after a slow taper program.

Currently, medication groups used for prophylactic migraine treatment include β-adrenergic blockers, antidepressants, calcium channel antagonists, serotonin antagonists, and anticonvulsants. It is believed that these groups all interact with serotonergic neural systems, by either binding to 5-HT$_2$ or 5-HT$_{1C}$ receptor sites, "down-regulating" the 5-HT$_2$ receptor, or modulating the discharge of serotonergic neurons (Peroutka, 1990a,b).

β-Adrenergic Blockers

The β blockers, the most widely used class of drugs in prophylactic migraine treatment, are 60 to 80% effective in producing a greater than 50% reduction in attack frequency. Rabkin et al. (1966) serendipitously discovered propranolol's effectiveness in headache treatment in patients who were being treated for angina. Many controlled studies (for review see Andersson and Vinge, 1990) have shown that propranolol, metoprolol, timolol, nadolol, and atenolol reduce the attack frequency in patients with migraine with and without aura (Diamond and Medina, 1976; Weber and Reinmuth, 1972).

Pindolol (Ekbom and Lundberg, 1972; Sjaastad and Stensrud, 1972), alprenolol (Ekbom, 1975), oxprenolol (Ekbom and Zetterman, 1977), and acebutolol (Nanda et al., 1978) have not been found to be effective migraine prophylaxis drugs. These drugs, which are partial agonists, exert intrinsic sympathomimetic activity, and this property may make them seem ineffective (Fanchamps, 1985). However, some studies fail to show propranolol's effectiveness (Holdorff et al., 1977). Because all of the negative studies are small and of low power, the possibility that beneficial effects have escaped detection cannot be excluded. In fact, pindolol (Anthony et al., 1972) and practolol (Sales and Bada, 1975) were found to be effective in open-label studies.

No absolute correlation has been found between propranolol's dose and its clinical efficacy (Andersson and Vinge, 1990). Pascual et al. (1989) reported that low-dose propranolol was effective in two thirds of their patients, but one third required high-dose propranolol, demonstrating individual patient variability.

A recent meta-analysis of 53 studies (2,403 treated patients) revealed that, on average, propranolol yielded a 44% reduction in migraine activity compared to a 14% reduction in migraine activity with placebo. Variations in propranolol dose levels across studies were unrelated to the magnitude of the propranolol treatment effect. Overall, one out of six patients discontinued propranolol treatment (Holroyd et al., 1991).

The relative efficacy of the different β blockers has not been clearly established, and most studies show no significant difference between drugs. Tfelt-Hansen et al. (1984) showed no difference between timolol and propranolol, and Sudilovsky et al. (1987) showed nadolol to be superior to propranolol. Gerber et al. (1991) found metoprolol to be more effective than propranolol; both β blockers were more effective at higher doses, and both were more effective than nifedipine, which was more effective than placebo. Propranolol is as effective as methysergide (Behan and Reid, 1980), clonidine, naproxyn (Andersson and Vinge, 1990), and amitriptyline (Zeigler et al., 1987). The choice of β blocker should be based on specific properties such as β_1 selectivity, convenience of drug formulation, and idiosyncratic drug effectiveness. Raskin (1988) believes that individual patient sensitivity may be relevant; therefore, before giving up on β blockers as a group it may be worthwhile to utilize combined or alternate trials.

The mechanism of action of β blockers is not certain, but it appears that their antimigraine effect is due to inhibition of β_1-mediated mechanisms (Ablad and Dahlof, 1986). Some have postulated that a membrane-stabilizing effect might be responsible for propranolol's effectiveness, because Stensrud and Sjaastad (1976) showed that d-propranolol (which is not a β blocker) was effective in migraine prophylaxis. Tfelt-Hansen (1986) reanalyzed their data using conventional statistical methodology and could not demonstrate any effect for d-propranolol, suggesting that the effect of propranolol is due to β blockade.

β Blockade results in inhibition of norepinephrine release by blocking prejunctional β receptors. In addition, it results in a delayed reduction in tyrosine hydroxylase activity (the rate-limiting step in norepinephrine synthesis) in the superior cervical ganglia. In the brainstem, a delayed reduction of locus ceruleus neuron firing rate has been demonstrated in the rat after propranolol administration (Ablad and Dahlof, 1980). This could explain the delay in the prophylactic effect of the β blockers.

The action of β blockers most likely is central and could be mediated by: (1) inhibiting central β receptors, interfering with the vigilance-enhancing adrenergic pathway; (2) interacting with 5-HT receptors (but not all β blockers bind to the 5-HT receptors); and (3) cross-modulation of the serotonin system (Koella, 1985; Silberstein and Silberstein, 1990).

Schoenen et al. (1986) have shown that contingent negative variation (CNV), an event-related slow negative scalp potential, is significantly increased and its habituation reduced in patients with untreated common migraine. CNV normalizes after treatment with β blockers, consistent with central adrenergic hyperactivity in migraine. Migraineurs with elevated CNV scores have a much better response to β blocker therapy (80% effective) than migraineurs with a low or normal score (22% effective), suggesting that the CNV may predict the response to β blocker treatment (Schoenen et al., 1986).

Migraineurs exhibit an enhanced centrally mediated secretion of epinephrine after exposure to light (Stoica and Enulescu, 1990); this returns to normal after treatment with propranolol.

β Blockers clinically useful in the treatment of migraine consist of both the nonselective blocking agents (propranolol, nadolol, and timolol) and the selective β_1 blockers (metoprolol and atenolol).

All β blockers can produce behavioral side effects such as drowsiness, fatigue, lethargy, sleep disorders, nightmares, depression, memory disturbance, and hallucinations, indicating that they all affect the CNS. In animals, β blockers reduce spontaneous motor activity, counteract amphetamine-induced hyperactivity, and produce slow-wave and paradoxical sleep disturbances. The central effect of β blockers is used to treat anxiety (Koella, 1985). Common side effects include gastrointestinal complaints and decreased exercise tolerance. Less common are orthostatic hypotension, significant bradycardia, impotence, and aggravation of intrinsic muscle disease. Propranolol has been reported to have an adverse effect on the fetus (Featherstone, 1983a). Congestive heart failure, asthma, and insulin-dependent diabetes are contraindications to the use of nonselective β blockers.

Case reports (Bardwell and Trott, 1987; Gilbert, 1982; Kumar and Cooney, 1990; Prendes, 1980) have suggested that propranolol might be implicated in the development of migrainous infarction or in increasing visual symptoms in patients with migraine with aura. However, Kangasniemi et al. (1987), in a double-blind, placebo-controlled study, found that metoprolol was clearly effective in prophylaxis of migraine with aura. Hedman et al. (1988) looked at the modification of the aura symptoms by metoprolol. During metoprolol treatment there were fewer migraine attacks, and those that occurred were less severe. There was no change in the total visual and nonvisual aura symptoms, but scintillations and paresthesias were more common and speech disturbances were less frequent. At this time it appears that β blockers are not absolutely contraindicated in migraine with aura unless a clear stroke risk is present. The reported adverse reactions to propranolol may be either coincidental or idiosyncratic, but the actual risk is uncertain.

Treatment with β blockers must be individualized following the principles of prophylactic therapy. If the first β blocker is ineffective or has significant side effects, it may be worthwhile to try a second β blocker. Some authors have commented on continued improvement (Rosen, 1983) and lack of rebound after discontinuation of propranolol (Diamond et al., 1982). However, it seems more reasonable to slowly taper β blockers, because abruptly stopping them can cause increased headache (Kangasniemi et al., 1987) and the withdrawal symptoms of tachycardia and tremulousness (Frishman, 1987).

Propranolol (*Inderal*) is a nonselective β blocker with a half-life of 4 to 6 hours, also available in an effective long-acting formulation (Inderal LA) (Diamond et al., 1987; Pradalier et al., 1989). The therapeutically effective dose of propranolol ranges from 40 to 400 mg/day, with no correlation between propranolol and 4-hydroxypropranolol plasma levels and headache relief (Cortelli et al., 1985). The short-acting form can be given three to four times a day and the long-acting form once or twice a day (we recommend twice a day). The patient should start with Inderal 60 LA, 40 mg/day in divided doses, and slowly increase to tolerance.

Nadolol (*Corgard*) is a nonselective β blocker with a long half-life. It is less lipid soluble than propranolol and has fewer CNS side effects. The dose ranges from 20 to 160 mg/day given once daily or in split doses. Some authorities prefer nadolol to propranolol because it has fewer side effects (Sudilovsky et al., 1987).

Timolol (*Blocadren*) is a nonselective β blocker with a short half-life. The dose ranges from 20 to 60 mg/day in divided doses.

Atenolol (*Tenormin*) is a selective β_1 blocker with fewer side effects than propranolol. The dose ranges from 50 to 200 mg/day once daily.

Metoprolol (*Lopressor*) is a selective β_1 blocker with a short half-life. The dose ranges from 100 to 200 mg/day in divided doses.

Antidepressants

Tricyclic antidepressants (TCAs) and atypical antidepressants (AAs) (fluoxetine, trazadone) increase the availability of synaptic norepinephrine or 5-HT by inhibiting high-affinity reuptake. Monoamine oxidase inhibitors (MAOIs) block the degradation of the catecholamines. Some antidepressants are more potent inhibitors of norepinephrine, and others of 5-HT, reuptake. The therapeutic action of antidepressant treatment was initially believed to be a consequence of increased synaptic norepinephrine and 5-HT. However, this hypothesis does not account for the temporal discrepancy between the rapid drug-induced effects on amine uptake, which occur within hours; the antidepressant effects, which take 2 to 3 weeks; and prophylactic headache response, which takes 3 to 10 days. In addition, reuptake inhibitors such as amphetamine or cocaine are not effective antidepressants or prophylactic headache drugs (Heninger and Charney, 1987).

The most consistent neurochemical finding with antidepressant treatment (including the TCAs, AAs, MAOIs, and electroconvulsive therapy) is a decrease in β-adrenergic receptor density and norepinephrine-stimulated cyclic adenosine monophosphate response. Increased α_1 receptor system sensitivity is not seen as consistently with antidepressant treatment. Long-term antidepressant treatment decreases 5-HT_2 receptor binding and imipramine-binding sites (related to the 5-HT uptake system) but does not change 5-HT_1 receptor binding. A strong interaction exists between the norepinephrine and 5-HT systems. Antidepressant treatment β receptor down-regulation is dependent on an intact 5-HT system, and lesions of the norepinephrine system block the decrease in 5-HT_2 receptor binding (Heninger and Charney, 1987).

The decrease in 5-HT_2 receptor binding sites does not correlate with a decrease in function; in fact, there may be enhanced physiologic responsiveness. If one records the electrical activity of neurons following the iontophoretic application of 5-HT, one finds the response is enhanced following antidepressant treatment, suggesting that an enhancement of the second messenger system has occurred. In addition, antidepressant treatment decreases the sensitivity of the presynaptic 5-HT autoreceptors, thereby enhancing 5-HT release (Heninger and Charney, 1987).

TCA up-regulates the γ-aminobutyric acid (GABA) B receptor, down-regulates the histamine receptor, and enhances the neuronal sensitivity to substance P. Some TCAs are 5-HT_2 receptor antagonists.

The mechanism of headache prophylaxis with antidepressant treatment (TCAs, AAs, and MAOIs) is uncertain but does not result from treating masked depression. Antidepressants are useful in treating many chronic pain states (Mendel et al., 1986), including headache independent of the presence of depression, and the response occurs sooner than the expected antidepressant effect (Couch et al., 1976; Kishore-Kumar et al., 1990; Panerai et al., 1990). (Most clinical studies have concentrated on pain and headache other than migraine.) In animal pain models, antidepressants potentiate the effects of coadministered narcotics (Feinmann, 1985). The clinically effective antidepressants in headache prophylaxis either inhibit 5-HT reuptake or are antagonists at the 5-HT_2 receptors (Richelson, 1990).

The TCAs most commonly used for migraine (and tension-type) headache prophylaxis include amitriptyline, nortriptyline, doxepin, and protriptyline. Most TCAs have not been vigorously evaluated in migraine prophylaxis; their use is based on anecdotal or uncontrolled reports (Raskin, 1988). Couch et al. (1976) found amitriptyline to be effective in an open study. Zeigler et al. (1987), in a placebo-controlled, double-blind crossover study, found amitriptyline as effective as propranolol and superior to placebo; this benefit was independent of depression. Although Pies (1983) found trazodone, an atypical non-TCA that is a highly selective 5-HT reuptake inhibitor, to be effective in a patient with features of both migraine and tension-type headache, most investigators, including ourselves, rarely find it effective. Trazodone is metabolized to m-chlorophenylpiperazone (m-CPP), a known migraine precipitant, perhaps by being a 5-HT_{1C} receptor agonist (Brewerton et al., 1988). Plasma levels of m-CPP in patients on trazodone are 40% that of the parent drug (Curzon et al., 1990).

Fluoxetine, a new, atypical, non-TCA, is a potent specific 5-HT uptake inhibitor with minimal antihistaminic and antimuscarinic activity. Fluoxetine has fewer anticholinergic side effects than the TCAs. It produces less weight gain and even, in some cases, weight loss. It has fewer cardiovascular side effects than the TCAs (Abramowicz, 1990a). Anecdotal reports (Markley et al., 1991), a small placebo-controlled study (Adly et al., 1992), and our experience seem to indicate its benefit in migraine prophylaxis. Some researchers have reported that fluoxetine does not improve or may worsen headache (Solomon and Kunkel, 1990). A larger placebo-controlled, double-blind study of fluoxetine is underway.

Pharmacology of the TCAs
There is wide individual variation in the absorption, distribution, and excretion of the TCAs, with a 10- to 30-fold variation in individuals' drug metabolism. A therapeutic window may exist above which the TCAs are ineffective, but this has been evaluated only for nortriptyline treatment of depression. The presence of a therapeutic window and the wide variation in TCA metabolism necessitates individualized dosing and monitoring of TCA plasma levels. TCAs are lipid soluble, with a high volume of distribution, and avidly bind to plasma proteins. The antihistamine and antimuscarinic activity of the TCAs accounts for many of their side effects (Richardson and Richelson, 1984).

Principles of TCA and AA Use.
The patient should be started on a low dose of the chosen TCA at bedtime. If the TCA is too sedating, the patient can be switched from a tertiary TCA (amitriptyline, doxepin) to a secondary TCA (nortriptyline, protriptyline). If patients develop insomnia or nightmares, the TCA can be given in the morning. The TCA dose range is wide and must be individualized. Bipolar patients can become manic on antidepressants. Fluoxetine can be given as a single dose in the morning. It is less sedating than the TCAs, and some patients may require a hypnotic for sleep induction.

Side effects of TCAs are common. Most of these involve antimuscarinic effects and cerebral intoxication, but cardiac toxicity and orthostatic hypotension can occur. Antimuscarinic side effects include dry mouth, metallic taste, epigastric distress, constipation, dizziness, tachycardia, palpitations, blurred vision, and urinary retention. Paradoxically, excess sweating can also occur. Trazodone alone among the TCAs can cause priapism, and rarely amitriptyline will cause inappropriate secretion of antidiuretic hormone. Any antidepressant treatment may change depression to hypomania or frank mania (particularly in bipolar patients). Ten percent of patients may develop tremors, and confusion or delirium may occur, particularly in older patients who are more vulnerable to the muscarinic side effects. Antidepressant treatments may also reduce the seizure threshold (Baldessarini, 1990). TCAs should be used with caution in patients with glaucoma (Lieberman and Stoudemire, 1987).

Tertiary amines. Amitriptyline (Elavil, Endep) is a tertiary amine tricyclic that is sedating and has antimuscarinic activity. Patients with coexistent depression are more tolerant and require higher doses of amitriptyline. The dose ranges from 10 to 400 mg/day, starting at a dose of 10 to 25 mg at bedtime.

Doxepin (Sinequan, Adapin) is a sedating tertiary amine TCA. The dose ranges from 10 to 300 mg/day, starting at a dose of 10 mg at bedtime.

Secondary amines. Nortriptyline (Pamelor, Aventyl) is a secondary amine that is less sedating than amitriptyline. Nortriptyline is a major metabolite of amitriptyline. If insomnia develops the drug can be given earlier in the day or in divided doses. The dose ranges from 10 to 150 mg/day, starting at a dose of 10 to 25 mg at bedtime.

Protriptyline (Vivactil) is a secondary amine similar to nortriptyline. The dose ranges from 10 to 150 mg/day, starting at a dose of 10 mg a day.

Atypical antidepressants. Fluoxetine (Prozac) is an atypical antidepressant that is a specific serotonergic uptake inhibitor. Side effects in general are less than with the TCAs. The most common side effects associated with fluoxetine include anxiety, nervousness, insomnia, drowsiness, fatigue, tremor, sweating, anorexia, nausea, vomiting, and dizziness or lightheadedness. Headache was noted in 20.3% of patients on fluoxetine; however, it was also noted in 19.9% of patients on placebo (Barnhart, 1991a). The dose ranges from 10 to 60 mg/day, starting at a dose of 20 mg in the morning. The combination of fluoxetine and non-MAOI antidepressants can be beneficial in treating refractory depression (Weilburg et al., 1989) and, in our experience, resistant cases of migraine.

The other antidepressants—surmontil, imipramine, desipramine, ascendin, ludiomil, and buproprion—can be tried in resistant cases, particularly if complicated by depression.

Monoamine oxidase inhibitors. The MAOI phenelzine (Nardil), at a dose of 15 mg three times a day, was shown (in an open study) to be effective in 80% of 25 patients who were resistant to other forms of treatment (including cyproheptadine and methysergide) (Anthony and Lance, 1969). Many authorities find that phenelzine can be extremely effective in migraine prophylaxis when simpler treatments fail (Lance, 1986; Raskin, 1988).

MAO exists in two subtypes: MAO-A, which preferentially deaminates norepinephrine and 5-HT, and MAO-B, which preferentially deaminates dopamine. Phenelzine is a nonspecific inhibitor of MAO-A and -B. L-Deprenyl is a selective MAO-B inhibitor that may be effective in the treatment of Parkinson disease (Murphy et al., 1984).

The dose of Nardil ranges from 30 to 90 mg/day in divided doses. All patients on MAOI-A must be on a restricted diet and avoid the use of certain medications to prevent hypertensive crisis. Alcohol, foods with a high tyramine content (aged cheese, pickled fish, fermented sausage, avocados, bananas, pods of broad beans, chicken livers, Chinese food), meperidine, and sympathomimetics, including Midrin, must be avoided (Davidson et al., 1984; Raskin, 1988; Tollefson, 1983).

The most common side effects of MAOIs include insomnia, orthostatic hypotension, constipation, increased perspiration, weight gain, peripheral edema, and, less commonly, inhibition of ejaculation or reduced libido. Insomnia can be reduced by giving most of the medication early in the day. Hypertensive crisis may be avoided by having the patient take the MAOI 3 to 4 hours before or after eating or take the entire dose at bedtime as gut MAO activity rapidly returns to normal (Raskin, 1988). Sublingual nifedipine has been used to treat hypertensive crisis when it occurs in MAOI users (Clary and Schweitzer, 1987).

The MAOI and amitriptyline combination has been reported to be relatively safe and effective in the treatment of refractory depression when the two drugs are started concurrently (Lader, 1983; Raskin, 1983; Saper, 1989). Some headache experts have used this combination in the treatment of refractory migraine (Raskin, 1988; Saper, 1989). Combination therapy may decrease the risk of hypertensive crisis (Pare et al., 1982), but severe reactions, including hyperthermia, delirium, and seizures, have been reported (White and Simpson, 1984). The newer AAs such as fluoxetine must not be combined with an MAOI, since fatal outcome has been reported. One must wait 5 weeks after stopping fluoxetine before starting an MAOI, and 2 to 3 weeks after stopping an MAOI before starting fluoxetine.

Calcium Channel Blockers

The calcium antagonists are a group of chemically heterogeneous drugs developed as cardiovascular agents. There was no appreciation of their actions as calcium (Ca^{2+}) channel blockers until Fleckstein (1971) discovered that their actions could be reversed competitively by Ca^{2+}. The Ca^{2+} antagonists belong to four different chemical groups: dihydropyridines (nifedipine, nimodipine, nicardipine); phenylalkylamines (verapamil); benzothiazepines (diltiazem); and diphenylpiperazines (flunarazine) (Greenberg, 1986).

Ca^{2+}, in combination with a calcium-binding protein such as calmodulin or troponin, regulates many functions, including muscle contraction, neurotransmitter and hormone release, and enzyme activity. The extracellular concentration of Ca^{2+} is high; the intracellular concentration of free Ca^{2+} is 10,000-fold smaller. The concentration gradient is established by membrane pumps and the sequestering of free Ca^{2+} in the cell. When stimulated, the cell can open Ca^{2+} channels in the plasma membrane or release intracellular stores of Ca^{2+}. Ca^{2+} antagonist drugs principally interfere with the entry of Ca^{2+} through voltage-sensitive channels (Greenberg, 1987; Snyder and Reynolds, 1985).

Voltage-sensitive Ca^{2+} channels have been divided into three subtypes, termed L, N, and T, based on conductances and sensitivity to voltage. Only the L-type channel is sensitive to the commercially available Ca^{2+} channel blockers, many of which bind to separate distinct sites on the L channel. The dihydropyridines all bind to a common site and in addition may inhibit cyclic nucleotide phosphodiesterase. This dual capacity may contribute to their marked effect on vascular relaxation (Murad, 1990).

Ca^{2+} antagonist receptors in the brain are primarily associated with selected synaptic areas and not with blood vessels. Ca^{2+} antagonists block the release of 5-HT from brain slices stimulated with dihydropyridine Ca^{2+} agonists (Snyder and Reynolds, 1985). Intracerebral vessels appear to depend exclusively on extracellular Ca^{2+} to induce contraction. Nimodipine has been shown to be effective in preventing delayed spasm following subarachnoid hemorrhage, probably as a result of both neural and vascular influences (Peroutka, 1983).

The mechanism of action of the Ca^{2+} antagonists in migraine prophylaxis is uncertain. They were introduced into the treatment of migraine on the assumption that they prevent hypoxia of cerebral neurons, contraction of vascular smooth muscles, and inhibition of Ca^{2+}-dependent enzymes involved in prostaglandin formation. Perhaps it is their ability to block 5-HT release, interfere with neurovascular inflammation, or interfere with the initiation and propagation of spreading depression (flunarizine) that is critical (Wauquier et al., 1985).

Andersson and Vinge (1990) have reviewed the Ca^{2+} antagonists used to treat migraine. Flunarazine has the best documented efficacy, but adverse side effects may limit its usefulness. Available documentation for verapamil is promising, and that for nifedipine and diltiazem less so. The documentation for nimodipine is conflicting. In randomized controlled trials, Solomon et al. (1983) and Markley et al. (1984) found that verapamil reduced headache frequency and duration but not intensity. In an open study, Meyer et al. (1984) found verapamil effective in reducing the frequency of migraine with aura but not migraine without aura. These and two additional open studies were reviewed by Solomon (1989), who concluded that overall verapamil was of "benefit" in 79% of patients. Verapamil at a dose of 320 mg/day may be more effective than at a dose of 240 mg/day (Solomon, 1985, 1989).

Nifedipine reduced the frequency and severity of migraine in patients with Raynaud phenomenon, but could provoke migraine in women treated for dysmenorrhea (Sandahl et al., 1979). Jonsdottir et al. (1987) reported symptomatic improvement in 65% of patients with common migraine and in 77% of those with classic migraine. McArthur et al. (1989), in a placebo-controlled parallel study (24 patients treated for up to 12 weeks), found no benefit from nifedipine.

Side effects were frequent (54%) and included dizziness, edema, flushing, headache, and mental symptoms.

Diltiazem (60 to 90 mg four times a day) was effective in two small open studies (Riopelle and McCans, 1987; Smith and Schwartz, 1984). Nimodipine has been found by Gelmers (1983), Havanka-Kanniainen et al. (1985), and Stewart et al. (1988) to be effective in reducing the frequency and severity of migraine attacks. Ansell et al. (1988) found no benefit. The Migraine-Nimodipine European Study (MINES) multicenter trial found the drug to be ineffective in the treatment of migraine both with aura (MINES, 1989b) and without (MINES, 1989a). Because the placebo response rate in both studies was high, the effectiveness of nimodipine is still uncertain (Leone et al., 1990).

Flunarizine is not available in the United States. In many placebo-controlled studies, it has been shown to be more effective than placebo and as effective as pizotofen, propranolol, and metoprolol (Andersson and Vinge, 1990). Nicardipine, in a placebo-controlled, double-blind study, was shown to be effective in reducing headache frequency, duration, and intensity in 30 patients with migraine without aura (Bussone et al., 1987; Leandri et al., 1990).

Side effects of the Ca^{2+} antagonists are dependent on the drug, and include dizziness and headache (particularly with nifedipine), depression, vasomotor changes, tremor, gastrointestinal complaints (including constipation), peripheral edema, orthostatic hypotension, and bradycardia. Patients frequently report an initial increase in headache. Headache improvement frequently requires weeks of treatment (Meyer et al., 1985; Meyer and Hardenberg, 1983).

Verapamil (Calan, Isoptin) is available as a 40-, 80-, or 120-mg tablet or as a 120-, 180-, or 240-mg sustained-release preparation. The patient should be started at a dose of 80 mg two to three times a day with a maximum of 640 mg/day in divided doses. The sustained-release preparation of verapamil can be given once or twice a day, but unreliable absorption reduces reliability. The most common side effect is constipation; dizziness, nausea, hypotension, headache, and edema are less common. Bioavailability is 20%. The absorbed drug is tightly protein bound. Peak plasma levels occur in 5 hours; the half-life ranges from 2.5 to 7.5 hours (McGoon et al., 1982).

Diltiazem (Cardizem) is available in 30-, 60-, 90-, and 120-mg tablets. The patient should be started at a dose of 30 mg two to three times a day, with a maximal dose of 360 mg/day in divided doses. Side effects are infrequent: hypotension, antrioventricular block, and headaches are occasionally seen. Bioavailability is 50%; the drug is tightly protein bound.

Nifedipene (Procardia) is available in 10- or 20-mg capsules. The starting dose of 10 mg/day can be increased to a maximum of 120 mg/day in divided doses. Side effects are common, and include hypotension, headache, nausea, and vomiting. Bioavailability is 50%; almost all the drug is protein bound.

Nimodipine (Nimotop) is available in 30-mg capsules. The dose is 30 to 60 mg four times a day. Side effects are infrequent.

Flunarizine (Sibellium) is not available in the United States. The dose is 5 to 10 mg/day. The most prominent side effects include weight gain, somnolence, dry mouth, dizziness, hypotension, and occasional extrapyramidal reactions.

Anticonvulsants

Anticonvulsant medication has been recommended for migraine prophylaxis, particularly in childhood (Barlow, 1984; Prensky, 1987). Some researchers believe that anticonvulsants are more effective in children who have paroxysmal EEGs (Rapoport et al., 1989), but others believe they are effective regardless of the EEG (Prensky, 1987). All anticonvulsants except valproic acid and phenobarbital may interfere with the efficacy of the oral contraceptives (Coulam and Annagers, 1979; Hanston and Horn, 1985).

Phenobarbital

Barlow (1984) recommends phenobarbital for younger patients. Forsythe and Hockaday (1988) believe that double-blind trials are necessary to establish the efficacy of the antiepileptic drugs in view of their adverse effects on learning and behavior. In our experience, phenobarbital is a useful adjunct during detoxification from short-acting barbiturates (Saper, 1990a; Silberstein et al., 1990).

Phenytoin

Barlow (1984) believes phenytoin is effective in the treatment of childhood migraine, as do Prensky (1987) and Millichapp (1978). Raskin (1988) believes that there is a subpopulation of patients in whom it may be effective. Robbins (1989) reported a case of a patient with post-traumatic headache with scintillating scotoma that responded to phenytoin. We believe that phenytoin may be effective in some patients.

Carbamazepine

Carbamazepine was found to be effective in one study (Rompel and Bauermeister, 1970) but not another (Anthony et al., 1972). Carbamazepine and valproate are effective in the treatment of mania (Baldessarini, 1990). In our experience, carbamazepine (Tegretol), 600 to 1,200 mg/day (beginning at 100 mg twice a day), can be effective in the prophylactic treatment of migraine, particularly in those patients with coexisting mania or hypomania. Monitoring of plasma levels and white blood count is essential.

Valproic Acid

Valproic acid possesses anticonvulsant activity in a wide variety of experimental epilepsy models. Valproate at high concentrations increases GABA levels in synaptosomes, perhaps by inhibiting its degradation; enhances the postsynaptic response to GABA; and, at lower concentrations, increases potassium conductance, producing neuronal hyperpolarization. Valproate turns off the firing of the 5-HT neurons of the dorsal raphe, which are implicated in controlling head pain (Raskin, 1990b). Disordered GABA metabolism during migraine has been reported (Welch et al., 1975). Imbalance in the plasma concentrations of GABA, an inhibitory amino acid, and glutamic acid, an excitatory amino acid, has also been observed (Ferrari et al., 1990).

Recent studies suggest the efficacy of valproate in the prophylaxis of headache, including migraine. Sorensen (1988), in an open study, found divalproex sodium (600 mg daily) effective in patients with refractory migraine. Mathew (1990c) found it to benefit patients suffering from chronic daily headache (transformed migraine). Hering and Kuritzky (1992) found it effective in the treatment of migraine in a placebo-controlled, double-blind study of 29 patients, 86.2% of whom had a good result. No serious side effects were reported. Our clinical experience confirms the efficacy of valproate. A large multicentered double-blind, controlled study has confirmed its effectiveness (Saper et al., 1993).

Valproic acid is a simple eight-carbon, two-chain fatty acid with 80% bioavailability after oral administration. It is highly protein bound, with an elimination half-life between 8 and 17 hours. Side effects include sedation, hair loss, tremor, and changes in cognitive performance. Transient nausea, vomiting, and indigestion can occur. The most serious side effect is hepatotoxicity, which requires monitoring of liver function studies. Fatal hepatic dysfunction is a rare idiosyncratic reaction, most often seen in children with a severe seizure disorder and mental retardation (Dreifuss et al., 1987). Hyperammonemia can occur and is usually asymptomatic. Thrombocytopenia and coagulation abnormalities are rare (Rimmer and Richens, 1985).

Valproic acid (Depakene) is available as 250-mg capsules and as a syrup (250 mg/5 ml).

Divalproex sodium is a stable coordination complex composed of sodium valproate and valproic acid in a 1:1 molar ratio. Depakote is an enteric-coated form of divalproex sodium available as 125-, 250-, and 500-mg capsules and a sprinkle formulation. Starting with 500 to 750 mg/day in divided doses, the dose should be slowly increased while monitoring serum levels (the usual therapeutic level is from 50 to 100 mg/ml). The maximum recommended dose is 60 mg/kg/day. Liver function tests should be obtained before and periodically after initiating therapy, especially during the first 6 months (Penry and Dean, 1989).

Serotonin Antagonists

Methysergide

Methysergide (Sansert) is a semisynthetic ergot $5-HT_2$ receptor antagonist that displays affinity for the $5-HT_1$ receptor; its chronic administration blocks the development of neurogenic inflammation (Moskowitz, 1990). Methysergide is an effective migraine prophylactic drug in 60% or more of migraineurs (Curran and Lance, 1964; Curran et al., 1967); this benefit may be greater in patients with migraine with aura (Drummond, 1985).

Side effects of methysergide include transient muscle aching, claudication, abdominal distress, nausea, weight gain, and hallucinations. Frightening hallucinatory experiences after the first dose are not uncommon (Curran et al., 1967). Curran and Lance (1964) have treated leg claudication with vasodilators with some enhancement of methysergide's effectiveness, suggesting that its action on headache is not a result of vasoconstriction.

The major complication of methysergide is the rare (1:5,000) development of retroperitoneal, pulmonary, or endocardial fibrosis (Elkind et al., 1968; Graham, 1967; Buff et al., 1989). To prevent this complication, a medication-free interval of 3 to 4 weeks following each 5- to 6-month course of continuous treatment is recommended. However, Raskin (1988) believes that the fibrotic reaction is not dependent on dose or time but is idiosyncratic and that methysergide can be used continually if one takes the precautions of careful cardiac auscultation, semiannual or annual chest radiographs, and yearly abdominal computerized tomography scan with enhancement or magnetic resonance imaging. If methysergide is discontinued, it may be ineffective when restarted, but it may again be effective months or years later.

The dose ranges from 4 to 8 mg/day, starting at a dose of 1 to 2 mg/day; occasional patients require 14 mg/day (Raskin, 1988). Contraindications include coronary artery disease, peripheral vascular disease, cerebrovascular disease, hypertension, and pregnancy (Curran et al., 1967).

Ergonovine

Ergonovine is an ergot alkaloid 5-HT antagonist that may be an effective migraine preventive drug (Raskin, 1988). Gallagher (1989) found it useful in the treatment of menstrual migraine. Side effects are uncommon and include nausea, abdominal pain, and aching legs. The dose is 0.2 to 0.4 mg three to four times a day. Contraindications include Prinzmetal angina, peripheral vascular disease, asthma, and pregnancy.

Ergonovine is no longer commercially available. We have used *methylergonovine maleate* (*Methergine*), a principal metabolite of methysergide and a 5-HT antagonist, in place of ergonovine. The dose is 0.2 to 0.4 mg three to four times a day. Side effects and contraindications are the same as for ergonovine.

Cyproheptadine

Cyproheptadine, an antagonist at the $5-HT_2$, histamine H_1, and muscarinic cholinergic receptors, is widely used in the prophylactic treatment of migraine in children (Barlow, 1984; Forsythe and Hockaday, 1988; Raskin, 1988). Curran and Lance (1964) found cyproheptadine more effective than placebo but less effective than methysergide. Raskin (1988) believes it is an effective drug in adults.

Cyproheptadine (Periactin) is available as 4-mg tablets. The total dose ranges from 12 to 36 mg/day (given two to three times a day or at bedtime). Common side effects are sedation and weight gain; dry mouth, nausea, lightheadedness, ankle edema, aching legs, and diarrhea are less common. Cyproheptadine may inhibit growth in children (Smyth and Lazurus, 1974).

Pizotifen (*Sandomigran*), a $5-HT_2$ receptor antagonist structurally similar to cyproheptadine, is not available in the United States. Controlled and uncontrolled studies in Europe (reviewed by Peatfield, 1986) have shown this drug to be of benefit in 40 to 79% of patients. The usual dose is 3.0 mg at bedtime. Side effects include drowsiness and weight gain (Capildeo and Rose, 1982).

Miscellaneous Prophylactic Drugs

Clonidine

Clonidine is an imidazoline that activates α_2-adrenergic receptors. Clonidine inhibits the firing of locus ceruleus neurons (the major source of noradrenergic neurons) induced by opiate withdrawal by activating presynaptic inhibitory α_2

receptors. This is the basis of clonidine's clinical effectiveness in treating opiate (Aghajanian, 1978; Bakris et al., 1982), alcohol, and cigarette withdrawal (Baumgartner and Rowen, 1987) and in controlling menopausal hot flashes (Nagamani et al., 1987).

Clonidine's effectiveness in migraine treatment of adults and children is equivocal (Bredfeldt et al., 1989; Kallanranta et al., 1977; Ryan and Ryan, 1975; Sills et al., 1982; Hakkarainen et al., 1980). Raskin (1988) and Peatfield (1986) believe it is of no value. The clonidine patch may be a useful adjunct in detoxifying patients who are overusing analgesics or ergotamine (Dalessio, 1991).

Clonidine (Catapres) is available as 0.1-, 0.2-, and 0.3-mg tablets and as a patch delivering 0.1 mg (TTS #1), 0.2 mg (TTS #2), and 0.3 mg (TTS #3) per day. The dose ranges from 0.1 to 0.2 mg/day.

Calcitonin

Calcitonin is a single-chain polypeptide hypocalcemic hormone secreted by the thyroid gland. Salmon calcitonin (100 IU/day) is effective in treating pain, perhaps by increasing the circulating levels of β-endorphin, adrenocorticotropic hormone, and cortisol (Ustdal et al., 1989). Salmon calcitonin given IM (Gennari et al., 1986) or by nasal spray (Micieli et al., 1988) and an analogue of eel calcitonin given IM (Patti et al., 1987) are proposed as effective in migraine prophylaxis.

Captopril

Captopril (Capoten) is an angiotensin-converting enzyme (ACE) and enkephalinase inhibitor that also inhibits the breakdown of bradykinin. In an open study, Sicuteri (1981) found captopril effective in 11 of 11 hypertensive patients and in 12 of 24 normotensive patients, perhaps by inhibiting the degradation of enkephalins. Minervini and Pinto (1987), in a small double-blind study, found captopril more effective than placebo.

The total dose ranges from 25 to 150 mg given in divided doses two or three times a day. Side effects are uncommon and include proteinuria, hypotension, angioedema, skin rash, and loss of taste. Cough unresponsive to medication occurs in 5 to 20% of patients treated with ACE inhibitors (Abramowicz, 1991). Birth defects have been reported in children born to women using ACE inhibitors.

Papaverine

Papaverine, a vasodilator chemically related to verapamil, has been shown to be effective in a number of small series of patients (Poser, 1974; Raskin, 1988; Sillanpaa and Koponen, 1978; Vijayan, 1977). The total dose ranges from 300 to 600 mg/day. The drug is rapidly absorbed and well tolerated. Side effects include nausea, drowsiness, vertigo, and constipation. A rare eosinophilic hepatitis has been reported.

Lithium

Lithium is effective in the treatment of cluster headache. Based on the analogy to cluster, Medina (1982) found lithium carbonate effective in treating cyclic migraine, a disorder in which patients have bouts of migrainous headaches separated by headache-free periods. Lithium may be a particularly useful adjunctive medication in bipolar or manic patients. Side effects include hand tremor, polyuria, thirst, and ankle edema. Long-term complications include hypothyroidism, oliguric renal failure, and diabetes insipidus. The dose of lithium is 900 to 1,800 mg/day, titrated to give a serum level between 0.75 and 1.25 mg/liter. Combined use with verapamil can cause adverse responses (lithium toxicity) at standard doses. Doses of lithium must be substantially reduced when given with verapamil, even when the blood level is in the therapeutic range (Price and Giannini, 1986; Price and Shalley, 1987).

Feverfew

Feverfew (*Tanacetum parthenium*) is a medicinal herb used in self-treatment of migraine. A pilot study of 17 migraineurs who ate fresh feverfew leaves daily was undertaken at the City of London Migraine Clinic. Patients were given capsules of freeze-dried feverfew or placebo. Those receiving placebo had a tripling in the frequency of migraine attacks. Patients on placebo reported increased nervousness, tension headaches, insomnia, or joint stiffness constituting a "post-feverfew syndrome" (perhaps another example of rebound). Feverfew has side effects, including mouth ulceration and a more widespread oral inflammation with loss of taste. The mechanism of action of feverfew in migraine is uncertain. Feverfew is rich in sesquiterpene lactones, especially parthenolide, which may be a nonspecific norepinephrine, 5-HT, bradykinin, prostaglandin, and acetylcholine antagonist. The long-term safety and effectiveness and biologic variation in sesquiterpene lactone content of feverfew are of concern (Johnson et al., 1985).

Use of Symptomatic Agents for Migraine Prophylaxis

Aspirin

O'Neill and Mann (1979) and Masel et al. (1980), in double-blind studies, found that aspirin (650 mg/day) decreased headache frequency. In a double-blind trial of low-dose aspirin (325 mg every other day) in 22,071 U.S. male physicians (Physician Health Study), Buring et al. (1990) found a 20% reduction in headache frequency. Although this is statistically significant, it may not be clinically significant. Furthermore, daily aspirin use may lead to aspirin overuse and the development of rebound headaches. Aspirin in low doses clearly is indicated for the prophylaxis of myocardial infarction and transient ischemic attacks. We would use aspirin only in patients with prolonged or nonvisual aura, as part of a treatment program.

NSAIDs

Some NSAIDs may be effective in migraine prophylaxis. These include sodium naproxen, naproxin, fenoprofen, metoprofen, and tolfenamic acid (Pradalier et al., 1988). Some headache disorders (chronic paroxysmal hemicrania, hemicrania continua) are defined by their responsiveness to indomethacin (Bordini et al., 1991; Sjaastad and Dale, 1976; Sjaastad and Spierings, 1984). Although NSAIDs are effective, they must be used with caution because of their adverse effects on gastrointestinal and renal function.

Ergotamine

The prophylactic use of ergotamine is discouraged. The exception is in women with primarily menstrual migraine, who can use ergotamine at the time of vulnerability without the danger of developing rebound headache.

Dihydroergotamine

Some studies have shown that an oral programmed release form of DHE (DHE methanesulfonate, DHE retard) at a dose of 5 mg twice a day is effective in the prophylactic treatment of migraine (Centonze et al., 1983; Fontanari et al., 1983; Martucci et al., 1983; Mastrosimone and Iaccarino, 1983). DHE retard is not available in the United States.

SPECIAL SITUATIONS

Treatment of Menstrual Migraine

Sixty percent of women have attacks of migraine associated with menses, and 13% have their attacks exclusively with menses. The initial treatment should be the same as that for nonmenstrual migraine (Digre and Damasio, 1987; Edelson, 1985; Silberstein, 1984). Because menstrually related migraine typically occurs at the same time of month or in association with symptoms that herald its occurrence, increasing the dose of prophylactic medication perimenstrually or using intermittent prophylaxis may control these resistant menstrual headaches (Epstein et al., 1975; Raskin, 1988). Women who have migraine exclusively with their menses can be treated by the perimenstrual use of a combination of preventive or symptomatic medication (Silberstein and Merriam, 1991).

Popular but ineffective treatments include diuretics and vitamins. Diuretics help with fluid retention but not with menstrually related migraine (Lundberg, 1986; Reid and Yen, 1981). The efficacy of pyridoxine to treat both premenstrual syndrome (PMS) and menstrual migraine has not been established in double-blind studies (Hagen et al., 1985; Williams et al., 1985).

The inhibition of prostaglandin production, which may be enhanced in menstrual migraine, may account for the effectiveness of the NSAIDs (Chan, 1983; Vardi et al., 1979). NSAIDs are effective if given in adequate doses symptomatically or prophylactically 1 to 2 days before the expected onset of headache and continued for the duration of vulnerability (Robinson et al., 1977; Sargent et al., 1985). If the first NSAID is ineffective, other classes of NSAIDs should be tried (Table 5–5).

Ergotamine and its derivatives can be used preventively at the time of menses without significant risk of developing ergot dependence if not used frequently during other times of the month (Edelson, 1985; Raskin, 1988; Silberstein, 1984). Ergotamine tartrate, at bedtime or twice a day, is an effective prophylactic agent (Raskin, 1988). Ergotamine in combination with belladonna and phenobarbital (Bellergal) may be useful in treating both headache and PMS (Robinson et al., 1977). Ergonovine maleate (an ergot derivative) is no longer available; we use methylergonovine instead. It is effective when given perimenstrually, but this benefit may decrease with time (Gallagher, 1989). DHE (D'Alessandro et al., 1983; Facchinetti et al., 1983) given perimenstrually in slow-release oral forms was effective in 16 of 20 patients in one open study. DHE given IM or IV, or soon by nasal spray, may be extremely effective to prevent and/or terminate menstrual migraine (Silberstein et al., 1990).

If an attack of severe menstrual migraine cannot be controlled by the use of NSAIDs and ergots, analgesics in combination with narcotics may be used (Silberstein, 1984). If these do not terminate the attack, additional recommendations include corticosteroids, major tranquilizers (chlorpromazine, haloperidol, thiothixene), or a course of IV DHE (Silberstein et al., 1990).

Successful hormonal therapy of menstrual migraine has been reported using estrogens (DeLignieres et al., 1986), estrogen antagonists (Calton and Burnett, 1984), prolactin release inhibitors (Freeman et al., 1990), and estrogens in combination with progesterone or testosterone (Dalton, 1973). Progesterone alone (injection, pills, or suppositories) is not effective in the treatment of headache or other symptoms of PMS (Freeman et al., 1990), despite many favorable anecdotal reports (Bancroft and Backstrom, 1985; Dalton, 1973).

The decrease in estrogen levels during the late luteal phase of the menstrual cycle triggers migraine (Somerville, 1972b). Estrogen replacement prior to menstruation has been used to prevent migraine (Somerville, 1975). In a double-blind crossover study, DeLignieres et al. (1986) used percutaneous estradiol gel perimenstrually with significant (96.3% versus 30.8%) headache reduction. In a double-blind trial of percutaneous estradiol gel, Dennerstein et al. (1988) reported similar excellent results. Magos et al. (1983), in an open study and to a lesser extent in a double-blind study (Magos et al., 1986), found estradiol implants, only available investigationally in the United States, and cyclic progesterones to be effective in menstrual migraine.

Somerville (1975) attempted prophylaxis of menstrual migraine with estradiol implants. These implants did not produce stable plasma estrogen levels and caused severe menstrual disturbance, loss of periodicity of headaches, and unpredictable headache improvement. In contrast, the cutaneous gel (DeLignieres et al., 1986) and the estradiol implant used by Magos et al. (1986) provide stable blood estrogen levels. The estradiol cutaneous patch (Estraderm) provides a stable plasma estrogen level and has anecdotally been reported to be as effective as the gel or implants (Abramowicz, 1986; Judd, 1987).

Combinations of estrogens and progestogens in the form of oral contraceptives may be appropriate for some patients with intractable menstrual migraine, particularly when it is associated with severe dysmenorrhea (Kappius and Goolkasian, 1987). Raskin (1988) reported anecdotally that perimenstrual use of a synthetic oral estrogen (0.05 mg ethinylestradiol), in combination with an androgen (2 mg methyltestosterone), was effective in 22 of 36 patients.

Danazol, an androgen derivative, suppresses the pituitary–ovarian axis by binding to androgen and progestin receptors, and by inhibiting ovarian steroidogenesis. It may be effective in the prophylaxis of menstrual migraine when given at a dose of 200 to 600 mg/day, started before the expected onset of the headache and continued through the menses (Calton and Burnett, 1984; Powles, 1986;

Table 5–6 Treatment of menstrual migraine

1. Nonsteroidal anti-inflammatory drugs (NSAIDs)
2. Ergotamine and its derivatives
3. Perimenstrual use of standard prophylactic drugs
4. Short course of corticosteroids or major tranquilizers
5. Hormonal therapy
   Estrogens (with or without androgens or progestogen)
   Synthetic androgens (Danazol)
   Antiestrogen (Tamoxifen)
   Dopamine agonists (Bromocriptine)

Sarno et al., 1987). Increased headache has been reported after the first dose, and the development of pseudotumor cerebri has been reported (Saper, 1987a).

Tamoxifen (Nolvadex) (O'Dea and Davis, 1990; Wentz, 1985), an antiestrogen, may be effective in resistant menstrual migraine. Tamoxifen binds to a cytosol estrogen receptor. Its long-acting nuclear retention time results in estrogen antagonism by down-regulation of an estrogen receptor and inhibition of messenger RNA transcription. A dose of 5 to 15 mg/day for days 7 to 14 of the luteal cycle has given significant relief of menstrual headache without side effects.

Bromocriptine (Parlodel) (Andersch et al., 1978; Andersen et al., 1977; Ylostalo et al., 1982), a dopamine D_2 receptor agonist, is an inhibitor of prolactin release. A dose of 2.5 to 5 mg/day during the luteal phase of the menstrual cycle may decrease the premenstrual symptoms of breast engorgement, irritability, and headache.

The sequential approach to the treatment of menstrual migraine appears in Table 5–6.

Menopausal Migraine

The normal menopause results from depletion of ovarian follicles that can be stimulated to ovulate. Plasma sex steroid hormone levels are low, and gonadotropin levels are elevated. The postmenopausal period is associated with both early and late symptoms (Utian, 1987a, 1987b). Hot flushes, a vasomotor change, correlate with bursts of activity in hypothalamic pacemaker neurons, leading to pulses of luteinizing hormone (Ravnikar, 1990; Rebar and Spitzer, 1987). Hormonal replacement with estrogens alone or in combination with progestins is often used to treat symptoms and prevent osteoporosis (Shoemaker et al., 1977).

Headache management can be difficult in women who require estrogen replacement therapy for menopausal symptoms but develop headaches as a result of the therapy. Several empirical strategies may be utilized. Reducing the dose of estrogen or changing the type of estrogen from a conjugated estrogen to pure estradiol, synthetic ethinyl estradiol, or a pure estrone may significantly reduce headache. Aylward et al. (1974), in a controlled, double-blind crossover trial of menopausal women, found that oral estropipate decreased the frequency and intensity of headache, whereas ethinyl estradiol increased headache.

Changing from interrupted to continuous administration may be very effective if the headaches are associated with estrogen withdrawal. These techniques may be combined. Kudrow (1975) reported a 58% improvement in headache control through a reduced, continuous dose of estrogen.

Parenteral estrogens, with or without adjunct hormones, can be effective. Greenblatt and Bruneteau (1974), who studied postmenopausal women with oral estrogen–induced headache, found their headache could be improved by switching from oral to parenteral estrogens (estradiol) and adding androgens (testosterone). The estradiol cutaneous patch (Estraderm), which provides a physiologic ratio of estradiol to estrone and a steady state concentration of estrogen, anecdotally has been associated with fewer headache side effects, but this has not been proven in any controlled study (Abramowicz, 1986; Judd, 1987). We recommend concurrent gynecologic consultation with all hormonal manipulations.

Treatment of Headache in Children

Treatment should begin by reassuring the family that the child has a benign condition that will most likely improve within 6 months independent of treatment. The child should have a regular bedtime and a reasonable meal schedule, and an activity overload should be avoided (Silberstein, 1990). Provoking factors should be identified and eliminated. Biofeedback and relaxation, either alone or as an adjunct to pharmacotherapy, are perhaps more effective in children than adults (Labbe, 1988).

Pharmacologic treatment begins with simple analgesics. Because of the risk of Reye syndrome, if there is any suspicion of systemic illness in children younger than 15, acetaminophen is the drug of choice (Forsythe and Hockaday, 1988; Silberstein, 1984). Guidelines for the use of combination analgesics are the same as those for adults, with modification of the dose based on age and weight.

Ergot derivatives are usually not recommended for younger children (Congdon and Forsythe, 1979; Forsythe and Hockaday, 1988). However, many pediatric neurologists are now using DHE alone or with metoclopramide or promethazine to treat intractable headache in children and adolescents. Linder (1991) has treated patients between the ages of 6 and 16 with IV DHE and promethazine, and reported an 80% success rate. Treatment of adolescents with IV DHE and metoclopramide achieved a success rate of 90% (Silberstein et al., 1990).

The decision to use preventive (prophylactic) therapy is influenced by the frequency, duration, and intensity of the migraine attacks and the response to simple analgesics. Severe, frequent attacks, especially if complicated by neurologic symptoms, warrant preventive treatment. Since migraine in children has a high remission rate, tapering preventive medication and giving the child a drug holiday should be considered if he or she has been in remission for 3 or more months (Barlow, 1984).

The basis of preventive medication use in children is mainly empiric (Bille et al., 1977). There are few well-controlled, double-blind preventive medication studies in children, and the results are frequently contradictory (Barlow, 1984; Forsythe and Hockaday, 1988; Hanson, 1988). The same preventive medications are used in children as in adults. The most commonly used medications, based on anecdotal report, include phenytoin (Raskin, 1988), propranolol (Forsythe et al., 1984; Ludvigsson, 1974; Olness et al., 1987), amitriptyline (Noronha, 1985; Sorge et al., 1982), and cyproheptadine, which is safe, can be given at bedtime, and may be more effective in younger children (Barlow, 1984; Lavenstein, 1991). All should be used with caution. One TCA (desipramine) has been reported to cause sudden death in children (Abramowicz, 1990b).

Treating Migraine during Pregnancy

Ideally, no pharmacotherapy should be administered during pregnancy. Patients should be informed that the headache will probably terminate during and after the second trimester, and the best course to follow is to try to bear the discomfort until then. However, because of the intractable nature of the symptoms and the possible accompanying dehydration and prostration, which may themselves produce a risk factor, it is sometimes necessary for medications to be administered.

There are no studies that establish the safety of any agent, although clinical experience suggests some are relatively safe. For occasional, periodic headache, many clinicians rely on acetaminophen with codeine or codeine alone. Increased frequency of headaches may provide justification for prophylaxis. β-Adrenergic blockers, such as propranolol or others (Rayburn and Lavin, 1986), can be used if absolutely necessary, although adverse effects have been reported (Featherstone, 1983a).

Severe, acute attacks that warrant parenteral therapy should be treated in a hospital. IV fluids and other conservative measures, such as ice applications, may be sufficient. A narcotic can be used in a limited fashion for severe pain.

It is advisable, even when these modest measures are taken, but particularly if the condition warrants more aggressive pharmacotherapy, that the patient and spouse be properly informed that the use of drugs during pregnancy poses risks that may range from fetal deformity to fetal and even maternal death. The use of such drugs has a possible justification, but the decision is not that of the physician alone. Written consent and acknowledgment (informed consent) by both the patient and spouse is necessary. It is advisable that treatment not proceed without this written arrangement, which fully delineates the justification and risks inherent in such treatment.

REFERENCES

Ablad, B. and C. Dahlof (1986). Migraine and β-blockade: Modulation of sympathetic neurotransmission. *Cephalalgia* 6(Suppl. 5):7–13.

Abramowicz, M. (ed.) (1986). Transdermal estrogen. *Med. Lett. Drugs Ther.* 28: 119–120.

Abramowicz, M. (ed.) (1990a). Fluoxetine (Prozac) revisited. *Med. Lett. Drugs Ther.* *32*:83–85.

Abramowicz, M. (1990b). Sudden death in children treated with a tricyclic antidepressant. *Med. Lett. Drugs Ther. 32*:53.

Abramowicz, M. (ed.) (1991). Drugs for hypertension. *Med. Lett. Drugs Ther. 33*:33–38.

Adly, C., J. Straumanis and A. Chesson (1992). Fluoxetine prophylaxis of migraine. *Headache 32*:101–104.

Aellig, W.H. (1984). Investigation of the venoconstrictor effect of 8' hydroxydihydroergotamine, the main metabolite of dihydroergotamine, in man. *Eur. J. Clin. Pharmacol. 26*:239–242.

Aghajanian, G.K. (1978). Tolerance of locus coeruleus neurones to morphine and suppression of withdrawal response by clonidine. *Nature 276*:186–188.

Albibi, R. and R.W. McCallum (1983). Metoclopramide: Pharmacology and clinical application. *Ann. Intern. Med. 98*:86–95.

Alvarez, W.C. (1934). The present day treatment of migraine. *Mayo Clin. Proc. 9*:22.

Alvarez, W.C. (1940). Can one cure migraine in women by inducing menopause? Report on forty-two cases. *Mayo Clin. Proc. 15*:380–382.

American Psychiatric Association (1987). *Diagnostic and Statistical Manual of Mental Disorders,* 3rd ed., rev. American Psychiatric Press, Inc., Washington, DC.

Amery, W.K., J. Waelkens, and I. Caers (1986a). Dopaminergic mechanisms in premonitory phenomena. In *The Prelude to the Migraine Attack* (W.K. Amery and A. Wauquier, eds.), pp. 64–77. Bailliere Tindall, London.

Amery, W.K., J. Waelkens, and V. Van den Bergh (1986b). Migraine warnings. *Headache 26*:60–66.

Andermann, F. (1987). Clinical features of migraine-epilepsy syndrome. In *Migraine and Epilepsy* (F. Andermann and E. Lugaresi, eds.), pp. 3–30. Butterworth, Boston.

Andersch, B., L. Hahn, C. Wendestam et al. (1978). Treatment of premenstrual syndrome with bromocriptine. *Acta Endocrinol. 88*(Suppl 216):165–174.

Andersen, A.N., J.F. Larsen, O.R. Steenstrup et al. (1977). Effect of bromocriptine on the premenstrual syndrome. A double-blind clinical trial. *Br. J. Obstet. Gynaecol. 84*:370–374.

Andersen, A.R., P. Tfelt-Hansen, and N.A. Lassen (1987). The effect of ergotamine and dihydroergotamine on cerebral blood flow in man. *Stroke 18*:120–123.

Andersson, K. and E. Vinge (1990). β-adrenoceptor blockers and calcium antagonists in the prophylaxis and treatment of migraine. *Drugs 39*(3):355–373.

Andersson, P.G. (1988). Ergotism—the clinical picture. In *Drug-Induced Headache* (H.C. Diener and M. Wilkinson, eds.), pp. 16–19. Springer-Verlag, Berlin.

Ansell, E., T. Fazzone, R. Festenstein et al. (1988). Nimodipine in migraine prophylaxis. *Cephalalgia 8*:269–272.

Anthony, M. and J.W. Lance (1969). Monoamine oxidase inhibition in the treatment of migraine. *Arch. Neurol. 21*:263–268.

Anthony, M., J.W. Lance, and B. Somerville (1972). A comparative trial of prindolol, clonidine and carbamazepine in the interval therapy of migraine. *Med. J. Aust. 6*:1343–1346.

Aylward, M., F. Holly, and R.J. Parker (1974). An evaluation of clinical response to piperazine oestrone sulphate (''Harmogen'') in menopausal patients. *Curr. Med. Res. Opin. 2*:417–423.

Bakris, G.L., P.D. Cross, and J.E. Hammarstein (1982). The use of clonidine for the management of opiate abstinence in a chronic pain patient. *Mayo Clin. Proc. 57*: 657–660.

Baldessarini, R.J. (1990). Drugs and the treatment of psychiatric disorders. In *Goodman and Gilman's The Pharmacological Basis of Therapeutics,* 8th ed. (A.G. Gilman, T.W. Rall, A.S. Nies, and P. Taylor, eds.), pp. 383–435. Pergamon Press, New York.

Bancroft, J. and T. Backstrom (1985). Premenstrual syndrome. *Clin. Endocrinol. (Oxf.)* 22:313–336.

Bardwell, A. and J. Trott (1987). Stroke in migraine as a consequence of propranolol. *Headache 27:*381–383.

Barlow, C.F. (1984). *Headaches and Migraine in Children.* Lippincott, Philadelphia.

Barnhart, E.R. (ed.) (1991a). *Physicians' Desk Reference,* 45th ed. Medical Economics Inc., Oradell, NJ.

Barnhart, E.R. (ed.) (1991b). *Physicians' Desk Reference for Nonprescription Drugs,* 12th ed. Medical Economics, Inc., Oradell, NJ.

Baumgartner, C., P. Wessely, C. Bingol et al. (1989). Longterm prognosis of analgesic withdrawal in patients with drug-induced headaches. *Headache 29:*510–514.

Baumgartner, G.R. and R.C. Rowen (1987). Clonidine vs chlordiazepoxide in the management of acute alcohol withdrawal syndrome. *Arch. Intern. Med. 147:* 1223–1226.

Bayless, T.M., B. Rothfeld, C. Massa et al. (1975). Lactose and milk intolerance: Clinical implications. *N. Engl. J. Med. 292:*1156–1159.

Beaver, W.T. (1984). Combination analgesics. *Am. J. Med. 77:*38–53.

Behan, P.O. and M. Reid (1980). Propanalol in the treatment of migraine. *Practitioner 224:*201–204.

Belgrade, M.J., L.J. Ling, M.B. Schleevogt et al. (1989). Comparison of single-dose meperidine, butorphanol, and dihydroergotamine in the treatment of vascular headache. *Neurology 39:*590–592.

Bell, R., D. Montoya, A. Snualb, and M.A. Lee (1990). A comparative trial of three agents in the treatment of acute migraine headache. *Ann. Emerg. Med. 19:* 1079–1082.

Berde, B. and E. Stuermer (1978). Introduction to the pharmacology of ergot alkaloids and related compounds as a basis of their therapeutic application. In *Ergot Alkaloids and Related Compounds* (B. Berde and H.O. Schild, eds.), pp. 1–28. Springer-Verlag, Berlin.

Bickerstaff, E.R. (1975). *Neurological Complications of Oral Contraceptives.* Clarendon Press, Oxford.

Bickerstaff, E.R. (1987). Migraine variants and complications. In *Migraine: Clinical and Research Aspects* (J.N. Blau, ed.), pp. 55–75. Johns Hopkins University Press, Baltimore.

Bille, B. (1962). Migraine in school children. *Acta Pediatr. 51*(Suppl. 136):13–147.

Bille, B. (1989). Migraine in children: Prevalence, clinical features and a 30-year followup. In *Migraine and Other Headaches* (M.D. Ferrari and X. Lataste, eds.), pp. 29–38. Parthenon, Park Ridge, NJ.

Bille, B., J. Ludvigsson, and G. Sanner (1977). Prophylaxis of migraine in children. *Headache 17:*61–63.

Bix, K.J., D.J. Pearson, and S.J. Bentley (1984). A psychiatric study of patients with supposed food allergy. *Br. J. Psychiatry 145:*121–126.

Blau, J.N. (1980). Migraine prodromes separated from the aura: Complete migraine. *BMJ 281:*658–660.

Blau, J.N. (1982). Resolution of migraine attacks: Sleep and the recovery phase. *J. Neurol. Neurosurg. Psychiatry 45:*223–226.

Blau, J.N. (1984). Migraine pathogenesis: The neural hypothesis reexamined. *J. Neurol. Neurosurg. Psychiatry 47:*437–442.

Blau, J.N. (1987). Adult migraine: The patient observed. In *Migraine: Clinical and Research Aspects* (J.N. Blau, ed.), pp. 3–30. Johns Hopkins University Press, Baltimore.

Bordini, C., F. Antonaci, L.J. Stovner et al. (1991). "Hemicrania continua": A clinical review. *Headache 31:*20–26.

Boyle, R., P.O. Behan, and J.A. Sutton (1990). A correlation between severity of migraine and delayed emptying measured by an epigastric impedance method. *Br. J. Clin. Pharmacol. 30:*405–409.

Bradshaw, P. and M. Parsons (1965). Hemiplegic migraine, a clinical study. *Q.J. Med. 133:*65–85.

Bredfeldt, R.C., J.E. Sutherland, and J.E. Kruse (1989). Efficacy of transdermal clonidine for headache prophylaxis and reduction of narcotic use in migraine patients. A randomized crossover trial. *J. Fam. Pract. 29:*153–156.

Brewerton, T.D., D.L. Murphy, E.A. Mueller, and D.C. Jimerson (1988). Induction of migrainelike headaches by the serotonin agonist *m*-chlorophenylpiperazine. *Clin. Pharmacol. Ther. 43:*605–609.

Brooks, P.M. and R.O. Day (1991). Nonsteroidal antiinflammatory drugs—differences and similarities. *N. Engl. J. Med. 324:*1716–1725.

Buff, D.D., M.B. Bogin, and L.L. Faltz (1989). Retroperitoneal fibrosis: A report of selected cases and a review of the literature. *N.Y. State J. Med. 9:*511–516.

Buring, J.E., R. Peto, and C.H. Hennekens (1990). Low-dose aspirin for migraine prophylaxis. *JAMA 264:*1711–1713.

Bussone, G., S. Baldini, G. D'Andrea et al. (1987). Nimodipine versus flunarizine in common migraine: A controlled pilot trial. *Headache 27:*76–79.

Buzzi, M.G. and M.A. Moskowitz (1990). The antimigraine drug, sumatriptan (GR43175), selectively blocks neurogenic plasma extravasation from blood vessels in dura mater. *Br. J. Pharmacol. 99:*202–206.

Cady, R.K., J.K. Wendt, J.R. Kirchner et al. (1991). Treatment of acute migraine with subcutaneous sumatriptan. *JAMA 265:*2831–2835.

Caers, L.I., F. DeBeukelaar, and W.K. Amery (1987). Flunarizine, a calcium-entry blocker, in childhood migraine, epilepsy, and alternating hemiplegia. *Clin. Neuropharmacol. 10:*162–168.

Callaham, M., and N. Raskin (1986). A controlled study of dihydroergotamine in the treatment of acute migraine headache. *Headache 26:*168–171.

Calton, G.J. and J.W. Burnett (1984). Danazol and migraine. *N. Engl. J. Med. 310:* 721–722.

Campbell, S. (1975). Double-blind psychometric studies on the effects of natural estrogens on post-menopausal women. In *The Management of the Menopause and Post-Menopausal Years* (S. Campbell, ed.), pp. 149–158. University Park Press, Baltimore.

Campbell, W.B. (1990). Lipid-derived autocoids: Eicosanoids and platelet-activating factor. In *Goodman and Gilman's The Pharmacological Basis of Therapeutics,* 8th ed., (A.G. Gilman, T.W. Rall, A.S. Nies, and P. Taylor, eds.), pp. 600–617. Pergamon Press, New York.

Capildeo, R. and F.C. Rose (1982). Single-dose pizotifen, 1.5 mg nocte: A new approach in the prophylaxis of migraine. *Headache 22:*272–275.

Casaer, P. (1989). Alternating hemiplegia in childhood. In *Migraine and Other Headaches* (M.D. Ferrari and X. Lataste, eds.), pp. 39–51. Parthenon, Park Ridge, NJ.

Cedars, M.I. and H.L. Judd (1987). Nonoral routes of estrogen administration. *Obstet. Gynecol. Clin. North Am. 14:*269–298.

Centonze, V., E. Attolini, L. Santoiemma et al. (1983). DHE retard for prophylactic therapy of migraine: Efficacy and tolerability. *Cephalalgia 3*(Suppl. 1):179–184.

Centonze, V., D. Magrone, M. Vino et al. (1990). Flunarizine in migraine prophylaxis: Efficacy and tolerability of 5 mg and 10 mg dose levels. *Cephalalgia 10:*17–24.

Chan, W.Y. (1983). Prostaglandins and nonsteroidal antiinflammatory drugs in dysmenorrhea. *Annu. Rev. Pharmacol. Toxicol. 23:*131–149.

Clary, C. and E. Schweitzer (1987). The treatment of MAOI hypertensive crisis with sublingual nifedipine. *Clin. Psychiatry 48:*249–250.

Collaborative Group for the Study of Stroke in Young Women (1975). Oral contraceptives and stroke in young women. *JAMA 231:*718–722.

Congdon, P.J. and W.I. Forsythe (1979). Migraine in childhood: A study of 300 children. *Dev. Med. Child Neurol. 21:*209–216.

Coope, J. (1975). Double-blind cross-over study of estrogen replacement therapy. In *The Management of the Menopause and Post-Menopausal Years* (S. Campbell, ed.), pp. 159–172. University Park Press, Baltimore.

Cortelli, P., T. Sacquegna, F. Albani et al. (1985). Propranolol plasma levels and relief of migraine. *Arch. Neurol. 42:*46–48.

Couch, J.R., D.K. Ziegler, and R. Hassanein (1976). Amitriptyline in the prophylaxis of migraine: Effectiveness and relationship of antimigraine and antidepressant effects. *Neurology 26:*121–127.

Coulam, C.B. and J.R. Annagers (1979). New anticonvulsants reduce the efficacy of oral contraception. *Epilepsia 20:*519–525.

Cullberg, J. (1972). Mood changes and menstrual symptoms with different gestagen/estrogen combinations: A double-blind comparison with a placebo. *Acta Psychiatr. Scand. Suppl. 236:*259–276.

Curran, D.A., H. Hinterberger, and J.W. Lance (1967). Methysergide. *Res. Clin. Stud. Headache 1:*74–122.

Curran, D.A. and J.W. Lance (1964). Clinical trial of methysergide and other preparations in the management of migraine. *J. Neurol. Neurosurg. Psychiatry 27:* 463–469.

Curzon, G., G.A. Kennett, K. Shah, and P. Whitton (1990). Behavioural effects of *m*-chlorophenylpiperazine (*m*-CPP), a reported migraine precipitant. In *Migraine, A Spectrum of Ideas* (M. Sandler and G. Collins, eds.), pp. 173–181. Oxford Medical Publications, Oxford, England.

D'Alessandro, R., G. Gamberini, A. Lozito, and T. Sacquegna (1983). Menstrual migraine: Intermittent prophylaxis with a timed-release pharmacological formulation of dihydroergotamine. *Cephalalgia 3*(Suppl. 1):158.

Dalessio, D.J. (ed.) (1980). *Wolff's Headache and Other Head Pain,* 4th ed. Oxford University Press, Oxford, England.

Dalessio, D.J. (ed.) (1987). *Wolff's Headache and Other Head Pain,* 5th ed. Oxford University Press, Oxford, England.

Dalessio, D.J. (1991). The clonidine (Catapres) protocol. *Headache Q. 2:*133–134.

Dalton, K. (1973). Progesterone suppositories and pessaries in the treatment of menstrual migraine. *Headache 13:*151–159.

Davidson, J., W.W.K. Zung, and J.I. Walker (1984). Practical aspects of MAO inhibitor therapy. *J. Clin. Psychiatry 45:*81–84.

DeLignieres, B., M. Vincens, P. Mauvais-Jarvis et al. (1986). Prevention of menstrual migraine by percutaneous oestradiol. *BMJ 293:*1540.

Dennerstein, L., C. Morse, G. Burrows et al. (1988). Menstrual migraine: A double-blind trial of percutaneous estradiol. *Gynecol. Endocrinol. 2:*113–120.

Deonna, T.W. (1988). Paroxysmal disorders which may be migraine or may be confused with it. In *Migraine in Childhood* (J.M. Hockaday, ed.), pp. 75–87. Butterworth, Boston.

Diamond, S., and D.J. Dalessio (1982). Drug abuse in headache. In *The Practicing Physician's Approach to Headache,* 3rd ed., pp. 114–121. Williams & Wilkins, Baltimore.

Diamond, S., L. Kudrow, J. Stevens, and D.B. Shapiro (1982). Long-term study of propranolol in the treatment of migraine. *Headache 22:*268–271.

Diamond, S. and J.L. Medina (1976). Double blind study of propranolol for migraine prophylaxis. *Headache 16:*24–27.

Diamond, S., G.D. Solomon, F.G. Freitag, and N.D. Mehta (1987). Long-acting propranolol in the prophylaxis of migraine. *Headache 27:*70–72.

Diener, H., W.D. Gerber, S. Geiselhart et al. (1988). Short- and long-term effects of withdrawal therapy in drug-induced headache. In *Drug-Induced Headache* (H. Diener and M. Wilkinson, eds.), pp. 133–145. Springer-Verlag, Berlin.

Digre, K. and H. Damasio (1987). Menstrual migraine: Differential diagnosis, evaluation, and treatment. *Clin. Obstet. Gynecol. 30:*417–430.

Dreifuss, F.E., N. Santilli, D.H. Langer et al. (1987). Valproic acid hepatic fatalities: A retrospective review. *Neurology 37:*379–385.

Drummond, P.D. (1985). Effectiveness of methysergide in relation to clinical features of migraine. *Headache 25:*145–146.

Drummond, P.D. (1986). A quantitative assessment of photophobia in migraine and tension headache. *Headache 26:*465–469.

Drummond, P.D. (1987). Scalp tenderness and sensitivity to pain in migraine and tension headache. *Headache 27:*45–50.

Drummond, P.D. and Lance, J.W. (1984). Clinical diagnosis and computer analysis of headache symptoms. *J. Neurol. Neurosurg. Psychiatry 47:*128–133.

Dumuis, A., M. Sebben, E. Monferini et al. (1991). Azabicycloalkylbenzimidazolone derivatives as a novel class of potent agonists at the 5-HT$_4$ receptor positively coupled to adenylate cyclase in brain. *Arch. Pharmacology 343:*245–251.

Edelson, R.N. (1985). Menstrual migraine and other hormonal aspects of migraine. *Headache 25:*376–379.

Edmeads, J. (1988). Emergency management of headache. *Headache 28:*675–679.

Egger, J., J. Wilson, C.M. Carter et al. (1983). Is migraine food allergy? *Lancet 2:* 865–869.

Ehrenberg, B.L. (1991). Unusual clinical manifestations of migraine and "the borderland of epilepsy" reexplored. *Semin. Neurol. 11:*118–127.

Ekbom, K. (1975). Alprenolol for migraine prophylaxis. *Headache 15:*129–132.

Ekbom, K. and P.O. Lundberg (1972). Clinical trial of LB-56 (*d,* 1-4-(2-hydroxy-3-isopropylaminopropoxy) indol): An adrenergic β-receptor blocking agent in migraine prophylaxis. *Headache 12:*15–17.

Ekbom, K. and M. Zetterman (1977). Oxprenolol in the treatment of migraine. *Acta Neurol. Scand. 56:*181–184.

Elkind, A.H., A.P. Friedman, A. Bachman et al. (1968). Silent retroperitoneal fibrosis associated with methysergide therapy. *JAMA 206:*1041–1044.

Ensink, F. (1991). Subcutaneous sumatriptan in the acute treatment of migraine. *J. Neurol. 238:*S66–S69.

Epstein, M.T., J.M. Hockaday, and T.D.R. Hockaday (1975). Migraine and reproductive hormones throughout the menstrual cycle. *Lancet 1:*543–548.

Facchinetti, F., G. Sances, A. Volpe et al. (1983). Hypothalamus pituitary-ovarian axis in menstrual migraine: Effects of dihydroergotamine retard prophylactic treatment. *Cephalalgia 3*(Suppl. 1):159–167.

Fanchamps, A. (1985). Why do not all β-blockers prevent migraine? *Headache 25*:61–62.

Featherstone, H.J. (1983a). Fetal demise in a migraine patient on propranolol. *Headache 23*:213–214.

Featherstone, H.J. (1983b). Low dose propranolol therapy for aborting acute migraine. *West. J. Med. 138*:416–417.

Feinmann, C. (1985). Pain relief by antidepressants: Possible modes of action. *Pain 23*: 1–8.

Ferguson, A. (1990). Food sensitivity or self-deception? *N. Engl. J. Med. 323*:476.

Ferrari, M.D. and J. Odnik (1989). Urinary excretion of biogenic amines in migraine and tension headache. In *New Advances in Headache Research* (F.C. Rose, ed.), pp. 85–88. Smith-Gordon & Co., London.

Ferrari, M.D., J. Odnik, K.D. Bos et al. (1990). Neuroexcitatory plasma amino acids are elevated in migraine. *Neurology 40*:1582–1586.

Fields, H. (1991). Depression and pain: A neurobiological model. *Neuropsychiatry Neuropsychol. Behav. Neurol. 4*:83–92.

Fisher, C.M. (1980). Late-life migraine accompaniments as a cause of unexplained transient ischemic attacks. *Can. J. Neurol. Sci. 7*:9–17.

Fisher, C.M. (1986). Late-life migraine accompaniments—further experience. *Stroke 17*:1033–1042.

Fisher, C.M. (1988). Analgesic rebound headache refuted. *Headache 28*:666.

Fleckenstein, A. (1971). Specific inhibitors and promotors of calcium action in the excitation-contraction coupling of heart muscle and their role in the prevention or production of myocardial lesions. In *Calcium and the Heart* (P. Harris and L. Opie, eds.), pp. 135–188. Academic Press, London.

Fontanari, D., L. Perulli, F. Conte et al. (1983). Planned release dihydroergotamine in common migraine and "tension-vascular headache": Multicentre clinical trial. *Cephalalgia 3*(Suppl. 1):189–191.

Forbes, J.A., W.T. Beaver, K.F. Jones et al. (1991). Effect of caffeine on ibuprofen analgesia in postoperative surgery pain. *Clin. Pharmacol. Ther. 49*:674–684.

Forsythe, I. and J.M. Hockaday (1988). Management of childhood migraine. In *Migraine in Childhood and Other Non-Epileptic Paroxysmal Disorders* (J.M. Hockaday, ed.), pp. 63–74. Butterworth, Boston.

Forsythe, W.I., D. Gillies, and M.A. Sills (1984). Propranolol ("Inderal") in the treatment of childhood migraine. *Dev. Med. Child Neurol. 26*:737–741.

Fozard, J.R. and J.A. Gray (1989). 5-HT$_{1C}$ receptor activation: A key step in the initiation of migraine? *Trends Pharmacol. Sci. 10*:307–309.

Freeman, E., K. Rickels, S.J. Sondheimer, and M. Polansky (1990). Ineffectiveness of progesterone suppository treatment for premenstrual syndrome. *JAMA 264*: 349–353.

Friedman, A.P., K.H. Finley, and J.R. Graham (1962). Classification of headache. *Arch. Neurol. 6*:173–176.

Frishman, W.H. (1987). Beta adrenergic blocker withdrawal. *Am. J. Cardiol. 59*: 26F–32F.

Fuller, G.N. and R.J. Guiloff (1990). Propranolol in acute migraine: A controlled study. *Cephalalgia 10*:229–233.

Gallagher, R.M. (1986). Emergency treatment of intractable migraine. *Headache 26*: 74–75.

Gallagher, R.M. (1989). Menstrual migraine and intermittent ergonovine therapy. *Headache 29*:366–367.

Gelmers, H.J. (1983). Nimodipine, a new calcium antagonist, in the prophylactic treatment of migraine. *Headache 23*:106–109.

Gennari, C., M.S. Chierichetti, S. Gonnelli et al. (1986). Migraine prophylaxis with salmon calcitonin: A cross-over double-blind, placebo-controlled study. *Headache 26:*13–16.

Gerber, W.D., H. Diener, E. Scholz, and U. Niederberger (1991). Responders and non-responders to metoprolol, propranolol and nifedipine treatment in migraine prophylaxis: A dose-range study based on time-series analysis. *Cephalalgia 11:* 37–45.

Gilbert, G.J. (1982). An occurrence of complicated migraine during propranolol therapy. *Headache 22:*81–83.

Goadsby, P.J. and A.L. Gundlach (1991). Localization of ^{3}H-dihydroergotamine-binding sites in the cat central nervous system: Relevance to migraine. *Ann. Neurol. 29:* 91–94.

Gold, M.S., A.C. Pottash, D.R. Sweeney et al. (1980). Opiate withdrawal using clonidine, a safe, effective, and rapid nonopiate treatment. *JAMA 243:*343–346.

Goldner, J.A., and L.P. Levitt (1987). Treatment of complicated migraine with sublingual nifedipine. *Headache 27:*484–486.

Goldstein, M. and T.C. Chen (1982). The epidemiology of disabling headache. *Adv. Neurol. 33:*377–390.

Goldzieher, J.W., L.E. Moses, E. Averkin et al. (1971). A placebo-controlled double-blind crossover investigation of the side effects attributed to oral contraceptives. *Fertil. Steril. 22:*609–623.

Graham, J. (1967). Cardiac and pulmonary fibrosis during methysergide therapy for headache. *Am. J. Med. Sci. 254:*1–12.

Graham, J.R. (1968). Headache and cranial neuralgias. In *Handbook of Clinical Neurology,* Vol. 5 (P.J. Vinken and G.W. Bruyn, eds.), pg. 54. Elsevier, New York.

Greenberg, D.A. (1986). Calcium channel antagonists and the treatment of migraine. *Clin. Neuropharmacol. 9:*311–328.

Greenberg D.A. (1987). Calcium channels and calcium channel antagonists. *Ann. Neurol. 21:*317–330.

Greenblatt, R.B. and D.W. Bruneteau (1974). Menopausal headache—psychogenic or metabolic? *J. Am. Geriatr. Soc. 283:*186–190.

Griffin, M.R., J.M. Piper, J.R. Daugherty et al. (1991). Nonsteroidal anti-inflammatory drug use and increased risk for peptic ulcer disease in elderly persons. *Ann. Intern. Med. 114:*257–263.

Hachinski, V., J.W. Norris, J. Edmeads, and P. Cooper (1978). Ergotamine and cerebral blood flow. *Stroke 9:*594–596.

Hachinski, V.C.C., J. Porchawka, and J.C. Steele (1973). Visual symptoms in the migraine syndrome. *Neurology 23:*570–579.

Hagen, I., B. Nesheim, and T. Tuntland (1985). No effect of vitamin B-6 against premenstrual tension: A controlled clinical study. *Acta Obstet. Gynecol. Scand. 64:* 667–670.

Hakkarainen, H., E. Hokkanen and T. Kallanranta (1980). Does clonidine have a role in treating migraine? *Upsala J. Med. Sci. Suppl. 31:*16–19.

Hansen, S.L., L. Borelli-Miller, P. Strange et al. (1990). Ophthalmoplegic migraine: Diagnostic criteria, incidence of hospitalization and possible etiology. *Acta Neurol. Scand. 81:*54–60.

Hanson, R.R. (1988). Headaches in childhood. *Semin. Neurol. 8:*51–60.

Hanston, P.O., and J.R. Horn (eds.) (1985). *Drug Interaction Newsletter 5:*7–10.

Havanka-Kanniainen, H., E. Hokkanen, and V.V. Myllyla (1985). Efficacy of nimodipine in the prophylaxis of migraine. *Cephalalgia 5:*39–43.

Headache Classification Committee of the International Headache Society (1988). Classification and diagnostic criteria for headache disorders, cranial neuralgia, and facial pain. *Cephalalgia 8*(Suppl. 7):1–96.

Hedman, C., A.R. Andersen, P.G. Andersson et al. (1988). Symptoms of classic migraine attacks: Modifications brought about by metoprolol. *Cephalalgia 8:* 279–284.

Heninger, G.R. and D.S. Charney (1987). Mechanism of action of antidepressant treatments: Implications for the etiology and treatment of depressive disorders. In *Psychopharmacology: The Third Generation of Progress* (H.Y. Meltzer, ed.), pp. 535–544. Raven Press, New York.

Henry, P., J.F. Dartigues, M.P. Benetier et al. (1985). Ergotamine- and analgesic-induced headaches. In *Migraine* (C. Rose, ed.), pp. 197–205. London.

Hering, R. and A. Kuritzky (1992). Sodium valproate in the prophylactic treatment of migraine: A double-blind study versus placebo. *Cephalalgia 12:*81–84.

Hockaday, J.M. (1988a). Definitions, clinical features, and diagnosis of childhood migraine. In *Migraine in Childhood* (J.M. Hockaday, ed.), pp. 5–24. Butterworth, Boston.

Hockaday, J.M. (1988b). Equivalents of childhood migraine. In *Migraine in Childhood* (J.M. Hockaday, ed.), pp. 54–62. Butterworth, Boston.

Hockaday, J.M. and R.W. Newton (1988). Migraine and epilepsy. In *Migraine in Childhood* (J.M. Hockaday, ed.), pp. 885–104. Butterworth, Boston.

Holdorff, B., M. Sinn, and G. Roth (1977). Propranolol in der migraineprophylaxe. *Med. Klinik 72:*1115–1120.

Holroyd, K.A., D.B. Penzien, and G.E. Cordingley (1991). Propranolol in the management of recurrent migraine: A meta-analytic review. *Headache 31:*333–340.

Hosking, G. (1988). Special forms: Variants of migraine in childhood. In *Migraine in Childhood* (J.M. Hockaday, ed.), pp. 35–53. Butterworth, Boston.

Humphrey, P.P.A., W. Feniuk, and M.J. Perren (1990). Antimigraine drugs in development: Advances in serotonin receptor pharmacology. *Headache 30*(Suppl. 1):12.

Hupp, S.L., L.B. Kline, and J.J. Corbett (1989). Visual disturbances of migraine. *Surv. Ophthalmol. 33:*221–236.

Insel, P. (1990). Analgesic-antipyretics and antiinflammatory agents: Drugs employed in the treatment of rheumatoid arthritis and gout. In *Goodman and Gilman's The Pharmacological Basis of Therapeutics,* 8th ed. (A.G. Gilman, T.W. Rall, A.S. Nies, and P. Taylor, eds.), pp. 638–681. Pergamon Press, New York.

Isler, H. (1982). Migraine treatment as a cause of chronic migraine. In *Advances in Migraine Research and Therapy* (F.C. Rose, ed.), pp. 159–164. Raven Press, New York.

Isler, H. (1986). Frequency and time course of premonitory phenomena. In *The Prelude to the Migraine Attack* (W.K. Amery and A. Wauquier, eds.), pp. 44–53. Bailliere Tindall, London.

Iversen, H.K., M. Langemark, P.G. Andersson et al. (1990). Clinical characteristics of migraine and episodic tension-type headache in relation to old and new diagnostic criteria. *Headache 30:*514–519.

Jaffe, J.H. (1985). Drug addiction and drug abuse. In *The Pharmacological Basis of Therapeutics,* 7th ed (A.G. Gilman, T.W. Rall, A.S. Nies, and P. Taylor, eds.), pp. 522–573. Pergamon Press, New York.

Jensen, K., P. Tfelt-Hansen, M. Lauritzen, and J. Olesen (1986). Classic migraine: A prospective recording of symptoms. *Acta Neurol. Scand. 73:*359–362.

Jewett, D.L., G. Fein, and M.H. Greenberg (1990). A double-blind study of symptom provocation to determine food sensitivity. *N. Engl. J. Med. 323:*429–433.

Johnson, E.S., N.P. Kadam, D.M. Hylands, and P.J. Hylands (1985). Efficacy of feverfew as prophylactic treatment of migraine. *BMJ 291:*569–573.

Jones, J., D. Sklar, J. Dougherty, and W. White (1989). Randomized double-blind trial of intravenous prochlorperazine for the treatment of acute headache. *JAMA 261:* 1174–1185.

Jonsdottir, B.A., J.S. Meyer, and R.L. Rogers (1987). Efficacy, side effects and tolerance compared during headache treatment with three different calcium blockers. *Headache 27:*364–369.

Judd, H. (1987). Efficacy of transdermal estradiol. *Obstet. Gynecol. 156:*1326–1331.

Kallanranta, T., H. Hakkarainen, E. Hokkanen, and T. Tuovinen (1977). Clonidine in migraine prophylaxis. *Headache 17:*169–172.

Kangasniemi, P., A.R. Andersen, P.G. Andersson et al. (1987). Classic migraine: Effective prophylaxis with metoprolol. *Cephalalgia 7:*231–238.

Kanto, J., H. Allonen, K. Koski et al. (1981). Pharmacokinetics of dihydroergotamine in healthy volunteers and in neurological patients after a single intravenous injection. *Int. J. Clin. Pharmacol. Ther. Toxicol. 19:*127–130.

Kappius, R.E.K. and P. Goolkasian (1987). Group and menstrual phase effect in reported headaches among college students. *Headache 27:*491–494.

Katz, A.M., W.D. Hager, F.C. Messineo, and A.J. Pappano (1984). Cellular actions and pharmacology of the calcium channel blocking drugs. *Am. J. Med. 77(2b):*2–10.

Kishore-Kumar, R., M.B. Max, S.C. Schafer et al. (1990). Desipramine relieves postherpetic neuralgia. *Clin. Pharmacol. Ther. 47:*305–312.

Klapper, J.A. and J.S. Stanton (1991). The emergency treatment of acute migraine headache; a comparison of intravenous dihydroergotamine, dexamethasone, and placebo. *Cephalalgia 11*(Suppl. 11):159–160.

Koehler, S.M. and A. Glaros (1988). The effect of aspartame on migraine headache. *Headache 28:*10–13.

Koella, W.P. (1985). CNS-related (side-)effects of β-blockers with special reference to mechanisms of action. *Eur. J. Clin. Pharmacol. 28*(Suppl.):55–63.

Kudrow, L. (1975). The relationship of headache frequency to hormone use in migraine. *Headache 15:*36–49.

Kudrow, L. (1982). Paradoxical effects of frequent analgesic use. *Adv. Neurol. 33:* 335–341.

Kumar, K.L. and T.G. Cooney (1990). Visual symptoms after atenolol therapy for migraine. *Ann. Intern. Med. 112:*712–713.

Kupersmith, M.J., W.K. Hass, and N.E. Chase (1979). Isoproterenol treatment of visual symptoms in migraine. *Stroke 10:*299–305.

Kuritzky, A., Ziegler, K.E. and R. Hassanein (1981). Vertigo, motion sickness and migraine. *Headache 21:*227–231.

Labbe, E.E. (1988). Childhood muscle contraction headache: Current issues in assessment and treatment. *Headache 28:*430–434.

Lader, M. (1983). Combined use of tricyclic antidepressants and monoamine oxidase inhibitors. *J. Clin. Psychiatry 44:*20–24.

Lake, A.E., J.R. Saper, S. Madden, and C. Kreeger (1990). Inpatient treatment for chronic daily headache: A prospective long-term outcome. *Headache 30:* 299–300.

Lambert, G.A., A. Zagami, and J.W. Lance (1986). Physiology and pharmacology of cervical spinal cord elements activated by stimulation of the dura mater. *Soc. Neurosci. Abstr. 12:*230.

Lance, J.W. (1982). *Mechanisms and Management of Headache,* 4th ed. Butterworth, Boston.

Lance, J.W. (1986). The pharmacotherapy of migraine. *Med. J. Aust. 144:*85–88.

Lance, J.W. (1988). The controlled application of cold and heat by a new device (Migralief apparatus) in the treatment of headache. *Headache 28:*458–461.

Lance, J.W. (1990). A concept of migraine and the search for the ideal headache drug. *Headache 30*(Suppl. 1):17.

Lance, J.W. and M. Anthony (1966). Some clinical aspects of migraine. *Arch. Neurol. 15*:356–361.

Lane, P.L., B.A. McLellan, and C.J. Baggoley (1989). Comparative efficacy of chlorpromazine and meperidine with dimenhydrinate in migraine headache. *Ann. Emerg. Med. 18*:360–365.

Lane, P.L. and R. Ross (1985). Intravenous chlorpromazine—preliminary results in acute migraine. *Headache 25*:302–304.

Lataste, X. (1989). Dihydroergotamine nasal spray. In *Migraine and Other Headaches* (M.D. Ferrari and X. Lataste, eds.), pp. 249–260. Parthenon, Park Ridge, NJ.

Lauritzen, M. (1986). Spreading cortical depression as a mechanism of the aura in classic migraine. In *The Prelude to the Migraine Attack* (W.K. Amery and A. Wauquier, eds.), pp. 134–141. Bailliere Tindall, London.

Lavenstein, B. (1991). A comparative study of cyproheptadine, amitriptyline, and propranolol in the treatment of preadolescent migraine. *Cephalalgia 11*(Suppl. 1): 122–123.

Leandri, M., S. Rigardo, R. Schizzi, and C.U. Parodi (1990). Migraine treatment with nicardipine. *Cephalalgia 10*:111–116.

Leão, A.A.P. (1944). Spreading depression of activity in the cerebral cortex. *J. Neurophysiol. 7*:359–390.

Leone, M., F. Frediani, G. Patruno et al. (1990). Is nimodipine useful in migraine prophylaxis? Further considerations. *Headache 30*:363–365.

Levine, B.D., K. Yoshimura, T. Kobayashi et al. (1987). Dexamethasone in the treatment of acute mountain sickness. *N. Engl. J. Med. 321*:1707–1719.

Levy, D.E. (1988). Transient CNS deficits: A common, benign syndrome in young adults. *Neurology 38*:831–836.

Lieberman, E. and A. Stoudemire (1987). Use of tricyclic antidepressants in patients with glaucoma: Assessment and appropriate precautions. *Psychosomatics 28*: 145–148.

Linder, S.L. (1991). Treatment of acute childhood migraine headaches. *Cephalalgia 11*(Suppl. 11):120–121.

Littlewood, J.T., V. Glover, P.T.G. Davies et al. (1988). Red wine as a cause of migraine. *Lancet 1*:558–559.

Ludvigsson, J. (1974). Propranolol used in prophylaxis of migraine in children. *Acta Neurol. Scand. 50*:109–115.

Lundberg, P.O. (1986). Endocrine headaches. In *Handbook of Clinical Neurology,* Vol. 48 (F.C. Rose, ed.), pp. 431–440. Elsevier, New York.

MacDonald, A., Forsythe, I., and C. Wall (1989). Dietary treatment of migraine. In *Headache in Children and Adolescents* (G. Lanzi, U. Balottin, and A. Cernibori, eds.), pp. 333–338. Elsevier, New York.

Magos, A.L., M. Brincat, and J.W.W. Studd (1986). Treatment of the premenstrual syndrome by subcutaneous oestradiol implants and cyclical oral norethisterone: Placebo-controlled study. *BMJ292*:1629–1633.

Magos, A.L., K.J. Zilkha, and J.W.W. Studd (1983). Treatment of menstrual migraine by oestradiol implants. *J. Neurol. Neurosurg. Psychiatry 46*:1044–1046.

Manzoni, G.C., F. Granella, G. Malferrari et al. (1989). An epidemiological study of headache in children aged between 6 and 13. In *Headache in Children and Adolescents* (G. Lanzi, U. Balottin, and A. Cernibori, eds.), pp. 185–188. Elsevier, New York.

Markley, H.G., J.C.D. Cheronis, and R.W. Piepho (1984). Verapamil in prophylactic therapy of migraine. *Neurology 34*:973–976.

Markley, H.G., P.A. Gasser, M.E. Markley, and S.M. Pratt (1991). Fluoxetine in prophylaxis of migraine: Clinical experience. *Cephalalgia 11*(Suppl. 11):164–165.

Martucci, N., V. Manna, P. Mattesi et al. (1983). Ergot derivatives in the prophylaxis
of migraine: A multicentric study with a timed-release dihydroergotamine formulation. *Cephalalgia 3*(Suppl. 1):151–155.

Masel, B.E., A.L. Chesson, B.H. Peters et al. (1980). Platelet antagonists in migraine
prophylaxis: A clinical trial using aspirin and dipyridamole. *Headache 20*:13–18.

Mastrosimone, F. and C. Iaccarino (1987). Progress in migraine: Treatment with dihy-
droergotamine-retard. *Cephalalgia 7*(Suppl. 1):168–170.

Mathew, N.T. (1990a). Abortive versus prophylactic treatment of migraine—a reappraisal. *Headache 30*:238–239.

Mathew, N.T. (1990b). Drug-induced headache. *Neurol. Clin. 8*:903–912.

Mathew, N.T. (1990c). Valproate in the treatment of persistent chronic daily headache.
Headache 30:301.

Mathew, N.T., U. Reuveni, and F. Perez (1987). Transformed or evolutive migraine.
Headache 27:102–106.

Mathew, N.T., E. Stubits, and M. Nigam (1982). Transformation of migraine into daily
headache: Analysis of factors. *Headache 22*:66–68.

McArthur, J.C., K. Marek, A. Pestronk et al. (1989). Nifedipine in the prophylaxis
of classic migraine: A crossover, double-masked, placebo-controlled study of
headache frequency and side effects. *Neurology 39*:284–286.

McGoon, M.D., R.E. Vlietstra, D.R. Holmes, and J.E. Osborn (1982). The clinical use
of verapamil. *Mayo Clin. Proc. 57*:495–510.

McHenry, L.C. (1969). *Garrison's History of Neurology.* Charles C Thomas, Springfield, IL.

Medina, J.L. (1982). Cyclic migraine: A disorder responsive to lithium carbonate. *Psychosomatics 23*:625–637.

Mendel, C.M., R.F. Klein, D.A. Chappell et al. (1986). A trial of amitriptyline and
fluphenazine in the treatment of painful diabetic neuropathy. *JAMA 255*:637–639.

Metys, J., J. Metysova, and R. Soucek (1990). Do tricyclic migraine prophylactics share
pharmacological profile of antidepressant drugs? *Actas Nerv. Super. 32*:233–234.

Meyer, J.S. (1985). Calcium channel blockers in the prophylactic treatment of vascular
headache. *Ann. Intern. Med. 102*:395–397.

Meyer, J.S., R. Dowell, N.T. Mathew, and J. Hardenberg (1984). Clinical and hemodynamic effects during treatment of vascular headaches with verapamil. *Headache
24*:313–321.

Meyer, J.S. and J. Hardenberg (1983). Clinical effectiveness of calcium entry blockers in
prophylactic treatment of migraine and cluster headaches. *Headache 23*:266–277.

Meyer, J.S., M. Nance, M. Walker et al. (1985). Migraine and cluster headache treatment
with calcium antagonists supports a vascular pathogenesis. *Headache 25*:
358–367.

Micieli, G., A. Cavallini, E. Martignoni et al. (1988). Effectiveness of salmon calcitonin
nasal spray preparation in migraine treatment. *Headache 28*:196–200.

Migraine-Nimodipine European Study Group (1989a). European multicenter trial of nimodipine in the prophylaxis of classic migraine (migraine with aura). *Headache
29*:639–642.

Migraine-Nimodipine European Study Group (1989b). European multicenter trial of nimodipine in the prophylaxis of common migraine (migraine without aura). *Headache 29*:633–638.

Miller, F.W. and T.J. Santoro (1985). Nifedipine in the treatment of migraine headache
and amaurosis fugax in patients with systemic lupus erythematosus. *N. Engl. J.
Med. 311*:921.

Millichapp, J.G. (1978). Recurrent headaches in 100 children. *Childs Brain 4*:95–105.

Minervini, M.G. and K. Pinto (1987). Catopril relieves pain and improves mood depression in depressed patients with classical migraine. *Cephalalgia 7*(Suppl. 6): 485–486.

Moffett, A.M., M. Swash, and D.F. Scott (1974). Effect of chocolate: A double-blind study. *J. Neurol. Neurosurg. Psychiatry 37*:445–448.

Moskowitz, M.A. (1990). Basic mechanisms in vascular headache. *Neurol. Clin. 8*: 801–815.

Muller-Schweinitzer, E. (1984). Pharmacological actions of the main metabolites of dihydroergotamine. *Eur. J. Clin. Pharmacol. 26*:699–705.

Murad, F. (1990). Drugs used for the treatment of angina: Organic nitrates, calcium-channel blockers, and β-adrenergic antagonists. In *Goodman and Gilman's The Pharmacological Basis of Therapeutics,* 8th ed. (A.G. Gilman, T.W. Rall, A.S. Nies, and P. Taylor, eds.), pp. 764–783. Pergamon Press, New York.

Murphy, D.L., N.A. Garrick, C.S. Aulakh, and R.M. Cohen (1984). New contributions from basic science to understanding the effects of monoamine oxidase inhibiting antidepressants. *J. Clin. Psychiatry 45*:37–43.

Murray, W.J. (1964). Evaluation of aspirin in treatment of headache. *Clin. Pharmacol. Ther. 5*:21–25.

Nagamani, M., M.E. Kelver, and E.R. Smith (1987). Treatment of menopausal hot flashes with transdermal administration of clonidine. *Am. J. Obstet. Gynecol. 156*:561–565.

Nanda, R.N., R.H. Johnson, J. Gray et al. (1978). A double-blind trial of acebutolol for migraine prophylaxis. *Headache 18*:379–381.

Nilsson, L. and L. Solvell (1967). Clinical studies on oral contraceptives—a randomized, double-blind, crossover study of 4 different preparations (Anovlar[R] mite, Lyndiol[R] mite, Ovulen[R], and Volidan[R]). *Acta Obstet. Gynecol. Scand. 46*(Suppl. 8): 3–31.

Noronha, M.J. (1985). Double-blind randomized crossover trial of timolol in migraine prophylaxis in children. *Cephalalgia 5*(Suppl. 3):174–175.

O'Dea, P.K. and E.H. Davis (1990). Tamoxifen in the treatment of menstrual migraine. *Neurology 40*:1470–1471.

Olesen, J. (1978). Some clinical features of the acute migraine attack. An analysis of 750 patients. *Headache 18*:268–271.

Olesen, J., A. Aebelholt, and B. Veilis (1979). The Copenhagen acute headache clinic: Organization, patient material and treatment results. *Headache 19*:223–227.

Olesen, J., and L. Edvinsson (eds.) (1988). *Basic Mechanisms of Headache.* Elsevier, New York.

Olness, K., J.T. MacDonald, and D.L. Uden (1987). Comparison of self-hypnosis and propranolol in the treatment of juvenile classic migraine. *Pediatrics 79*:593–597.

O'Neill, B.P. and J.D. Mann (1979). Aspirin prophylaxis in migraine. *Lancet 2:* 1179–1181.

Packard, R.C. (1979). What does the headache patient want? *Headache 19*:370–374.

Panerai, A.E., G. Monza, P. Movilia et al. (1990). A randomized, within-patient, crossover, placebo-controlled trial on the efficacy and tolerability of the tricyclic antidepressants chlorimipramine and nortriptyline in central pain. *Acta Neurol. Scand. 82*:34–38.

Pare, C.M.B., N. Kline, C. Hallstrom, and T.B. Cooper (1982). Will amitriptyline prevent the "cheese" reaction of monoamine-oxidase inhibitors? *Lancet 9*:183–186.

Pascual, J., J.M. Polo, and J. Berciano (1989). The dose of propranolol for migraine prophylaxis. Efficacy of low doses. *Cephalalgia 9*:287–291.

Patten, J.P. (1991). Clinical experience with oral sumatriptan: A placebo-controlled dose-ranging study. *J. Neurol. 238:*S62–S65.

Patti, F., U. Scapagnini, F. Nicoletti et al. (1987). A short-term trial of an analogue of eel-calcitonin in headache. *Headache 27:*334–339.

Pearce, J.M.S. (1984). Migraine: A cerebral disorder. *Lancet 2:*86–89.

Peatfield, R. (1986). Drugs acting by modification of serotonin function. In *Headache,* pp. 129–131. Springer-Verlag, Berlin.

Peatfield, R.C. (1987). Can transient ischemic attacks and classical migraine always be distinguished? *Headache 27:*240–243.

Penry, J.K. and J.C. Dean (1989). The scope and use of valproate in epilepsy. *J. Clin. Psychiatry 50:*17–22.

Peroutka, S.J. (1983). The pharmacology of calcium channel antagonists: A novel class of anti-migraine agents? *Headache 23:*278–283.

Peroutka, S.J. (1990a). Developments in 5-hydroxytryptamine receptor pharmacology in migraine. *Neurol. Clin. 8:*829–838.

Peroutka, S.J. (1990b). The pharmacology of current anti-migraine drugs. *Headache 30*(Suppl. 1):12.

Peters, B.H., C.J. Fraim, and B.E. Masel (1983). Comparison of 650 mg aspirin and 1000 mg acetaminophen with each other, and with placebo in moderately severe headache. *Am. J. Med. 76:*36–42.

Pfaffenrath, V., W. Oestreich, and W. Haase (1990). Flunarizine (10 and 20 mg) i.v. versus placebo in the treatment of acute migraine attacks: A multi-centre double-blind study. *Cephalalgia 10:*77–81.

Pies, R. (1983). Trazodone and intractable headaches. *J. Clin. Psychiatry 44:*317.

Portenoy, R.K. (1990). Chronic opioid therapy in non-malignant pain. *J. Pain Symptom Management 5*(Suppl.):46–61.

Poser, C.M. (1974). Papaverine in prophylactic treatment of migraine. *Lancet 2:*1290.

Powles, T.J. (1986). Prevention of migrainous headaches by tamoxifen. *Lancet 2:*1344.

Pradalier, A., A. Clapin, and J. Dry (1988). Treatment review: Non-steroid anti-inflammatory drugs in the treatment and long-term prevention of migraine attacks. *Headache 28:*550–557.

Pradalier, A., G. Serratrice, M. Collard et al. (1989). Long-acting propranolol on migraine prophylaxis: Results of a double-blind, placebo-controlled study. *Cephalalgia 9:*247–253.

Prendes, J.L. (1980). Consideration on use of propranolol in complicated migraine. *Headache 20:*93–95.

Prensky, A.L. (1987). Migraine in children. In *Migraine: Clinical and Research Aspects* (J.N. Blau, ed.), pp. 31–53. Johns Hopkins University Press, Baltimore.

Prezewlocki, P., Z. Hollt, T. Duka et al. (1979). Long-term morphine treatment decreases endorphin levels in rat brain and pituitary. *Brain Res. 174:*341–357.

Price, W.A. and A.J. Giannini (1986). Neurotoxicity caused by lithium-verapamil synergism. *J. Clin. Pharmacol. 26:*717–719.

Price, W.A. and J.E. Shalley (1987). Lithium-verapamil toxicity in the elderly. *J. Am. Geriatr. Soc. 35:*177–179.

Rabkin, R., D.P. Stables, N.W. Levin, and M. Suzman (1966). The prophylactic value of propranolol in angina pectoris. *Am. J. Cardiol. 18:*370–383.

Rapoport, A.M. (1992). The diagnosis of migraine and tension-type headache, then and now. *Neurology 42:*11–15.

Rapoport, A.M., F.D. Sheftell, and B. Gordon (1989). The successful treatment of migraine with anticonvulsant medication in patients with abnormal EEGs. *Headache 29:*309.

Rapoport, A.M. and R.E. Weeks (1988). Characteristics and treatment of analgesic rebound headache. In *Drug-Induced Headache* (H. Diener and M. Wilkinson, eds.), pp. 162–167. Springer-Verlag, Berlin.

Raskin, N.H. (1981). Chemical headaches. *Annu. Rev. Med. 32:*63–71.

Raskin, D.E. (1983). Combined tricyclic and MAOI treatment of depressed patients. *Am. J. Psychiatry 140:*10.

Raskin, N.H. (1986). Repetitive intravenous dihydroergotamine as therapy for intractable migraine. *Neurology 36:*995–997.

Raskin, N.H. (1988). *Headache,* 2nd ed. Churchill Livingstone, New York.

Raskin, N.H. (1990a). Conclusions. *Headache 30*(Suppl. 1):24.

Raskin, N.H. (1990b). Modern pharmacotherapy of migraine. *Neurol. Clin. 8:*857–865.

Raskin, N.H. (1990c). Treatment of status migrainosis. *Headache 30*(Suppl. 2):550–553.

Raskin, N.H. and R.K. Schwartz (1980). Icepick-like pain. *Neurology 30:*203–205.

Ratinahirana, H., Y. Darbois, and M.G. Bousser (1990). Migraine and pregnancy: A prospective study in 703 women after delivery. *Neurology 40:*437.

Ravnikar, V. (1990). Physiology and treatment of hot flushes. *Obstet. Gynecol. 75*(Suppl.):3S–8S.

Rayburn, W.F. and J.P. Lavin (1986). Drug prescribing for chronic medical disorders during pregnancy: An overview. *Am. J. Obstet. Gynecol. 155:*565–569.

Rebar, R.W. and I.B. Spitzer (1987). The physiology and measurement of hot flushes. *Am. J. Obstet. Gynecol. 156:*1284–1288.

Reid, R.L., and S.S.C. Yen (1981). Premenstrual syndrome. *Am. J. Obstet. Gynecol. 139:*85–104.

Richardson, J.W. and E. Richelson (1984). Antidepressants: A clinical update for medical practitioners. *Mayo Clin. Proc. 59:*330–337.

Richelson, E. (1990). Antidepressants and brain neurochemistry. *Mayo Clin. Proc. 65:* 1227–1236.

Rimmer, E.M. and A. Richens (1985). An update on sodium valproate. *Pharmacotherapy 5:*171–182.

Riopelle, R. and J.L. McCans (1982). A pilot study of the calcium channel antagonist diltiazem in migraine syndrome prophylaxis. *Can. J. Neurol. Sci. 9:*269.

Robbins, L. (1989). Post-traumatic headache with scintillating scotoma treated with phenytoin (Dilantin). *Headache 29:*515–516.

Robinson, K., K.M. Huntington, and M.G. Wallace (1977). Treatment of the premenstrual syndrome. *Br. J. Obstet. Gynaecol. 84:*784–788.

Rompel, H. and P.W. Bauermeister (1970). Aetiology of migraine and prevention with carbamazepine (Tegretol). *S. Afr. Med. J. 44:*75–80.

Rosen, J.A. (1983). Observations on the efficacy of propranolol for the prophylaxis of migraine. *Ann. Neurol. 13:*92–93.

Rothner, A.D. (1983). Diagnosis and management of headache in children and adolescents. *Neurol. Clin. 1:*511–526.

Ryan, R.E. (1974). A study of Midrin in the symptomatic relief of migraine headache. *Headache 14:*33–42.

Ryan, R.E. and R.E. Ryan, Jr. (1975). The effects of clonidine in the prophylactic treatment of migraine. *Headache 15:*199–212.

Sacks, O. (1985). *Migraine: Understanding a Common Disorder.* University of California Press, Berkeley.

Saito, K., S. Markowitz, and M.A. Moskowitz (1988). Ergot alkaloids block neurogenic extravasation in dura mater: Proposed action in vascular headaches. *Ann. Neurol. 24:*732–737.

Sales, F., and J.L. Bada (1975). Practolol and migraine. *Lancet 1:*742.

Salmon, M.A. (1983). Diagnosis of abdominal migraine in children. In *Migraine in Childhood* (J. Wilson, ed.), pp. 1–2. The Medicine Publishing Foundation, Oxford.

Sandahl, B., U. Ulmsten, and K. Andersson (1979). Trial of the calcium antagonist nifedipine in the treatment of primary dysmenorrhea. *Arch. Gynecol. Obstet. 227:* 147–151.

Sanders, S.W., N. Haering, H. Mosberg, and H. Jaeger (1986). Pharmokinetics of ergotamine in healthy volunteers following oral and rectal dosing. *Eur. J. Clin. Pharmacol. 30:*331–334.

Saper, J.R. (1983). *Headache Disorders: Current Concepts in Treatment Strategies.* Wright-PSG, Littleton MA.

Saper, J.R. (1986). Changing perspectives on chronic headache. *Clin. J. Pain 2:*19–28.

Saper, J.R. (1987a). Danazol and headaches. *Top. Pain Management 3:*11.

Saper, J.R. (1987b). Ergotamine dependency—a review. *Headache 27:*435–438.

Saper, J.R. (1989). Chronic headache syndromes. *Neurol. Clin. 7:*387–412.

Saper, J.R. (1990a). Chronic headache syndromes. *Neurol. Clin. 8:*891–901.

Saper, J.R. (1990b). Chronic opioid Rx for non-malignant pain? *Top. Pain Management 5:*45.

Saper, J.R., T. Johnson, and M. VanMeter (1983). "Mixed headache," a chronic headache complex. A study of 500 patients. *Headache 23:*143.

Saper, J.R. and J.M. Jones (1986). Ergotamine tartrate dependency: Features and possible mechanisms. *Clin. Neurophamacol. 9:*244–256.

Saper, J.R., N. Mathew, and S.D. Silberstein (1993). Safety and efficacy of Divalproex in the prophylaxis of migraine headaches: A multicenter double-blind placebo-controlled trial. *Neurology* (submitted).

Sargent, J., P. Solbach, H. Damasio et al. (1985). A comparison of naproxen sodium to propranolol hydrochloride and a placebo control for the prophylaxis of migraine headache. *Headache 25:*320–324.

Sarno, A.P., E.J. Miller, and E.G. Lundblad (1987). Premenstrual syndrome: Beneficial effects of periodic, low-dose Danazol. *Obstet. Gynecol. 70:*33–36.

Saxena, P.R. and M.D. Ferrari (1989). 5-HT$_1$-like receptor agonists and the pathophysiology of migraine. *Trends Pharmacol. Sci. 10:*200–204.

Schaumberg, H.H., R. Byck, R. Gerstl, and J.H. Mashman (1969). Monosodium L-glutamate: Its pharmacology and role in the Chinese restaurant syndrome. *Science 163:*826–828.

Schiffman, S.S., C.E. Buckley, and M.A. Sampson. (1987). Aspartame and susceptibility to headache. *N. Engl. J. Med. 317:*1181–1185.

Schmidt, R. and A. Fanchamps (1974). Effect of caffeine on intestinal absorption of ergotamine in man. *Eur. J. Clin. Pharmacol. 7:*213–216.

Schoenen, J., A. Maertens de Noordhout, M. Timsit-Berthier, and M. Timsit (1986). Contingent negative variation and efficacy of β-blocking agents in migraine. *Cephalalgia 6:*231–233.

Scholz, E., H. Diener, and S. Geiselhart (1988). Drug-induced headache—does a critical dosage exist? In *Drug-Induced Headache* (H. Diener and M. Wilkinson, eds.), pp. 29–43. Springer-Verlag, Berlin.

Scholz, M., and M. Hoffert (1987). Low dose nifedipine is no better than vehicle in abortive treatment of classic migraine headache. Presented at the 5th World Congress on Pain, IASP, Hamburg.

Schran, H.F., and F.L.S. Tse (1985). Pharmacokinetics of dihydroergotamine following subcutaneous administration in humans. *Int. J. Clin. Pharmacol. Ther. Toxicol. 23:*1–4.

Selby, G. and J.W. Lance (1960). Observations on 500 cases of migraine and allied vascular headache. *J. Neurol. Neurosurg. Psychiatry 23:*23–32.

Shoemaker, E.S., J.P. Forney, and P.C. MacDonald (1977). Estrogen treatment of post-menopausal women. *JAMA 238:*1524–1530.

Sicuteri, F. (1981). Enkephalinase inhibition relieves pain syndromes of central dysnociception (migraine and related headache). *Cephalalgia 1:*229–232.

Sicuteri, F., A. Testi, and B. Anselmi (1961). Biochemical investigations in headache: Increase in 5-hydroxindoleacetic acid excretion during migraine attacks. *Int. Arch. Allergy Appl. Immunol. 19:*55–58.

Silbergeld, S., N. Brast, and E.P. Noble (1971). The menstrual cycle: A double-blind study of symptoms, mood and behavior, and biochemical variables using enovid and placebo. *Psychosom. Med. 33:*411–428.

Silberstein, S.D. (1984). Treatment of headache in primary care practice. *Am. J. Med. 77*(3A):65–72.

Silberstein, S.D. (1990). Twenty questions about headaches in children and adolescents. *Headache 30:*716–724.

Silberstein, S.D. (1991). Appropriate use of abortive medication in headache treatment. *Pain Management 4:*22–28.

Silberstein, S.D. and G.R. Merriam (1991). Estrogens, progestins, and headache. *Neurology 41:*786–793.

Silberstein, S.D., E.A. Schulman, and M.M. Hopkins (1990). Repetitive intravenous DHE in the treatment of refractory headache. *Headache 30:*334–339.

Silberstein, S.D. and M.M. Silberstein (1990). New concepts in the pathogenesis of headache. *Pain Management 3:*297–303, 334–342.

Silberstein, S.D., and J.R. Silberstein (1992). Analgesic/ergotamine rebound headache: Prognosis following detoxification and treatment with repetitive IV DHE. *Headache 32:*252.

Sillanpaa, M. (1983). Changes in the prevalence of migraine and other headaches during the first seven school years. *Headache 23:*15–19.

Sillanpaa, M. and M. Koponen (1978). Papaverine in the prophylaxis of migraine and other vascular headache in children. *Acta Paediatr. Scand. 67:*209–212.

Sills, M., P. Congdon, and I. Forsythe (1982). Clonidine and childhood migraine: A pilot and double-blind study. *Dev. Med. Child Neurol. 24:*837–841.

Simkins, R.T., N. Tepley, G.L. Barkley, and K.M.A. Welch (1989). Spontaneous neuromagnetic fields in migraine: Possible link to spreading cortical depression. *Neurology 39*(Suppl. 1):325.

Sjaastad, O. and I. Dale (1976). A new(?) clinical headache entity: Chronic paroxysmal hemicrania. 2. *Acta Neurol. Scand. 54:*140–159.

Sjaastad, O. and E.L.H. Spierings (1984). "Hemicrania continua": Another headache absolutely responsive to indomethacin. *Cephalalgia 4*(Suppl. 1):65–70.

Sjaastad, O. and P. Stensrud (1972). Clinical trial of a beta receptor blocking agent (LB 46) in migraine prophylaxis. *Acta Neurol. Scand. 48:*124–128.

Smith, R. and A. Schwartz (1984). Diltiazem prophylaxis in refractory migraine. *N. Engl. J. Med. 310:*1327–1328.

Smyth, G.A. and L. Lazarus (1974). Suppression of growth hormone secretion by melatonin and cyprohetadine. *J. Clin. Invest. 54:*116–121.

Snyder, S.H. and I.J. Reynolds (1985). Calcium-antagonist drugs: Receptor interactions that clarify therapeutic effects. *N. Engl. J. Med. 313:*995–1002.

Solomon, G.D. (1985). Comparative efficacy of calcium antagonist drugs in the prophylaxis of migraine. *Headache 25:*368–371.

Solomon, G.D. (1989). Verapamil in migraine prophylaxis—a five-year review. *Headache 29:*425–427.

Solomon, G. and R. Kunkel (1990). Effects of fluoxetine on premenstrual syndrome in chronic headache sufferers. *Headache 30:*301.

Solomon, G.D., J.G. Steel, and L.J. Spaccavento (1983). Verapamil prophylaxis of migraine: A double-blind, placebo-controlled study. *JAMA 250*:2500–2502.

Solomon, S. and R.B. Lipton (1991). Criteria for the diagnosis of migraine in clinical practice. *Headache 31*:384–387.

Somerville, B.W. (1972a). A study of migraine in pregnancy. *Neurology 22*:824–828.

Somerville, B.W. (1972b). The role of estradiol withdrawal in the etiology of menstrual migraine. *Neurology 22*:355–365.

Somerville, B.W. (1975). Estrogen-withdrawal migraine. *Neurology 25*:239–244.

Sorensen, K.V. (1988). Valproate: A new drug in migraine prophylaxis. *Acta Neurol. Scand. 78*:346–348.

Sorensen, P.S., K. Hansen, and J. Olesen (1986). A placebo-controlled, double-blind, cross-over trial of flunarizine in common migraine. *Cephalalgia 6*:7–14.

Sorge, F., P. Barone, L. Steardo, and M.R. Romano (1982). Amitriptyline as a prophylactic for migraine in children. *Acta Neurol. 5*:362–367.

Sorge, F., R. DeSimone, E. Marano et al. (1988). Flunarizine in prophylaxis of childhood migraine. A double-blind, placebo-controlled, crossover study. *Cephalalgia 8*: 1–6.

Sorge, F., M. Nolano, E. DeStasio et al. (1989). Recurrent abdominal pain, headache and periodic syndrome: Need of a multidisciplinary approach. In *Headache in Children and Adolescents* (G. Lanzi, U. Balottin, and A. Cernibori, eds.), pp. 39–42. Elsevier, New York.

Soyka, D., Z. Taneri, W. Oestreich, and R. Schmidt (1989). Flunarizine IV in the acute treatment of common or classical migraine attacks—a placebo-controlled double-blind trial. *Headache 29*:21–27.

Speed, W.G. (1989). Closed head injury sequelae: Changing concepts. *Headache 29*: 643–647.

Spierings, E.L.H. (1984). The role of arteriovenous shunting in migraine. In *The Pharmacological Basis of Migraine Therapy* (W.K. Amery, J.V. Van Nueten, and A. Wauquier, eds.), pp. 36–49. Pitman, London.

Spierings, E.L.H. (1989). Treatment of the migraine attack. In *Migraine and Other Headaches* (M.D. Ferrari and X. Lataste, eds.), pp. 241–248. Parthenon, Park Ridge NJ.

Stensrud, P. and O. Sjaastad (1976). Short term trial of propranolol in racemic form (Inderal), d-propranolol and placebo in migraine. *Acta Neurol. Scand. 53*: 229–232.

Stewart, D.J., A. Gelston, and A. Hakim (1988). Effect of prophylactic administration of nimodipine in patients with migraine. *Headache 28*:260–262.

Stoica, E. and O. Enulescu (1990). Propranolol corrects the abnormal catecholamine response to light during migraine. *Eur. Neurol. 30*:19–22.

The Subcutaneous Sumatriptan International Study Group (1991). Treatment of migraine attacks with sumatriptan. *N. Engl. J. Med. 325*:316–321.

Sudilovsky, A., A.H. Elkind, R.E. Ryan et al. (1987). Comparative efficacy of nadolol and propranolol in the management of migraine. *Headache 27*:421–426.

Symon, D.K., and G. Russell (1989). The general paediatrician's view of migraine—a review of 250 cases. In *Headache in Children and Adolescents* (G. Lanzi, U. Balottin, and A. Cernibori, eds.), pp. 61–66. Elsevier, New York.

Takeshima, T., S. Nishikawa, and K. Takahashi (1988). Sublingual administration of flunarizine for acute migraine: Will flunarizine take the place of ergotamine? *Headache 28*:602–606.

Tfelt-Hansen, P. (1986). Efficacy of β-blockers in migraine. *Cephalalgia 6*(Suppl. 5): 15–24.

Tfelt-Hansen, P., J. Olesen, A. Aebelholt-Krabbe et al. (1980). A double-blind study of metoclopramide in the treatment of migraine attacks. *J. Neurol. Neurosurg. Psychiatry 43*:369–371.

Tfelt-Hansen, P., B. Standnes, P. Kangasniemi et al. (1984). Timolol vs propranolol vs placebo in common migraine prophylaxis: A double-blind multicenter trial. *Acta Neurol. Scand. 69*:1–8.

Tillgren, N. (1947). Treatment of headache with dihydroergotamine tartrate. *Acta Med. Scand. Suppl. 196*:222–228.

Tokola, R. and E. Hokkanen (1978). Propranolol for acute migraine. *BMJ 2*:1089.

Tollefson, G.D. (1983). Monoamine oxidase inhibitors: A review. *J. Clin. Psychiatry 44*: 280–288.

Troost, B.T., L.E. Mark, and J.C. Maroon (1979). Resolution of classic migraine after removal of an occipital lobe arteriovenous malformation. *Ann. Neurol. 5*: 199–201.

Ustdal, M., P. Dogan, A. Soyeur, and S. Terzi (1989). Treatment of migraine with salmon calcitonin: Effects on plasma β-endorphin, ACTH, and cortisol levels. *Biomed. Pharmacother. 43*:687–691.

Utian, W.H. (1974). Oestrogen, headache and oral contraceptives. *S. Afr. Med. J. 48*: 2105–2108.

Utian, W.H. (1987a). Overview on menopause. *Am. J. Obstet. Gynecol. 156*:1280–1283.

Utian, W.H. (1987b). The fate of the untreated menopause. *Obstet. Gynecol. Clin. North Am. 14*:1–11.

Van den Bergh, V., W.K. Amery, and J. Waelkens (1987). Trigger factors in migraine: A study conducted by the Belgian migraine society. *Headache 27*:191–196.

Van Meter, M. and J.R. Saper (1981). An inpatient headache unit: Development, direction, and struggles. *Headache 21*:126.

Vardi, J., J.M. Rabey, and M. Streifler (1979). Prostaglandins and their synthesis inhibitors in migraine. In *Practical Applications of Prostaglandins and Their Synthesis Inhibitors* (S.M.M. Karin, ed.), pp. 139–148. University Park Press, Baltimore.

Vijayan, N. (1977). Brief therapeutic report: Papaverine prophylaxis of complicated migraine. *Headache 17*:159–162.

Volans, G.N. (1978). Research review: Migraine and drug absorption. *Clin. Pharmacokinet. 3*:313–318.

Waelkens, J., I. Caers, and W.K. Amery (1986). Effects of therapeutic measures taken during the premonitory phase. In *The Prelude to the Migraine Attack* (W.K. Amery and A. Wauquier, eds.), pp. 78–83. Bailliere Tindall, London.

Ward, N., C. Whitney, D. Avery, and D. Dunner (1991). The analgesic effects of caffeine in headache. *Pain 44*:141–155.

Waters, W.E. (1986). *Headache* (Series in Clinical Epidemiology). Wright-PSG, Littleton, MA.

Wauquier, A., D. Ashton, and R. Marranes (1985). The effects of flunarizine in experimental models related to the pathogenesis of migraine. *Cephalalgia 5*(Suppl. 2): 119–120.

Weber, R.B. and O.M. Reinmuth (1972). The treatment of migraine with propranolol. *Neurology 22*:366–369.

Weilburg, J.B., J.F. Rosenbaum, J. Biederman et al. (1989). Fluoxetine added to non-MAOI antidepressants converts nonresponders to responders: A preliminary report. *J. Clin. Psychiatry 50*:447–449.

Welch, K.M.A., E. Chabi, K. Bartosh et al. (1975). Cerebrospinal fluid gamma aminobutyric acid levels in migraine. *BMJ 3*:516–517.

Welch, K.M.A., G. D'Andrea, N. Tepley et al. (1990). The concept of migraine as a state of central neuronal hyperexcitability. *Neurol. Clin. 8*:817–828.

Wendorff, J. (1989). Symptomatic and idiopathic headaches in four years of practice in our neuropediatric department. In *Headache in Children and Adolescents* (G. Lanzi, U. Balottin, and A. Cernibori, eds.), pp. 55–60. Elsevier, New York.

Wentz, A.C. (1985). Management of the menopause. In *Novak's Textbook of Gynecology*, 11th ed. (H.W. Jones, A.C. Wentz, and L.S. Burnett, eds.), pp. 397–442. Williams & Wilkins, Baltimore.

White, K. and G. Simpson (1984). The combined use of MAOIs and tricyclics. *J. Clin. Psychiatry 45*:67–69.

Whitty, C.W.M. (1967). Migraine without headache. *Lancet 2*:283–285.

Whitty, C.W.M. (1986). Familial hemiplegic migraine. In *Handbook of Clinical Neurology, Vol. 48, Headache* (F.C. Rose, ed.), pp. 141–153. Elsevier, New York.

Whitty, C.W.M. and J.M. Hockaday (1968). Migraine: A follow-up study of 92 patients. *BMJ 1*:735–736.

Wilkinson, M. (1986). Clinical features of migraine. In *Handbook of Clinical Neurology, Vol. 48, Headache* (F.C. Rose, ed.), pp. 117–133. Elsevier, New York.

Wilkinson, M. (1988a). Introduction. In *Drug-Induced Headache* (H. Diener and M. Wilkinson, eds.), pp. 1–2. Springer-Verlag, Berlin.

Wilkinson, M. (1988b). Treatment of migraine. *Headache 28*:659–661.

Williams, M.J., R.I. Harris, and B.C. Dean (1985). Controlled trial of pyridoxine in the premenstrual syndrome. *J. Int. Med. Res. 1*:174–179.

Wyllie, W.G. and B. Schlesinger (1933). The periodic group of disorders in childhood. *Br. J. Child. Dis. 30*:349–351.

Ylostalo, P., A. Kauppila, J. Puolakka et al. (1982). Bromocriptine and norethisterone in the treatment of premenstrual syndrome. *Obstet. Gynecol. 58*:292–298.

Yuill, G.M., W.R. Swinburn, and L.A. Liversedge (1972). A double-blind crossover trial of isometheptene mucate compound and ergotamine in migraine. *Br. J. Clin. Pract. 26*:76–79.

Zammarano, C.B., E. Quaranti, M.C. Miceli, and D. Poli (1989). A statistical analysis of the distribution of the clinical patterns of migraine. In *Headache in Children and Adolescents* (G. Lanzi, U. Balottin, and A. Cernibori, eds.), pp. 67–74. Elsevier, New York.

Ziegler, D.K. (1985). The headache symptom: How many entities? *Arch. Neurol. 42*:273–277.

Ziegler, D.K. (1987). The treatment of migraine. In *Wolff's Headache and Other Head Pain*, 5th ed. (D.J. Dalessio, ed.), pp. 87–111. Oxford University Press, New York.

Ziegler, D.K. and R.S. Hassanein (1990). Specific headache phenomena: Their frequency and coincidence. *Headache 30*:152–156.

Ziegler, D.K., A. Hurwitz, R.S. Hassanein et al. (1987). Migraine prophylaxis: A comparison of propranolol and amitriptyline. *Arch. Neurol. 44*:486–489.

6

Cluster Headache: Diagnosis, Management, and Treatment

LEE KUDROW

Cluster headache is a severe unilateral, brief duration headache that occurs in bouts and is frequently associated with ipsilateral nasal stuffiness, rhinorrhea, lacrimation, and conjunctival injection. It was first described by Eulenburg (1874) and Romberg (1840), independently, and later by Harris (1926). It is often referred to as "migrainous neuralgia," after Harris (1936). Horton et al. (1939), however, popularized the condition when they described it as a new syndrome. Ekbom (1947) was the first to report the periodic nature of cluster headache. This "clustering" pattern, noted by Kunkle et al. (1954), gave the term "cluster headache" to the disorder (Table 6–1).

CLASSIFICATION

Cluster headache was first classified as a primary headache disorder by the Ad Hoc Committee on the Classification of Headache in 1962. Its nomenclature was reaffirmed by the Migraine Research Group of the World Federation of Neurology in 1969 and most recently refined by the Headache Classification Committee of the International Headache Society in 1988 (Table 6–2). The latter classification excluded variants such as cluster–vertigo (Gilbert, 1965, 1970), cluster–migraine (Medina and Diamond, 1977), and cluster–tic syndrome (Green and Apfelbaum, 1978; Hornabrook, 1964; Kunkel and Dohn, 1974; Lance and Anthony, 1971b; Watson and Evans, 1985). These variants were reduced to "cluster headache–like syndromes." Excluded also from the current nomenclature is "symptomatic cluster headache." Although some or all of these variants will likely reappear in subsequent classification attempts, their descriptions are omitted from this review.

Table 6–1 Cluster headache eponyms, misnomers, and other appellations

Authors	Date	Eponyms	Other names
Romberg	1840	Description only	
Möllendorff	1867		Red migraine
Eulenburg	1878		Angioparalytic hemicrania
Sluder	1910	Sluder's syndrome	Sphenopalatine neuralgia
			Lower-half headache
Bing	1913	Bing's headache	Erythroprosopalgia
		Bing's syndrome	
Harris	1926		Migrainous neuralgia
Harris	1936		Ciliary neuralgia
Vail	1932		Vidian neuralgia
Gardner et al.	1947		Greater superficial
			petrosal neuralgia
Horton et al.	1939	Horton's headache	Erythromelalgia
	1952	Horton's syndrome	Histaminic cephalgia
Kunkle et al.	1952		Cluster headache

Reproduced with permission from Kudrow, L. (1979). Cluster headache: Diagnosis and management. *Headache* 19:143.

DEFINITION

There are two major types of cluster headache (subtypes or variations are not discussed here). The *episodic type* is the most common, constituting 80% of all cases. Episodic cluster headache is defined by periods of susceptibility to headache, called "cluster periods," alternating with periods of refractoriness called "remissions."

Chronic cluster headache is a term used when remissions have not occurred for at least 12 months. Other characteristics of chronic cluster, such as increased frequency of attacks and decreased responsiveness to prophylactic drug therapy, distinguish it from episodic cluster. A lack of remissions since onset of disease defines primary cluster headache. Secondary chronic headache patients have in the past experienced remissions, but subsequently become chronic (Ekbom and Olivarius, 1971). Despite the distinction between primary and secondary chronic cluster, there appears to be little difference—either therapeutically or prognostically—between the two types.

Table 6–2 International Headache Society classification of cluster headache

Cluster headache	3.1
Periodicity undetermined	3.1.1
Episodic	3.1.2
Chronic	3.1.3
Primary chronic	3.1.3.1
Secondary chronic	3.1.3.2
Chronic paroxysmal hemicrania	3.2
Cluster headache-like syndrome	3.3

Chronic paroxysmal hemicrania, or Sjaastad syndrome, was first described in 1974 (Sjaastad and Dale, 1974). At this time it is considered by many to be a variant of cluster headache. There appear to be sufficient differences, however, to consider chronic paroxysmal hemicrania quite separately from cluster headache (Sjaastad et al., 1980).

CLINICAL PICTURE

Cluster periods, those periods during which attacks occur, generally last between 6 and 12 weeks. Remission periods have an average duration of approximately 12 months. There may be considerable variation. Attacks occur with a frequency of approximately one to three times a day, each lasting about 45 minutes. They are unilateral, oculotemporal or oculofrontal in location, excruciating in severity, and boring and nonthrobbing in character. The associated symptoms are also unilateral and consist of lacrimation, rhinorrhea or nasal stuffiness, and a partial Horner syndrome that includes unilateral ptosis and miosis. The frequency with which partial Horner syndrome is observed during cluster attacks has been reported separately by Ekbom (1970a), Lance (1978), and Kudrow (1979) (Table 6–3).

Characteristically, vasodilator medications such as nitroglycerin and histamine will induce cluster attacks. Ekbom (1968) was able to induce an acute cluster attack in all his subjects diagnosed as having cluster headache using 1 mg of nitroglycerin sublingually. Often, but not always, alcohol induces an acute cluster attack while the patient is in an active cluster period. Attacks are commonly induced on awakening from a nap in the afternoon or from sleep during the night, most commonly approximately 90 minutes after falling asleep.

The Cluster Attack

The cluster attack is stereotyped by specific signs, symptoms, emotions, and behavior. The following is a firsthand account of such an episode (Kudrow, 1980, pp. 25–27):

> Following a period of perhaps several hours of feeling quite elated and energetic, I experienced a fullness in my ears, somewhat more on the right side than the left, having a character similar to that which occurs during rapid descent in an airplane

Table 6–3 Frequency of ptosis and/or miosis in cluster headache clinic populations

Investigators	Year	Temporary	Permanent
Ekbom	1970	69	5.7 (ptosis)
			6.7 (miosis)
Lance and Anthony	1971	32	Rare
Kudrow	1981	60	0.5

Reproduced with permission from Kudrow, L. (1982). Cluster headache: Clinical, mechanistic, and treatment aspects. *Panminerva Med. 24*:47.

or elevator. I then became aware of a dull discomfort, an extension of ear fullness at the base of my skull—further extending over the entire head, on both sides, though somewhat more on the right. At this point, two or three minutes have elapsed; seemingly short but long enough for me to know that a "cluster" has indeed begun and will ultimately get worse. Such anticipation causes me considerable consternation regarding any decision to continue my activities, or cancel plans and find a place to be alone; giving way to a slowly increasing anxiety, fear, panic and withdrawal. I become aware of myself "listening" for changes in my head. Is the cluster prematurely aborting itself, progressing further, or unchanging? A sudden stab, only fleeting, strikes my temple, then again—somewhere near the apex of my skull and upper molars in my face, always on the right side. It strikes me again, deep into the skull base, and as quickly, changes location to a small area above my eyebrow. My nose is stuffed and yet runs simultaneously. If I could sneeze I feel the attack would end. Yet in spite of all tricks, I find myself unable to induce sneezing. While the sharp stabs continue in this fashion, a slow crescendo of dull pain presents itself in an area of a hand's length and breadth over the eye and temporal region. The pain area narrows into a smaller area, and yet, as if magnified, enlarges in intensity. I find myself bending my neck downward, though slightly, as if my head is being gently pushed from behind. My neck, up to the base of my skull, is tight and feels as if I was wearing a neck collar. I feel compelled to remove my tie and loosen my shirt collar even though I know that it will not offer me even a modicum of relief.

In an effort to alter this persistent discomfort, I drop my head between my legs while seated. My face and eyes seem to fill with fluid, but the pain persists and remains unchanged. Despite my suntan, as I look into the mirror, a gaunt, sickly, pale face peers back. My right lid is only slightly drooping and the white of my eye is charted with many red vessels, giving the eye an overall color of pink. Right and left pupils appear equal and constricted, as is usual for light-eyed people. Having difficulty standing in one place too long, I leave the mirror to continue alternating my pacing and sitting.

As usual, I am struck with the additional fear that the pain will never end, but dismiss it as impossible, since even if that were the case, I would surely kill myself.

The pain, now located somewhere behind my eye and slightly above it, worsens. The pain is best described as a "force" pushing with such incredible power through my eye that my head appears to be moving backward, yielding to its resistance. The "force" wanes and waxes, but the duration of successive exacerbations seem to increase. The cluster attack is at its peak which is celebrated by an outpouring of tears from only my right eye. I have now been in cluster for thirty-five minutes—ten minutes at its peak.

My wife peeks into the room where I hold forth. I look up and see her expression of pity, frustration, and helplessness. She sees my tortured face as I have seen it in the mirror at this stage before; a drooling mouth, agape, gray face wet on one side, an almost closed eyelid; and smelling of pain and anguish. She closes the door and leaves, feeling hurt for me, anger for the stupidity of medical science, and guilt—since deep within her mind is the suspicion that she is the cause for my suffering.

I cry for her, but cry more for myself. The pain is so incredible. Suddenly I am overwhelmed by a fury. I lift a chair high over my head and crash it to the floor. With a doubled fist I strike the wall. The pain persists.

Waning periods soon become longer in duration and I allow myself to suspect that the peak is behind me—but cautiously, since I have been too often disappointed.

Indeed, the pain is ending. The descent from the mountain is rapid. The "force" is gone. Only severe pain remains. My nose and eye continue to run. The road back, as with all travel, covers the same territory, but faster. Stabbing, easily tolerated pain is felt. Then gone. Dull, aching fullness, neck stiffness, all disappear, replaced in turn by a welcome sensation of pins and needles over the right scalp area—similar to the way one's leg feels after it has been "asleep." Thus my head has awakened after a nightmare of torment.

Eye and nose dry, I let out a sigh. I collect my pile of wet tissues that are strewn all over the floor and deposit them in a wastepaper basket. The innocent chair, now uprighted, I rub my slightly bruised fist.

Thus, having ended the battle and cleaned up its field, I open the door and enter my pain-free world . . . until tomorrow.

Prevalence

The prevalence rate of cluster headache in the general population is unknown. Estimates have been offered, however, based on populations in headache clinics (Table 6–4). These have varied from rates of 0.04% (Heyck, 1975) to 1.5% (Kudrow, 1980).

Sex, Age, and Race

Cluster headache is predominantly a male disorder. Male-to-female ratios of clinic populations range from 4.5:1 to 6.7:1 (Ekbom, 1970a; Friedman and Mikropoulos, 1958; Kudrow, 1980; Lance and Anthony, 1971b; Lovshin, 1961). The mean age of onset, approximately 27 to 30 years, varies little between clinic populations (Ekbom, 1970a; Friedman and Mikropoulos, 1958; Kudrow, 1980). The range varies widely, however, from the age of 1 year (Kudrow, 1980) to the late 60s (Table 6–5).

Lovshin (1961) reported that black patients appeared to be overrepresented within the Cleveland Clinic's population of patients with cluster headache. Our own clinic survey supports this finding (Kudrow, 1980).

Table 6–4 Several reports on the prevalence of cluster headache and migraine

Authors	No. of patients		Migraine-cluster ratio
	Migraine	Cluster	
Lieder	52	4	13.0:1
Carroll	89	16	5.6:1
Balla and Walton	399	28	14.3:1
Ekbom	400	16	25.0:1
Lance et al.	612	13	47.1:1
Heyck	1890	48	39.4:1
Friedman	2667	237	11.3:1
Kudrow	2835	425	6.7:1

Reproduced with permission from Kudrow, L. (1979). Cluster headache: Diagnosis and management. *Headache* *19:*144.

Table 6–5 Male–female ratio and mean age at onset of cluster headache

Authors	Date	No. of patients	Onset Age	Onset Range	M:F Ratio
Friedman and Mikropoulos	1958	50	28	11–44	4.5:1
Ekbom	1970	105	27.5	10–61	5.6:1
Lance and Anthony	1971	60		8–62	6.5:1
Kudrow	1979	425	29.6	1–63	5.1:1

Reproduced with permission from Kudrow, L. (1979). Cluster headache: Diagnosis and management. *Headache* 19:144.

Periodicity

The cluster period is characterized by susceptibility to attack; spontaneous and provoked attacks are limited to this time span. It applies only to patients with episodic cluster headache. Ekbom (1970b) reported a frequency of one to two times a year in approximately 70% of patients. In another survey (Kudrow, 1980), the mean duration of cluster periods was found to be 3 months, with a range of 2 to 4 months, in 84% of patients. These results were consistent with those of other reports (Ekbom, 1970a; Friedman and Mikropoulos, 1958; Lance, 1978).

Ekbom (1970b) suggested that highest cluster period frequencies occurred in spring and autumn. Lance (1978) did not find this to be the case. The distribution of cluster period frequency was found to be equally divided among all four seasons in his series.

More recently, a cyclic periodicity of cluster periods was confirmed (Kudrow, 1987b; Kudrow et al., 1990). Approximately 400 patients who recorded 900 cluster periods were evaluated prospectively over a 10-year period. The frequency of cluster periods was found to be related to photoperiod changes (length of daylight), increasing with shortening or lengthening photoperiods. Cluster period frequency peaks occurred within 2 weeks following the longest and shortest days of the year (July and January) and decreased within 2 weeks following the changing of the clocks for Daylight Savings and Standard times. The proposed mechanisms for these observations is discussed below.

Rhythmicity of cluster headache attacks within cluster periods has also been noted. Attacks that occur 24 hours apart frequently recur at the same time. Attacks that occur twice a day are generally 12 hours apart but, more importantly, at the same time of the day.

Remission Periods

Remissions are spontaneously occurring periods during which attacks do not occur—either spontaneously or provoked. According to Ekbom (1970a), the average duration of remission periods was less than 2 years. Records from 428 patients at the California Medical Clinic for Headache revealed that 19.2% experienced remissions of between 1 and 6 months, 47.7% between 7 and 12 months, 14.3% for 2 years, and the remainder longer than 2 years' duration (Kudrow, 1980).

Physical Characteristics

Graham (1969) noted that a great many individuals with cluster headache had specific facial features. He described a "leonine" appearance, deep skin furrows (especially the nasolabial and glabellar folds), and forehead wrinkles. There appears to be narrowing of the palpebral fissures, asymmetric skin wrinkles, telangiectasia, and "orange-peel" thick skin; overall, the appearance is similar to that of an alcoholic (Table 6–6). Graham stated, however, that some of his patients who were nondrinkers had the typical cluster facies (personal communication, 1974). He found that, although women had none of these characteristics, they were somewhat masculine looking. We have noted similar appearances among some of our women patients with cluster headache. Moreover, we have found that some of our male patients had characteristics more descriptive of acromegaly in appearance (Kudrow, 1979).

On the average, males with cluster headache are 3 inches taller than matched male controls (Kudrow, 1974; Schele et al., 1978). In our clinic population, hazel eye color occurred three times more frequently than in controls. Patients with cluster headache smoked more cigarettes per day than controls. Use of alcohol was significantly greater in the cluster group. Hemoglobin levels have been reported to be higher among patients with cluster headache (Graham et al., 1970; Kudrow, 1974), although, in a more recent survey, no significant differences in hemoglobin were found between cluster and control groups (Kudrow, 1980).

Associated Disorders

An increased incidence of peptic ulcer disease has been reported by Ekbom (1970b), Graham (1972), and others. We found a 21% incidence of duodenal ulcer disease in our male cluster population—twice that of controls (Kudrow, 1976b).

Table 6–6 Physical characteristics often observed among males with cluster headache

Facial
Ruddy complexion
Deep furrows
"Orange-peel" skin
Telangiectasia
Narrowed palpebral fissures
Asymmetric creases
Broad chin, skull
Leonine appearance
General
Rugged appearance
Tall, trim
Obesity rare
Hazel eye color (1/3)

Reproduced with permission from Kudrow, L. (1979). Cluster headache: Diagnosis and management. *Headache 19*:145.

Table 6-7 Incidence (%) of various disorders in cluster headache compared with noncluster and general population groups

Group	Migraine M	Migraine F	Ulcer (M)	CHD (M)	HBP (M)
Cluster	10.9	52.4	21.0	7.6	3.4
Noncluster			10.7*	3.6	8.6
U.S. population	4.0	16.0*	10.0*	3.0	10.0

* $p < 0.5$.

Reproduced with permission from Kudrow, L. (1979). Cluster headache: Diagnosis and management. *Headache* 19:145.

Key to abbreviations: CHD, coronary heart disease; HBP, high blood pressure.

The incidence of coronary artery disease among our cluster patients was higher than that of controls, but not significantly. Graham believes that a significant difference would have been reached had our cluster and control groups been older (personal communication, 1976). Hypertension was negatively associated with the cluster headache group. This low frequency, however, was not significant.

The incidence of migraine among women with cluster was over 50%, consistent with the results of Lance and Anthony (1971a). Among males with cluster, a higher but not significantly higher frequency of migraine was found (Kudrow, 1976b) (Table 6-7).

Personality and Psychopathology

Contrary to earlier reports, Minnesota Multiphasic Personality Inventory studies by Kudrow and Sutkus (1979) and others (Andrasik et al., 1982; Cuypers et al., 1981) have not demonstrated a greater frequency of neuroses or other psychopathology in cluster headache populations, when compared to controls.

DIFFERENTIAL DIAGNOSIS

Only a few conditions can possibly be confused with cluster headache. These include chronic paroxysmal hemicrania, migraine, trigeminal neuralgia, temporal arteritis, pheochromocytoma, and Raeder's paratrigeminal syndrome (Table 6-8).

Chronic Paroxysmal Hemicrania

Chronic paroxysmal hemicrania (CPH) was first described by Sjaastad and Dale (1974). Sjaastad (1987) reported that he had been personally informed of approximately 80 cases worldwide; thus, CPH remains a rare entity. According to Russell (1984), the mean CPH attack frequency was found to be 14 attacks per day, ranging from 4 to 38 per day. The mean duration of attacks was 15 minutes, with a range of 3 to 46 minutes.

Table 6–8 Differential diagnosis

Disorder	Frequency	Duration	Location	Intensity	Quality	Other findings
Cluster	1–3/day	30–90 min	Unilateral, oculofrontal, temporal	Excruciating	Nonthrobbing, boring	Unilateral lacrimation, rhinorrhea, conjunctival injection, partial horner, can't lie down
CPH	4–38/day	3–46 min	Unilateral oculofrontal, temporal	Severe	Nonthrobbing, boring	Unilateral lacrimation, rhinorrhea, conjunctival injection, partial horner, not restless
Migraine	1–3/month	6–30 hr	Unilateral 60%	Severe	Throbbing 80%	Nausea 85%, Vomiting 40%, Photophobia >85%, Sonophobia
Trigeminal neuralgia	Several/day	Seconds to minutes	Unilateral, 5th nerve distribution	Severe	Electric, lancinating, nonthrobbing	Trigger zones on face
Temporal arteritis	Persistent		Unilateral, temporal	Severe	Burning, throbbing, nonthrobbing	Chewing claudication, tender and torturous temporal artery, elevated ESR, polymyalgia
Pheochromocytoma	Daily to monthly	Less than 1 hr	Bilateral, occipital	Severe in supine position	Throbbing	Sweating, pallor, tachycardia with rise in blood pressure
Raeder syndrome	Persistent	Persistent	Unilateral supraocular	Severe	Burning, throbbing, nonthrobbing	Partial horner syndrome

Although CPH has been considered a chronic disorder, as the term implies, a prechronic state has been described (Pelz & Mersky, 1982; Sjaastad, 1987; Sjaastad et al., 1980). An episodic type of paroxysmal hemicrania was recently reported (Kudrow et al., 1987). CPH differs from cluster headache in that attacks are more frequent, shorter in duration, and associated with less restlessness. Most importantly, CPH is completely responsive to indomethacin and unresponsive to anticluster prophylactic medications (Sjaastad, 1987).

Migraine

Characteristically, migraine attacks occur with a frequency of one to three times a month, often associated with menstrual periods. Each attack may last from 1 to 3 days with some variation; pain develops slowly over a period of several hours. In 80% of cases the headache is unilateral, involving the region of the temporal artery and extending over the hemicranial area. Often, the pain is described as throbbing and is associated with nausea, vomiting, photophobia and sonophobia. Not infrequently, strong odors are poorly tolerated during the headache phase. Paresthesias, hot-and-cold sensations, orthostatic lightheadedness, and anorexia may also be experienced. In migraine with aura, a visual prodrome lasting approximately 30 minutes precedes the headache phase.

Trigeminal Neuralgia

Trigeminal neuralgia occurs with equal frequency in men and women, generally in older age groups. The pain of trigeminal neuralgia is characterized as severe, razor sharp, electriclike, or cutting. It is precipitated by the touching of trigger zones on the face, ipsilaterally. These zones are most commonly found in an area around the nasolabial folds, but may occur anywhere from the chin to the forehead. Activation of the trigger site may result from the slightest touch, including even a gentle breeze across the face. Most frequently, the act of eating, chewing, or shaving triggers the attack. The attack begins with a slight sensation of gentle jabbing over the involved site followed by a sensation of lightning tics that last from seconds to minutes. The attack may begin abruptly without warning sensations. Among other differentiating features, attacks of trigeminal neuralgia are not likely to occur in the middle of the night, awakening the patient from sleep, as seen in cluster headache (Dalessio, 1969).

Temporal Arteritis

Temporal arteritis generally affects older age groups. The arteries most typically affected are the superficial, temporal, vertebral, and ophthalmic. Other arteries, such as the internal carotid and the central retinal, are also affected, although less frequently. The disease is self-limiting but may cause blindness if untreated. In approximately 50% of cases, a nonspecific aching or stiffness of the neck, shoulders, or hip girdle precedes the onset of head pain by several months (polymyalgia rheumatica). The head pain is described as persistent, waxing and waning throughout the day, unilateral in location, and related to the distribution of the superficial temporal artery. It is severe, burning, and throbbing in the early course of the disease and nonthrobbing later. The superficial temporal artery is generally tender on palpation and reveals a marked firmness and tortuosity. Claudication on chewing is frequently experienced and is an important feature. The sedimentation rate is generally markedly elevated. The finding of giant cells on temporal artery biopsy is diagnostic of this condition (Horton et al., 1932; Huston et al., 1978).

Pheochromocytoma

The paroxysmal hypertensive episode seen in pheochromocytoma is associated with release of catecholamine followed by head pain, pallor, tachycardia, and profuse sweating. The pain may be described as paroxysmal, rapid in onset, and severe. It often awakens the patient during the early morning hours and is commonly induced during exertion. Headaches are characterized as throbbing and almost always bilateral and occipital in location. Coughing, sneezing, bending, and straining may aggravate the pain. Attacks may occur with a daily to monthly frequency, generally lasting less than 1 hour (Thomas et al., 1966).

Raeder's Paratrigeminal Syndrome

The pain of Raeder syndrome is persistent and may last from weeks to months. During the first 2 weeks the patient is likely to be awakened in the middle of the night with severe unilateral pain of a burning, throbbing, or nonthrobbing character. Late in the course, the pain is less severe but continuous. Drooping of the ipsilateral eyelid associated with miosis is an accompanying feature. Anhydrosis is not a typical feature of this disorder. Several features causing confusion with cluster headache include partial Horner syndrome, severe and burning ipsilateral supraorbital pain, and pain awakening the patient in the middle of the night. Unlike cluster headache, however, the duration of pain is constant (Raeder, 1924; Vijayan and Watson, 1978).

GENETICS AND FAMILY HISTORY

The frequency of familial migraine among patients with cluster headaches differs little from that of control populations. Reports have varied from 15 to 34% (Ekbom, 1970a; Kudrow, 1980; Kunkle et al., 1954; Lance, 1978). The frequency of familial cluster headache among patients with cluster headache in our series was only 3.4% (Kudrow, 1980). A search for human leukocyte antigen (HLA) specificity in a population of 25 male patients with cluster headache revealed no significant differences for HLA frequency (Kudrow, 1978b). This negative finding was corroborated by Cuypers and Altenkirch (1979). In contrast to these reports, Martelletti et al. (1984) reported a decreased frequency of antigen HLA-B14 in their cluster headache population.

MECHANISMS

Vascular and Hemodynamic Changes

Following their initial observations of patients with cluster headache, Horton et al. (1939) concluded that dilation of the external carotid artery caused the symptoms of cluster headache. Furthermore, Horton (1952) believed that this dilation was mediated by intrinsic blood histamine. He noted that during the attack patients often exhibited enlarged temporal arteries, compression of which relieved the pain. He also observed an ipsilateral flush during the attacks associated with an increase in skin temperature of 1 to 2°C. It should be noted, however, that Ekbom and Kudrow (1979) have not found flushing to be a characteristic of cluster headache; in fact, ipsilateral pallor was more frequently observed.

Because of the retro-orbital location of pain, investigations in recent years turned to possible changes in the internal carotid artery. Broch et al. (1970) could find no blood flow changes between contralateral and ipsilateral internal carotid arteries after placing flowmeters on those vessels during cluster attacks. It should be noted that placement of the flowmeter probes was quite proximal (1 cm above the carotid sinus) and thus the probes conceivably could have been insensitive to more distal carotid artery changes.

Sjaastad et al. (1974) measured cutaneous blood flow by an isotope washout method on symptomatic and contralateral sides of the forehead in six patients during attack and interval phases of cluster attack periods. Although the lowest cutaneous blood flow values were found on the ipsilateral side during attacks, differences were not significant. Conversely, dynamic tonometry revealed increased pulse-synchronous amplitudes on the symptomatic side during attacks. The researchers concluded that, although this evidence did not allow for deductions regarding total blood flow through the eye, vasoconstriction occurring in more distal segments of the intraocular vessels could induce proximal vasodilation in an effort to overcome increased resistance to blood flow.

Contrary to these observations, during a fortuitous angiographic examination of a patient experiencing an acute attack of cluster headache, Ekbom and Greitz (1970) noted a segmental luminal narrowing of the ipsilateral internal carotid artery in the region of the carotid canal. They also found a significant dilation of the ipsilateral ophthalmic artery. In view of Ekbom and Greitz's findings, we studied supraorbital and frontal artery blood flow changes in patients with cluster headache using Doppler flow velocity examinations and facial thermography (Kudrow, 1979). Our Doppler flow velocity result, later corroborated by Nattero et al. (1980), revealed decreased supraorbital artery flow velocity ipsilaterally. Facial thermography consistently revealed decreased temperatures over the supraorbital area (Kudrow, 1979), corroborating the thermographic findings of Friedman and Wood (1976) and Lance and Anthony (1971b). Doppler flow velocity patterns in cluster headache, however, remain contradictory. Changes between ipsilateral and contralateral supraorbital arteries among patients were reported to be higher ipsilaterally (Schroth et al., 1983) or not significantly different (Russell and Lindegaard, 1985).

Cerebral blood flow (CBF) appears to be increased during an attack of cluster headache. Norris et al. (1976) first reported increased values for CBF in a patient during an attack. Sakai and Meyer (1978), in a rather extensive study, presented their findings on CBF. During the cluster attack there was a significant increase in CBF in both hemispheres, but more so in the contralateral hemisphere. In contrast, Henry et al. (1978) could not demonstrate CBF changes in three patients with cluster headache. More recently, Aebelholt-Krabbe et al. (1984) found an increased regional CBF in central, basal, and parietotemporal regions during attacks.

Increased CBF in cluster headache has been explained as an impairment of autoregulatory responses (Sakai and Meyer, 1978), reactive hyperemia (Norris et al., 1976), or a pain-related activity (Aebelholt-Krabbe et al., 1984). Sakai and Meyer (1979) lent further support to the hypothesis of impaired autoregulatory activity by demonstrating an impaired response to carbon dioxide and increased response to oxygen.

Impaired Sympathetic Neuronal Activity

The vascular changes described above may reflect autonomic nervous system dysfunction in the pathogenesis of cluster headache. Direct evidence of impaired central sympathetic activity has been reported.

In their now classic pupillometric study, Fanciullacci et al. (1982) demonstrated impaired sympathetic neuronal activity during patients' cluster periods, between attacks. Following instillation of 2% tyramine solution to the eyes of cluster patients and control subjects, they found significant impairment of midriatic responses in the ipsilateral pupil when compared to the contralateral side. Their results were corroborated by Salvesen et al. (1987) and Boccuni et al. (1984). The latter authors, having found electrocardiographic evidence of hyperventilation-provoked asynchronous repolarization, further suggested that impaired sympathetic neuronal activity was not limited to pupillary responses (Boccuni et al., 1984).

Facial sweating patterns were also found to be abnormal among cluster headache patients when compared to controls. Saunte et al. (1983) reported that, in a population of cluster patients, thermal stimulation by heat and exercise during cluster periods but between attacks demonstrated a decreased sweating response ipsilaterally. Pilocarpine administration, however, caused ipsilaterally increased sweating, suggesting a denervation, hypersensitivity response. Contrary to most other systems, a hypersensitivity response due to sympathetic denervation of sweat glands would suggest preganglionic involvement.

Biochemical and Hormonal Changes

Consistent with the suspicions of Horton (1952) that histamine played a major role in cluster headache, Sjaastad (1970) found an increased urinary output of histamine in three of six patients during cluster attacks. Subsequently, Sjaastad and Sjaastad (1977) determined urinary excretion of labeled histamine and its metabolites in cluster headache following oral and subcutaneous administration of radioactive histamine. With the exception of one patient who was diagnosed as having chronic paroxysmal hemicrania, the results in all patients were normal. Anthony and Lance (1971) obtained blood histamine levels from 20 patients with cluster headache during 22 attacks. Histamine levels were found to be higher during headache periods than during preheadache periods in 19 of 22 attacks. The mean increase was 20.5%, a highly significant difference. The importance of these changes in histamine levels is questionable, however, because in a series of patients later studied by Anthony et al. (1978), the frequency of cluster attacks was not decreased after prophylactic administration of H_1 and H_2 receptor antagonists. Similar negative results were obtained in a more recent multicenter study by Graham, Kudrow, and Diamond (unpublished results, 1980) in which a total of 60 patients with cluster headache treated prophylactically with H_1 and H_2 receptor blockers showed no significant improvement compared with those treated with placebos.

The role of histamine in cluster headache has recently been reappraised. Hardebo et al. (1980) demonstrated an enhanced dilatory response of large extracranial arteries to in vivo histamine. Appenzeller et al. (1978, 1981) suggested a role for histamine in the attack phase of cluster headache. They found morphologic evidence of mast cell degranulation in temporal skin biopsies from cluster headache patients. Mast cells were found to be in proximity to cutaneous nerves. Their findings suggested extrusion of histamine in proximity to cutaneous neurovascular bundles. The results of their study were later corroborated by some investigators (Dimitriadou et al., 1990; Liberski and Mirecka, 1984; Liberski and Prusinski, 1982), but unconfirmed by others (Aebelholt-Krabbe & Rank, 1985; Cuypers et al., 1980).

Plasma testosterone and luteinizing hormone levels were found to be significantly reduced in a population of patients with cluster headache during cluster periods compared with periods of remission (Kudrow, 1976a, 1977b). These results were interpreted to suggest hypothalamus–pituitary involvement. Subsequently, Nelson (1978) reported that testosterone values were abnormally low in 22% of patients with cluster headache but that approximately the same frequency of abnormal values was found in patients with migraine with aura. Klimek (1982) further corroborated low testosterone levels in patients with cluster headache but found that plasma testosterone levels were similarly depressed in patients with trigeminal neuralgia and reticular pain syndromes. He concluded that the lowering of plasma testosterone levels observed in patients with cluster headaches is more a function of pain than of a process involving hypothalamic–pituitary axis dysfunction. Lower testosterone levels in cluster headache patients were further reported by Romiti et al. (1982). They concluded that decreased plasma testosterone levels in cluster headache patients may have reflected disordered rapid eye movement (REM) states.

Chronobiologic Changes

Altered plasma testosterone levels among cluster headache patients suggested involvement of hypothalamic–pituitary pathways, which stirred the interest of neuroendocrinologists with particular reference to chronobiology. Change or loss in circadian rhythmicity was subsequently reported for plasma testosterone (Facchinetti et al., 1986), prolactin (Polleri et al., 1982; Waldenlind and Gustafsson, 1987), melatonin (Chazot et al., 1984; Waldenlind et al., 1984), β-endorphins (Nappi et al., 1985), cortisol (Nappi et al., 1981; Ferrari et al., 1983; and Waldenlind et al., 1987), and blood pressure and temperature (Ferrari et al., 1979). Support for a hypothalamus–pituitary role in cluster headache was reported by Bussone et al. (1988) and Leone et al. (1990), who had demonstrated a significantly reduced thyrotropin response to thyrotropin-releasing hormone, solely during cluster periods.

   It would appear, therefore, that the cluster headache period may be characterized by disturbance in circadian rhythmicity of neuroendocrine substances, and its cyclic occurrence may be due to circannual rhythm dysfunction (Kudrow, 1987b; Kudrow et al., 1990). The locus of these changes may reside in hypothalamic suprachiasmatic nuclei.

NERVOUS SYSTEM PATHWAYS

The Cluster Attack

Kunkle (1959) proposed that cluster headache attacks may result from parasympathetic storms involving the 7th and 10th cranial nerves. Indeed, he found acetylcholinelike substances in the cerebrospinal fluid in 4 of 14 patients with cluster headaches. Gardner et al. (1947) were also of the opinion that cluster headaches resulted from parasympathetic activation, specifically mediated through the greater superficial petrosal nerve. Section of the greater superficial petrosal nerve resulted in partial success in 50% of patients and an excellent outcome in 25%. Stowell (1970) suggested that cluster headaches were produced by efferent impulses from the greater superficial petrosal nerve arising in the parasympathetic nuclei of the hypothalamus. He further reported that section of the greater superficial petrosal nerves in 28 patients with cluster headache had a successful outcome in 12. Recurrence, however, was noted in 53.6% of the patients within 3 years postoperatively. One patient in whom Sachs (1968) sectioned the nervus intermedius remained free of clusters during a 10-year follow-up period.

The role of the trigeminal nerve in the pathogenesis of cluster headache was introduced simultaneously by Moskowitz (1984), Sicuteri et al. (1984, 1985), and Hardebo (1984). Moskowitz (1984) suggested that cluster attacks may be mediated by a neurogenic inflammatory response in the trigeminal ganglia. The painful site, he proposed, may be in the cavernous sinus. Involvement of this anatomic site is supported by observations in symptomatic cluster headache. Lesions responsible for this type of cluster headache have been found in or near the cavernous sinus (Greve and Mai, 1988; Herzberg et al., 1975; Mani and Deeter, 1982; Tfelt-Hansen et al., 1982; Thomas, 1975).

Sicuteri et al. (1983, 1985) presented evidence for substance P and allied neurotransmitters as biochemical mediators that may provoke a rostral spread of neuronal activity in the trigeminal nerve. Indeed, somatastatin, an inhibitor of substance P, was purported to alleviate cluster attacks (Sicuteri et al., 1984).

Dimitriadou et al. (1990) suggested a compatible role for the seemingly disparate findings for cluster attack pathogenesis. They postulated that acetylcholine released from parasympathetic nerve endings would stimulate release of histamine from mast cells, causing an antidromic response in trigeminal nerve terminals with release of substance P, resulting in further degranulation of mast cells, inflammatory response, and pain.

The Cluster Period

Bruyn et al. (1976) hypothesized that cluster headache attacks are associated with central α-adrenergic paroxysms (both excitatory and inhibitory).

Kudrow (1983) proposed that the carotid body may play a major role in the pathogenesis of cluster headache. Throughout the course of the cluster period, it may be that chemoreceptor activity is blunted by central inhibition of sympathetic and dysinhibition of parasympathetic efferent pathways arising in the hypothalmus. The major manifestation of these changes would probably occur during sleep, exaggerating the physiologic depression of respiration associated with sleep. Thus, sleep apnea and hypoxemia may result and may indeed be associated features of the cluster period. In the presence of impaired peripheral receptor responsivity, events such as REM-associated inhibition of respiratory muscle function, non-REM bradycardia, hypoventilation, vasodilators, and altitude hypoxia may cause hypoxemia. It was further suggested that these events precede and herald the onset of the cluster attack. When oxygen desaturation exceeds threshold limits of chemoreceptor activity, chemoreceptors would be unusually excited, as seen in denervation supersensitivity responses. This may be the consequence of the buildup of stored chemoreceptor-activating neuro-transmitters. This proposal also presumes that inhibitory mechanisms of chemoreceptor activity may be blocked.

On activation of the chemoreceptors, afferent impulses reach the nucleus solitarius in the medulla and, through interconnections, are further transmitted to the respiratory center, dorsal motor nucleus, and salivary nucleus. This may result in efferent stimulation of the motor nerves of respiration via reticulospinal pathways in the spinal cord and of the vagus and seventh cranial nerves, respectively.

This hypothesis has gained support from recent studies. In a polysomnographic study of episodic and chronic cluster headache patients, Kudrow et al. (1984) demonstrated a higher than expected frequency of sleep apnea associated with hypoxemia. Cluster attacks awakening the patients during this study were preceded by hypoxemic events, usually during REM states. In a subsequent study, it became apparent that the duration of relative hypoxemia in relationship to attack onset was more important than the magnitude of hypoxemia. In a recent study (Kudrow and Kudrow, 1990), oxygen saturation was monitored before and after administration of nitroglycerin in patients during active cluster periods and during remission periods and in nonheadache subjects. Arterial oxygen saturation (SaO_2) values decreased in all groups following nitroglycerin administration, returning to baseline within 30 minutes in control and remission patients. In the active cluster group, however, significantly decreased SaO_2 values persisted for a mean duration of 20 minutes longer, culminating in cluster headache attacks. These results suggested, as the hypothesis predicted, that persistent relative hypoxemia may have been due to impairment of compensatory chemoreceptor autoregulation and may characterize the cluster period. Recently, evidence for blunted chemoreceptor activity was presented by Zhao et al. (1990). In a group of patients and control subjects, the authors instructed patients to breathe a mixture of 12% oxygen and 88% nitrogen for 30 minutes. The subjects were monitored for oxygen saturation for 30 minutes. At the end of the test, patients in active cluster periods showed significantly less reduction of SaO_2 than controls. These results were interpreted as reflecting an abnormality in central regulation and/or chemoreceptor sensitivity.

TREATMENT OF CLUSTER HEADACHE

The successful treatment of cluster headache is governed by principles differing little from those that apply to most medical disorders. Patient education, prophylactic medication, and symptomatic treatment are paramount.

Patient Education

For many patients, the painful experience of the cluster headache attack and the anticipation of future attacks are enough to provoke a state of anxiety and anguish that persists throughout the cluster period. It should be communicated that most attacks may now be prevented within the cluster period by prophylactic measures or may be readily aborted. The cluster period itself, however, can be neither prevented nor shortened.

In the natural course of this disorder, as suggested by one study (Kudrow, 1982), approximately one third of patients who have been subject to cluster headache for 20 years or longer may experience a complete remission. In another third of patients, after 20 years attacks may be so mild as to obviate the need for medication, and, in the final third, the pattern of attacks may remain unchanged.

In all cases, patients should be instructed to avoid afternoon naps and alcoholic beverages, including wine and beer. Alcohol, in most instances, induces acute attacks during an active cluster period but not during remission. Patients should be warned to avoid prolonged exposure to volatile substances such as solvents, gasoline, or oil-based paints during cluster periods. Dietary influences, with the exception of alcohol, appear to have little importance in cluster headache.

Bursts of anger, prolonged anticipatory anxiety, and excessive physical activity should be avoided because cluster attacks are apt to occur during the relaxation period that follows. Prolonged experience of anger, hurt, rage, or frustration during cluster periods often is associated with a new onset of a cluster period (Kudrow, 1980).

Altitude hypoxemia at levels above 5,000 feet may induce attacks during cluster periods. Attacks frequently occur during airplane travel because the pressurization in most planes is equilibrated to approximately 7,000 to 8,000 feet. Cluster attacks expected during ski trips at higher altitudes may be prevented by oral administration of acetazolamine, 250 mg twice a day for 4 days, starting 2 days before altitude is reached.

Finally, patients may be advised that the onset of cluster periods often follows a long period of sleep alteration—that is, changes in the sleep–wake cycle. Such changes may result from vacation trips, work-shift changes, new occupations, postsurgical periods, and completion of university studies. As mentioned earlier, cluster periods may also begin following prolonged periods of anger, rage, worry, or frustration. Although many variables are associated with changes in life-style, alterations of sleep–wake patterns that often accompany these changes may be the most important.

Prophylactic Treatment

Attacks that occur only during sleep hours may be prevented by the administration of ergotamine tartrate, 2 mg orally, 1 to 2 hours before bedtime. Such attacks are often REM stage related (Dexter and Riley, 1975; Kudrow et al., 1984) and are likely to appear 90 minutes after sleep onset.

It has been our experience with a rather large population of cluster headache patients using ergotamine for prolonged periods of time that ergotamine rebound attacks are unlikely to occur with a daily dosage of 2 mg, nor is ergotism likely with this ergotamine dosage in a healthy cluster population. It should be noted, however, that ergotamine is contraindicated in the presence of peripheral vascular disease, cardiovascular disease, and cerebrovascular atheromatous disease. Additional contraindications include pregnancy, liver or renal disease, serious infection, and postsurgical periods.

Attacks that occur during various times of the day may be prevented by the prophylactic use of agents such as methysergide, verapamil, lithium, or prednisone. The proper selection of prophylactic agents depends on the health of the patient, compatibility with other medications, and history of untoward reactions. Combined drug regimens should be guided by cluster headache type, patient's age, timing of attacks, and history of treatment resistance (Figure 6–1).

Episodic Cluster Headache

For episodic cluster headache patients under 30 years of age, and for those who have suffered their first occurrence and as yet remain unclassified, the prophylactic treatment of choice is methysergide. Methysergide is most effec-

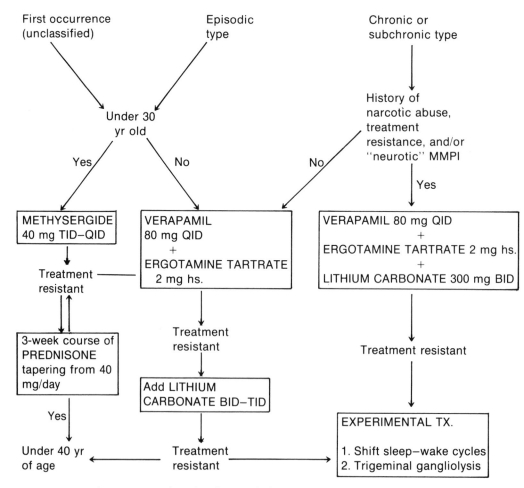

Figure 6–1. Algorithm for prophylactic treatment of cluster headache.

tive in the early course of disease and least effective during later cluster periods. Its efficacy rate has been established at approximately 65% (Friedman and Elkind, 1963; Kudrow, 1978b). The most common side effects are gastrointestinal disturbance, paresthesias of the lower extremities, and leg pain. In the presence of such symptoms, discontinuance is recommended. Complications include retroperitoneal, endomyocardial, or pulmonary fibrosis, as reported by Graham (1965), Graham and Parnes (1965), and Kunkel (1971). Contraindications are similar to those for ergotamine.

In patients over 30 years of age who have experienced several cluster periods, and in patients under 30 years of age who are resistant to methysergide, our treatment of choice is verapamil, 80 mg four times a day, spaced evenly throughout waking hours. In our experience, the addition of ergotamine, 2 mg 1 hour before bedtime, captures an additional 15 to 20% of patients. The efficacy of verapamil prophylaxis was first reported by Meyer and Hardenberg (1983) and subsequently corroborated by Gabel and Spierings (1989). The beneficial action of verapamil, a calcium channel blocker, remains unexplained in cluster headache. Determination of its specific site of action in cluster headache is complicated by the wide distribution of calcium entry channels throughout the somatic, neuronal, and vascular systems. In our experience, constipation is the major side effect. In addition, approximately 5 to 8% of our younger patients experience girdle pain, which appeared to be muscular by description.

Treatment resistance to the above regimen may be overcome by the addition of lithium carbonate, 300 mg twice a day. Ekbom (1974) was the first to report the beneficial effects of lithium prophylaxis in cluster headache. Encouraged by these results, our clinic evaluated the efficacy of lithium in 32 patients over a 32-week period (Kudrow, 1977a). Of 28 patients completing this study, 42% obtained improvement ranging between 60 and 90%. Fifty-four percent obtained a greater than 90% improvement, and only one patient was considered unimproved. Subsequent studies by Mathew (1978), Savoldi et al. (1983), and Ekbom (1981) reported similar results. In doses of 900 mg/day or more, tremor is a common side effect. Concomitant use of diuretics or severely restricted sodium diets are contraindicated; the lithium ion competes with intracellular sodium and may lead to toxicity. Toxicity may be further avoided by preventing blood levels above 1 mg/dl.

In our experience, the combined use (triple therapy) of verapamil, ergotamine, and lithium provides significant prophylaxis for over 90% of episodic cluster headache patients. In cases of treatment resistance to triple therapy in patients over 40 years of age and among those patients resistant to methysergide, a 3-week course of prednisone is recommended. Prednisone is prescribed at 40 mg/day in divided doses for a period of 5 days and is tapered off over a period of 3 weeks. It is contraindicated in patients with hypertension, peptic ulcer disease, diabetes, current infection, and diverticulosis. Before Jammes's controlled study (1975) of prednisone prophylaxis in cluster headache, the use of steroids and their efficacy had been reported in the medical literature (Friedman and Mikropoulos, 1958; Graham, 1976; Horton, 1952; MacNeal, 1978). In our own series of 77 patients with episodic cluster headache (Kudrow, 1978a), therapy with prednisone produced a marked relief in 76.6%, partial improvement in 11.7%, and no significant improvement in 11.7%. Of 15 patients with chronic cluster headache, 40% had obtained marked improvement.

Chronic and Subchronic Cluster Headache

In a recent study, approximately 50% of subchronic and chronic cluster patients were reported to be treatment resistant (Kudrow, 1987). Subchronic cluster headache was defined to include cases in which remissions were shorter than 5 months. Minnesota Multiphasic Personality Inventory studies revealed that 50% of subchronic and chronic patients had elevated scores for either depression or hysteria and for addiction-proneness as well; these characteristics are associated with treatment resistance (Kudrow, 1987a).

In the absence of characteristics that would predict treatment resistance, the recommended course of treatment is as described for episodic cluster headache. For potentially treatment-resistant patients, a combination of verapamil, ergotamine tartrate, and lithium carbonate is recommended (triple therapy).

Continued treatment resistance despite the above recommendations is a rare occurrence and should alert the clinician to possible narcotic abuse. In the absence of narcotic abuse, experimental approaches may be considered. In an open-labeled prophylactic study, Hering and Kuritsky (1989) successfully treated 11 of 15 cluster headache patients with sodium valproate, 600 to 2,000 mg daily, prophylactically. No correlation was found between efficacy and valproate plasma levels. Treatment was reported to be well tolerated except for mild nausea in three patients. The authors suggested that sodium valproate may act as a γ-aminobutyric acid mimetic agent on interneurons of the hypothalamic suprachiasmatic nucleus.

An experimental approach aimed at shortening cluster periods is currently being studied at the California Medical Clinic for Headache. It entails exposure to bright light stimulation in an effort to reset circadian pacemakers by shifting sleep–wake cycles. Other chronobiology-dependent disorders have been successfully treated in this manner (Czeisler et al., 1989; Lewy et al., 1987; Richardson et al., 1981). The most efficacious surgical approach has been reported by Mathew and Hurt (1985). A significant success rate among treatment-resistant patients was attained by radiofrequency trigeminal gangliolysis. Complications of this procedure may include sensory and secretomotor changes and/or anesthesia dolorosa.

Symptomatic Treatment

Oxygen inhalation is the most effective and safest method of aborting acute cluster headaches (Anthony, 1981; Fogan, 1985; Kudrow, 1981). The technique for achieving maximal success in this regard is as follows:

1. Oxygen inhalation should be initiated at the onset of the attack.
2. The patient should assume a sitting position leaning slightly forward.
3. The oxygen flow rate should be set at 7 liters/minute.
4. Patients should be warned against hyperventilating, which may paradoxically limit oxyhemoglobin saturation. A high level of oxygen satura-

tion (98 to 99%) must be sustained for several minutes to achieve relief of attacks (Kudrow & Kudrow, 1990).
5. The delivery system should include a facial mask rather than a nasal cannula.

The mechanism by which oxygen inhalation interrupts the cluster attack has been suggested by Kudrow (1983) and subsequently demonstrated by Kudrow and Kudrow (1990) to be related to preattack oxygen desaturation.

Where ergotamine is preferred, sublingual preparations are recommended. They should be used at the very onset of the attack. Sublingual preparations may be repeated only once or twice after 15-minute intervals. In general, daily use of ergotamine should be limited to a maximum of 2 mg/24-hour period. In an emergency room situation or office setting, parenteral administration of ergotamine may be indicated if oxygen is either unavailable or ineffective. Dihydroergotamine (DHE-45), 1 mg intramuscularly, is preferred. Ergotamine tartrate, 0.5 mg intramuscularly, is also effective. Other symptomatic medications include 5% cocaine hydrochloride (Barre, 1982) or 4% lidocaine (Kittrelle et al., 1985) administered intranasally with the head tilted back and turned toward the ipsilateral side. The effect of these agents appears to be limited by the patient's intranasal anatomy, proper administration, and tolerance. The benefit is probably due to local anesthetic effects on either the sphenopalatine ganglion or nerve endings in mucosal tissue (Kittrelle et al., 1985).

Management of CPH

As reported by Sjaastad (1987), the treatment of choice for CPH is indomethacin, 200 mg daily in divided doses. The response is complete and indeed diagnostic of this condition. In our experience, 75 to 100 mg/day in divided doses has been successful in all cases. Furthermore, indomethacin may be decreased to low maintenance levels of approximately 25 mg/day in many patients. Guidelines for treating children with CPH are lacking with the exception of a recent case report of a 9-year-old boy who had CPH since age 6 (Kudrow and Kudrow, 1989). The child was successfully treated prophylactically with baby aspirin, 162 mg twice daily, maintained for 3 months. Attacks have not occurred over a 4-year follow-up period since discontinuation of aspirin.

REFERENCES

Ad Hoc Committee on Classification of Headache (1962). *JAMA 179:*717–718.
Aebelholt-Krabbe, A., L. Henriksen, and J. Olesen (1984). Tomographic determination of cerebral blood flow during attacks of cluster headache. *Cephalalgia 4:*17–23.
Aebelholt-Krabbe, A. and F. Rank (1985). Histological examinations of the superficial temporal artery in patients suffering from cluster headache. *Cephalalgia 5*(Suppl. 3):282–283.
Andrasik, F., E.B. Blanchard, J.G. Arena et al. (1982). Cross-validation of the Kudrow-

Sutkus MMPI classification system for diagnosing headache type. *Headache 22:* 2–5.

Anthony, M. (1981). Treatment of attacks of cluster headache with oxygen inhalation. *Clin. Exp. Neurol. 18:*195.

Anthony, M. and J.W. Lance (1971). Histaminic and serotonin in cluster headache. *Arch. Neurol. 25:*225–231.

Anthony, M., G.D.A. Lord, and J.W. Lance (1978). Controlled trials of cimetadine in migraine and cluster headache. *Headache 18:*261–264.

Appenzeller, O., W. Becker, and A. Ragaz (1978). Cluster headache. Ultrastructural aspects. *Neurology 28:*371.

Appenzeller, O., W.J. Becker, and A. Ragaz (1981). Cluster headache. Ultrastructural aspects and pathogenetic mechanisms. *Arch. Neurol. 38:*302–306.

Barre, F. (1982). Cocaine as an abortive agent in cluster headache. *Headache 22:*69–73.

Boccuni, M., G. Morace, U. Pietrini et al. (1984). Coexistence of pupillary and heart sympathergic asymmetries in cluster headache. *Cephalalgia 4:*9–15.

Broch, A., I. Hørven, H. Nornes et al. (1970). Studies of cerebral and ocular circulation in a patient with cluster headache. *Headache 10:*1–13.

Bruyn, G.W., B.K. Bootsma, and H.L. Klawans (1976). Cluster headache and bradycardia. *Headache 16:*11–15.

Bussone, G., F. Frediani, M. Leone et al. (1988). TRH test in cluster headache. *Headache 7:*43–54.

Chazot, G., B. Claustrat, J. Brun et al. (1984). A chronobiological study of melatonin, cortisol, growth hormone and prolactin secretion in cluster headache. *Cephalalgia 4:*213–220.

Cuypers, J. and H. Altenkirch (1979). HLA antigens in cluster headache. *Headache 19:* 228–229.

Cuypers, J., H. Altenkirch, and S. Bunge (1981). Personality profiles in cluster headache and migraine. *Headache 21:*21–24.

Cuypers, J., K. Westphal, and S.T. Bunge (1980). Mast cells in cluster headache. *Acta. Neurol. Scand. 61:*327–329.

Czeisler, C.A., R.E. Kronauer, J.S. Allan et al. (1989). Bright light induction of strong (type O) resetting of the human circadian pacemaker. *Science 244:*1328–1333.

Dalessio, D.J. (1969). A reappraisal of the trigger zones of tic douloureux. *Headache 9:* 73–76.

Dexter, J.D. and T.L. Riley (1975). Studies in nocturnal migraine. *Headache 15:*51–62.

Dimitriadou, V., P. Henry, B. Brochet et al. (1990). Cluster headache: Ultrastructural evidence for mast cell degranulation and interaction with nerve fibres in the human temporal artery. *Cephalalgia 10:*221–228.

Ekbom, K. (1968). Nitroglycerin as a provocative agent in cluster headache. *Arch. Neurol. 19:*487–493.

Ekbom, K. (1970a). A clinical comparison of cluster headache and migraine. *Acta Neurol. Scand. Suppl. 41:*1–48.

Ekbom, K. (1970b). Pattern of cluster headache with a note on the relation to angina pectoris and peptic ulcer. *Acta Neurol. Scand. 46:*225–237.

Ekbom, K. (1974). Litium vid kroniska symptom av cluster headache. *Preliminart Meddelande Pousc. Med. 19:*148–156.

Ekbom, K. (1981). Lithium for cluster headache: Review of the literature and preliminary results of long-term treatment. *Headache 21:*132–139.

Ekbom, K. and T. Greitz (1970). Carotid angiography in cluster headache. *Acta Radiol. (Diagn.) (Stockh.) 10:*177–186.

Ekbom, K. and L. Kudrow (1979). Facial flush in cluster [editorial]. *Headache 19:*47.

Ekbom, K. and B. de F. Olivarius (1971). Chronic migrainous neuralgia-diagnostic and therapeutic aspects. *Headache 11*:97–101.

Ekbom, K.A. (1947). Ergotamine tartrate orally in Horton's "histaminic cephalgia" (also called Harris' "ciliary neuralgia"). *Acta Psychiatr. Scand. Suppl. 46:* 106–113.

Eulenburg, A. (1874). *Lehrbuch der nervenkrankheiten 2. Au Fl. II Teil*, p. 264. Hirschwald, Berlin.

Facchinetti, F., G. Nappi, C. Cicoli et al. (1986). Reduced testosterone levels in cluster headache: A stress-related phenomenon. *Cephalalgia 6*:29–34.

Fanciullacci, M., U. Pietrini, G. Gatto et al. (1982). Latent dysautonomic pupillary lateralization in cluster headache. A pupillometric study. *Cephalalgia 2*:135–144.

Ferrari, E., C. Canepari, P.A. Bossolo et al. (1983). Changes of biological rhythms in primary headache syndromes. *Cephalalgia 3*(Suppl. 1):58–68.

Ferrari, E., E. Martignon, A. Vailati et al. (1979). Chronobiological aspects of cluster headache. Effects of lithium therapy. In *Headache* (F. Savoldi and G. Nappi eds.), pp. 152–160 Palladio Editore, Pavia, Italy.

Fogan, L. (1985). Treatment of cluster headache. A double-blind comparison of oxygen v air inhalation. *Arch. Neurol. 42*:362–363.

Friedman, A.P. and A.H. Elkind (1963). Appraisal of methysergide in treatment of vascular headaches of migraine type. *JAMA 184*:125–130.

Friedman, A.P. and H.E. Mikropoulos (1958). Cluster headache. *Neurology 8*:653–663.

Friedman, A.P. and E.H. Wood (1976). Thermography in vascular headache. In *Medical Thermography* (S. Uema, ed.), pp 80–84. Brentwood Publishers, Los Angeles.

Gabel, I.J. and E.L.H. Spierings (1989). Prophylactic treatment of cluster headache with verapamil. *Headache 29*:167–168.

Gardner, W.J., A. Stowell, and R. Dutlinger (1947). Resection of the greater petrosal nerve in the treatment of unilateral headache. *J. Neurosurg. 4*:105–114.

Gilbert, G.J. (1965). Meniere's syndrome and cluster headaches: Recurrent paroxysmal vasodilatation. *JAMA 191*:691.

Gilbert, G.J. (1970). Cluster headache and cluster vertigo. *Headache 9*:195.

Graham, J.R. (1965). Possible renal complications of Sansert (methysergide) therapy for headache. *Headache 5*:12–14.

Graham, J.R. (1969). Cluster headache. Presentation at the International Symposium on Headache, Chicago.

Graham, J.R. (1972). Cluster headache. *Headache 11*:175–185.

Graham, J.R. (1976). Cluster headache. In *Pathogenesis and Treatment of Headache* (O. Appenzeller, ed.), pp. 93–108. Spectrum, New York.

Graham, J.R. and L.R. Parnes (1965). Possible cardiac and renovascular complications of Sansert therapy. *Headache 5*:14–18.

Graham, J.R., A.Z. Rogado, M. Rahman, and I.V. Gramer (1970). Some physical, physiological and psychological characteristics of patients with cluster headache. In *Background to Migraine* (A.L. Cochrane, ed.), pp. 38–51. Heinemann, London.

Green, M. and R.I. Apfelbaum (1978). Cluster-tic syndrome. *Headache 18*:112.

Greve, E. and J. Mai (1988). Cluster headache-like headaches: A symptomatic feature? A report of three patients with intracranial pathologic findings. *Cephalalgia 8:* 79–82.

Hardebo, J.E. (1984). The involvement of trigeminal substance P neurons in cluster headache. An hypothesis. *Headache 24*:294–304.

Hardebo, J.E., A. Aebelholt-Krabbe, and F. Gjerris (1980). Enhanced dilatory response to histamine in large extracranial vessels in chronic cluster headache. *Headache 20*:316–320.

Harris, W. (1926). *Neuritis and Neuralgia.* Oxford University Press, London.

Harris, W. (1936). Ciliary (migrainous) neuralgia and its treatment. *BMJ 1:*457–460.

Headache Classification Committee of the International Headache Society. (1988). Classification and diagnostic criteria for headache disorders, cranial neuralgias and facial pain. *Cephalalgia 8*(Suppl. 7):1–96.

Henry, P.Y., J. Vernhiet, J.M. Orgogozo et al. (1978). Cerebral blood flow in migraine and cluster headaches. *Res. Clin. Stud. Headache 6:*10–16.

Hering R. and A. Kuritsky (1989). Sodium valproate in the treatment of cluster headache: An open clinical trial. *Cephalagia 9:*195.

Herzberg, L., J.A.R. Lenman, G. Victoratos, and F. Fletcher (1975). Cluster headache associated with vascular malformations. *J. Neurosurg. Psychiatry 38:*648–649.

Heyck, H. (1975). In *Der Kopschmerz,* 4th ed., p. 114. George Thieme Verlag, Stuttgart.

Hornabrook, R.W. (1964). Migrainous neuralgia. *N. Z. Med. J. 63:*774.

Horton, B.T. (1952). Histaminic cephalgia. *Lancet 2:*92–98.

Horton, B.T., A.R. MacLean, and W.M. Craig (1939). A new syndrome of vascular headache: Results of treatment with histamine: Preliminary report. *Mayo Clin. Proc. 14:*257–260.

Horton, B.T., T.B. Magath, and G.E. Brown (1932). An undescribed form of arteritis of the temporal vessels. *Proc. Staff Meet. Mayo Clin. 7:*700–701.

Huston, K.A., G.G. Hunder, J.T. Lie et al. (1978). Temporal arteritis. A 25-year epidemiologic, clinical, and pathologic study. *Ann. Intern. Med. 88:*162–167.

Jammes, J.L. (1975). The treatment of cluster headache with prednisone. *Dis. Nerv. Syst. 36:*375–376.

Kittrelle, J.P., D.S. Grouse, and M. Seybold (1985). Cluster headache. Local anaesthetic abortive agents. *Arch. Neurol. 42:*496–498.

Klimek, A. (1982). Plasma testosterone levels in patients with cluster headache. *Headache 22:*162–164.

Kudrow, D.B. and L. Kudrow (1989). Successful aspirin prophylaxis in a child with chronic paroxysmal hemicrania. *Headache 29:*280–281.

Kudrow, L. (1974). Physical and personality characteristics in cluster headache. *Headache 13:*197–201.

Kudrow, L. (1976a). Plasma testosterone levels in cluster headache: Preliminary results. *Headache 16:*28–31.

Kudrow, L. (1976b). Prevalence of migraine, peptic ulcer, coronary heart disease and hypertension in cluster headache. *Headache 16:*66–69.

Kudrow, L. (1977a). Lithium prophylaxis for chronic cluster headache. *Headache 17:*15–18.

Kudrow, L. (1977b). Plasma testosterone and LH levels in cluster headache. *Headache 17:*91–92.

Kudrow, L. (1978a). Comparative results of prednisone, methysergide, and lithium therapy in cluster headache. In *Current Concepts in Migraine Research* (R. Greene, ed.), pp. 159–163. Raven Press, New York.

Kudrow, L. (1978b). HL-A antigens in cluster headache and classical migraine. *Headache 18:*167–168.

Kudrow, L. (1979). Thermographic and Doppler flow asymmetry in cluster headache. *Headache 19:*204–208.

Kudrow, L. (1980). *Cluster Headache: Mechanisms and Management,* pp. 10–150. Oxford University Press, London.

Kudrow, L. (1981). Response to cluster headache attacks to oxygen inhalation. *Headache 21:*1–4.

Kudrow, L. (1982). Natural history of cluster headache. Part 1. Outcome of drop-out patients. *Headache 22:*203–206.

Kudrow, L. (1983). A possible role of the carotid body in the pathogenesis of cluster headache. *Cephalalgia 3*:241–247.

Kudrow, L. (1987a). Subchronic cluster headache. *Headache 27*:197–200.

Kudrow, L. (1987b). The cyclic relationship of natural illumination to cluster period frequency [abstract]. *Cephalalgia* (Suppl. 6):76–77.

Kudrow, L., G. Cornélissen, and F. Halberg (1990). Population study of 3- and 6-monthly changes in cluster headache onsets. *Proceedings of the 2nd World Conference on Clinical Chronobiology,* Monte Carlo, p. 15.

Kudrow, L., P. Esperanca, and N. Vijayan (1987). Episodic paroxysmal hemicrania. *Cephalalgia 7*:197–201.

Kudrow, L., and D.B. Kudrow (1990). Association of sustained oxyhemoglobin desaturation and onset of cluster headache attacks. *Headache 30*:474–480.

Kudrow, L., D.J. McGinty, E.R. Phillips, and M. Stevenson (1984). Sleep apnea in cluster headache. *Proceedings of the 12th Scandinavian Migraine Society Meeting,* Helsinki, June 17–18, p. 56.

Kudrow, L. and B.J. Sutkus (1979). MMPI pattern specificity in primary headache disorders. *Headache 19*:18–24.

Kunkle, E.C. (1959). Acetylcholine in the mechanism of headaches of the migraine type. *Arch. Neurol. Psychiatry 84*:135.

Kunkle, E.C., J.B. Pfeiffer, Jr., W.M. Wilhoit et al. (1954). Recurrent brief headache in "cluster" pattern. *Trans. Am. Neurol. Assoc. 77*:240.

Kunkel, R.S. (1971). Fibrotic syndromes with chronic use of methysergide. *Headache 11*:1–5.

Kunkel, R.S. and D.F. Dohn (1974). Surgical treatment of chronic migrainous neuralgia. *Cleve. Clin. Q. 41*:189–192.

Lance, J.W. (1978). *Mechanisms and Management of Headache,* 3rd ed. Butterworth, London.

Lance, J.W. and M. Anthony (1971a). Migrainous neuralgia or cluster headache? *J. Neurol. Sci. 13*:401–414.

Lance, J.W. and M. Anthony (1971b). Thermographic studies in vascular headache. *Med. J. Aust. 1*:240.

Leone, M., G. Patruno, A. Vescovi, and G. Bussone (1990). Neuroendocrine dysfunction in cluster headache. *Cephalalgia 10*:235–239.

Lewy, A.J., R.L. Sacks, L.S. Miller, and T.M. Hoban (1987). Antidepressant and circadian phase-shifting effects of light. *Science 235*:352–354.

Liberski, P.P. and B. Mirecka (1984). Mast cells in cluster headache. Ultrastructure, release pattern and possible pathogenetic significance. *Cephalalgia 4*:101–106.

Liberski, P.P. and A. Prusinski (1982). Further observations on the mast cells over the painful region in cluster headache patients. *Headache 22*:115–117.

Lovshin, L.L. (1961). Clinical caprices of histaminic cephalgia. *Headache 1*:3–6.

MacNeal, P.S. (1978). Useful therapeutic approaches to the patient with "problem headache." *Headache 18*:26–30.

Mani, S. and J. Deeter (1982). Arteriovenous malformation of the brain presenting as a cluster headache—a case report. *Headache 22*:184–185.

Martelletti, M.D., A. Romiti, M.F. Gallo et al. (1984). HLA-B14 antigen in cluster headache. *Headache 24*:152–154.

Mathew, N.T. (1978). Clinical subtypes of cluster headache and response to lithium therapy. *Headache 25*:166.

Mathew N.T. and W. Hurt (1985). Radiofrequency trigeminal gangliolysis in the treatment of chronic intractable cluster headache. *Headache 25*:166.

Medina, J.L. and S. Diamond (1977). The clinical link between migraine and cluster headache. *Arch. Neurol. 34*:470.

Meyer, J.S. and B.A. Hardenberg (1983). Clinical effectiveness of calcium entry blockers in prophylactic treatment of migraine and cluster headaches. *Headache 23:* 266–277.

Moskowitz, M.A. (1984). The neurobiology of vascular head pain. *Ann. Neurol. 16:* 157–168.

Nappi, G., F. Facchinetti, G. Bono et al. (1985). Lack of β-lipotropin circadian rhythmicity in episodic cluster headache: A model for chronopathology. In *Updating in Headache* (V. Pfaffenrath, P-O. Lundberg, and O. Sjaastad, eds.), pp. 269–275. Springer-Verlag, Berlin.

Nappi, G., E. Ferrari, A. Polleri et al. (1981). Chronobiological study of cluster headache. *Chronobiologia 2:*140.

Nattero, G., L. Savi, and G. Pisanti (1980). Doppler flow velocity in cluster headache. *International Congress, Headache, '80,* Florence, Italy.

Nelson, R.F. (1978). Testosterone levels in cluster and non-cluster migrainous headache patients. *Headache 18:*265–267.

Norris, J.W., V.C. Hachinski, and P.W. Cooper (1976). Cerebral blood flow changes in cluster headache. *Acta Neurol. Scand. 54:*371–374.

Pelz, M. and H. Merskey (1982). A case of pre-chronic paroxysmal hemicrania. *Cephalalgia 2:*47–50.

Polleri, A., G. Nappi, G. Murialdo et al. (1982). Changes in the 24-hour prolactin pattern in cluster headache. *Cephalalgia 2:*1–7.

Raeder, J.G. (1924). "Paratrigeminal" paralysis of oculo-pupillary sympathetic. *Brain 47:*149–158.

Richardson, G.S., R.M. Coleman, J.C. Zimmerman et al. (1981). Chronotherapy: Resetting the circadian clock of patients with delayed sleep phase insomnia. *Sleep 4:* 1–21.

Romberg, M.H. (1840). *A Manual of Nervous Diseases of Man* (E.H. Sievering, trans.). London Sydenham Society, London.

Romiti, A., P. Martelletti, M.F. Gallo, and M. Giacovazzo (1982). Low plasma testosterone levels in cluster headache. *Cephalalgia 3:*41–44.

Russell, D. (1984). Chronic paroxysmal hemicrania: Severity, duration, and time of occurrences of attack. *Cephalalgia 4:*53–56.

Russell, D. and K.-F. Lindegaard (1985). Cluster headache: Doppler examination of the extracranial arteries. *Cephalalgia 5*(Suppl. 3):276–277.

Sachs, E., Jr. (1968). The role of the nervous intermedius in facial neuralgia: Report of four cases with observations on the pathways for taste, lacrimation, and pain in the face. *J. Neurosurg. 23:*54–60.

Sakai, F. and J.S. Meyer (1978). Regional cerbral hemodynamics during migraine and cluster headaches measured by the 133 Xe inhalation method. *Headache 18:* 122–132.

Sakai, F. and J.S. Meyer (1979). Abnormal cerebrovascular reactivity in patients with migraine and cluster headache. *Headache 19:*257–266.

Salvesen, R., A. Bogucki, M.M. Wysocka-Bakowska et al. (1987). Cluster headache, pathogenesis: A pupillometric study. *Cephalalgia 7:*273–284.

Saunte, C., D. Russell and O. Sjaastad (1983). Cluster headache: On the mechanisms behind attack-related sweating. *Cephalalgia 3:*175–185.

Savoldi, F., G. Bono, G.C. Manzoni et al. (1983). Lithium salts in cluster headache treatment. *Cephalalgia 3*(Suppl. 1):79–84.

Schele, R., B. Ahlborg, and K. Ekbom (1978). Physical characteristics and allergy history in young men with migraine and other headaches. *Headache 18:*80–86.

Schroth, G., W.D. Gerber, and H.D. Langohr (1983). Ultrasonic Doppler flow in migraine and cluster headache. *Headache 23:*284–288.

Sicuteri, F., M. Fanciullacci, P. Geppetti et al. (1985). Substance P mechanism in cluster headache: Evaluation in plasma and cerebrospinal fluid. *Cephalalgia 5:*143–149.

Sicuteri, F., P. Geppetti, S. Marabini, and F. Lembeck (1984). Pain relief by somatostatin in attacks of cluster headache. *Pain 18:*359–365.

Sicuteri, F., L. Raino, and P. Geppetti (1983). Substance P and endogenous opioids: How and where they could play a role in cluster headache. *Cephalalgia 3*(Suppl. 1):143–145.

Sjaastad, O. (1970). Kinin-OG histaminiunders ø kelser ved migrene. In *Kliniske Aspecter i Migrene Forshningen,* pp. 61–69. Norlundes Bogtrykkeri, Copenhagen.

Sjaastad, O. (1987). Chronic paroxysmal hemicrania: Clinical aspects and controversies. In *Migraine: Clinical, Therapeutic, Conceptual and Research Aspects* (J.N. Blau, ed.), pp. 135–152. Chapman and Hall, London.

Sjaastad, O., R. Apfelbaum, W. Caskey et al. (1980). Chronic paroxysmal hemicrania (CPH): The clinical manifestations: A review. *Ups. J. Med. Sci. Suppl. 31:*27–33.

Sjaastad, O. and I. Dale (1974). Evidence for a new (?) treatable headache entity. *Headache 14:*105–108.

Sjaastad, O., K. Rootwelt, and I. Hørven (1974). Cutaneous blood flow in cluster headache. *Headache 13:*173–175.

Sjaastad, O. and Ø.V. Sjaastad (1977). Histamine metabolism in cluster headache and migraine. *J. Neurol. 216:*105–117.

Stowell, A. (1970). Physiologic mechanisms and treatment of histaminic or petrosal neuralgia. *Headache 9:*187–194.

Tfelt-Hansen, P., O.B. Paulsen, and A. Krabbe (1982). Invasive adenoma of the pituitary gland and chronic migrainous neuralgia. A rare coincidence or a causal relationship? *Cephalalgia 2:*25–28.

Thomas, A.L. (1975). Periodic migrainous neuralgia associated with an arteriovenous malformation. *Postgrad. Med. J. 51:*460–461.

Thomas, J.G., E.D. Rooke, and W.F. Kvale (1966). The neurologist's experience with pheochromocytoma: A review of 100 cases. *JAMA 197:*754.

Vijayan, N. and C. Watson (1978). Pericarotid syndrome. *Headache 18:*244–254.

Waldenlind, E., K. Ekbom, Y. Friberg et al. (1984). Decreased nocturnal serum melatonin levels during active cluster headache periods. *Opusc. Med. 29:*109–112.

Waldenlind, E. and S.A. Gustafsson (1987). Prolactin in cluster headache: Diurnal secretion, response to thyrotropin-releasing hormone. *Cephalalgia 7:*43–54.

Waldenlind, E., S.A. Gustafsson, K. Ekbom, and L. Wetterberg (1987). Circadian secretion of cortisol and melatonin in cluster headache during active cluster periods and remission. *J. Neurol. Neurosurg. Psychiatry 50:*207–213.

Watson, P. and R. Evans (1985). Cluster-tic syndrome. *Headache 25:*123–126.

World Federation of Neurology's Research Group on Migraine and Headache. (1969). *J. Neurol. Sci. 9:*202.

Zhao, J.M., J. Schaanning, and O. Sjaastad (1990). Cluster headache: The effect of low oxygen saturation. *Headache 30:*656–659.

7

Chronic Paroxysmal Hemicrania and Similar Headaches

OTTAR SJAASTAD

CHRONIC PAROXYSMAL HEMICRANIA

Chronic paroxysmal hemicrania (CPH), first described by Sjaastad and Dale (1974), is a rare headache disorder. In a recent literature review reports of only 84 patients were found (Antonaci and Sjaastad, 1989), but the unreported number of diagnosed and treated cases is probably several times this number.

Clinical Appearance

CPH has many features in common with cluster headache. Both are severe unilateral headaches without side alternation associated with ipsilateral nasal stuffiness/rhinorrhea, lacrimation, and conjunctival injection. Neither headache is associated with visual auras such as scotomas or scintillations. Nocturnal attacks are characteristic of both, and the mean age of onset is around 30 to 34 years. For these reasons, both have been grouped under the common designation "cluster headache syndrome" (Headache Classification Committee of the International Headache Society, 1988; Sjaastad, 1989).

Nevertheless, it is presently believed that CPH represents a distinct entity for several reasons (Sjaastad and Dale, 1976). In contrast to patients with cluster headache, (1) females are predominantly affected (70%); (2) the attack frequency is much higher, with a mean of 10.8 attacks per 24 hours (range, 1 to 40); and (3) indomethacin has a prompt, dramatic, lasting, and rather selective effect. There are other differences between CPH and cluster headache. Attacks of CPH are shorter (mean 13.3 ± 7.6 minutes) than cluster headache attacks (49.0 ± 35.5 minutes) (Russell, 1984), and CPH attacks may be "mechanically precipitated": approximately 10% of CPH patients may bring on attacks by flexing and rotating the neck.

The clustering of attacks may not be a major distinction between CPH and cluster headache. In cluster headache, the episodic form of cluster headache was discovered first. In some patients, episodic cluster headache is transformed into a chronic cluster (the *secondary* chronic form). In CPH, the chronic stage was discovered first. Later, it was shown that there may be a stage prior to the chronic stage with only periodic symptoms (Sjaastad, 1979)—that is, a noncontinuous or remitting stage that may occasionally be permanent. Thus, the terminology is different between cluster headache and CPH because of the sequence of discovery of the various subforms. Nevertheless, the phenomena may be essentially the same in both headaches. Even in the chronic stage of CPH there is a clear fluctuation in attack severity—a "modified cluster pattern" (Sjaastad, 1986, 1987).

Many patients do not have a prechronic stage (Bogucki et al., 1984; Sjaastad and Dale, 1976); these patients are *primary* chronic cases. Patients who reach the chronic stage (i.e., >6 months with continuous headache attacks) may remain in that stage for protracted periods. Of 84 patients in the literature, 20% remained in the remitting stage, 22% had undergone a transition from the remitting stage to the chronic stage, and 58% had been chronic from the onset (Antonaci and Sjaastad, 1989). The remitting stage may be more prominent than is presently believed.

CPH pain can be excruciatingly severe, but there is a continuous fluctuation between severe and moderate attacks. In the worst periods, there may be a continuous, sore feeling in the usually painful areas (i.e., the ocular–periocular areas, the forehead, the temporal area, the neck, the shoulders, and the aural–retroaural areas) between attacks. Maximum pain usually occurs in the frontal area. The pain usually has a piercing, boring, or clawlike character, but in the initial stages, especially in precipitated attacks, it may be pulsating.

This headache can be eliminated by continuous administration of adequate doses of indomethacin (Sjaastad and Dale, 1974). The dosage is easily titrated and may vary greatly, both between individuals and in the same individual at different times (i.e., from <25 to 250 mg/day), depending on the severity of the attacks. Although a slight interictal sore feeling may persist with this therapy, the severe paroxysmal attacks are eliminated. Indomethacin is remarkably well tolerated. Although it may cause dyspepsia, we have not had to stop treating any of our patients. If dyspepsia does occur, indomethacin suppositories and a histamine H_2 receptor blocking agent can be used.

Differential Diagnoses

CPH may be confused with other unilateral headaches and other indomethacin-responsive headaches. CPH responds to indomethacin absolutely; presently only one other headache is known to do so: *hemicrania continua* (Sjaastad and Spierings, 1984). Hemicrania continua is characterized by a steadily continuing headache; especially in the early stages of this disorder, however, separate, long-lasting pain episodes may dominate. The headache is moderate and usually not accompanied by autonomic phenomena (Bordini et al., 1991).

The other indomethacin-responsive headaches only partly respond to indomethacin and differ from CPH in their clinical pattern. *"Jabs and jolts" syndrome* (Sjaastad, 1979) is characterized by short-lived pains (usually lasting for

1 or 2 seconds, although occasionally somewhat longer) appearing either in multiple locations or strictly localized. Jabs and jolts may occur alone or with other headache disorders, such as migraine, cluster headache, and hemicrania continua. The term "jabs and jolts" corresponds to the new term "idiopathic stabbing headache" (Headache Classification Committee of the International Headache Society, 1988) and "ice pick pain" (described by Raskin and Schwartz, 1980), which frequently is associated with migraine and is not absolutely indomethacin responsive. "Exertional headache" also partially responds to indomethacin.

Chronic, unilateral headaches without sideshift, not responding to indomethacin, include the following differential diagnostic possibilities: cluster headache, cervicogenic headache, and migraine. The duration of pain, accompanying symptoms, sex, and other associated factors simplify the differential diagnosis (see Chapter 8, Table 8–1, and Chapter 6).

The recently described unilateral headache syndrome, "*SUNCT*," should be considered in the differential diagnosis (Sjaastad et al., 1989). Three adult men with a long history of strictly unilateral periocular pain, occurring in paroxysms lasting 15 to 60 seconds and occurring up to 5 to 30 times per hour, were described. Associated symptoms included conjunctival injection, tearing, forehead sweating, and rhinorrhea, all on the symptomatic side. Attacks were precipitated by chewing or moving the head. An episodic and a chronic form exist, and the headache is refractory to all drug treatment, including indomethacin.

Pathogenesis

Intraocular pressure and pulse-synchronous (corneal indentation pulse) amplitudes increase during the attack phase compared with the preattack phase, and clearly more so on the symptomatic than on the nonsymptomatic side (Hørven and Sjaastad, 1977; Hørven et al., 1989). The abruptness with which this occurs strongly indicates that the pressure increase is due to intraocular vasodilation. The corneal temperature also increases, most markedly on the symptomatic side, consistent with the vasodilation theory.

A quantitative study of various autonomic variables concerning organs anatomically close to the eye has demonstrated abnormalities such as bilaterally increased nasal secretion and lacrimation during attacks, most marked on the symptomatic side. Forehead sweating was increased on the symptomatic side in some, but not all, cases. Forehead sweating clearly increased on both sides following heating in CPH—as opposed to what usually occurs in cluster headache. The forehead sweating patterns in cluster headache and CPH also differed after pilocarpine administration (Sjaastad, 1986). This indicates that there are fundamental differences in the pathogenesis of CPH and cluster headache.

To find out whether these changes are confined to autonomic parameters pertaining to the anterior parts of the head or the face, cerebral blood flow, via electromagnetic flowmetry and intra-arterial xenon method, and intra-arterial blood pressure were measured during and between attacks. No definite attack-inducing changes were found (Sjaastad, 1986).

Attacks can be abruptly precipitated by applying pressure to certain particularly sensitive points in the neck or by neck flexion. In only a few seconds, tears appear and the intraocular pressure is increased on the symptomatic side. Obstructing the flow in the common or internal carotid artery on the symptomatic side does not initiate an attack, nor does rubbing these arteries. The pathway from the neck to the eye therefore appears to be neurogenic, not vascular.

In some precipitated attacks, the pain onset may be delayed by 30 seconds or more, preceded by ipsilateral forehead sweating. Thus autonomic phenomena (e.g., the sweating) are not caused by the pain. Evidence also suggests that the pain is not caused by the autonomic phenomena. If atropine is administered systemically prior to attacks, the autonomic phenomena (i.e., sweating, nasal secretion, and lacrimation) are markedly decreased or abolished but the pain persists. A dichotomy between pain and autonomic phenomena can thus be obtained.

Although the neck seems to play a significant part in attack generation, there also seems to be a clear influence of central mechanisms. Nocturnal attacks appear in close connection with the rapid eye movement sleep phase. It is difficult to reconcile these phenomena with a solitary "peripheral" mechanism; thus an additional "central" dysregulation is strongly suggested.

CPH can probably be viewed as a disorder closely related to, but nevertheless distinct from, cluster headache because of its different clinical pattern, different treatment, and perhaps different pathogenesis (Sjaastad, 1992).

ATYPICAL CLUSTER HEADACHE AND "INDOMETHACIN-RESPONSIVE HEADACHE"

The term "atypical cluster headache" was first used (Hørven and Sjaastad, 1977) to describe patients exhibiting a symptomatology strongly reminiscent of cluster headache but with atypical clinical features. In the reported cases, the supplementary tests—intraocular pressure, corneal indentation pulse amplitude, and corneal temperature measurements—clearly indicated a link to ordinary cluster headache. Three patients had CPH, one had cluster and retrobulbar neuritis, and two had less clear-cut attacks of cluster headache. In addition, these latter two cases (both men) exhibited atypical traits, such as marked interparoxysmal electroencephalographic changes. No attempt has been made to classify these cases more subtly.

This term has lost precision in recent years. In some series, more than half of the patients did not have unilateral headache, nocturnal attacks were not part of the picture, and nausea and vomiting occurred more frequently than lacrimation. In these series, the link, if any, to cluster headache is fragmentary. The usage of this term in connection with such ill-defined and vague headaches is ill conceived and should be abandoned. Used in the original way, this term may still be admissible.

Several types of headache respond to indomethacin, some fully (CPH and hemicrania continua) and others only partially (jabs and jolts syndrome and exertional headache). The two headache forms with full indomethacin response, hemicrania continua and CPH, differ distinctly clinically. CPH logically belongs to the cluster headache syndrome (Sjaastad, 1986, 1987, 1992). The headaches that only partly respond to indomethacin do not appear to belong in this category, and this may also apply to hemicrania continua. The response to indomethacin, the unilaterality of pain, and the female preponderance are features common to hemicrania continua and CPH, but this may not be sufficient to justify a grouping of the two.

REFERENCES

Antonaci, F. and O. Sjaastad (1989). Chronic paroxysmal hemicrania (CPH): A review of the clinical manifestations. *Headache 29:*648–656.

Bogucki, A., R. Szymanska, and W. Braciak (1984). Chronic paroxysmal hemicrania: Lack of pre-chronic stage. *Cephalalgia 4:*187–189.

Bordini, C., F. Antonaci, L.J. Stovner et al. (1991). "Hemicrania continua": A clinical review. *Headache 31:*20–26.

Headache Classification Committee of the International Headache Society (1988). Classification and diagnostic criteria for headache disorders, cranial neuralgia, and facial pain. *Cephalalgia 8*(Suppl. 7):1–96.

Hørven, I., D. Russell, and O. Sjaastad (1989). Ocular blood flow changes in cluster headache and chronic paroxysmal hemicrania. *Headache 29:*373–376.

Hørven, I. and O. Sjaastad (1977). Cluster headache syndrome and migraine. Ophthalmological support for a two-entity theory. *Acta Ophthalmol. (Copenh.) 55:*35–50.

Raskin, N.H. and R.K. Schwartz (1980). Icepick-like pain. *Neurology 30:*203–205.

Russell, D. (1984). Chronic paroxysmal hemicrania: Severity, duration and time of occurrence of attacks. *Cephalalgia 4:*53–56.

Sjaastad, O. (1979). Chronic paroxysmal hemicrania (CPH). The clinical picture. In *Proceedings of the Scandinavian Migraine Society 10th annual meeting* (G. Kärrlander and P.-O. Lundberg, eds.), p. 10. Uppsala, Sweden.

Sjaastad, O. (1986). Chronic paroxysmal hemicrania. In *Handbook of Clinical Neurology* (P.J. Vinken, G.W. Bruyn, and H.L. Klawans, eds.), pp. 257–266. Elsevier, Netherlands.

Sjaastad, O. (1987). Chronic paroxysmal hemicrania: Recent developments. *Cephalalgia 7:*179–188.

Sjaastad, O. (1989). Chronic paroxysmal hemicrania (CPH): Nomenclature as far as the various stages are concerned. *Cephalalgia 9:*1–2.

Sjaastad, O. (1992). *The Cluster Headache Syndrome.* W.B. Saunders, Philadelphia.

Sjaastad, O. and I. Dale (1974). Evidence for a new (?) treatable headache entity. *Headache 14:*105–108.

Sjaastad, O. and I. Dale (1976). Evidence for a new (?) clinical headache entity "chronic paroxysmal hemicrania" 2. *Acta Neurol. Scand. 54:*140–149.

Sjaastad, O. and E.L.H. Spierings (1984). "Hemicrania continua": Another headache absolutely responsive to indomethacin. *Cephalalgia 4:*65–70.

Sjaastad, O., C. Saunte, R. Salvesen et al. (1989). Shortlasting, unilateral neuralgiform headache attacks with conjunctival injection, tearing, sweating, and rhinorrhea. *Cephalalgia 9:*147–156.

8

Cervicogenic Headache

OTTAR SJAASTAD

It is generally believed that, although headache may originate in the cervical spine or the neck, this is a rare phenomenon. Our studies of chronic paroxysmal hemicrania (CPH), a strictly unilateral headache, led us to believe that headache might be closely associated with disorders of the neck (Sjaastad et al., 1982). In the early 1980s, we began to recognize a group of patients with a side-locked, unilateral headache who, like patients with CPH, could precipitate attacks mechanically but who had a temporal pattern distinct from those of cluster headache and CPH. We believe that this headache probably originates in the neck, and refer to it as cervicogenic headache (Sjaastad et al., 1984). We have seen a large number of such patients, and they form a rather homogeneous picture. Most are female and relatively young (the mean age of onset is around 30), with clinical symptoms and signs referable to the neck.

CLINICAL MANIFESTATIONS

The pain of cervicogenic headache is usually non-throbbing unilateral, without side alternation, and located in the temporal, frontal, and ocular areas (Fredriksen et al., 1987; Sjaastad et al., 1983). Although the pain frequently begins in the neck, it is not limited to the neck or face. When severe, the pain may be bilateral, but it is most severe on the original side. An attack can last hours to days, and the interval between pain attacks varies from days to weeks. Eventually, the pain may become chronic. A number of patients experience ipsilateral, diffuse shoulder and arm pain; this is important diagnostically. Neck movements are usually restricted and crepitation may be present.

Most patients are able to provoke identical attacks by Valsalva maneuvers, moving the neck, or keeping the head in a locked, awkward position for a prolonged period. Awkward nocturnal positioning of the head may give rise to morning headaches. As in CPH, attacks may be precipitated by firm digital pressure on the symptomatic side of the neck on tender trigger points located over the C_2 root and the greater occipital nerve. Associated ipsilateral phenomena are occasionally seen concurrently: tinnitus, moderate facial flushing, reduced vision, and lid edema, particularly of the lower lid. During severe attacks, migrainous phenomena such as nausea, loss of appetite, vomiting, and phono- and photophobia may occur. Dizziness and difficulty swallowing may occasionally occur.

EVIDENCE FOR CERVICAL ORIGIN

Some evidence suggests a causal relationship between cervical disorders and cervicogenic headache: sustained, awkward neck movements or trigger point pressure precipitate attacks; stiffness and neck pain occur with movements; and the range of motion of the neck is reduced and crepitation occurs. Vague, annoying ipsilateral shoulder, arm, and hand pain occur. These findings suggest the presence of a unilateral cervical disorder. Furthermore, ipsilateral local anesthetic blocks of the C_2 (and at times C_3) roots during the symptomatic periods results in complete or partial pain relief (Hunter and Mayfield, 1949; Sjaastad et al., 1983), especially in patients with a history of trauma. Anesthetic blocks of the greater occipital nerve reduces or removes the pain in cervicogenic headache, whereas it has little or no influence on the pain of migraine (Bovin and Sand, 1992). Hunter and Mayfield (1949) cut the second sensory cervical root intraspinally on the symptomatic side, and the pain disappeared completely. This improvement seemed to be long lasting (F. H. Mayfield, personal communication, 1985). Unfortunately, these relevant findings seem to have been neglected. Hunter and Mayfield's patients were similar to ours in most respects. Headache attacks were recurring, unilateral without sideshift, and of varying duration. They started in the suboccipital region and spread forward to the vertex and eye area and, when severe, to the entire head, but maintained a higher intensity on the original side. There was occasional vomiting and giddiness, tenderness on the occipital/suboccipital area, ipsilateral tinnitus, nasal stuffiness, and facial flushing. Age of onset, female preponderance, visual disturbances, and swallowing difficulties were not mentioned.

Because many structures in the neck or occipital region could be the source of this headache, we have deliberately avoided the use of the term "vertebragenic," which would imply that the pain originates from a lesion in the vertebra. In our opinion, the more neutral term "cervicogenic" headache is correct. Cervicogenic indicates the region where the headache originates but does not pinpoint the structures primarily affected. The term "migraine cervicale" should be abandoned because it implies a variety of migraine. The term "cervical headache" may convey the impression that the pain is located in the cervical area and not that the pain originates in the neck, and this is not what we mean to convey.

Cervicogenic headache, as we have defined it (Sjaastad et al., 1990), is unilateral. Although bilateral cases exist, they are probably cases that exhibit "unilaterality on both sides," and may be more frequent than presently believed. At the present time, unilateral cases may be diagnosed with reasonable certainty, but this is not true for bilateral cases. At this stage, cervicogenic headache patients presenting with bilateral headache are difficult to differentiate from cases of tension-type headache and migraine without aura. The diagnostic error may become unallowably high, and might discredit the whole field. For the time being, bilateral cases should be separated from unilateral cases, at least in scientific approaches.

DIFFERENTIAL DIAGNOSIS

Cervicogenic headache must be differentiated from other unilateral headaches. Cervicogenic headache clearly differs from cluster headache and CPH in attack duration, frequency, severity, response to medication, and supplementary test findings (Table 8–1). In groups of patients, there is clear difference between these disorders; in the individual, however, differential difficulties may arise. In chronic cluster, when the characteristic cluster phenomenon is lacking, the differential diagnostic problems may be considerable. In fact, Hunter and Mayfield's cases (1949) have been misinterpreted as cluster headache. Cervicogenic headache may be difficult to distinguish clinically from hemicrania continua (Bordini et al., 1991); hemicrania continua, unlike cervicogenic headache, is absolutely responsive to indomethacin.

Separating cervicogenic headache from "migraine without aura" is probably most difficult. Emphasis should be placed on symptoms and signs pertaining

Table 8–1 Differential diagnostic aspects of cervicogenic headache versus cluster headache and chronic paroxysmal hemicrania

	Cluster headache	CPH	Cervicogenic headache
Sex	85–90% males	Female preponderance (approx 70%)	>2/3 females
Attack duration	+ +	+	+ + +
Frequency of attacks	1–3/day	10/day (mean)	1–3 per 1 or more weeks[a]
Severity of pain	+ + +	+ + +	+(+)
Mechanical precipitation	−	+ +	+ + +
Horner-like syndrome	+(−)	−	−
Effect of indomethacin	−	+ + +	(+)
Effect of lithium	+ + +	− [b]	−
Ergotamine effect	+ +	−	−
Corneal indentation pulse amplitude and intraocular pressure increase during attack	+	+(+)	−

[a] Eventually the pain may become chronic.
[b] CPH patients even deteriorate on lithium.

to the neck: reduced range of motion in the neck; ipsilateral, diffuse shoulder and arm pain; and the ability to precipitate attacks either by external neck pressure or by certain sustained neck movements. To diagnose cervicogenic headache, the unilaterality without sideshift and the ipsilateral associated phenomena are important. The visual disturbances in migraine proper are frequently bilateral and homonymous. The visual disturbances in cervicogenic headache are monocular and ipsilateral. Scintillating scotomata, seen in migraine with aura, have not been described in cervicogenic headache. Migraine may not always change sides between attacks (Graham, 1968). Migraine usually starts in the frontotemporal area; cervicogenic headache always starts in the neck or posterior parts of the head. Pain relief following anesthetic blockade of the greater occipital nerve, although a crucial feature in cervicogenic headache, is rarely, if at all, seen in migraine.

We are faced with a group of patients who probably differ from migraine patients and should be categorized separately. Cervicogenic headache differs from other universally accepted headache types. Employing our present criteria (Sjaastad et al., 1990) shows that this headache is much more prevalent than is popularly believed.

ETIOLOGY AND PATHOGENESIS

The etiology and pathogenesis of the cervicogenic headache are poorly understood. The cervicogenic headache group is not a homogeneous one from an etiologic/pathogenetic viewpoint. Hypothetically, the uncovertebral joints (Krogdahl and Torgersen, 1940) could play a role in the pathogenesis of this headache, although the pathogenesis in some cases may be more complicated (Jansen and Spoerri, 1984; Jansen et al., 1989). New surgical approaches are being evaluated to treat this headache. We believe that the "syndrome sympathique cervical posterieur" of Barré (1926) and migraine cervicale (Bärtschi-Rochaix, 1968) have clinical features similar to those of our cases. We are not convinced that their cases represent distinct, homogeneous groups of patients. The patients described by Hunter and Mayfield (1949) are more similar to ours.

Headache of cervical origin—"cervicogenic headache"—is still a controversial issue. Some of the controversies have been sorted out; others remain to be resolved in the future.

Editor's Note

Cervicogenic headache was originally described by Ottar Sjaastad, the author of this chapter. As stated by the author, this is still a controversial headache. This headache presently seems to be accepted in many headache centers around the world. For that reason also, it is included in this book. It has, however, so far not been accepted in the International Headache Society classification.

Sjaastad's patients have a uniform headache profile consisting of unilateral headaches without sideshift; the headaches may be infrequent, but are longlasting with no clustering of attacks. Signs of neck involvement and precipitation by neck movements or trigger point pressure are crucial to the diagnosis. Associated "migraine features" (nausea, vomiting, phonophobia, irritability, blurring vision) are not common. Pfaffenrath (1989) would add failure to respond to indomethacin to differentiate cervicogenic headache from chronic paroxysmal hemicrania. Many patients with cervicogenic headache have trigger points that, when stimulated, produce headache. Greater occipital nerve blockade frequently produces relief. Many patients with cervicogenic headache have a history of head or neck trauma, but their radiographs are not different from those of matched controls.

Edmeads (1978) has argued that cervicogenic headaches are a subset of migraine without aura. Cervicogenic headache meets many of the International Headache Society criteria for migraine (unilateral headache, nausea/vomiting, phono/photophobia). Familial occurrence is no longer used as a diagnostic criterion for migraine. Lack of side alternation of attacks is observed in 20% of migraine patients (see Chapter 5). For this reason, the lack of side alternation in cervicogenic headache does not distinguish it from migraine without aura in an absolute way.

Whether cervicogenic headache is a unique disorder or a variety of migraine without aura (and with a cervical trigger) is uncertain at this time.

REFERENCES

Barré M. (1926). Sur un syndrome sympathique cervical posterieur et sa cause frequente: 1. Arthrite cervicale. *Rev. Neurol. 33:*1246–1248.

Bärtschi-Rochaix, W. (1968). Headache of cervical origin. In *Handbook of Clinical Neurology, Vol 5: Headache and Cranial Neuralgias* (P.J. Vinken and G.W. Bruyn, eds.), pp. 192–203. North Holland Publishing Co., Amsterdam.

Bordini, C., F. Antonaci, L.J. Stovner et al. (1991). "Hemicrania continua": A clinical review. *Headache 31:*20–26.

Bovin, G. and T. Sand (1992). Cervicogenic headache, migraine without aura and tension-type headache: Diagnostic blockade of greater occipital and supra-orbital nerves. *Pain 51:*43–48.

Edmeads, J. (1978). Headaches and head pains associated with diseases of the cervical spine. *Med. Clin. North Am. 62:*533–544.

Fredriksen, T.A., H. Hovdal, and O. Sjaastad (1987). "Cervicogenic headache": Clinical manifestation. *Cephalalgia 7:*147–160.

Graham, J.R. (1968). Migraine. Clinical aspects. In *Handbook of Clinical Neurology, Vol. 5: Headache and Cranial Neuralgias* (P.J. Vinken and G.W. Bruyn, eds.), pp. 45–58. North Holland Publishing Co., Amsterdam.

Hunter, C.R. and F.H. Mayfield (1949). Role of the upper cervical roots in the production of pain in the head. *Am. J. Surg. 48:*743–751.

Jansen, J., E. Markakis, B. Rama, and J. Hildebrandt (1989). Hemicranial attacks or permanent hemicrania—a sequel of upper cervical root compression. *Cephalalgia 9:*123–130.

Jansen, J. and O. Spoerri (1984). Atypical frontoorbital pain and headache—due to compression of upper cervical roots. In *Updating in Headache* (V. Pfaffenrath, P.O. Lundberg, and O. Sjaastad, eds.), pp. 14–16. Springer, Berlin.

Krogdahl, T. and O. Torgersen (1940). Die "Unco-Vertebralgelenke" und die "Arthroses deformans uncovertebralis." *Acta Radiol. 21:*231–262.

Pfaffenrath, V. (1989). Cervicogenic headache and its differential diagnosis. In *Migraine and Other Headaches* (M.D. Ferrari and X. Lataste, eds.), pp. 161–177. Parthenon, Park Ridge, NJ.

Sjaastad, O., T.A. Fredriksen, and V. Pfaffenrath (1990). Cervicogenic headache: Diagnostic criteria. *Headache 30:*725–726.

Sjaastad, O., D. Russell, C. Saunte, and I. Hørven (1982). Chronic paroxysmal hemicrania. VI. Precipitation of attacks. Further studies on the precipitation mechanisms. *Cephalalgia 2:*211–214.

Sjaastad, O., C. Saunte, and H. Breivik (1984). Chronisch-paroxysmale Hemikranie. Eine Sonderform des Zervikogenen (vertebragenen) Kopfschmerzes? In *Primäre Kopfschmerzen. Pathogenese, Diagnostic und Therapie* (V. Pfaffenrath, A. Schrader, and I.S. Neu, eds.), pp. 9–16. MMV Medizin Verlag, München.

Sjaastad, O., C. Saunte, H. Hovdal et al. (1983). "Cervicogenic" headache. An hypothesis. *Cephalalgia 3:*249–256.

9

Headache Associated with Chemicals, Toxins, Systemic Infections, and Metabolic Disorders (Toxic Vascular Headache)

JOHN STIRLING MEYER
DONALD J. DALESSIO

A large number of systemic conditions are associated with bilateral and symmetric, throbbing headache. There is a great deal of evidence that these headaches reflect painful dilation of the cephalic vasculature of the brain and scalp combined. This subject is reviewed in detail here, including certain classic experiments performed by Harold Wolff and his colleagues, because they remain basic for understanding the pathogenesis of head pain of vascular etiology.

The most common type of vascular headache, familiar to almost everyone, is that which accompanies fever and which usually becomes more intense as the fever rises. This headache is almost certainly due to congestion of the vessels of the brain and scalp. During stepwise hyperthermia in the monkey, both internal ($+42\%$) and external ($+25\%$) carotid blood flow progressively increases as body temperature is raised from 36 to 41°C (Meyer and Handa, 1967). Cerebral oxidative metabolism likewise increases and is the cause of increased blood flow and delirium that eventually will result if temperature continues to rise. It has also been shown that, in human patients treated with fever therapy, cerebral blood flow (CBF) increases if effective fever is produced (Heyman et al., 1950). This subject is discussed in more detail later. Other common causes of toxic vascular headaches include hangover after excessive alcohol ingestion, respiratory and metabolic acidosis, hypoxia, hypoglycemia, and reactions to many medications. In all of these conditions clinical or experimental evidence shows increased CBF or cephalic blood flow that documents the accompanying cerebrovascular congestion, and this is the essential cause of vascular headache. These common forms of headache are discussed later.

Histamine, which is released into the circulation in many allergic and toxic states, increases CBF and causes a predictable headache in almost all subjects. Conversely, antihistaminics decrease the CBF (Amano and Meyer, 1982a) and tend to alleviate toxic vascular headache, as do many cerebral vasoconstrictor agents, including aspirin, indomethacin, and other nonsteroidal anti-inflammatory agents. Because histamine has been considered an important etiologic metabolite in relation to a majority of toxic vascular headaches, it has been studied extensively as a model of vascular headache, particularly by Harold Wolff; this is discussed later in this chapter.

Another biologic substance that predictably produces characteristic pounding headaches of the vascular type is the prostaglandin PGI_2, or prostacyclin. This ubiquitous vascular prostaglandin is metabolized from arachidonic acid by means of the enzyme cyclo-oxygenase by all vascular endothelia. Prostacyclin is the most potent cerebral vasodilator substance known. It greatly increases cephalic blood flow, and inhibition of its synthesis by nonsteroidal anti-inflammatory agents, such as indomethacin, greatly reduces CBF and relieves vascular headache (Amano and Meyer, 1982b). Intravenous administration of prostacyclin rapidly produces a typical pulsatile and pounding vascular headache, associated with nausea and vomiting (Szczeklik and Gryglewski, 1979).

Cephalic hyperemia seems to accompany toxic vascular headaches, and it appears similar to the cephalic hyperemia accompanying migraine headaches (Kobari et al., 1990). Whether this is causal in nature or secondary to activation of the brain by pain itself, or is due to both factors, remains an unsettled question of considerable interest. Available information suggests that both factors operate in cerebral hyperemia, which provides an objective marker that pain in the head is present. Changes in CBF measured by positron emission tomography in awake, healthy human volunteers subjected to painful heating of the right forearm indicated that specific and highly localized areas of the cortex are actively involved in pain perception (Talbot et al., 1991). Four contralateral areas of the left cerebral cortex were activated with hyperemia during right limb pain. These were in Brodmann's area 24 and the parietal cortex; the limbic cortex, which probably regulates the emotional reaction to pain, was activated at the same time. In migraine and toxic vascular headache, the cephalic hyperemia is more widespread.

CLINICAL USE OF HISTAMINE AS AN EXPERIMENTAL MODEL OF TOXIC VASCULAR HEADACHE

Harold Wolff and his associates, as well as several other eminent physicians and neurosurgeons in the 1930s, used the intravenous infusion of 0.1 mg/minute of histamine as an experimental model for inducing and studying toxic vascular headache among human volunteers. Since it is not at all certain that institutional review boards nowadays would approve comparable protocols, requiring the induction of experimental toxic headache by histamine injection in human patients and volunteers while continuously recording cerebrospinal fluid pressure by means of a spinal needle placed via lumbar puncture and also recording superficial temporal artery pulsations, Wolff's classic work is summarized here. This type of toxic vascular headache was discovered because intravenous histamine was injected for tests of gastric function, which were in vogue at that time, and the histamine injection was regularly accompanied by bilateral head pain.

The response of the human vascular system to histamine infusion was accompanied by reductions of the blood pressure from around 130/70 mm Hg to approximately 70/30 mm Hg for several minutes followed by a prompt rebound of blood pressure to normal levels, or slightly above them, when the histamine infusion was discontinued. This was accompanied by the onset of an intense, diffuse headache of 6 to 8 minutes' duration at the time when intracranial pulsations and pressure were greatly increased.

It was also observed in human subjects during neurosurgical procedures, where it was possible to examine the pial vessels during headache under local anesthesia, as well as among experimental animal models, that intravenous injections of histamine dilated both the cerebral arteries and veins. It was postulated, therefore, that the toxic headache produced by intravenous histamine was vascular in nature. Indeed, some physicians advocated repeated infusions of histamine in those suffering from vascular headaches, particularly cluster headaches, in an attempt to desensitize these individuals from "histamine cephalalgia," which was thought for a time to be the cause of many vascular headaches. This approach to treatment with histamine desensitization has generally been abandoned.

After injections of histamine the amplitude of intracranial pulsations increased (Pickering and Hess, 1933; Weiss et al., 1932; Wolff, 1948). The dynamic effects of cardiac systole on dilated cerebral arterial walls increased, as did CBF; intracranial and venous pulsations also increased as the blood pressure was restored to normal. The head pain was absent, as the blood pressure temporarily fell, and CBF temporarily decreased as a result of a brief loss of impaired cerebral autoregulation. All the above events were measured in cats as well as human volunteers by Wolff and associates.

It was concluded that the increased amplitude of intracranial pulsations after histamine injection increases the stretch of the walls of the dilated intracranial vessels with each cardiac systole, although the vasodilation itself was not sufficient to increase the amplitude of intracranial pulsations during the interval of decreased blood pressure. However, intense cerebral vasodilation in the presence of a normal or raised blood pressure increased both CBF and intracranial pulsations, with accompanying arterial and venous distention. These are important considerations when it is recalled that the dural veins and sinuses and the larger pial and cerebral vessels are important pain-sensitive structures.

When the cerebrospinal fluid pressure was increased to 500 or 600 ml of water by infusion of normal saline under pressure into the lumbar subarachnoid space, the histamine headache was promptly relieved. Inhalation of 5 to 10% carbon dioxide in 95% oxygen, however, produced similar increases in intracranial pulsations as did histamine, with a sensation of fullness in the head, but no headache was reported (Meyer et al., 1966). Wolff was of the opinion that histamine distended the walls of the cerebral vessels, particularly the pial vessels, which greatly increased the number of sensory (afferent) impulses arising from the nerves that innervate them (Bronk, 1935) when the blood pressure was restored to normal. This unusual flood of afferent impulses was considered to be responsible for the head pain. The fact that inhalation of 10% carbon dioxide produced similar intracranial pulsations without headache has never adequately been explained.

Wolff, working with Schumacher et al. (1940), then proceeded to use intravenous infusions of histamine to analyze the neural pathways concerned with the toxic vascular headache induced by this method, comparing results with the headache induced by injecting air into the subarachnoid space for pneumoencephalography, used at the time for diagnostic purposes because computerized tomography and magnetic resonance imaging of the brain were not then available. Infiltrating the nerves of the scalp on one side of the head did not alter the severe, generalized headache produced by histamine injection or by pneumoencephalography. Wolff and Schumacher concluded that superficial sensation of the scalp did not mediate these types of headache.

When the circulation of the scalp was occluded by a tight bandage, Wolff and Schumacher concluded that the headache induced by histamine was not entirely abolished, confirming earlier work by Pickering and Hess (1933), although Wolff and Schumacher's patients reported that some modification of the intensity of the headache did result from this unpleasant procedure. Wolff and Schumacher used a sphygmomanometer cuff wrapped around the head that was inflated above systolic blood pressure. When the cuff was inflated, the histamine headache was diminished or indistinguishable from the head discomfort produced by the tight headband itself. When the cuff was rapidly deflated, the histamine headache again became apparent with its former intensity.

Previously, Hardy et al. (1940) had reported that the threshold for sensation of one pain is raised by the introduction of a second pain, suggesting that the diminution of headache by a tight head bandage may be due, in part, to the pain caused by the bandage itself rather than obstructing the scalp arteries and preventing painful vasodilation. Wolff and co-workers were also able to show that, during histamine headache, manual obliteration of the superficial temporal artery reduced, but did not obliterate, the head pain, nor did unilateral ligation of the superficial temporal artery alter the bilateral head pain caused by histamine injection.

Surgical manipulation of the exposed superficial temporal artery was reported as painful, and this type of induced pain was referred to the upper teeth and temporal regions and orbit on the same side. After injection of 0.1 mg histamine phosphate into the temporal artery, there was severe pain in the ipsilateral temporal area more widespread than occurred when the temporal artery was manipulated. This was followed by unilateral flushing of the face and forehead, with intense unilateral dull and throbbing headache. The temporoparietal regional pain then became bilateral and disappeared about 3.5 minutes after the injection.

Among seven patients studied by Wolff at the New York Hospital who had ligation and section of the middle meningeal arteries with destruction of their periarterial nerves, intravenous injection of histamine produced the usual bilateral and symmetric headache, which led him to conclude that the middle meningeal artery and the dural arteries are not major contributors to the pain of histamine headache. Northfield (1938) made his own separate observations in

England that supported this conclusion. After injection of histamine into the internal carotid artery in six of Northfield's patients, homolateral headache occurred in five cases and no headache in one, but injection of histamine into the external carotid artery in six cases produced no headache in five and faint generalized headache in one.

Wolff concluded (Wolff, 1938, 1987), by a process of elimination, that the cerebral arteries are the chief sources of histamine headache because:

1. The cerebral vessels, particularly those near the base of the brain, have afferent nerves providing pain sensations (Levine and Wolff, 1932).
2. Cerebral vasodilation is invariably observed following injection of histamine.
3. Histamine headache is abolished by elevating the intracranial pressure, thereby minimizing vasodilation (Clark et al., 1938a,b; Pickering and Hess, 1933; Wolff, 1948).
4. Local anesthesia of the scalp does not diminish histamine headache.
5. Anesthetizing the extracranial arteries does not diminish histamine headache.
6. Compressing the arteries of the scalp probably reduces the intensity of the histamine headache by counterirritation produced by the compressing headband, which is painful.
7. There is a lack of appreciable decrease in histamine headache on one side following ligation of the middle meningeal or the temporal artery, or both arteries, on that side.
8. Development of homolateral histamine headache follows the injection of histamine into the internal carotid artery but not into the external carotid artery.

Wolff stated, "The evidence thus far adduced indicates that many cranial arteries participate in headache but the cerebral arteries are the chief contributors to the pain of histamine headache and determine its intensity" (1987).

Wolff then tested to find which of the cerebral arteries are implicated in generalizing head pain. He noted that the major vessels of the circle of Willis at the base of the brain and the proximal portions of the main arteries of the circle have all been demonstrated to be pain sensitive by electrically stimulating them during exposure of the brain for surgical procedures carried out under local anesthesia. The resulting head pain is intense, definite, and constantly localized. The small branches of these arteries become progressively insensitive as they spread over the convexity of the brain or become intracerebral in location.

Stimulation of the internal carotid and of the anterior, middle and posterior cerebral arteries causes pain within, behind, or over the eye as far medially as the midline and as far laterally as the temporal regions. Stimulation of the basilar artery and its pontine and internal auditory arteries causes pain behind the ears. Faradic stimulation of the vertebral and basilar arteries and the posterior interior cerebellar arteries causes pain in the occipital and suboccipital regions. Histamine headaches are also distributed over the sum of the areas just described.

Pain Pathways Involved in Histamine Headaches

Wolff and colleagues then induced headaches by the intravenous injection of histamine in subjects who had previously had sections of various cranial and cervical nerves. In these clinical investigations, anatomic inferences as to which pathways had been interrupted were based, whenever possible, on surgical visualization of the nerves sectioned rather than on the resulting areas of analgesia (Ray, 1954).

Based on common knowledge concerning the distribution of pain fibers to the skin over the head and neck, the assumption was made that the head as high as the vertex is supplied by the fifth cranial nerve and that the back of the head and neck are supplied chiefly from the second and third cervical nerves. Analgesia in these regions was due to destruction of the aforementioned pathways or their nuclei or ganglia. Although other afferent pathways are believed to carry pain fibers from the head, such as the upper cervical and 11th and 12th cranial nerves supplying the occiput and the 7th, 9th, and 10th cranial nerves supplying the region in and behind the ear, interruption of these pathways did not result in demonstrable analgesia.

In normal persons, Pickering and Hess (1933) and Wolff (1948) reported that intravenous injection of histamine produced symmetric headache involving the forehead just above the orbits, the temples, the vertex and both occipital regions. For Wolff's experimental studies, subjects with unilateral analgesia were chiefly employed so that the normal side served as a control. The following assumptions were made: if headache failed regularly to be induced in an analgesic area on one side of the head but occurred regularly in the corresponding area of the opposite intact side, the absence of headache on the analgesic side was due to interruption of the afferent pathways conducting pain impulses that were interpreted, by the subject studied, as headache in that region of the head (Schumacher et al., 1940).

Results were as follows: Partial section of the sensory root of the fifth cranial nerve did not alter the pattern of histamine headache. Complete section of the sensory root of the fifth cranial nerve with hemianalgesia of the face and scalp resulted in absence of head pain in the frontotemporal zones in the region of analgesia. Similar observations had been reported previously by Pickering (1939), Pickering and Hess (1933) and Northfield (1938). In one patient with a lesion of the brainstem and upper part of the cervical region of the cord resulting in hemianalgesia of the head, histamine injection caused unilateral headache sparing the hemianalgesic side of the head. In one patient with occipital hemianalgesia that had resulted from syringomyelia, injection of histamine produced headache on the unaffected side, but on the analgesic side of the back of the head pain was absent.

The above evidence suggests that the upper cervical nerves are afferent pathways for the painful impulses responsible for occipital headache. This question was tested by stimulating the arteries of the posterior fossa with faradic current, which causes pain in the occiput among patients undergoing neurosurgical operations for control of pain. Stimulation of the vertebral artery and the posterior interior cerebellar artery caused pain in the occiput and suboccipital regions, and stimulation of the basilar and internal auditory artery caused pain behind the ear. Section of the first three cervical nerves and branches of the 9th and 10th cranial nerves abolished pain when these arteries of the posterior fossa were stimulated. Section of the 7th cranial nerve for removal of acoustic neuroma did not abolish the cephalalgia induced by histamine injection, nor did section of the glossopharyngeal nerve for glossopharyngeal neuralgia. Likewise, two patients who had extensive sectioning bilaterally of the cervical portion of the sympathetic trunks had typical histamine headaches after injection of histamine. These findings by Wolff and Ray are consonant with earlier reports from England by Northfield (1938) and Pickering and Hess (1933), but not with the surgical reports of two patients reported by Dandy (1931) in Baltimore, who claimed termination of severe hemicrania in two patients by resecting the inferior cervical and first thoracic sympathetic ganglia on the side of the head pain.

In summary, the classic work of Harold Wolff and others suggests that important afferent pathways for head pain, particularly for the vascular type of headache produced experimentally by histamine injection, are mediated by the sensory roots of the 5th cranial nerve, sensory roots of the upper three cervical nerves, and the 9th and 10th cranial nerves. However, the afferent pathways are numerous, and ascribing the sensation of headache to one or another nerve is an unjustified simplification.

HEADACHES RESULTING PRIMARILY FROM DISTENTION OF CEREBRAL AND PIAL ARTERIES

Headache Associated with Infection and Fever

Septicemia, bacteremia, and fever are commonly associated with headache. It is unlikely, however, that the agent responsible for the fever is identical to that resulting in the headache. The most intense, prolonged headaches associated with infections are those that accompany typhoid fever, typhus fever, and influenza. The headache is dull, deep, aching, and generalized, but is often worse, especially at the beginning, in the back of the head. It is increased in intensity by bodily effort. It is often worse in the latter part of the day, especially if the patient is ambulatory, or when the patient is most exhausted or prostrated. The intensity of pain is decreased by manual compression of the common carotid artery. It is not modified appreciably by ergotamine tartrate, except possibly toward the end of the period of the headache.

A 19-year-old laboratory technician, who daily manipulated both murine and scrub typhus virus at her work, entered the hospital complaining of severe headache with occasional fever. Six days before admission she developed a moderately severe occipital headache. During the intervening 5 days this headache was of increasing intensity, recurred daily, was worse in the late afternoon and evening, and persisted through the night. It was usually absent the following morning. At the time of the headache her face was flushed. The headache was of a throbbing, aching quality, made worse by turning the head, by bending over, or by bodily effort. It became generalized, and was often most intense in the frontal region, especially during the 3 days before admission. The headache was not affected by acetylsalicylic acid, 0.6 g, but was appreciably diminished by codeine phosphate, 60 mg. The patient had no stiff neck, nausea, or vomiting. She was able to work until the day of hospitalization, and the fierce headache was out of all proportion to the general constitutional symptoms and signs. She had a moderate leukopenia and a temperature of 38.5°C. Two rose-colored macules were found under each breast.

Seven months before this illness the patient had been inoculated with both murine and scrub typhus vaccine. Three days after her hospital admission, or 9 days after onset, the headache spontaneously ended, and she became symptom free. Tests of antibody titer established the diagnosis of murine typhus fever. (Wolff, 1987)

It was possible to observe in experimental animals, prepared so that the pial vessels could be visualized through a skull window, that the intravenous injection of foreign protein (typhoid vaccine) was followed by cerebral vasodilation. Such vasodilation was sometimes, but not always, associated with fever. Because of the use of barbiturates in inducing anesthesia, which was necessary to the experiment, fever was inconstantly obtained. No change in the pressure of the cerebrospinal fluid was observed, although sometimes the pressure became slightly higher. The vasodilation was usually extreme, and it was suggested that headache would probably follow such a state.

Because it has been observed that the fever induced by the intravenous administration of typhoid vaccine is frequently associated with headache or with sensations of fullness in the head, the relation of the cranial arteries to the headache was experimentally investigated in observations of patients who were undergoing fever therapy for chorea or rheumatoid arthritis (Schumacher et al., 1940).

Method. A tambour was placed on the temporal artery, a needle introduced into the lumbar sac, and the pulsations simultaneously recorded as heretofore described. After a suitable control period, during which records were made, an appropriate amount (25,000,000 to 1,000,000,000 bacteria per cubic centimeter) of typhoid vaccine was administered intravenously. If no chill or rise in temperature took place within 60 or 90 minutes, a second and smaller amount was given. Estimates of the state of the headache, determinations of the blood pressure, and records of the pulsations of the cerebrospinal fluid and the temporal artery were made at frequent intervals throughout the procedure.

Results. Twelve such experiments were performed. Because of the many hours of immobilization necessary for a complete record of the beginning and the end of the cycle of fever and the consequent discomfort to patients with arthritis, experiments completely satisfactory from a technical point of view were not obtained. However, the observations were adequate and consistent and permitted inferences (Figure 9–1).

Onset of a headache or a sensation of fullness in the head was found in all instances to follow increased amplitude of pulsations of the cerebrospinal fluid and of the temporal artery. Spontaneous lessening of the headache closely paralleled the decrease in amplitude of these pulsations, and as the amplitude of the pulsations again increased, the headache became more severe. With the ultimate decline in

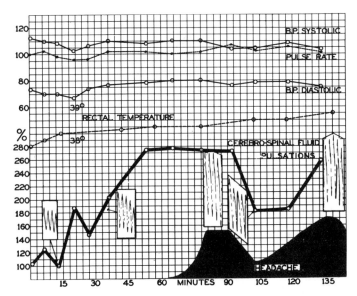

Figure 9–1. Relation of the headache associated with intravenous injection of typhoid vaccine to the amplitude of pulsations of the cerebrospinal fluid. The onset, increase, and decrease in intensity of the headache paralleled the amplitude of pulsations of the cerebrospinal fluid. A spontaneous remission in the severity of the headache paralleled the decrease in the amplitude of pulsations of the cerebrospinal fluid.

amplitude of the pulsations the headache ended. The pressure of the cerebrospinal fluid was at all times within the usual physiologic limits. (Wolff, 1987)

Observations of the temporal artery and the cerebrospinal fluid showed that here, too, the spontaneous increase and decrease of the headache paralleled the amplitude of pulsations.

The similarity between the pyrexial headache and those induced by histamine was previously noted. The amplitude of pulsations of the cerebrospinal fluid in headache induced by fever and by histamine was greatly increased, in contrast with that in migraine headache, in which there was no increase in amplitude. Pickering and Hess (1933) added the observation that increasing the cerebrospinal fluid pressure by means of a manometer attached to a needle in the lumbar subarachnoid space reduced fever headache.

The fact that increasing the intracranial pressure decreased the intensity of the headache indicates that the mechanism of the headache in fever and that of the headache following injection of histamine are similar, and that in both the intracranial arteries are the chief contributors to the pain. It is likely that the headache associated with acute infections, fever, sepsis, and bacteremia has such an explanation.

Although any fever or infection may be associated with headache, some of the common fevers and infectious diseases that have been linked with severe headache as [the] initiating or accompanying symptom, but that in themselves have no special identifying characteristics, are as follows:

Those of bacterial origin include: pneumonia, septicemia, tonsillitis and adenoiditis, scarlet fever, chorea, typhoid fever, paratyphoid fever, undulant fever (brucellosis), tularemia, bubonic plague, [and] Haverhill fever.

Those of probable viral origin include: acute coryza, influenza, herpes simplex, measles, mumps, smallpox, poliomyelitis, yellow fever, dengue, rabies, rubella, [and] infectious mononucleosis.

Those of rickettsial origin include: typhus fever, trench fever, and oroya fever.

Headache with each attack of malarial fever may be intense.

Accessory evidence that dilatation of intracranial vessels accompanies some acute systemic infections is provided by observations of changes in the force required to produce headache by rapid head movement during the illness. It has been noted, for example, that during a 3-week period of recurrent chills and fever induced by therapeutic tertian malaria, the threshold to jolt headache (expressed in g units) fell from a control level of 6.9 to values as low as 1.6 g. This depression of threshold was not entirely dependent upon the presence of high body temperature, for it varied independently of the height of the fever.

Similarly, in another patient, a lowered threshold to jolt headache could be demonstrated during the first stage of an acute nasopharyngitis accompanied by malaise and lethargy, and during an attack of acute gastroenteritis, also with systemic symptoms, and presumably of the winter viral type. (Wolff, 1987).

"Hangover" Headache

As mentioned earlier, there is a good deal of evidence that hangover headache resulting from excessive alcohol ingestion belongs in the category under discussion. Although CBF is increased in acute alcoholic intoxication, the mechanism of the headache that follows, usually in the morning after alcohol intoxication, is complicated. So-called impurities in alcoholic beverages may also have significant pharmacodynamic effects, but their relevance to hangover headache is difficult to define. Although ethyl alcohol causes cerebral vessels to dilate and CBF to increase, the period of maximum alcohol concentration in the blood does not necessarily correlate with the severity of headache. The headache is usually most severe when the alcohol concentration in the blood is reduced or minimal. However, alcohol is well known as a precipitator of migraine and cluster headache, possibly because of increased prostacyclin synthesis, and aspirin, indomethacin, and other nonsteroidal anti-inflammatory agents, all of which are potent cerebral vasoconstrictors, usually lessen hangover headaches. Repeated trials with the experimental administration of 60 to 90 ml of 95% ethyl alcohol have not been followed by headache, even in those who suffer from frequent vascular headaches. Other cerebral vasoconstrictors, such as 100% oxygen inhaled by face mask and hyperventilation, benefit hangover headache, which supports the view that cerebral vasodilation plays a part in the head pain.

Intake of alcohol under laboratory conditions, however, is quite different from social drinking. The discipline imposed by experimental situations precludes the excitement that accompanies its use in a party setting. It appears, therefore, as though the action of the alcohol in inducing headache is indirect, although it is likely that the headache results from cranial vasodilation. The throbbing quality, the increase in intensity with elevation of blood pressure or sudden head movement, and the decline in intensity on carotid artery compression that sometimes follows the administration of vasoconstrictor agents, such as caffeine by mouth or ergotamine tartrate by intravenous injection, support this view. It is unlikely that edema of the brain is relevant to the headache.

> The common observation that hangover headache is readily aggravated by head movement offers suggestive evidence for dilatation of intracranial vessels as a factor in this type of headache. Accelerometer measurements in one patient revealed that jolts of 4.0 to 4.2 g would intensify his usual right temporal hangover headache, whereas on symptom-free days jolts of 5.5 g or much higher would be required to induce headache. (Wolff, 1987)

It is suggested that the vasodilator type of headache results not only from the pharmacodynamic action of alcohol and impurities on cranial vessels, but also from the effects on the subject of late hours, loss of sleep, excitement of social intercourse (talking, singing, and laughing), sustained effort and exhaustion, loss of restraint, and perhaps some remorse. In short, it is associated with psychobiologic factors akin to those operating in certain other types of vascular headaches. However, because hangover headache is by no means a rare phenomenon and can be produced for experimental purposes so readily, it presents an inviting problem for further study.

It has been demonstrated that oral fructose increases the rate of alcohol metabolism in the healthy human (Pawan, 1968). Mean blood alcohol levels are lower after the ingestion of fructose, using the subject as his or her own control. Thirty grams of fructose will increase the rate of metabolism of alcohol by 15 to 30%. No other sugars have this effect on alcohol metabolism, including glucose, galactose, and sucrose. Large amounts of vitamins, including the B-complex vitamins, ascorbic acid, vitamin E, and the like, do not affect the rate of alcohol metabolism in the healthy human. This being the case, it is possible to reduce the intensity and frequency of hangover headache by employing fructose, either therapeutically or prophylactically.

The mechanism of action of fructose is uncertain. However, alcohol dehydrogenase is the rate-limiting enzyme in the degradation of alcohol, and this is dependent, to a considerable extent, on the availability of the hydrogen acceptor nicotinamide adenine dinucleotide (NAD). It is suggested that fructose stimulates the conversion of NADH to NAD, which allows the rate of alcohol metabolism to be partially accelerated.

Postseizure Headache

The headache that follows an epileptic attack with loss of consciousness, with or without convulsive movements, is a generalized, moderately intense, throbbing pain, usually of several hours' duration. It is noted when the patient regains consciousness, is often associated with a desire to sleep, and may be absent when the patient awakes.

The human brain has been repeatedly observed during the convulsive seizure. An initial pallor may be noted just preceding and during the first part of the fit. However, whether or not initial pallor is noted, the latter part of the fit and the postfit stage are always accompanied by widespread vasodilation of cerebral vessels. The dilated vessels are first cyanotic and then bright red.

Because this bright red dilated phase persists for several hours, it is suggested that this cerebral artery dilation is the basis of the postepileptic headache.

Measurements of CBF in humans, as well as in experimental animals, support the view that cerebral congestion is responsible for postseizure headaches (Meyer and Portnoy, 1959; Meyer et al., 1966). During the seizures, cerebral metabolism and blood flow are greatly increased, cerebral autoregulation is lost, and marked acidosis and hyperemia of the brain result.

Headache Associated with Hypoxia

Experimentally induced cerebral hypoxemia (Wolff and Lennox, 1930), especially when coupled with an increase in carbon dioxide tension in the blood, results in extreme dilation of cerebral vessels, notably of the arteries and arterioles. This observation is probably related to the fact that some persons at high altitudes (Barcroft et al., 1922; Monge, 1942) complain of headache that persists for hours or days until physiologic adjustments have been achieved, or until the individual returns to a lower altitude. Such headaches are usually prevented by ingestion of acetazolamide prior to ascent to high altitude. Associated with the intense throbbing headache is a sensation of fullness of the head, hot flushes of the face, photophobia, injection of the ocular mucosa, and deep cyanosis. It is likely that such headaches are due to cerebrovascular distention.

> An intense, throbbing headache of hours' or days' duration is a striking feature in persons exposed for a shorter or longer period to carbon monoxide. That the headache is due to distention of pial and cerebral vessels is extremely likely. Thus, hypoxemia resulting from inhalation of carbon monoxide has a dilator effect on the cerebral vessels. When, for experimental purposes, dilute mixtures of carbon monoxide and air were given to animals, and the cerebral blood vessels observed through cranial windows, cerebral vasodilatation and increased cerebrospinal fluid pressure were noted. An increased cerebrospinal fluid pressure in man as well as in animals has also been demonstrated, the result, probably, of vasodilation and a change in permeability of the blood vessel walls. (Wolff, 1987)

It has also been shown in humans that, during brief hypoxia, CBF increases remarkably (Meyer et al., 1969; Kudrow, 1980), so that vascular headache is a predictable outcome of more prolonged hypoxia.

Headache Associated with Ischemic Hypoxia

It has been demonstrated in animals that, after sudden localized or generalized cerebral ischemia, when collateral or general circulation was re-established, extreme cerebral vasodilation and increased CBF comparable to the so-called reactive hypermia of muscle and skin occur. This situation has also been called "luxury perfusion" because cerebral perfusion is in excess of tissue demand (Lassen, 1966). Reactive hyperemia of the brain has also been demonstrated to occur in humans after cerebral ischemic hypoxia resulting from temporary vascular occlusion, and these patients frequently complain of headache (Meyer et al., 1965; Fisher, 1968). Headache occurring in patients with cerebrovascular disease also may be due to serotonin release, which has been invoked in the pathogenesis of migraine (Edmeads, 1979).

Headache Associated with High Altitude

Appenzeller (1972) pointed out that headache may be associated with acute mountain sickness, acute pulmonary edema of altitude, and chronic mountain sickness in well-acclimatized subjects. Altitude headache is uncommon below 8,000 feet, appears with increasing frequency at higher elevations, and above 12,000 feet is more or less universal in persons not acclimatized to altitude (Table 9–1).

Altitude headache often appears hours after exposure to low oxygen tension and is not relieved by administration of oxygen. The headache is assumed to be related to vasodilation and/or brain edema and is aggravated by maneuvers that increase intracranial pressure, such as coughing, straining at stool, head jolting, and particularly exertion. Persons with altitude headache are uncomfortable when lying down. Papilledema and retinal hemorrhages have been observed in some patients with acute mountain sickness.

Experimentally induced cerebral hypoxemia, especially when coupled with an increase in carbon dioxide tension in the blood, results in extreme dilation of cerebral vessels, notably of the arteries and arterioles. This observation probably is related to the fact that some persons at high altitudes complain of headache that persists for hours or days until physiologic adjustments have been achieved, or until the individual returns to a lower altitude (Barcroft, 1925; Barcroft et al., 1922; Houston, 1976; Leufaut and Sullivan, 1970). Associated with the intense throbbing headache is a sensation of fullness of the head, hot flushes of the face, photophobia, injection of the ocular mucosa, and deep cyanosis. It is likely that such headaches are due in part to cerebrovascular distention.

Table 9–1 Headache and hypoxia: Neurologic signs and symptoms

Altitude in meters (feet)	Symptoms	Alveolar PO$_2$ (mm Hg)	Headache
3,048 (10,000)	Impairment of recent memory, judgment, and ability to perform complex calculations; increased heart rate and pulmonary ventilation	60	Frequent in unacclimatized subjects
3,658 (12,000)	Dyspnea, impaired ability to perform complex tasks, headache, nausea, decreased visual acuity	52	Frequent in all
4,573 (15,000)	Decrease in auditory acuity, constriction of visual fields, impaired judgment, irritability; exercise can lead to unconsciousness	46	Frequent in all
5,486 (18,000)	Decrements in personality and intellect; threshold for loss of consciousness in resting unacclimatized individuals after seveal hours' exposure	40	Universally present
6,096 (20,000)	Handwriting illegible in conscious subjects	33	Universally present
6,706 (22,000)	Almost all individuals unconscious after sufficient exposure time	30	Universally present

Singh et al. (1960) have investigated headache associated with acute mountain sickness. Lumbar punctures in 34 subjects exposed to high altitude demonstrated a significant increase in cerebrospinal fluid pressure, and in one patient
a biopsy of the brain revealed brain edema. Manifestations usually develop 8
to 24 hours after arrival at the high altitude and remit over 4 to 8 days. The
syndrome is thus distinguished from hypoxia per se, or from chronic mountain
sickness, by virtue of its time of onset, duration, and course.

Mental symptoms are frequently associated with altitude headache. If the
ascent is slow, sensations of exhilaration and well-being are often described.
As altitude increases, more serious mental problems develop. Mental tasks
become difficult, and irritability and depression are common. To quote Barcroft
(1922):

> Alcohol affects different persons in different ways; so on my journeying in high
> altitudes I have seen most of the symptoms of alcoholism reproduced. I have seen
> men vomit, I have seen them quarrel, I have seen them become reckless, I have
> seen them become morose. I have seen one of the most disciplined of men fling his
> arms about on the ledge of a crevasse to the great embarrassment of the guide. I
> have seen the most loyal companion become ill-tempered and abusive to the point
> at which I feared international complications would arise. (Wolff, 1987)

These symptoms can be relieved to some degree by careful and gradual ascent,
to allow acclimatization. Acetazolamide, given 250 mg every 8 hours before
and during exposure to altitude, may reduce manifestations of acute mountain
sickness. Furosemide, 80 mg every 12 hours, has also been suggested. For
some, the symptoms are unrelieved and descent to a lower altitude is necessary.

Decompression Headache

Arterial hypoxia, not contaminated by hypercapnea, occurs in those exposed
to high altitudes and in those in decompression chambers. Decompression sickness appears when a sudden change in the pressure of ambient gases, to which
the subject has become equilibrated, occurs. A sudden reduction in pressure of
45% is usually sufficient to cause symptoms.

The symptoms produced by rapid decompression are caused primarily by
the formation of nitrogen gas bubbles in blood and fatty tissues. Nitrogen does
not diffuse readily and is not used in body metabolism. Thus, when body fluids
and tissues saturated with nitrogen are suddenly exposed to a lower pressure,
bubbles of nitrogen gas form that lodge in small blood vessels and fatty tissues,
because nitrogen is five times more soluble in oil than in water (Behnke, 1965).

Similar problems occur in aviators during rapid ascent, at about 30,000 feet.
This phenomenon is altered by breathing 100% oxygen or an oxygen–helium
mixture, before flight, to partially wash nitrogen out of the body. When this is
done, rapid ascent to 40,000 feet can be accomplished. In a pressurized cabin,
of course, these problems are minimized.

Most decompression sickness now occurs in sports divers, and all patients
seen by the authors have been in this category. The neurologic complications
can be striking (Erde and Edmonds, 1975; Kidd and Elliott, 1975). As shown in

Table 9–2 Neurologic manifestations of decompression

Site	Manifestations
Central (brain)	Blurred vision, scintillating scotomata, visual field defects, bilateral throbbing headache, vertigo, speech disturbance, confusion, hemiparesis, hemisensory defects, focal or generalized seizures
Spinal cord	Low back, radicular pain, often bilateral, and girdling, commonly in upper lumbar region; paraparesis, loss of bladder and sphincter control, hypoesthesias, sensory levels; paraplegia may occur

Table 9–2, both the spinal cord and brain are affected. Bilateral throbbing headache occurs frequently and at times may be the only symptom of decompression sickness. The headache is often indistinguishable from migraine with aura. A migraine attack after decompression may require recompression therapy, because it may be indistinguishable from arterial gas embolism to the brain.

Treatments for both high-altitude and decompression sickness are generally preventive. Descent from altitude will abolish some manifestations but may only retard others. Thus, aviators who have experienced decompression sickness should not be re-exposed even to low altitudes of flight for 72 to 96 hours, since re-expansion of nitrogen bubbles already present in fatty tissues may exacerbate their signs and symptoms.

Adequate recompression therapy is the only specific treatment for decompression sickness. At times this may require prolonged recompression, for more than several days. All other measures can be considered as ancillary, including the use of 100% oxygen and methods to retard or prevent brain edema (dexamethasone, 8 to 10 mg every 4 to 6 hours, and intravenous injection of mannitol or dextran).

Headache Associated with Anemia

Anemia associated with hypoxemia induces headache by causing dilation of the intracranial vessels. According to Graham (1959), anemia resulting from sudden loss of blood is more likely to be followed by headache than that due to slow loss, but even in chronic states of anemia, when the hemoglobin falls below 7.0 g, headache may follow. Anemia is associated with cerebral vasodilation and increased CBF directly proportional to the degree of anemia (Kee and Wood, 1987). Nevertheless, except in the case of acute blood loss or hemolysis, anemia, with levels of hemoglobin above 11 g, is rarely in itself the cause of headache.

Hemolytic crises, whether due to congenital or acquired hemolytic anemia, transfusion reactions, sickle cell disease, Mediterranean anemia, paroxysmal hemoglobinemia, and favus bean poisoning; polycythemia vera and polycythemia secondary to hypoxia experienced with chronic pulmonary disease; congenital heart lesions; high altitude; and chronic exposure to carbon monoxide may, because of the vasodilation they induce, result in headache.

In addition to the cerebral oxygen deficit caused by the various anemias, similar deprivation occurs in the course of circulatory collapse, impaired pulmonary ventilation, pulmonary infiltration, pulmonary artery obstruction, and shunting cardiovascular anomalies.

Nitrite Headache

The headache experimentally induced by amyl nitrite was studied in five subjects (Wolff, 1929). Inhalation of amyl nitrite produced a prompt fall in both systolic and diastolic blood pressure. Headache was experienced when the blood pressure had returned toward the previous level, with increase in the amplitude of pulsations of the cranial arteries. The headache subsequently disappeared, with return of the pulsations to the initial level.

Some individuals exposed to nitrites, either as medicament, in food, or in industry, complain of headache (Evans, 1912; Laws, 1910). Such headaches are of a dull aching quality and are usually accompanied by a flushed face (Henderson and Raskin, 1972). Gradually increasing tolerance to nitrites by those exposed to them usually results after a time in spontaneous reduction or elimination of headache. A too-sudden increase in the amount of nitrites absorbed, beyond the tolerance of the subject, is commonly followed by a recrudescence of the headache. Reduction in amount or withdrawal of the agent is then followed by recession of the headache. It is reported that the use of vasoconstrictors such as ephedrine and benzedrine has been followed by elimination of nitrite headaches or a reduction in their intensity. This statement is difficult to accept without suitable evidence, because, as shown above, even the powerful constrictor effect of ergotamine tartrate is nullified by the nitrite dilator action. Moreover, no control series of subjects with such headaches who received only placebos has been studied.

Headache Caused by Chemical Agents, with and without Anemic Cerebral Vasodilation

Chief among these headaches are those caused by carbon monoxide. Acetanilid, when used in excess, may cause headache by converting hemoglobin to methemoglobin, with resultant hypoxemia. In addition to the methemoglobinemia and sulfhemoglobinemia such as follows the ingestion of nitrates, sulfonamides, aniline compounds, acetanilid, and phenacetin are those headaches that occur in the acute stage of poisoning from ethyl alcohol, carbon tetrachloride, benzene, arsenic, lead, anticholinesterase, insecticides, and the nitrates, including nitroglycerin. Apresoline, thorazine, and calcium channel blockers, by virtue of their vasodilating action, may produce headache in some patients. Withdrawal of cerebral active drugs such as ergotamin, amphetamine, caffeine, and methysergide from those who have been using them in excess for long periods may precipitate severe headache. A common situation in patients with chronic cluster and migraine headaches is habitual use of ergotamine with resulting ergotamine withdrawal headaches when the drug is discontinued. This results in a vicious cycle of daily headaches, which is best treated by total withdrawal of ergotamine.

Headache with Electrolyte Disturbance Due to Ill-Defined Factors

Headache may also be associated with states of dehydration and disturbed electrolyte balance—that is, excess loss of fluid and electrolytes in the course of diarrhea, vomiting, postoperative fistulas, heat exhaustion, diuresis, and removal of ascitic fluid.

Caffeine Withdrawal Headache

Pharmacologically, caffeine is a cerebral vasoconstrictor, and withdrawal presumably results in excessive cerebral vasodilation and vascular congestion. In studies of two subjects, caffeine withdrawal headache has been shown to have many features suggesting that the pain arises from distention of intracranial, and possibly extracranial, arteries. Like the headache induced by histamine given intravenously, caffeine withdrawal headache is reduced in intensity by sustained straining or jugular compression, is readily accentuated by jolt movements of the head, and is eliminated during exposure to centrifugal force of 2.0 g in the head-to-seat direction.

"Hunger" or Hypoglycemic Headache

When a meal is missed or postponed, the subsequent hypoglycemia in persons subject to migraine may induce headache. Headache may also occur as a symptom of impending insulin shock in diabetics and patients with islet cell tumors of the pancreas. Headache as a manifestation of hypoglycemia may be a feature in patients suffering from hypopituitarism, adrenocortical insufficiency, hypothyroidism, and liver disease. Von Brauch (1957) called attention to the fact that headache may occur with hypoglycemic states. An important implication from this and other papers on the subject is that a serious change in the internal environment of the organism, such as occurs with low oxygen, high carbon dioxide, low sugar, or acidosis, that threatens survival of the neuron evokes extreme cerebral vasodilation. This then becomes the essential element in inducing the headache.

In a small series of subjects, Kunkle and Barker of the New York Hospital demonstrated that there is a relation between headache, food deprivation, the blood-sugar level, and threshold of jolt headache. Food deprivation, either with or without a fall of blood-sugar level, may be associated with lowering of the pain threshold. Thus, in one subject after 8 hours of fasting, the jolt headache threshold dropped from 7.0 to 5.1 g. In another subject, after insulin injected intravenously, when the blood-sugar level fell from 85 to 24 mg/100 cc, the threshold of jolt headache fell from 5.9 to 3.3 g. And inversely, after ingestion of 50 g of glucose, when the blood-sugar rose to normal (95 mg/100 cc) the threshold of jolt headache also rose to 6.3 g. These data further support the view that hunger headaches stem from pain-sensitive intracranial vessels.

Salzer (1960), who has examined and treated many patients with functional hyperinsulinism, describes a patient who had had resection of the right temporal artery for what was assumed to be a temporal arteritis of 2 years' duration. She also had had a laminectomy for removal of bony spurs impinging on the second cervical root—all without beneficial effect. A 6-hour glucose tolerance test revealed a blood-sugar fall to levels of 25 mg/100 ml at the fourth hour. The author, unfortunately, does not state if headache was precipitated during these periods of low glucose level! The patient was free of headache after a few weeks on a modified diet. (Wolff, 1987)

It is freely conceded that headache may result during some episodes of hyperinsulinism and during the hunger that results from missing a meal. Sometimes under these circumstances there is fatigue, tension, irritability, and mood changes. It is in such a setting that headache may develop. However, low blood sugar, or so-called functional hyperinsulinism, may be but one aspect of a patient's reaction to his or her difficult situation and not necessarily the direct mediator of the headache. Thus, granting that some persons with headache probably do develop a headache with low blood sugar levels, functional hyperinsulinism still cannot be considered a common primary cause of headache.

Treatment of Headaches Resulting from Distention of Cerebral and Pial Arteries

The headaches associated with fever, sepsis, bacteremia, anoxia, nitrites, and convulsions are modified by acetylsalicylic acid in 0.3- to 0.6-g amounts, and by codeine phosphate in 60-mg amounts; which agent should be used depends on the intensity of the pain. It is obvious, however, that the eradication of the underlying infection is most pertinent.

An increase in the oxygen content of the blood is followed by narrowing of cerebral and pial arteries (Wolff & Lennox, 1930). Hence, the breathing of high concentrations of oxygen may sufficiently oxygenate the blood that headache due to dilated intracranial arteries is diminished in intensity or eliminated. The headaches associated with carbon monoxide poisoning and other anoxemias, and the postseizure headache, may be modified by the inhalation of high concentrations of oxygen. For the same reason, patients with cluster headache who appear to have an unusually marked cerebral vasoconstrictive response to inhalation of 100% oxygen often report temporary but effective symptomatic relief of cluster headache during inhalation of 100% oxygen for 15 minutes (Sakai & Meyer, 1979).

MISCELLANEOUS VASCULAR HEADACHES

"Ice-Cream" or Cold Stimulus Headache

Raskin and Knittle (1976) have noted the tendency for "ice-cream headache" and orthostatic symptoms to occur in patients with migraine. This occurs provided the stimulus is cold enough, prolonged, and applied to the pharynx. Application of similar cold materials in the esophagus or stomach does not cause headache. The pain may be situated at the vertex and is often felt behind the eyes or in the frontal areas; it is almost always associated with the ingestion of ice cream, hence the name. Raskin and Knittle suggested that patients with migraine are particularly susceptible to ice-cream headache; they imply that this phenomenon is a biologic marker for migraine.

Postendarterectomy Hemicrania

Leviton et al. (1975) have described postendarterectomy hemicranial headache, a benign and self-limited condition occurring in patients 3 to 4 days after the operative procedure has been performed. The pain is hemicranial, throbbing, and indistinguishable from the usual migraine episode. It occurs primarily in those who have had migraine attacks prior to the carotid surgery. This disorder is perhaps due to a sudden increase in blood flow through a vascular system conditioned to low flow because of atherosclerosis, or to release of serotonin from platelet aggregation, at the site of surgical intervention (Edmeads, 1979).

Orgasmic Headache

A particular variety of exertional headache is associated with the physical activity of sexual intercourse, and hence the term "orgasmic headache." In 1974 Paulson and Klawans called attention to this variety of severe headache that appeared to occur in association with orgasm. They described 14 patients seen over the course of several years who had severe head pain either during or immediately after orgasm. The headache was often behind the eyes, bilateral or occipital, and of varying intensity, although usually rather short lived. The pain was almost always throbbing. Paulson and Klawans divided the patients into two groups on the basis of the presumed pathophysiology of the headache. Three patients were thought to have low spinal fluid pressure, which was documented in two, perhaps as a result of a tear in the subarachnoid membranes that occurred or was widened during the physiologic stress of coitus. The relationship of posture to pain in these patients was identical to that seen in patients with headache following lumbar puncture. In 11 other patients, Paulson and Klawans suggested that vascular factors were of pathophysiologic significance. Orgasmic headaches also occur in individuals with a history of migraine. The point of their paper was that the benign course of 14 patients differed from the usual impression that headaches associated with intercourse result from rupture or expansion of a vascular malformation or aneurysm.

In reply to this report, Lundberg and Osterman (1974) presented a brief report on the benign and malignant forms of headache associated with orgasm. They agreed with Paulson and Klawans that there is a benign but sometimes very troublesome and usually recurring type of vascular headache starting at the climax of sexual intercourse, and mentioned a number of such cases that had been followed for several years at the University of Uppsala. They pointed out, however, that bleeding associated with subarachnoid hemorrhage may occur at the time of intercourse; they described six patients in whom this had happened. Lundberg and Osterman emphasized that the occurrence of vomiting, disturbance of consciousness, stiff neck, and residual pain the day after the incident characterized the headache caused by subarachnoid hemorrhage and distinguished it from that of benign orgasmic cephalgia. Fisher (1968) reviewed his experience with 66 representative cases of subarachnoid hemorrhage caused by the rupture of saccular aneurysms; in 3 of these, the hemorrhage was associated with intercourse. Larger studies estimate that sexual intercourse was the

Table 9–3 Benign orgasmic headache

Researcher	Date	No. of patients	Manifestations	Sequelae
Paulson and Klawans	1974	14	Bilateral throbbing, low CSF in 3	No serious sequelae
Lundberg and Osterman	1974	50	Bilateral throbbing at climax	SAH in 6
Fisher	1968	60 with SAH	3 had onset at intercourse	
Levy	1981	1	Climax onset	Right hemiparesis, slow recovery
Dalessio	1974	4 (all male)	Bilateral brief throbbing at climax	No serious sequelae

Key to abbreviations: CSF, cerebrospinal fluid; SAH, subarachnoid hemorrhage.

circumstance for intracranial aneurysmal rupture in only 5% of cases (Adams et al., 1980).

Levy (1981) has described a 24-year-old male who suffered a stroke in the setting of sexual intercourse and orgasm. This patient developed a hemiparesis, without aphasia, and gradually recovered over the next month. He had a prior history of migraine. Levy suggests that this case represents an example of complicated migraine occurring in association with coitus. We have treated a middle-aged male, with a plaque of the left internal carotid artery, who dislodged a thrombus from the plaque during intercourse, resulting in headache, dysphasia, and right hemiparesis. Dalessio (1974) has examined four men with orgasmic headache. In all, the pain was bilateral, biooccipital, and throbbing in character. It generally occurred at climax, lasted approximately 1 hour, and was not associated with nausea, vomiting, photophobia, or speech and movement defects. Three of the four subjects had multiple episodes of this type. None had serious sequelae (Table 9–3).

Thus, it seems evident that there are benign and malignant forms of headache associated with intercourse or, in formal terms, orgasmic cephalgia. In most cases this is a benign syndrome. However, the alert clinician will be aware that a severe and disabling headache may result from bleeding at the time of intercourse as a result of rupture of a saccular aneurysm. The subsequent course of patients should differentiate the benign from the malignant forms of head pain. Where there is doubt, however, further neurologic studies are certainly indicated, particularly spinal puncture, computerized tomographic scan of the head, and/or contrast studies.

Effort (Exertional) Headache and Migraine

The etiology of effort headache is multifactorial. Many effort headaches are obviously those of classic migraine, particularly the headaches occurring after prolonged exertion, as in long-distance races. In most effort headaches, hypoxia does not play a role, although hypoxia is capable of extending and increasing the vascular headache produced by effort. Headache is a common complaint of the individual who exerts at high altitude, and it may be made worse by exposure to cold, breathlessness, dyspnea, and fatigue.

Exertional headache is an uncommon disorder in which head pain appears to be related to exertion or straining (Rooke, 1968). It commonly affects males in a broad age range from 10 to 70 years. Almost always, exertional headache is a benign, although disconcerting, symptom. Approximately 30% of patients are improved or free of this symptom within 5 years, and over 70% are free of headache within 10 years. Diamond (1977) has suggested that indomethacin, 75 mg/day, may be helpful in patients with this disorder.

Jokl (1965) was perhaps the first to note migraine occurring after exercise. His own description of this problem is graphic:

> During my freshman year in medical school I ran as an anchor man in the mile relay team of my university and the German track championships of Jena, Thuringia. We won by the smallest possible margin. I was then 17 years old and this was the first time I had been clocked in under fifty seconds. A few minutes after the race my happiness over the victory was interrupted by an attack of nausea, headache, prolonged weakness and vomiting. It lasted fifteen minutes whereupon it quickly subsided. None of my professors were able to explain this episode, nor could I find appropriate reference in any textbooks of physiology or medicine.

Jokl and Jokl (1977) noted several profound cases of effort migraine during the Olympic games in Mexico City and described these to one of the authors (Dalessio, 1974). The high altitude was an obvious predisposing factor, as was heat, humidity, and perhaps lack of training. Migraine after effort tended to occur with prolonged running rather than sprints. These highly conditioned athletes developed scotomata, unilateral retro-orbital pain, nausea, and vomiting, and in some cases a striking prostration occurred.

Rooke's (1968) series of benign exertional headache, encompassing 103 cases, includes some in which no significant exertion is described. Nonetheless, he finds only 10% in whom an organic disease was finally diagnosed. The majority of these persons were found to have a structural disorder at the base of the brain. None had aneurysm as the primary lesion.

Headache with effort implies that adequate physical activity has produced the requisite cephalgia. Mental effort, no matter how onerous, is not included here, nor should one include positional or movement headache (paroxysmal headache) in this category. Thus, for example, cough headache is omitted because the headache is almost always associated with the head movement that is a part of the cough. How much effort, then, causes headache? Arbitrarily, enough to double the resting pulse and sustained for at least 10 seconds, but ordinarily for minutes or hours. With this definition, a clear group of headache syndromes associated with physical activity emerges.

The personal experience of the authors with effort headache is limited to five long-distance runners. All had either a history of migraine or a family history of migraine. Migraine occurred during or after prolonged running at sea level in all cases. Two runners experienced episodic hemiparesis but none had any permanent defects (Table 9–4). Other patients with migraine report that exercise during a migraine attack makes the headache worse, and this has also

Table 9–4 Effort migraine in runners

Age	Sex	History of migraine	Family history of migraine	Scotomata/ field defects	Paresis/sensory defects	Permanent neurologic defects
26	M	Yes	Yes	Yes	Transient left paresis	No
19	M	Yes	Yes	Yes	Transient left paresis	No
50	M	No	Yes	Yes	Left sensory defect	No
18	M	No	Yes	Yes	Expressive aphasia; right hemiparesis, transient	No
32	M	Yes	Yes	Yes	Right hemiparesis, 1 hour	No

been our experience in interviewing many patients with migraine. This is accounted for by the fact that the normal ability of the brain to maintain a constant blood flow, a property called "autoregulation," is lost during a migraine attack (Sakai and Meyer, 1978). Hence, if blood pressure and cardiac output are increased by exercise during a migraine attack, CBF increases and the pounding headache is intensified.

SUMMARY

The intravenous injection of histamine results in dilation of the intracranial arteries, which, with normal systemic arterial pressure, causes increased CBF, cerebral vasodilation, and increased amplitude of intracranial pulsations. The intense headache associated with these changes has been studied as a means of analyzing other, nonexperimental headaches. The following conclusions were drawn:

   The intensity of the headache experimentally induced by histamine is proportional to the degree of dilation and stretch of the pial and dural vessels and perivascular tissue.
   Headache does not result from vascular dilation unless the intracranial vessels are sufficiently distorted. Carbon dioxide, when used as a vasodilator, is less effective than histamine in increasing the amplitude of intracranial pulsations and does not commonly produce headache.
   Headache experimentally induced by histamine does not depend on the integrity of sensation from the superficial tissues.
   The extracranial arteries play a minor role in contributing to the pain of headache experimentally induced by histamine.
   Cerebral arteries, principally the large arteries at the base of the brain, including the internal carotid, the vertebral, and the basilar artery and the proximal segments of their main branches, are chiefly responsible

for the quality and intensity of headache experimentally induced by histamine.

Although there may be other less important afferent pathways for the conduction of impulses interpreted as headache following injection of histamine, (1) the fifth cranial nerve on each side is the principal afferent pathway for headache resulting from dilation of the supratentorial cerebral arteries and felt in the frontotemporoparietal region of the head, and (2) the 9th and 10th cranial nerves and the upper cervical nerves are the most important afferent pathways for headache resulting from dilation of arteries of the posterior fossa and felt in the occipital region of the head.

Headaches that result primarily from distention of cerebral and pial arteries and resemble in mechanism the headache that follows the intravenous injection of histamine include the following: headaches associated with fever, bacteremia, side effects of drugs, and sepsis; headaches resulting from carbon monoxide poisoning; headaches that follow the industrial and therapeutic use of nitrites; headaches associated with polycythemia vera, chronic mountain sickness, and other hypoxemias; so-called hangover headache; and postseizure headache.

REFERENCES

Adams, H.P., D.D. Jergenson, N.F. Kassell, and A.L. Sahs (1980). Pitfalls in the recognition of subarachnoid hemorrhage. *JAMA 244:*794–796.

Amano, T. and J.S. Meyer (1982a). Cerebrovascular changes in patients with headache during antiserotoninergic treatment. *Headache 22:*249–255.

Amano, T. and J.S. Meyer (1982b). Prostaglandin inhibition and cerebrovascular control in patients with headache. *Headache 27:*52–59.

Appenzeller, O. (1972). Altitude headache. *Headache 12:*126–130.

Barcroft, J. (1925). *The Respiratory Functions of the Blood, Part II: Lessons from High Altitudes.* Cambridge University Press, London.

Barcroft, J.C., C.A. Binger, A.V. Bock et al. (1922). Observations upon the effects of high altitude on the physiological process of the human body, carried out in the Peruvian Andes, chiefly at Cerro de Pasco. *Phil. Trans. R. Soc. (Lond.) Ser. B. 211:*351.

Behnke, A.R. (1965). Problems in the treatment of decompression sickness (and traumatic air embolism). *Ann. N. Y. Acad. Sci. 117:*843–859.

Bronk, D.W. (1935). The nervous mechanism of cardiac-vascular control. *Harvey Lect.,* p. 245.

Clark, D., H.B. Hough, and H.G. Wolff (1936a). Experimental studies on headache: Observations on headache produced by histamine. *Arch. Neurol. Psychiatry 35:* 1054.

Clark, D., H.B. Hough, and H.G. Wolff (1936b). Experimental studies on headache: Observations on histamine headache. *Assoc. Res. Nerv. Dis. Proc. 15:*417.

Dalessio, D.J. (1974). Effort migraines. *Headache 14:*53.

Dandy, W.E. (1931). Treatment of hemicrania (migraine) by removal of the inferior cervical and first thoracic sympathetic ganglion. *Bull. Johns Hopkins Hosp. 48:* 357.

Diamond, S. (1977). Recurrent exertional headache. *JAMA 237:*580.

Edmeads, J. (1979). The headaches of ischemic cerebrovascular disease. *Headache 19:* 345–349.

Engel, G.L., J.P. Webb, E.B. Ferris et al. (1944). A migraine-like syndrome complicating decompression sickness. *War Med. 5:*304–314.

Erde, A.E. and C. Edmonds (1975). Decompression sickness: A clinical series. *J. Occup. Med. 17:*324.

Evans, E.S. (1912). A case of nitroglycerine poisoning. *JAMA 58:*550.

Fisher, M. (1968). Headaches in cerebral vascular disease. In *Handbook of Clinical Neurology.* Vol. 5 (P.J. Vinken and G.W. Bruyn, eds.), pp. 124–156. North Holland Press, Amsterdam.

Forbes, H.S., S. Cobb, and F. Fremont-Smith (1924). Cerebral edema and headache following carbon monoxide asphyxia. *Arch. Neurol. Psychiatry 11:*264.

Forward, S.A., M. Landowne, J.N. Follansbee, and J.E. Hansen (1968). Effect of acetazolamide on acute mountain sickness. *N. Engl. J. Med. 279:*839.

Graham, J.R. (1959). Headache in systemic disease. In *Headache: Diagnosis and Treatment* (A.P. Friedman and H.H. Merritt, eds.), Chap. 7. F.A. Davis, Philadelphia.

Hardy, J.D., H.G. Wolff, and H. Goodell (1940). Studies on pain. A new method for measuring pain threshold: Observations on spatial summation of pain. *J. Clin. Invest. 19:*649.

Heiss, W.D., B. Kufferle, I. Dewel et al. (1976). Cerebral blood flow and severity of mental dysfunction in chronic alcoholism. In *Cerebral Vascular Disease, 7th International Salzburg Conference,* pp. 89–93. George Thieme, Stuttgart.

Henderson, W.R. and N. Raskin (1972). Hot dog headache: Individual susceptibility to nitrite. *Lancet 2:*1162–1163.

Heyman, A., J.L. Patterson, Jr., and F.T. Nichols, Jr. (1950). The effects of induced fever on cerebral functions in neurosyphillis. *J. Clin. Invest. 29:*1335.

Houston, C.S. (1976). High altitude illness. *JAMA 236:*2193–2195.

Jokl, E. (1965). Indisposition after running. *Med. Dello Sport 5:*363.

Jokl, E. and P. Jokl (1977). Der Beltrag der Sportmedizin zur Klinischen Kardiologic—das Sporterz. In *Altern Leistungsfahigkeit Rehabilitation,* pp. 47–56. F.K. Schattauer Verlag, Munchen.

Kee, D.B. and J.H. Wood (1987). Influence of blood rheology on cerebral circulation. In *Cerebral Blood Flow* (J.H. Wood, ed.), pp. 173–185. McGraw-Hill, New York.

Kidd, D.J. and D.H. Elliott (1975). Decompression disorders in divers. In *The Physiology of Medicine of Diving and Compressed Air Work* (P.B. Bennett and O.H. Elliott, eds.), pp. 471–495. Williams & Wilkins, Baltimore.

Kobari, M., J.S. Meyer, M. Ichijo, and W.T. Oravez (1990). Cortical and subcortical hyperperfusion during migraine and cluster headache. *Neuroradiology 32:*4–11.

Kudrow, L. (1980). *Cluster Headache, Mechanisms and Management,* pp. 142–145. Oxford Medical Publications, Oxford University Press, New York.

Lassen, N.A. (1966). The luxury perfusion syndrome and its possible relation to acute metabolic audosis localized within the brain. *Lancet 2:*1113–1115.

Laws, C.E. (1910). The nitroglycerine head. *JAMA 54:*793.

Leufaut, C. and K. Sullivan (1970). Adaptation to high altitude. *N. Engl. J. Med. 284:* 1298.

Levine, M. and H.G. Wolff (1932). Afferent impulses from the blood vessels of the pia. *Arch. Neurol. Psychiatry 28:*140.

Leviton, A., L. Capland, and E. Salznan (1975). Severe headache after carotid endarterectomy. *Headache 15*:207–210.

Levy, D.K. (1981). Stroke and orgasmic cephalgia. *Headache 21*:12–14.

Lundberg, P.D. and P. Osterman (1974). The benign and malignant forms of orgasmic headache. *Headache 14*:164.

Meyer, J.S., F. Gotoh, and E. Favale (1965). Effects of carotid compression on cerebral metabolism and electroencephalogram. *EEG Clin. Neurophysiol. 19*:362–376.

Meyer, J.S., F. Gotoh, and M. Tomita (1966a). Acute respiratory acidemia. *Neurology 16*:463–474.

Meyer, J.S., F. Gotoh, and E. Favale (1966b). Cerebral metabolism during epileptic seizures in man. *EEG Clin. Neurophysiol. 21*:10–22.

Meyer, J.S. and J. Handa. (1967). Cerebral blood flow and metabolism during experimental hyperthermia (fever). *Minn. Med. 50*:37–44.

Meyer, J.S. and H.D. Portnoy (1959). Post-epileptic paralysis. *Brain 82*:162–185.

Meyer, J.S., T. Ryu, M. Toyoda et al. (1969). Evidence for a Pasteur effect regulatory cerebral oxygen and carbohydrate metabolism in man. *Neurology 19*:954–962.

Monge, C. (1942). Life in the Andes and chronic mountain sickness. *Science 95*:79.

Northfield, D.W.C. (1938). Some observations on headache. *Brain 61*:133.

Paulson, G.W. and H.L. Klawans (1974). Benign orgasmic headache. *Headache 13*:181.

Pawan, G.L.S. (1968). Vitamins, sugars, and ethanol metabolism in man. *Nature 220*: 374.

Pickering, G.W. (1939). Experimental observations on headache. *BMJ 1*:4087.

Pickering, G.W. and W. Hess (1933). Observations on the mechanism of headache produced by histamine. *Clin. Sci. 1*:77.

Raskin, N.H. and S.C. Knittle (1976). Ice cream headache and orthostatic symptoms in patients with migraine. *Headache 16*:222–225.

Ray, B.S. (1954). The surgical treatment of headache and atypical neuralgia. *J. Neurosurg. 2*:596.

Rooke, E.D. (1968). Benign exertional headache. *Med. Clin. North Am. 52*:801–808.

Sakai, F. and J.S. Meyer (1978). Regional cerebral hemodynamics curing migraine and cluster headaches measured by the ^{133}Xe inhalation method. *Headache 18*: 122–132.

Sakai, F. and J.S. Meyer (1979). Abnormal cerebrovascular reactivity in patients with migraine and cluster headache. *Headache 19*:257–266.

Salzer, H.M. (1960). Cephalgia; questions and answers. *JAMA 173*:146.

Schumacher, G.A., B.S. Ray, and H.G. Wolff (1940). Experimental studies on headache. Further analysis of histamine headache and its pain pathways. *Arch. Neurol. Psychiatry 44*:701.

Singh, L., P. Khanna, and M.G. Srivastava (1960). Acute mountain sickness. *N. Engl. J. Med. 280*:175–184.

Strauss, R.H. (1978). Diving medicine. *Am. Rev. Respir. Dis. 119*:1001–1023.

Szczeklik, A. and R.J. Gryglewski (1979). Actions of prostracyclin in man. In *Prostacyclin* (J.R. Vane and S. Bengstrom, eds.), pp. 383–408. Raven Press, New York.

Talbot, J.D., S. Marrett, A.C. Evans et al. (1991). Multiple representation of pain in human cerebral cortex. *Science 251*:1355–1358.

von Brauch, F. (1957). Hypoglycemic headache. *Dtsch. Med. Wochenschr. 76*:828.

Weiss, S., G.P. Robb, and L.B. Ellis (1932). The systemic effects of histamine in man, with special reference to the responses of the cardiovascular system. *Arch. Intern Med. 49*:360.

Wolff, H.G. (1929). The cerebral circulation: 11a. The action of acetylcholine. 11b. The action of the extract of the posterior lobe of the pituitary gland. 11c. The action of amylnitrite. *Arch. Neurol. Psychiatry 22*:686.

Wolff, H.G. (1938). Headache and cranial arteries. *Trans. Assoc. Am. Physicians 53:* 193.

Wolff, H.G. (1987). *Headache and other head pain,* (D.J. Dalessio, ed.), 5th ed., pp. 147–163. Oxford University Press, New York.

Wolff, H.G. and W.G. Lennox (1930). Cerebral circulation: 12. The effect on pial vessels of variation in the oxygen and carbon dioxide content of the blood. *Arch. Neurol. Psychiatry 23:*1097.

10

Tension-Type Headaches

SEYMOUR DIAMOND

When the International Headache Society (IHS) revised the headache classification system in 1988, it introduced the term "tension-type headache" to describe what was previously called tension headache, muscle contraction headache, psychomyogenic headache, stress headache, idiopathic headache, ordinary headache, and psychogenic headache (Headache Classification Committee of the IHS, 1988). Previously, "tension or muscle contraction headache" was defined by the Ad Hoc Committee on Classification of Headache of the National Institute of Neurological Diseases and Blindness (1962) as: "Ache or sensation of tightness, pressure, or constriction, widely varied in intensity, frequency, and duration, long-lasting, commonly occipital, and associated with sustained contraction of skeletal muscles, usually as a part of the individual's reaction during life stress" (Silberstein, 1993).

This description is vague, ambiguous, and not operational. The new definition by the IHS attempts to define tension-type headache more precisely and distinguish between patients with episodic tension-type headache and chronic tension-type headache (Silberstein and Silberstein, 1990). These subclassifications are based on the presence or absence of tenderness or increased electromyographic (EMG) activity. Although tension-type headache is no longer presumed to be caused solely by chronic muscle contraction, it may be associated with muscle tenderness and increased EMG activity. The new IHS criteria allow for the involvement of "muscle contraction" in a subset of patients without a priori assuming that this is the mechanism of tension-type headache (Silberstein, 1993).

Episodic tension-type headaches are defined (Headache Classification Committee of the IHS, 1988) as recurrent headaches lasting for 30 minutes to 7 days, with fewer than 15 headache days per month and at least two of the following pain characteristics:

1. Pressing/tightening (nonpulsating) quality
2. Mild or moderate intensity
3. Bilateral location
4. No aggravation by walking stairs or similar routine physical activity

In addition, both of the following conditions must be met: (1) no nausea or vomiting (anorexia may occur), and (2) photophobia and phonophobia are absent, or one but not the other is present.

Tension-type headache, the most prevalent form of headache, can occur at any age but is more common in adulthood. Using the new IHS criteria, Rassmussen et al. (1991) found a lifetime prevalence of tension-type headache in 69% of men and 88% of women. One-year prevalence rates were 63% in men and 86% in women. As with migraine, more women than men have tension-type headache (Friedman et al., 1964). Friedman's group found a positive family history in 40% of tension-type headache patients and 70% of migraineurs. This is lower than the lifetime prevalence of any headache in the population of over 90% (Rassmussen et al., 1991). This discrepancy is explained as follows. Many of Friedman's patients may have been experiencing the mixed headache syndrome, and the patients may have recollections of a family history limited to the severe, migraine-type headaches. Ziegler et al. (1972) reported a family history of episodic headache in 64% of all headache sufferers, with no increase in the percentage of a positive family history for migraineurs. Bakal and Kaganov (1979) reported similar findings. Friedman et al. (1964) found that headache onset was usually between 20 and 40 years of age. Because most patients had daily or constant headache, and only 15% had headache occurring less than once a week, this series was biased toward the more chronic patient (Silberstein, 1993).

Persons with episodic tension-type headaches usually seek relief with over-the-counter analgesics. A physician will only be consulted when the headaches do not respond to these simple analgesics or when they occur with an increased frequency and severity, causing diminished functioning in either an occupational or a social setting. Tension-type headache can manifest itself in relationship to stress, depression, anxiety, emotional conflicts, fatigue, repressed hostility, or simply creating an environment too great for the patient to handle.

Patients with tension-type headaches generally describe the pain as a steady, nonpulsatile ache. Other descriptions include viselike pressure, drawing, soreness, bitemporal or occipital tightness, and bandlike sensations about the head that may be termed a "hatband" effect. Patients may also complain of distinct cramping sensations, as if the neck and upper back were in a cast. It is usually mild to moderate in severity, in contrast to the moderate to severe pain observed in migraine. Some patients describe a feeling of constriction in the neck or jaw muscles (Olesen, 1988). The scalp may be extremely tender, and combing or brushing the hair or wearing a hat may elicit scalp soreness. Scalp tenderness is greater in headache patients (migraine or tension-type) during a headache than in nonheadache controls, is greatest at the site of the headache, and persists for several days after the headache subsides (Drummond, 1987).

The site of the headache varies, with pain frequently occurring at the forehead and temples or at the back of the head and neck. Patients may describe the pain as unilateral or bilateral, involving the frontal, temporal, occipital, or parietal regions or any combination of these sites (Friedman et al., 1964), and changing locations in half the attacks (Iversen et al., 1990). Unilateral headaches occurred in 10% of Friedman et al.'s patients, and headache that was strictly unilateral occurred in 13% of Hollnagel and Nørreland's patients (quoted in Olesen, 1988).

Although this headache may undergo frequent changes in severity and site, the pain, localized in one region, may continue with varying intensity for weeks, months, or even years. The pain's duration may be short and relieved by the patient changing position. Tension-type headache may be relieved by changing position, by limiting head, neck, and jaw movement, or by supporting the head.

In patients with episodic tension-type headache with an associated disorder of pericranial muscles, sharply localized "nodules" may be demonstrated in the pericranial or cervical muscles when the tender areas of the neck, head, and upper back are palpated during physical examination. In general, episodic tension-type headache sufferers have more muscle tenderness than headache-free controls, whether or not they are having a headache (Hatch et al., 1992). Pressure on contracted, tender muscles may increase headache intensity, cause pain radiation, and induce tinnitus, vertigo, and lacrimation. Shivering from exposure to the cold may aggravate the headache.

The role played by emotional factors in the pathogenesis of tension-type headaches has been the subject of much debate (Blanchard et al., 1989). Most investigators concur that pain and psychological factors do impact on each other (Adler et al., 1987; Mebane, 1990). Martin and his associates (1967) reviewed the psychiatric evaluations of 25 patients with muscle contraction headaches. They found no single psychological factor to be a provocateur of these headaches. Most of their patients demonstrated multiple conflicts, such as repressed hostility, sexual conflicts, and unresolved dependency needs. This study suggests that, in cases of tension-type headaches, somatization of anxiety in the form of either increased skeletal muscle tension or psychophysiologic expression is occurring. Family members may be performing an unconscious role in fostering the pain, because secondary gain is often present.

Chronic tension-type headaches may conceal a serious emotional disorder, such as depression. The patient will present with a persistent and vague headache for which no organic cause can be determined. For the patient, the physical symptoms are more socially acceptable than the anxiety or depressive symptoms; many patients are certain there is a somatic basis for their pain. The physician must be cognizant of other signs of depression, such as early morning fatigue, irritability, loss of energy or spontaneity, lack of interest, insomnia, or early morning awakening. The patient may have considered suicide.

Shulman (1992) noted that anxiety occurs as frequently as depression in pain patients. Headache may manifest in panic and phobic disorders. However, the most commonly observed anxiety state is a worried, apprehensive condition that frequently is demonstrated in depressed patients.

The relationship between these psychological factors and tension-type headaches has been challenged by other researchers (Bakal, 1982; Featherstone, 1985). Much of the controversy relates to the theories that migraine and tension-type headaches are extensions of each other (Ziegler and Hassanein, 1990). After 30 years of clinical observation, I believe that these are two distinct entities, although they may coexist in the same patient (mixed headache syndrome). The diagnostic dilemma is often blurred by the frequent habituation problems of patients experiencing daily headaches.

MECHANISM OF TENSION-TYPE HEADACHE

The mechanism of this type of headache was believed to be similar to that of chronic muscle contraction in any other part of the body. Local pathologic processes and their central influences were believed to be related to muscle spasm.

Many modern researchers (Lance et al., 1983) have observed that chronic tension-type headache may not be a result of disorders of the blood vessels and muscles. Instead, they may be affected by a chronic or intermittent disturbance of the monoaminergic, serotonergic, and endorphin function, involving the hypothalamus, brainstem, and spinal cord. This occurrence may be due to referral or a central pain phenomenon from the intermingling of major circuits of the brain and spinal cord.

Blau (1989) has attempted to divide chronic tension-type headache into two varieties. Type I is a constant, symmetric, bandlike pressure sensation in the head not affected by finger pressure, massage, heat, or cold, which Blau feels is associated with anxiety or depression. It should be noted that many of Blau's type I patients were abusing analgesics, and also may have experienced drug-induced headache. Type II is a localized, daily, fluctuating head pain associated with neck and pericranial muscle tenderness, and may correspond to tension-type headache associated with a disorder of pericranial muscles or headache related to a disorder of the cervical spine.

It is known that the excitatory effect of noxious stimulation of the soft structures of the head radiates centrally, causing the pain to be experienced at a site distant from the noxious stimulation. For example, when the condylar or basal region is stimulated by the injection of a hypertonic saline solution or by manual pressure in the region, the patient may experience orbital or frontal ache. The stimulation of the nuchal tissues may cause occipital headache. The pain caused by sustained contraction of skeletal muscle is triggered promptly by noxious stimulation and ends abruptly when the source of the stimulation is blocked by procaine.

EMG activity may be increased in some muscles in both episodic and chronic tension-type headache patients, as well as in patients with migraine. Pritchard (1989) measured frontal, occipital, and neck muscle EMG activity in subjects with migraine and tension-type headaches. The headache groups did not differ from controls in the headache-free state, but during a headache, occipital EMG activity was higher in the tension-type group than in the migraine headache sufferers.

Hatch et al. (1991), using an ambulatory EMG device, recorded the electrical activity from the neck muscles for 48 to 96 consecutive hours. Subjects noted their perceived levels of stress, pain, and negative affect. The EMG activity did not covary with stress, pain, or negative affect. This study showed no consistent muscle hyperactivity during a headache attack; however, *only* one muscle (neck) was sampled. Lichstein et al. (1991) found increased frontal EMG activity during the headache state in subjects with migraine and tension-type headache compared to headache-free controls and to the headache-free period, but these differences did not reach statistical significance.

Arena et al. (1991) measured EMG activity in trapezius and frontalis muscles in six positions (standing, bending from the waist, rising, sitting with back supported, sitting with back unsupported, and prone) and two states (headache and headache free) in subjects with tension-type headache. There was no effect of headache state, but tension-type headache sufferers had higher EMG activity in the trapezius muscle in the prone position compared to nonheadache controls.

Hatch et al. (1992), in a nonblinded study, looked at muscle tenderness and EMG activity in subjects with episodic tension-type headache, comparing them to headache-free controls during a headache-free state. Sixty-three percent of the headache subjects had tenderness in at least one (of eight) palpated muscles, compared to only 3% of controls. Only 11% of the headache sufferers had increased EMG activity, compared to 69% of the controls. Muscle tenderness was *not* found in all subjects, was found at only one or two muscle sites, and was of a relatively low level. There was no significant association between increased EMG activity and the presence of tenderness, although the subjects were headache free. No correlation was attempted between the presence of tenderness and the interval from the last headache. This is significant because scalp tenderness occurs during a headache and persists for up to 5 days (Drummond, 1987). This increased tenderness noted by Hatch and other workers could, in part, be a consequence of a prior headache.

Schoenen et al. (1987) have also looked at exteroceptive suppression of temporalis muscle EMG activity in headache (Figure 10–1). Motor control of the temporalis muscle can be assessed by studying the inhibition of voluntary jaw-closing EMG activity induced by stimulating the trigeminal nerve. Two successive exteroceptive suppressions (ES$_1$ and ES$_2$) (silent periods) are ob-

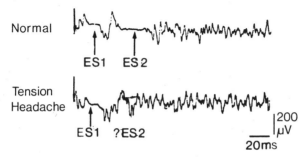

Figure 10–1. Exteroceptive suppression of temporalis muscle. Note absence of ES$_2$ in tension-type headache. (Reproduced with permission from Schoenen, J., B. Jamart, P. Gerard et al. (1987). Exteroceptive suppression of temporalis muscle activity in chronic headache. *Neurology 37*:1835.)

tained. ES_1 is mediated by an oligosynaptic neural net. ES_2 is mediated by a multisynaptic neural net, which is modulated by input from the limbic system, periaqueductal gray matter, amygdala, and hypothalamus. Whereas ES_1 is normal in headache, ES_2 is absent in 40% of patients with chronic tension-type headache and reduced in duration in 87%. In episodic tension-type headache, there may be a perimenstrual reduction in the ES_2 duration (Schoenen et al., 1991a) and a reduction of ES_2 duration (Wallasch et al., 1991), or its absence in others who may be more headache prone (Paulus et al., 1992).

Schoenen et al. (1991b) measured the response to biofeedback, anxiety scores, EMG activity, pain threshold, and ES_2 in 32 women with chronic tension-type headache, and found an abnormal EMG in 62.5% of the patients if three different muscles and three states (supine, standing, mental tasks) were tested. The EMG was abnormal in only 40% if only one muscle and one state were tested. If three muscles were tested, a decreased pain threshold was found in half; if only one muscle was tested, it was found in 34%. ES_2 duration was reduced in 87% of patients. They also found increased EMG or decreased pain thresholds in 72% of the patients, consistent with a diagnosis of chronic tension-type headache "associated with disorder of pericranial muscles." These findings were not observed in the remaining 28% of the patients, consistent with a diagnosis of chronic tension-type headache "unassociated with such a disorder." Headache severity, anxiety, ES_2, and response to biofeedback did not differ between these two groups, suggesting their separation may be artificial or a consequence of the headache (Silberstein, 1993).

BIOCHEMICAL CHANGES IN TENSION-TYPE HEADACHE

Platelets are the major source of serotonin in the blood and plasma, accounting for 98% of the circulating level. Platelet serotonin content in patients with chronic tension-type headache is significantly lower than in normal controls (Rolf et al., 1981). In addition, patients with chronic tension-type headache have mean levels of circulating plasma serotonin that are of the same order as in migrainous patients during a headache (Anthony and Lance, 1989). Patients with severe headache show abnormalities of cerebrospinal fluid β-endorphin and release of luteinizing hormone induced by naloxone (Silberstein and Merriam, 1991).

PSYCHOLOGICAL ASPECTS OF TENSION-TYPE HEADACHE

The headache is due to anxiety, stress, tension, or psychogenic determinants. As part of the medical history, a carefully detailed psychiatric inventory should be obtained. This should include details of the patient's marital relations, occupation, social relationships, life stresses, personality traits, habits, methods of coping with stressful situations, and sexual difficulties.

Adler et al. (1987) assert that suppressed anger was the most "problematic emotion for the tension headache patient". They noted that chronic tension headache could be viewed as a simultaneous manifestation of aggressive impulses and the defenses against them. Adults continually fight to control these emotions, out of fear and learned "civilized" behavior. In addition to headache, repressed anger may also be demonstrated as passive–aggressive and dependent behaviors, in order to control others and situations.

Anxiety

Patients with tension-type headache associated with anxiety will present with only one type of headache, which is daily and persistent. The severity is not disabling but will be described as annoying. Nausea and vomiting are not associated with this type of headache, and the acute headache is not preceded by a warning.

In identifying headaches associated with anxiety rather than depression, the initial interview is crucial. The patient with anxiety will cite job complaints, general anxiety, or being overwhelmed with too many tasks. Insomnia occurs frequently in these patients, in contrast to patients with depression, who complain of early or frequent awakening.

Treatment of chronic tension-type headaches associated with anxiety may be complex. It is essential that the physician reassure the patient about the cause of the headaches. This can be accomplished by attentive listening and demonstrating an interested attitude during the initial interview. Careful and thoughtful handling of the initial physical and neurologic examination is an integral part of the therapeutic approach. The majority of these patients can be managed effectively by the primary physician. However, in a few cases, referral for psychotherapy may be required.

Pharmacologic therapy of these patients must be addressed cautiously. The use of analgesics, tranquilizers, barbiturates, and ergot preparations should be avoided because of the possibility of iatrogenic habituation. Benzodiazepine therapy should not be undertaken in these patients. The prolonged nature of these headaches precludes the long-term use of benzodiazepine agents, because therapy may be necessary for several months.

Anxiolytic agents are indicated if stress or anxiety is identified as the source of these headaches. However, the physician must select a nonhabituating anxiolytic agent, such as buspirone. This agent is a 5-hydroxytryptamine (5-HT$_{1A}$) serotonin receptor partial agonist. The incidence of sedation associated with the use of buspirone is estimated at 10%, an incidence not significantly greater than placebo, which is considered to be 9%. Dependence on this agent has not been observed with prolonged therapy.

Depression

It has been estimated that, in family practice in the United Kingdom (Hodgkins, 1976), depression is the fourth most frequently diagnosed disorder. In the United States, it ranks 12th (Marsland et al., 1976). The presence of depression is often subtle and the diagnosis is frequently missed. Most physicians are probably able to recognize the classically depressed patient. This is the patient who walks into the office with a sad look, as well as slow speech and movement. This depressed person exhibits little interest in anything and sighs frequently (Editorial, 1971).

Two basic factors often provide insight for a possible depression. First, the physician should determine if there is a prior history of depression in the patient or family. The patient should be questioned about similar symptoms in relatives, friends, or self. Many will indicate previous occurrences of these symptoms. The patient may relate obscure symptoms that are actually depressive equivalents.

Second, the patient may relate the onset of the symptoms to a particular event. The depressive attacks may follow a wide variety of events the patient perceives as traumatic or feels as a personal loss. The event may be out of proportion to the severity of the resultant depression. A patient may relate the symptoms to some form of bodily injury, an illness, an injection, surgery, or a diagnostic examination. Also, the patient may emphasize that each of his or her symptoms results from this event. The incident that precipitated the headache or other depressive equivalents would not be compatible with the illness or as overwhelming as perceived. The patient usually feels weakened or maimed by the event.

If the depression is not subsequent to an illness or accident, it may follow some change in personal role, position, or socioeconomic status. Loss of a loved one often triggers normal depressed states. It can also initiate a malignant depression beyond the scope of the loss. The physician must consider the patient's history, which may reveal the loss to be very important within the personal scope of the individual. The loss may have a peculiar significance.

Clinical Findings

The depressed patient often presents with a wide variety of complaints that can be categorized as physical, emotional, and psychic. The physical complaints include chronic pain and headaches, sleep disturbances, severe insomnia and early awakening, appetite changes, and anorexia and rapid weight loss. A decrease in sexual activity may occur, ranging at times to impotence in males and amenorrhea or frigidity in females. Emotional complaints include feeling "blue," anxiety, and rumination over the past, present, and future. Finally, psychic complaints may include such statements as "morning is the worst time of the day," suicidal thoughts, and death wishes (Tables 10–1, 10–2, and 10–3).

A headache associated with depression is usually considered a tension-type headache. This headache consists of a steady, nonpulsatile ache, often distributed in a bandlike pattern around the head. It may be described as viselike, a steady pressure, a weight, a soreness, or a distinct cramplike sensation. They are capricious, bizarre, and follow no definite pattern as to location, although the occipital portion of the skull is frequently affected. Their duration is a distinguishing feature. A depressed person will describe the headache as lasting for years or throughout their life. A depressive headache is usually dull and generalized, characteristically worse in the morning and in the evening. This diurnal variation is the most distinctive characteristic of the headache and

Table 10–1 Physical complaints in depression

Complaint	Percentage of patients
Sleep disturbances	97
Early awakening	87
Headache	84
Dyspnea	76
Loss of weight	74
Difficulty falling asleep	73
Weakness and fatigue	70
Urinary frequency	70
"Spells"—dizziness	70
Appetite disturbances	70
Decreased libido	63
Cardiovascular disturbances	60
Sexual disturbances	60
Palpitations	59
Paresthesias	53
Nausea	48
Menstrual changes	41

Source: Reproduced with permission from Diamond, S. (1987). Depression and headache: A pharmacological perspective. In *Psychiatric Aspects of Headache* (C.S. Adler, S.M. Adler, and R.C. Packard, eds.), pp. 259–274. Williams & Wilkins, Baltimore.

Table 10–2 Emotional complaints in depression

Complaint	Percentage of patients
Blue; low spirits; sadness	90
Crying	80
Feelings of guilt, hopelessness, unworthiness, unreality	65
Anxiousness or irritability	65
Anxiety	60
Fear of insanity, physical disease, death; rumination over past, present, future	50

Table 10–3 Psychic complaints in depression

Complaint	Percentage of patients
"Morning is the worst time of day"	95
Poor concentration	91
No interest, no ambition	75
Indecisiveness	75
Poor memory	71
Suicidal thoughts; death wishes	35

has provided a correct diagnosis of severe depression when other features have been inconspicuous.

Certain details about the headache may indicate an underlying depression. The headaches of depressed patients usually appear at regular intervals in relation to daily life, occurring on weekends, Sundays, or holidays and on the first days of vacation or after exams. The greatest incidence of "nervous-type" headache occurs from 4:00 P.M. to 8:00 P.M. and from 4:00 A.M. to 8:00 A.M. These are usually the periods of the greatest and sometimes the most silent family crises. These headaches may occur early in the morning, when the depressed patient awakens and fantasies of conflict with family members or at work are manifested. In discussion with the depressed patient, we find that the headaches often occur when the patient leaves the relatively quiet atmosphere of the office for a weekend at home. The headache often coincides with interpersonal situations in which the sufferer feels compelled to appear comfortable, relaxed, and agreeable although he or she is struggling to repress resentment toward someone he or she is expected to love and respect.

Statistically, we have found that 84% of depressed patients indicated that headache was one of their complaints or their only complaint. In Table 10–1, the most frequently listed complaint with depression is sleep disturbance (Diamond, 1987). Of the patients that I or my colleagues examined, 97% presented with this complaint. In younger patients, there is less variation in sleep. The older individual experiences more difficulty with sleep. Sleep disturbances may manifest themselves as hypersomnia, insomnia, early awakening, or disturbing dreams. Early awakening is one of the more common sleep disturbances presenting with depression.

The emotional complaints characteristic of depression may vary, as reviewed in Table 10–2 (Diamond, 1987). The clue to depression is the introversion of the patient. Emotionally, the patient focuses on self and illness, repeatedly reviewing mistakes and misdeeds and deprecating himself or herself. Feelings of inadequacy and incompetence are common and persist in these people, and they look to the future with despair. Phobias and fears of a variable nature are common, such as fear of insanity, being alone in the house, changing jobs, or moving, all of which indicate depression. Irritability and hostility are common emotional symptoms.

In Table 10–3, a multitude of psychic complaints are presented (Diamond, 1987). An impairment in concentration or memory, loss of interest, difficulty in decision making, and despondency occur frequently in depression. These produce thoughts of suicide, ideas of reference, and delusions. A few patients will hallucinate. To the depressed patient, everything is an effort. Some people experience complete psychomotor retardation, and they have difficulty eating, sleeping, thinking, and dressing themselves. Daily tasks become major chores. Older people have serious memory defects and may have delusions of cancer or other incurable illnesses.

Depressed patients also will often present with somatic complaints. These symptoms will impact on various bodily functions. Table 10–4 illustrates certain indicators that implicate depression as the cause of these somatic complaints (Diamond, 1987). People with depressive illness may develop bodily symptoms,

Table 10–4   Clues that illness may be secondary to depression

1. Multiple complaints that do not fit a recognizable pattern.
2. Development of new symptoms as soon as others are helped.
3. Bad cooperation with treatment.
4. Symptoms that occur only in the presence of a certain individual, in a particular place, or at a certain time of year.
5. History of psychiatric problems.
6. The physician is confused and feels out of control of the patient.

and conversely people with painful organic diseases tend to become depressed. Too little attention is given to the depressive aspects of chronic pain and its treatment. The physical complaints dominate the situation so that the underlying depression tends to be overlooked.

The Biology of Depression

The biochemical determinants of depression have been researched heavily for the past 30 years. Much of our present knowledge comes from work completed in the mid-1950s (Maas, 1973). During that time, it was observed that tubercular patients treated with iproniazid developed euphoric states. It was later learned that iproniazid is a monoamine oxidase inhibitor and produces increasing levels of norepinephrine and serotonin in the brain and body tissue. About this time it was observed that a small percentage of patients being treated for hypertension with the rauwolfian alkaloids, such as reserpine, developed severe depression indistinguishable from endogenous depressions. These alkaloids were noted to deplete the brain of both biogenic amines. These observations evolved into our present theory of depression, which may be considered an illness involving multiple defects of neurotransmitters. However, these biogenic amines have not been fully explained.

The most popular biologic theories of depression hold that the disorder is associated with depletion of brain monoamine neurotransmitters such as serotonin and norepinephrine. Determining the most important substance in depression is controversial. Evidence is available to support both the norepinephrine and serotonin hypotheses (Feighner, 1982). Other neurotransmitters, such as dopamine and endorphin, may also be involved in depression (Fawcett, 1980). The discovery of endogenous, opiatelike substances in the brain, the endorphins and enkephalins, has significantly advanced our understanding of pain. Recent findings suggest that pain transmission in the central nervous system is controlled by an endorphin-mediated analgesia system. This system can be activated by several exogenous actions, including opioid substances, electrical stimulation, acupuncture, and even placebo (Basbaum and Fields, 1978; Fields, 1981; Mayer and Price, 1976; Snyder and Childers, 1979).

The importance of antidepressant drugs in pain control results from their effects on the synthesis and metabolism of serotonin and norepinephrine. Neurons have been found to contain serotonin and norepinephrine and are part of the brain's analgesia system (Diamond, 1983; Messing et al., 1975). Pain researchers are particularly interested in a descending serotonin pathway in the dorsal spinal cord, originating in the raphe nucleus, and an interlacing of norepinephrine and opioid neurons in the locus ceruleus (Diamond, 1983). Drugs that alter the synthesis or uptake of serotonin and/or norepinephrine—virtually all antidepressant agents—would be expected to play a role in the brain's regulation of pain. Serotonin antagonists have been known to influence both opiate- and stimulation-induced analgesia (Messing and Lytle, 1977). In animals, tricyclics produce analgesia directly (Saarnivaara and Mattila, 1974) or through potentiation of opiates (Malseed and Goldstein, 1979).

Diagnostic Measures

Several tests have been developed to evaluate depression and select the therapeutic agent to be used. The dexamethasone suppression test (DST) (Cobbin et al., 1979) basically involves administering a small amount of dexamethasone to the patient at midnight and measuring serum cortisol levels the following day. A subgroup of patients has been found with an endogenous depression who also exhibit nonsuppression. Most of these patients show normal suppression in the morning and nonsuppression later in the day. Approximately 45% of endogenously depressed individuals have an abnormal DST. Because the test is 96% specific for endogenous depression, an abnormal DST will occur in only 4 to 7% of patients with other psychiatric disorders, including schizophrenia, mania, personality disorders, and minor or neurotic depression.

If a patient has an abnormal response to the test, the physician must rule out organic illnesses that may cause an abnormal result. These include Cushing syndrome, pregnancy, and uncontrolled diabetes. The physician must also review the patient's current medications because many drugs alter the results. Currently, the DST is most valuable in monitoring the patient's response to therapy. Normalization of the DST appears to correlate with an improved clinical picture. Patients with an abnormal DST appear more likely to suffer from recurrent depressions than those patients who exhibit normal suppression. Studies are underway to determine if a patient's response to the DST can be used as a guide for drug therapy. Preliminary work indicates that the nonsuppressors have a better response to treatment. The relationship between the pituitary–adrenal axis and depression is currently unknown. The limbic system and cholinergic pathways have been implicated, but further research is required.

Diagnosing depression in chronic pain patients can be difficult because these patients tend to deny cognitive and affective symptoms, and vegetative complaints may be produced by pain (Blumer and Heilbronn, 1982). There is conflicting information on the ability of the DST to detect depression in chronic pain patients. Ward et al. (1992) studied the DST in both inpatients and outpatients with chronic pain. The inpatient group showed no association between DST suppression and major depression (81 patients, 13 with headaches). Nonsuppression was more prevalent in headache patients, occurring in 69% of the headache patients and 15% of the others. Inpatients with headache had a higher rate of depression (66%) than nonheadache patients (51%). Among the headache nonsuppressors, five of nine had a major depression. Among the suppressors, three of four had a major depression.

Another diagnostic test is the thyroid-stimulating hormone (TSH) response to thyrotropin-releasing hormone (TRH). A large percentage of endogenously depressed patients have a blunted TSH response to the administration of TRH. The mechanism for this blunted response is unknown, and the clinical value of this test has yet to be demonstrated.

The 3-methoxy-4-hydroxyphenylethyleneglycol (MHPG) urine test is used to evaluate the main metabolite of norepinephrine in the central nervous system. The urinary levels may demonstrate the norepinephrine metabolism (Blackwell, 1979; Cobbin et al., 1979; Maas, 1975). Subgroups of depressed patients have decreased MHPG in their urine, and other groups of depressed patients have normal or increased levels of MHPG.

Researchers have suggested that perhaps two groups of depression exist. In the first group, norepinephrine metabolism is disrupted and serotonin and dopamine systems are normal. The second group presents with a disorder of serotonin but not norepinephrine or dopamine. Studies revealed that low-MHPG depressives have a higher response to imipramine and desipramine as opposed to amitriptyline and nortriptyline. High-MHPG patients responded more effectively to amitriptyline or nortriptyline. Maas (1975) argued that low-MHPG patients had low norepinephrine but normal serotonin and high-MHPG patients had a low serotonin but normal norepinephrine repression.

The possibility of three distinct subgroups of depressive disorders has been suggested. The groups would be differentiated on the basis of low, intermediate, and high MHPG levels (Schatzberg et al., 1980, 1981, 1982). The patients with low MHPG demonstrated a clear response to imipramine or maprotiline, which may have decreased norepinephrine synthesis or release. Normal norepinephrine metabolism may occur in patients with intermediate subsensitive postsynaptic receptors and/or increased acetylcholine activity. To explain the disparate results from other studies, a three-group paradigm should be formulated. Low-MHPG patients have demonstrated relatively low levels of cerebrospinal fluid 5-hydroxyindoleacetic acid in other recent studies. A low-norepinephrine versus low-serotonin hypothesis would be disputed with these observations (Maas et al., 1982).

TREATMENT OF TENSION-TYPE HEADACHE

For the episodic tension-type headache, treatment is limited to abortive therapy, including over-the-counter analgesics or prescribed simple analgesics. These agents are usually helpful in relieving the pain. However, the importance of biofeedback training and counseling should be stressed if the headaches occur frequently.

The treatment of depression-associated tension-type headaches includes the use of the antidepressant agents. Tricyclics are usually the drugs of choice. This group includes amitriptyline, imipramine, desipramine, nortriptyline, doxepin, and protriptyline. The efficacy of these drugs has been shown in numerous studies (Ayd, 1971, 1980; Diamond, 1963, 1966; Diamond & Baltes, 1969). The

Table 10–5   Effects of antidepressants

Drug	Serotonin inhibition	Norepinephrine inhibition	Dopamine inhibition	Sedative effects	Anticholinergic effects
Amitriptyline	Moderate	Weak	Inactive	Strong	Strong
Desipramine	Weak	Potent	Inactive	Mild	Moderate
Doxepin	Moderate	Moderate	Inactive	Strong	Strong
Imipramine	Fairly potent	Moderate	Inactive	Moderate	Strong
Nortriptyline	Weak	Fairly potent	Inactive	Mild	Moderate
Protriptyline	Weak	Fairly potent	Inactive	None	Strong
Trimipramine	Weak	Weak	Inactive	Moderate	Moderate
Amoxapine	Weak	Potent	Moderate	Mild	Mild
Trazodone	Fairly potent	Weak	Inactive	Strong	Mild
Fluoxetine	Potent	Weak	Inactive	None	Mild–none
Bupropion HCl	Weak	Weak	Weak	None	None
Maprotiline	Weak	Moderate	Inactive	Moderate	Moderate

tricyclics are considered more effective in endogenous depression and less beneficial when the depressed patient has many accompanying neuroptic traits. The choice of tricyclic is not simple because each drug has unique characteristics, as reviewed in Table 10–5 (Diamond, 1977).

The most widely used tricyclic antidepressant in headache prophylaxis is amitriptyline, 25 to 300 mg daily. Other tricyclic agents frequently used in headache therapy include doxepin (10 to 150 mg daily), protriptyline (5 to 30 mg daily), nortriptyline (25 to 100 mg at bedtime), trimipramine (75 to 200 mg daily), and desipramine (25 to 150 mg daily). In selecting the tricyclic to be used in the treatment regimen, the presence of a sleep disturbance is a determining factor. Amitriptyline, doxepin, or nortriptyline in large, bedtime doses may be effective for those patients with early or frequent awakening. If the patient does not present with a sleep disturbance, desipramine or protriptyline should be considered. Protriptyline is the least sedating of this class of drugs, and the majority of the dose should be administered early in the morning.

Newer antidepressants are also available, such as trazodone, in doses of 75 to 300 mg daily. Trazodone has a very low profile for cardiovascular and anticholinergic effects, and drowsiness is the most commonly cited side effect. Persistent priapism has occasionally been reported with trazodone therapy (Scher et al., 1983). A bicyclic antidepressant, fluoxetine, has been the subject of much publicity because of its effectiveness in depression. The action of fluoxetine is much slower that of tricyclic antidepressants. However, it is less likely to produce the adverse effects frequently associated with the tricyclics. In headache therapy, fluoxetine is usually prescribed in doses up to 80 mg daily, in divided doses (Diamond, 1989). Maprotiline, another bicyclic, has effects similar to amitriptyline, doxepin, and nortriptyline.

One of the newest antidepressants available in the United States, bupropion hydrochloride, is not related to the tricyclics. It is administered in divided doses totaling 200 to 300 mg daily. Amoxapine is an antidepressant of the dibenzoxazepine class with marked dopamine effects. It is not indicated in the treatment of chronic tension-type headaches because of its reported adverse effects, tardive dyskinesia and neuroleptic malignant syndrome.

The monoamine oxidase inhibitors (MAOIs) are generally considered to be the second line of drugs for depression. They are not considered as efficacious as the tricyclics and are known to have more drug interactions. A patient on an MAOI must follow a special diet and avoid foods with tyramine (Table 10–6). The most commonly used MAOI is phenelzine sulfate (Robinson et al., 1973). MAOIs block the oxidative deamination of numerous monoamines, including epinephrine, norepinephrine, serotonin, and dopamine. According to prevailing theories, the amounts of these substances are increased in the brain and other tissues. The depression created by their deficiency is ameliorated or cured. Despite the precautions and fears with MAOIs, they are often found effective when the tricyclics fail. In studies comparing tricyclics and MAOIs (Ravaris et al., 1980), the MAOIs tended to exert a stronger antianxiety action whereas the tricyclics were more effective in reversing weight loss and improving sleep.

Combination therapy of a tricyclic and a MAOI simultaneously was previously verboten in practice. There had been isolated reports of hypertensive, hyperpyretic crises leading to death as a result of combination therapy. Standard practice was to initiate therapy with a tricyclic. If no improvement was noted within 4 to 6 weeks, the drug was discontinued, and after waiting 10 days to 2 weeks the MAOI was started. The two drugs were never given in combination. In 1971, Schuckit and his associates reviewed 25 reported cases of morbidity secondary to combination therapy. The results of that study indicated that the risks of combination therapy had been greatly exaggerated. Many of the complications reported could be attributed to drug overdose. Other symptoms could be related to the concomitant use of other drugs that act on the central nervous system. In the remaining cases, the tricyclic involved was imipramine and the MAOIs included iproniazid, tranylcypromine, isocarboxazid, pargyline, and phenelzine.

COEXISTENT MIGRAINE AND TENSION-TYPE HEADACHES (MIXED HEADACHE SYNDROME)

A discussion of tension-type headaches would be incomplete without a review of the diagnosis and treatment of the mixed headache syndrome. The Classification Committee of the IHS describes the mixed headache as coexisting migraine and tension-type headache (1988). The mixed headache patient is the case most frequently seen by the neurologist or headache specialist. This type of headache is comprised of the following symptomatology: (1) daily, continuous headache; (2) a hard or sick headache (migraine) occurring 1 to 10 times monthly; and (3) easy susceptibility to habituation to over-the-counter or prescribed analgesics and/or ergotamine tartrate (Mathew, 1981).

The relationship between migraine and depression has been examined. Garvey et al. (1984) reviewed the rate of occurrence of migraine in a group of patients with a depressive disorder. Their results demonstrated a higher incidence of migraine in depressed men than in the general population. A possible

Table 10–6 Diet for the headache patient on MAOIs

	Foods allowed	Foods to avoid
Beverage	Decaffeinated coffee, fruit juice, club soda, noncola soda (7UP, ginger ale); limit caffeine sources to 2 cups/day (coffee, tea, cola)	Chocolate, cocoa, alcoholic beverages, buttermilk
Meat, fish, poultry	Fresh or frozen: turkey, chicken, fish, beef, lamb, veal, pork Egg as meat substitute (limit 3 eggs/week) Tuna or tuna salad	Aged, canned, cured, or processed meat, including ham or game; pickled herring, salted and dried fish; chicken livers; bologna; fermented sausage; any food prepared with meat tenderizer, soy sauce, or brewer's yeast; any food containing nitrates, nitrites, or tyramine
Dairy products	Milk: homogenized, 2%, or skim Cheese: American, cottage, farmer, ricotta, cream, Velveeta Yogurt (limit ½ cup per day)	Cultured dairy products (buttermilk, sour cream); chocolate milk Cheese: bleu, Boursault, brick, Brie types, Camembert types, cheddar, Gouda, Stilton, Swiss (Emmentaler), Roquefort, mozzarella, Parmesan, provolone, Romano
Bread, cereal	Commercial bread, English muffins, melba toast crackers, RyKrisp, bagel All hot & dry cereals	Hot fresh homemade yeast bread, bread or crackers containing cheese; fresh yeast coffee cake, doughnuts, sourdough bread; any product containing chocolate or nuts
Potato or substitute	White potato, sweet potato, rice, macaroni, spaghetti, noodles	None
Vegetable	Any except those to avoid	Beans such as pole, broad, lima, Italian, fava, navy, pinto, garbanzo; snow peas, pea pods; sauerkraut, onions (except for flavoring), olives, pickles
Fruit	Any except those to avoid; limit citrus fruits to ½ cup per day; limit banana to ½ per day	Avocados, figs, raisins, papaya, passion fruit, red plums
Soup	Cream soups made from foods allowed in diet, homemade broths	Canned soup, soup or bouillon cubes, soup base with autolytic yeast or MSG (**Read Labels**)
Dessert	Fruit allowed in diet, any cake, pudding, cookies, or ice cream without chocolate or nuts, no yeast items, JELL-O	Chocolate ice cream, pudding, cookies, cake, or pies Mincemeat pie, nuts, peanut butter
Sweets	Sugar, jelly, jam, honey, hard candy	Chocolate candy or syrup, carob
Miscellaneous	Salt in moderation, lemon juice, butter or margarine, cooking oil, whipped cream, white vinegar & commercial salad dressings in small amounts	Pizza, cheese sauce, MSG in excessive amounts, yeast, yeast extract, meat tenderizer, Accent seasoned salt; mixed dishes (macaroni & cheese, beef stroganoff, cheese blintzes, lasagna), frozen TV dinners, marinated dishes

association between familial transmission of migraine and depression has been reviewed. Merikangas et al. (1988) compared a group of 133 patients with a major depression to 82 normal community controls, and interviewed 400 first-degree relatives of these two groups. They observed a significant association between migraine and depression in the depressed group and also in their relatives. The relatives of the controls also revealed a significant association between migraine and depression.

A "pain-prone" disorder has been proposed by Blumer and Heilbronn (1982) that would be considered a variant of depression. Their theory is based on the efficacy of antidepressants in the treatment of pain disorders. This type of disorder has also been identified as a "masked depression," which implies a psychiatric disorder (Feinmann, 1988).

When the diagnosis of coexisting migraine and tension-type headaches has been determined, the physician should avoid the use of sedation, tranquilizers, habituating analgesics, and narcotics to prevent addiction, which thereby perpetuates the problem. To prevent the rebound phenomenon, the use of ergotamine should be restricted to relief of the hard or sick headache. Ergots should never be prescribed on a daily basis. The use of caffeine-containing over-the-counter and prescription analgesics should be limited. The patient's intake of caffeine-containing beverages should also be restricted, with total daily consumption of caffeine limited to 200 to 300 mg.

For the acute relief of the daily headache, the nonsteroidal anti-inflammatory drugs (NSAIDs) may be beneficial. NSAIDs, such as ibuprofen, fenoprofen, naproxen sodium, diflunisal, and ketoprofen, have been used successfully in many mixed headache patients. The tricyclics or the MAOIs are the drugs of choice in the prophylactic treatment of the mixed headache syndrome. Pfaffenrath's group (1986) conducted a comparison study of time-released dihydroergotamine (DHE) and amitriptyline in the treatment of the mixed headache syndrome. Forty-one patients with mixed headaches were involved in the trial. By using headache diaries, data were collected 1 month prior to initiation of the study and for 2 months following discontinuation of treatment. In reducing headache intensity, amitriptyline was found more effective than DHE. However, the time-released DHE preparation was found significantly more effective in decreasing attacks of the "migraine" type.

For refractory cases, combination therapy consisting of a tricyclic antidepressant and an MAOI may be indicated. At our clinic, a review study was conducted on the use of MAOIs, alone or in combination with a tricyclic, in recidivist headache patients (Freitag et al., 1987). Improvement of greater than 50% was reported by 12 of 16 patients with mixed headaches. In using combination therapy, the physician should be familiar with the intricacies of these agents. This therapy should only be prescribed for the most recidivist patients.

The cautious addition of propranolol in the long-acting form may be considered in doses of 80, 120, and 160 mg on a daily basis. The once-daily administration of this drug enhances patient compliance. Occasionally, adding a NSAID to the therapeutic regimen may be helpful. The patient with the mixed headache syndrome may require a copharmacy approach with several agents. To ensure the successful treatment of chronic tension-type headaches and the mixed headache syndrome, the patient must receive continuity of care. Habituating analgesics must be avoided.

CERVICAL SPINE DISORDERS AND TENSION-TYPE HEADACHES

Headache is not limited to the head. Head pain may also be referred to and include the neck as a component of the pain syndrome. The patient may complain of pain in the upper cervical spine as part of both migraine and cluster headache syndromes. Disorders of the cervical spine may create localized pain but may also produce referred pain to the head. Migraine and cluster headaches as a cause of pain at the cervical spine have been described previously in this text. The following discussion focuses on disorders of the cervical spine as a cause of pain.

Structures and Mechanisms in Cervical Pain

There are multiple etiologies for pain involving the cervical spine. The mechanisms for such pain are numerous and, frequently, obscure. A review of the involved structures should enhance an understanding of the complexity of this problem.

Cervical nerves and roots, vertebral arteries, ligaments, periosteum, annulus fibrosus of the disks, and synovial joints are capable of producing pain. The second cervical nerve's sensory root produces the fibers that become the greater occipital nerve. This nerve provides the major sensory input from the posterior half of the head (Chouret, 1967; Edmeads, 1978). Irritation of the greater occipital nerve can produce headache. A variety of mechanisms can produce this condition, including inflammation (Dalessio, 1972), entrapment (Cameron, 1964), direct trauma, and compression between the atlas and the axis (Hunter and Mayfield, 1949). In addition, irritation of the sensory fibers of C_1 and C_2 may result in pain at both the neck and head. The role of C_3 and C_4 nerve root compression as a cause of head pain is not as well established (Braag and Rosner, 1975; Brain, 1963).

Occipital headache may result from inflammation, injury, or pressure on the occipital nerves, upper cervical spinal roots, dorsal horn, or sensory ganglion. The pain is a long-lasting, sustained, nonthrobbing ache of moderate intensity associated with muscle tenderness and may be difficult to differentiate from tension-type headache. Paresthesia or algesia of the tissues of the scalp and the skin of the neck is characteristic of occipital headache. If the cause of the disorder is postherpetic neuralgia, nerve or root section will probably not totally eliminate the pain. Infiltration of the sensory roots with local anesthetic may have a similar slight effect in reducing the pain intensity.

The distinction between occipital neuralgia and referred pain from the atlantoaxial or C_3 zygapophyseal joints must be established. At the latter site, there is usually more continuous pain with no sensory loss. To isolate this distinction, the second cervical ganglion may be blocked (Bogduk, 1981), or the tender area may be infiltrated locally with xylocaine and corticosteroids.

Occipital headache may be due to tumors of the upper cervical spine (meningiomas, neurofibromas, ependymomas), particularly if they are attached to or are adjacent to the first two or three nerve roots. This pain can resemble occipital neuralgia or an occipital tension-type headache. In addition to the pain, there is often a disturbance in sensory perception within the involved dermatomes. Magnetic resonance imaging is the diagnostic procedure of choice. Removal of the tumor, or rhizotomy when removal is impossible, eliminates or reduces the intensity of headache.

Cervicogenic headache is extremely controversial. It is described in greater detail in Chapter 8.

Occlusion of the vertebral arterial system in the neck has long been suspected to be a source for occipital headache (Yates and Hutchinson, 1961). Headache is a common complaint in patients with vertebrobasilar insufficiency (Grindal and Toole, 1975). The vertebral arteries are closely associated with the first six cervical vertebrae, rendering them susceptible to compression. Direct blows to the neck, attempted strangulation, aggressive cervical manipulation, or other neck trauma (Schneider and Crosby, 1959) may occasionally cause small tears in the intimal lining of the vertebral arteries. Subsequent development of thrombus formation may occur. The embolization that may ensue will produce various brainstem stroke syndromes, with the site dependent on the location of the emboli. In these cases, anticoagulant therapy must be started immediately. Compression of the vertebral arteries may occur with advanced osteophyte formation. However, the process by which this mechanism causes headache has not been fully explained. The sympathetic nerve supply that surrounds the vertebral arteries possibly affects the cerebral blood flow and thus may induce headache (Bartschi-Rochaix, 1968; Harper et al., 1972).

Bony anomalies of the craniovertebral junction may induce neck pain in 13 to 26% of affected cases (McRae, 1960, 1966, 1969). Anomalies such as occipitalization of the atlas, congenital atlantoaxial dislocation, and basilar invagination may produce pain. In many of these cases, flexion of the neck will trigger pain. The pain, which is localized to the suboccipital and occipital areas, is aggravated by the supine position (Edmeads, 1978). Congenital conditions, such as Dandy-Walker syndrome or Arnold-Chiari malformation, may cause cervical pain (Watkins, 1969) or exertional headache (Rooke, 1968).

Lesions of the skull and spine themselves, such as multiple myeloma, metastatic tumor, osteomyelitis, Potts disease, and Paget disease, can cause periosteal pain, producing protective muscle spasm. Paget disease can produce basilar impression and headache by producing cervical nerve root traction or by producing hydrocephalus (Edmeads, 1988).

Protective muscle spasm with radiographic evidence of cervical straightening is associated with a variety of cervical spine disorders, including a herniated cervical intervertebral disc. Unilateral neck-ache radiating to the occiput and at times to the temple and forehead may appear in patients with upper cervical facet joint disorders.

Headache Associated with Cervical Spondylosis

Brain et al., in 1963, first called attention to the headache and other clinical manifestations of cervical spondylosis. Brain and his colleagues defined cervical spondylosis as a degenerative disorder of the cervical spine, leading to narrowing of the intervertebral spaces and protrusion of the intervertebral discs.

With age, the water content of the intervertebral disc and annulus fibrosis progressively declines and there are simultaneous degenerative changes, beginning in the disc. The intervertebral space narrows and may be obliterated. There may be associated herniation of the disc through the annulus fibrosis, and osteophytes form on the vertebral body as well as the longitudinal wall, and may extend into the intervertebral foramina (Rowland, 1989). These changes can cause pressure on the spinal nerves in their foramina as well as pressure on the spinal cord. Because the disorder is degenerative rather than inflammatory, Brain et al. (1963) selected the term "spondylosis" rather than "spondylitis." Trauma, degeneration of the intravertebral discs with age, and a congenitally narrow canal are the main etiologic factors.

Cervical spondylosis is more common in men than women, and produces symptoms chiefly in the fifth and sixth decades. As a result of the morbid process, the nerve roots may be compressed in the foramina, now the site of a secondary formation of fibrous tissue, and undergo degeneration (Rowland, 1989). Nerve root involvement can produce paresthesias and radiculopathy. The cord is directly compressed and tethered by the adhesions around the nerve root, and normal neck movement causes continual mild injury. Blood supply may be affected by the compression of the spinal veins and the anterior spinal artery. Compression of the cervical cord or impairment of the blood supply to the cord with development of a spastic gait may be the most common symptom. Weakness, wasting, and fasciculations of the hands may occur. The cerebrospinal fluid may show a slight rise in protein, and when the neck is extended there may be a demonstrable obstruction on manometric tests. The process may be painless, or the patient may describe pain that encompasses the head and neck (Petersen et al., 1975).

Headache is a common accompaniment of cervical disc lesions. High cervical bony defects or root damage such as that caused by Paget disease, which involves the bones of the base of the skull and the upper cervical spine, are associated with headache (which may become frontal). Because most of the population over age 40 have radiologic changes of cervical spondylosis, but few have symptoms, it is important to not attribute headache to coexistent radiologically evident disease. However, 40% of patients with symptomatic (radiculopathy or myelopathy) cervical disc disease or spondylosis have headache as a major complaint (Edmeads, 1988). Pain in the cervical spine may occur through local inflammatory changes, referred radicular pain, or reflex spasm of the paraspinal muscles (Brain, 1963; Graham, 1964). This is the mechanism thought to be responsible for the headache associated with cervical spondylosis.

Spondylitic head pain begins as an ache in the morning and may progress to a more constant and nagging pain. The physical examination of the patient with moderate to advanced spondylosis will frequently reveal muscle spasm as well as suboccipital tenderness. Movement of the neck may be somewhat limited. Early in the course of therapy, an anti-inflammatory agent may be indicated. Conservative treatment consisting of immobilization with a cervical collar may eliminate the pain, rendering operative intervention unnecessary. Cervical traction may enhance pain relief. However, surgery (decompressive laminectomy) may be considered if the following are observed: spinal cord compression, significant root involvement, long tract signs such as motor weakness or reflex changes, or numbness.

Rheumatoid arthritis and ankylosing spondylitis are also associated with symptomatic involvement of the cervical spine. The major problem that occurs is atlantoaxial subluxation; contributing factors are inflammation, atlantoaxial bony dissolution, and stretching. Pain frequently occurs with subluxation. The patient often complains of a deep occipital ache, which increases in intensity as the head is flexed forward. A sharp pain may also occur. The pain may radiate to encompass the head in a hatband distribution, or the ache may localize to the temple or eye. Compression of the lower medulla and upper cervical cord may occur secondary to the increased mobility that is present, with the odontoid process being displaced backward into the spinal canal or foramen magnum. The headache may present with signs of cord compression, including paresthesias, long tract signs, or numbness. Pain secondary to inflammation may also occur with rheumatoid arthritis, presenting at the occiput and neck. Immobilization of the head or extension of the neck may temporarily relieve the condition. In refractory cases, surgery may be considered. Neck exercises and traction are not indicated.

Trauma to the Cervical Spine

Trauma to the neck may produce a variety of pain syndromes, ranging from a mild and self-limited condition to a prolonged pain problem involving the head and neck. Following the typical rear-end auto collision, the unsupported head and neck hyperextend. This hyperextension occurs within the first quarter-second. The muscle reflexes, the major protective mechanism for the neck, are unable to respond adequately in this short period. If head supports are properly fitted and correctly positioned in autos, there is a significant decrease in the incidence of hyperextension and the ensuing injuries.

In addition to hyperextension, hyperflexion or lateral flexion may occur following auto accidents or other traumas to the neck. The injuries incurred are not usually as extensive or serious as those precipitated by hyperextension because of the limited amount of flexion through which the head can progress (see Chapter 16).

The physical examination is usually normal during the initial 2 to 3 hours following neck trauma. However, after this initial period, anterior neck swelling and tenderness may be observed, particularly in acceleration–extension injuries, thus restricting neck movement. Trapezius spasm may also appear. The stiffness and decreased cervical range of motion will usually continue from days to weeks, with a gradual improvement. Headache is a common symptom in these injuries, along with tinnitus, pain in the cervical area, dizziness, vertigo, and visual disturbances. The patient may experience pain radiating down one or both arms, which results from nerve root pressure or spasm of the scalene muscles.

General treatment measures for soft tissue neck injuries include rest and protection of the neck. A soft cervical collar may offer relief. However, this treatment should be used on a limited basis and not continued after the healing period. Heat applied locally to the neck will relieve the muscle spasm. Physical therapy in its various forms may be employed and will usually enhance the comfort of the patient. Traction is contraindicated, because injured and inflamed muscles and ligaments would be stretched during this particular therapy. The cautious use of muscle relaxants may help (Hohl, 1983). After the spasm and tenderness regress, isometric exercises have been used successfully.

For many unfortunate patients, the symptoms will persist for a long period after the injury. Headache as well as neck pain and stiffness are the major continuing complaints. The physical examination on follow-up is usually normal, but neuropsychiatric testing is frequently abnormal (see Chapter 16). There is evidence that the initial injury to the neck may initiate the prolonged process of disk degeneration, demonstrated on follow-up cervical radiographic studies performed many years later. Greenfield and Ilfeld (1977) studied 179 consecutive patients with soft tissue injuries. These authors concluded that progress was much slower in those patients who presented initially with shoulder, arm, or back pain, in addition to the usual symptoms.

Reviewing follow-up reports of soft tissue neck injuries revealed that litigation is not a predictor of prolonged disability. Hohl and Hopp (1978) and Hohl (1974) indicated that injuries independent of the neck region appear to heal faster with fewer persisting symptoms. If litigation were the solitary reason for the symptomatology, these other injuries would also persist as long as the soft tissue neck injuries. Of Hohl's 266 patients, 45% continued to suffer significant symptoms for 2 years following final settlement of their litigation.

Pearce (1992) has noted that "whiplash injuries" are rarely observed in professional sportsmen. In an earlier report, Pearce (1989) noted that the major distinguishing characteristics of whiplash injuries are:

1. The unexplained high incidence in women.
2. The prolonged nature of symptoms and apparent disability in a significant, if small, subgroup of patients.
3. The common attendant symptoms of anxiety, fatigue, and irritability.
4. The uselessness of immobilization (collar) and analgesics, unlike with other physical sequelae of trauma.
5. The involvement of most sufferers in compensation claims in published series.

Although "whiplash" is a target of negative publicity, these acute neck sprains can be valid and may represent a serious injury.

Injury to the soft tissue of the anterior neck may produce headache. Traumatic dysautonomic cephalalgia has been described by Vijayan (1977). Symptoms include a unilateral vascular headache associated with pupillary dilation and facial swelling ipsilateral to the side of the injury. Vijayan proposed that the syndrome was caused by a stretching injury to the carotid arteries. Propranolol has been used successfully in the prophylaxis of this condition.

Thoracic outlet syndrome following neck trauma may present with obvious symptoms of subclavian artery aneurysm, gangrene, and brachial or subclavian artery thrombosis. In less distinct cases (Jamieson and Mersky, 1985), the clinical history and examination may be ambiguous and suggest a psychoneurotic disorder. Almost invariably, a triad of findings is present. These consist of neck, shoulder, and arm pain, postural discomfort of the arm, and paresthesias of the hand and finger. Only one fourth of the cases have postural effects or vascular changes. Although Adson sign may be present, other symptoms may facilitate diagnosis. These include tenderness over the brachial plexus or the margin of the trapezius, along with provocation of symptoms by military bracing of the arms or hyperabduction and extension of the arms.

REFERENCES

Ad Hoc Committee on Classification of Headache (1962). Classification of headache. *Arch. Neurol. 6:*13–16.

Adler C.S., S.M. Adler, and R.C. Packard (1987). *Psychiatric Aspects of Headache.* Williams & Wilkins, Baltimore.

Anthony, M. and J.W. Lance (1989). Plasma serotonin in patients with chronic tension headaches. *J. Neurol. Neurosurg. Psychiatry 52:*182–184.

Arena, J.G., S.L. Hannah, G.M. Bruno et al. (1991). Effect of movement and position of muscle activity in tension headache sufferers during and between headaches. *J. Psychosom. Res. 35:*187–195.

Ayd, F.J. (1971). Recognizing and treating depressed patients. *Mod. Med. 39:*80–86.

Ayd, F.J. (1980). Amitriptyline (Elavil) therapy for depressive reactions. *Psychosomatics 21.*

Bakal, D.A. (1982). *The Psychobiology of Chronic Headache.* Springer, New York.

Bakal, D.A. and J.A. Kaganov (1979). Symptom characteristics of chronic and non-chronic headache sufferers. *Headache 19:*285–289.

Bartschi-Rochaix, W. (1968). Headache of cervical origin. In *Clinical Neurology,* Vol. 5 (P.J. Vinken and G.W. Bruyn, eds.), pp. 192–201. North Holland Publishing, Amsterdam.

Basbaum A.I. and H.L. Fields (1978). Endogenous pain control mechanisms: Review and hypothesis. *Ann. Neurol. 4:*451–462.

Blackwell, B. (1979). MHPG in depression. *Psychiatr. Opinion,* July–August, pp. 28–32.

Blanchard E.B., C.A. Kirsch, K.A. Appelbaum, and J. Jaccard (1989). The role of psychopathology in chronic headache: Cause and effect. *Headache 29:*295–301.

Blau, J.N. (1989). Tension headaches: Clinical features and an attempt at clarification. In *Migraine and Other Headaches* (M.D. Ferrari and X. Lataste, eds.), pp. 65–71. Parthenon Publishing Group, NJ.

Blumer, D. and M. Heilbronn (1982). Chronic pain as a variant of depressive disease. *J. Nerv. Ment. Dis. 170:*381–394.

Bogduk, N. (1981). Local anesthetic block of the second cervical ganglion; a technique with application to cervical headache. *Cephalalgia 1:*41.

Braag, M.M. and S. Rosner (1975). Trauma of cervical spine as cause of chronic headache. *J. Trauma 15:*441–446.

Brain, W.R. (1963). Some unsolved problems of cervical spondylosis. *BMJ 1:*771–777.

Cameron, B.M. (1964). Cervical spine sprain headache. *Am. J. Orthop. 6:*9.

Chouret, E.E. (1967). The greater occipital neuralgia headache. *Headache 7:*33–34.

Cobbin, D., B. Requin-Blow, R.L. Williams et al. (1979). Urinary MHPG levels and tricyclic antidepressant drug selection. *Arch. Gen. Psychiatry 36:*1111–1115.

Dalessio, D.J. (1972). In *Wolff's Headache and Other Head Pain,* 3rd ed., pp. 552–555. Oxford University Press, New York.

Diamond, S. (1963). The use of amitriptyline hydrochloride in general practice. *Ill. Med. J. 123:*347–348.

Diamond, S. (1966). Double-blind controlled study of amitriptyline-perphenazine combination in medical office patients with depression and anxiety. *Psychosomatics 7:* 371–375.

Diamond, S. (1977). Nine experts review a FP's depression regimen. *Patient Care 11:* 42–77.

Diamond, S. (1983). Depression and headache. *Headache 23:*122–126.

Diamond, S. (1987). Depression and headache: A pharmacological perspective. In *Psychiatric Aspects of Headache* (C.S. Adler, S.M. Adler, and R.C. Packard, eds.), pp. 259–274. Williams & Wilkins, Baltimore.

Diamond, S. (1989). The use of fluoxetine in the treatment of headache. Letter to the editor. *Clin. J. Pain 5:*200–201.

Diamond, S. and B.J. Baltes (1969). The office treatment of mixed anxiety and depression with combination therapy. *Psychosomatics 10:*360–365.

Drummond, P.D. (1987). Scalp tenderness and sensitivity to pain in migraine and tension headache. *Headache 27:*45–50.

Editorial (1971). The great pretender. *Emerg. Med. 3:*21–27.

Edmeads, J.R. (1978). Headaches and head pains associated with diseases of the cervical spine. *Med. Clin. North Am. 62:*533–544.

Edmeads, J.R. (1988). The cervical spine and headache. *Neurology 38:*1874–1878.

Fawcett, J. (1980). Depression at the biochemical level. *Psychiatr. Ann. 109*(Suppl.): 362–368.

Featherstone, H.J. (1985). Migraine and muscle contraction headaches: A continuum. *Headache 25:*194–198.

Feighner, J.P. (1982). Pharmacological management of depression. *Fam. Pract. Recert. 4*(Suppl. 1):13–24.

Feinmann, C. (1988). The contribution of psychiatry. In *Headache: Problems in Diagnosis and Management* (A. Hopkins, ed.), pp. 271–304. W.B. Saunders, Philadelphia.

Fields, H.L. (1981). Pain II: New approaches to management. *Ann. Neurol. 9:*101–106.

Freitag, F.G., S. Diamond, and G.D. Solomon (1987). Antidepressants in the treatment of mixed headache: MAO inhibitors and combined use of MAO inhibitors and tricyclic antidepressants in the recidivist headache patient. In *Advances in Headache Research* (F.C. Rose, ed.), pp. 271–275. John Libbey & Co., Ltd., London.

Friedman, A.P., T.J.C. Von Storch, and H.H. Merritt (1964). Migraine and tension headaches. A clinical study: 2000 cases. *Neurology 4:*773.

Garvey, M.J., G.D. Tollefson, and C.B. Schaffer (1984). Migraine headaches and depression. *Am. J. Psychiatry 141:*986–988.

Graham, J.R. (1964). Treatment of muscle contraction headache. *Mod. Treatment 1:* 1399–1403.

Greenfield, J. and F.W. Ilfeld (1977). Acute cervical strain. Evaluation and short-term prognostic factors. *Clin. Orthop. 122:*196.

Grindal, A.B. and J.F. Toole (1975). Headaches and transient ischemic attacks. *Stroke 5:*603–606.

Harper, A.M., V.P. Deshmuth, O.V. Ronan et al. (1972). The influence of sympathetic nervous activity on cerebral blood flow. *Arch. Neurol. 27:*1–6.

Hatch, J.P., P.J. Moore, M. Cyr-Provost et al. (1992). The use of electromyography and muscle palpation in the diagnosis of tension-type headache with and without pericranial muscle involvement. *Pain 49:*175–178.

Hatch, J.P., T.J. Prihoda, P.J. Moore et al. (1991). A naturalistic study of the relationships among electromyographic activity, psychological stress, and pain in ambulatory tension-type headache patients and headache-free controls. *Psychosom. Med. 53:*576–584.

Headache Classification Committee of the International Headache Society (1988). Classification and diagnostic criteria for headache disorders, cranial neuralgias and facial pain. *Cephalalgia 8*(Suppl. 7):1–96.

Hodgkins, K. (1976). Educational implications of the Virginia study. *J. Fam. Pract. 3:* 1.

Hohl, M. (1974). Soft tissue injuries of the neck in automobile accidents; factors influencing prognosis. *J. Bone Joint Surg. 56A:*1675.

Hohl, M. (1983). Soft tissue neck injuries. In *The Cervical Spine* (R.W. Bailey, ed.), pp. 282–287. J.B. Lippincott, Philadelphia.

Hohl, M. and E. Hopp (1978). Soft tissue injuries of the neck II. Factors influencing prognosis. *Orthop. Trans. 2:*29.

Hunter, C.R. and F.H. Mayfield (1949). Role of the upper cervical nerve roots in the production of pain in the head. *Am. J. Surg 78:*743–749.

Iversen, H.K., M. Langemark, P.G. Andersson et al. (1990). Clinical characteristics of migraine and episodic tension-type headache in a relation to old and new diagnostic criteria. *Headache 30:*514–519.

Jamieson, W.G. and H. Mersky (1985). Representation of the thoracic outlet syndrome as a problem in chronic and psychiatric management. *Pain 22:*195–200.

Lance, J.W., G.A. Lambert, P.J. Goadsby, and J.W. Duckworth (1983). Brainstem influences on the cephalic circulation: Experimental data from cat and monkey of relevance to the mechanism of migraine. *Headache 23:*258–265.

Lichstein, K.L., S.M. Fischer, T.L. Eakin et al. (1991). Psychophysiological parameters of migraine and muscle-contraction headaches. *Headache 31:*27–34.

Maas, J. (1973). The biology of depression: Where we stand. *Psychiatry 5:*67–69.

Maas, J. (1975). Biogenic amines and depression. *Arch. Gen Psychiatry 32:*1357–1361.

Maas, J.W., J.H. Kocsis, C.D. Bowden et al. (1982). Pretreatment neurotransmitter metabolites and response to imipramine or amitriptyline treatment. *Psychol. Med. 12:*37–41.

Malseed, R.T. and F.J. Goldstein (1979). Enhancement of morphine analgesia by tricyclic antidepressants. *Neuropharmacology 18:*827–829.

Marsland, D.W., M. Wood, and F. Mayo (1976). Content of family practice. *J. Fam. Pract. 3:*1.

Martin, M.J., H.P. Rome, and W.M. Swensom (1967). Muscle contraction headache. A psychiatric review. *Res. Clin. Stud. Headache 1:*184.

Mathew, N.T. (1981). Prophylaxis of migraine and mixed headache. A randomized controlled study. *Headache 21:*105–109.

Mayer, D.J. and D.D. Price (1976). Central nervous system mechanisms of analgesia. *Pain 3*:1.

McRae, D.L. (1960). The significance of abnormalities of the cervical spine. Caldwell Lecture. *Am. J. Roentgenol. 84*:1–25.

McRae, D.L. (1966). The cervical spine and neurologic disease. *Radiol. Clin. North Am. 4*:145–158.

McRae, D.L. (1969). Bony abnormalities at the craniospinal junction. *Clin. Neurosurg. 16*:356–375.

Mebane, A.H. (1990). Antidepressant therapy for chronic pain syndromes. *Clin. Adv. Treat. Psychiatr. Dis. 4*:12–16.

Merikangas, K.R., N.J. Risch, J.R. Merikangas et al. (1988). Migraine and depression: Association and familial transmission. *J. Psychiatr. Res. 22*:119–129.

Messing, R.B. and L.D. Lytle (1977). Serotonin-containing neurons: Their possible role in pain and analgesia. *Pain 4*:1–21.

Messing, R.B., L. Phebus, L.A. Fisher et al. (1975). Analgesic effect of fluoxetine HCl (Lilly 110140), a specific uptake inhibitor for serotonergic neurons. *Psychopharmacol. Commun. 1*:511–521.

Olesen, J. (1988). Clinical characteristics of tension headache. In *Basic Mechanism of Headache* (J. Olesen and L. Edvinsson, eds.), pp. 9–14. Elsevier, Amsterdam.

Paulus, W., O. Baubüchi, A. Straube, and J. Schoenen (1992). Exteroceptive suppression of temporalis muscle activity in various types of headache. *Headache 32*: 41–44.

Pearce, J.M.S. (1989). Whiplash injury: A reappraisal. *J. Neurol. Neurosurg. Psychiatry 52*:1329–1331.

Pearce, J.M.S. (1992). Whiplash injury: Fact or fiction? *Headache Q. 3*:45–49.

Petersen, P.F., G.M. Austin, and L.A. Dayes (1975). Headaches associated with discogenic diseases of the cervical spine. *Bull. Los Angeles Neurol. Soc. 40*:96–100.

Pfaffenrath, V., U. Kellhamer, and W. Pollman (1986). Combination headache: Practical experience with a combination of a beta-blocker and an antidepressive. *Cephalalgia 1*(Suppl. 5):25–32.

Pritchard, D.W. (1989). EMG cranial muscle levels in headache sufferers before and during headache. *Headache 29*:103–108.

Rassmussen, B.K., R. Jensen, M. Schroll, and J. Olesen (1991). Epidemiology of headache in a general population—a prevalence study. *J. Clin. Epidemiol. 44*: 1147–1157.

Ravaris, C., C.L. Ravaris, D.S. Robinson et al. (1980). Phenelzine and amitriptyline in treatment of depression. A comparison of present and past studies. *Arch. Gen. Psychiatry 37*:1057–1080.

Robinson, D.S., A. Nies, C.L. Ravaris et al. (1973). The monoamine oxidase inhibitor, phenelzine, in the treatment of depressive-anxiety states. A controlled clinic trial. *Arch. Gen. Psychiatry 29*:407–413.

Rolf, L.H., G. Wiele, and G.G. Bruno (1981). 5-Hydroxytryptamine in platelets of patients with muscle contraction headache. *Headache 21*:10–11.

Rooke, E.D. (1968). Exertional headache. *Med. Clin. North Am. 52*:801–808.

Rowland, L.P. (1989). *Merritt's Textbook of Neurology*. Lea & Febiger, Philadelphia.

Saarnivaara, L. and M.J. Mattila (1974). Comparison of tricyclic antidepressants in rabbits. Antinociception and potentiation of the noradrenalin pressor responses. *Psychopharmacologia 35*:221–236.

Schatzberg, A.F., P.J. Orsulak, A.H. Rosenbaum et al. (1982). Toward a biochemical classification of depressive disorders V: Heterogeneity of unipolar depressions. *Am. J. Psychiatry 139*:471–475.

Schatzberg, A.F., A.H. Rosenbaum, P.J. Orsulak et al. (1980). Toward a biochemical classification of depressive disorders III: Pretreatment urinary MHPG levels as predictors of antidepressant response to imipramine. *Comm. Psychopharmacol. 4:*441–445.

Schatzberg, A.F., A.H. Rosenbaum, P.J. Orsulak et al. (1981). Toward a biochemical classification of depressive disorders IV: Pretreatment urinary MHPG levels as predictors of response to treatment with maprotiline. *Psychopharmacology 75:* 34–38.

Scher, M., J.N. Krieger, and S. Juergens (1983). Trazodone and priapism. *Am. J. Psychiatry 140:*1362–1363.

Schneider, R.C. and E.C. Crosby (1959). Vascular insufficiency of brain stem and spinal cord in spinal trauma. *Neurology 9:*643–656.

Schoenen, J., D. Bottin, J. Sulon et al. (1991a). Exteroceptive silent period of temporalis muscle in menstrual headaches. *Cephalalgia 11:*87–91.

Schoenen, J., P. Gerard, V. De Pasqua, and J. Sianard-Gainko (1991b). Multiple clinical and paraclinical analyses of chronic tension-type headaches associated or unassociated with disorder of pericranial muscles. *Cephalalgia 11:*135–139.

Schoenen, J., B. Jamart, P. Gerard et al. (1987). Exteroceptive suppression of temporalis muscle activity in chronic headache. *Neurology 37:*1834–1836.

Schuckit, M., E. Robins, J. Feighner et al. (1971). Tricyclic antidepressants and monoamine oxidase inhibitors. *Arch. Gen. Psychiatry 24:*509–514.

Shulman, B. (1992). Psychiatric management of the headache patient. In *The Practicing Physician's Approach to Headache,* 5th ed. (S. Diamond and D.J. Dalessio, eds.), pp. 217–223. Williams & Wilkins, Baltimore.

Silberstein, S.D. (1993). Tension-type and chronic daily headache. *Neurology* (in press).

Silberstein, S.D. and M.M. Silberstein (1990). New concepts in the pathogenesis of headache. Part II. Mechanisms and treatment. *Pain Management 3:*334–342.

Snyder, S.H. and S.R. Childers (1979). Opiate receptors and opioid peptides. *Annu. Rev. Neurosci. 2:*35–64.

Vijayan, N. (1977). A new post-traumatic headache syndrome. Clinical and therapeutic observations. *Headache 17:*19.

Wallasch, T.M., M. Reinecke, and H.D. Langohr (1991). EMG analysis of the late exteroceptive suppression period of temporal muscle activity in episodic and chronic tension-type headaches. *Cephalalgia 11:*109–112.

Ward, N.G., J.A. Turner, B. Ready, and S.J. Bigos (1992). Chronic pain, depression, and the dexamethasone suppression test. *Pain 48:*331–338.

Watkins, W.S. (1969). Paroxysmal headache due to the Chiari malformation. *Dis. Nerv. Syst. 30:*693–695.

Yates, P.O. and E.C. Hutchinson (1961). Cerebral infarction: The role of stenosis of the extracranial cerebral arteries. In *Medical Research Council Special Reports,* No. 30. H.M. Stationery Office, London.

Ziegler, D.K. and R.S. Hassanein (1990). Specific headache phenomena: Their frequency and coincidence. *Headache 30:*152–156.

Ziegler, D.K., R. Hassanein, and K. Hassanein (1972). Headache syndromes suggested by factor analysis of symptom variables in a headache prone population. *J. Chron. Dis. 25:*353–363.

11

Giant Cell Arteritis and Polymyalgia Rheumatica

DONALD J. DALESSIO
GARY W. WILLIAMS

Giant cell arteritis (GCA) is a febrile, often self-limiting disease that affects the aged of both sexes. It is characterized by painful inflammation of the temporal and other cranial arteries and generalized systemic signs and symptoms, including malaise, weakness, weight loss, anorexia, fever, and sweating (Huston et al., 1978). Other names for this arterial disease include temporal arteritis, granulomatous arteritis, and cranial arteritis. Of these several terms, the most descriptive is giant cell arteritis, which is probably employed least. Temporal arteritis is actually misleading because it implies localization of the inflammatory process to the superficial temporal arteries, whereas in the usual case the disease is widespread.

Criteria for the diagnosis of GCA have been published by the American College of Rheumatology. They include: (1) age ≥50 years at onset, (2) new onset of localized headache, (3) temporal artery tenderness or decreased temporal artery pulse, (4) elevated erythrocyte sedimentation rate (≥50 mm/hour by Westergren method), and (5) a positive temporal artery biopsy. These criteria were used to classify 214 patients with temporal arteritis and to distinguish them from 593 control patients with other forms of vasculitis. The presence of three of five of the criteria had a sensitivity of 93.5% and a specificity of 91.2%. If an elevated sedimentation rate was excluded as a criterion and scalp tenderness and jaw or tongue claudication substituted, the sensitivity was 95.3% and the specificity 90.7% (Hunder et al., 1990).

A related disease is polymyalgia rheumatica (PMR), characterized by complaints of pain and stiffness of the limbs and trunk, often associated with systemic signs of a nature similar to those of GCA described above. A significant number of patients with PMR, ranging from 5 to 30%, will eventually develop GCA during the course of their illness. This suggests that the two diseases are in fact one; the myalgias and synovitis of PMR may represent systemic manifestations of an underlying GCA.

LABORATORY FINDINGS

The laboratory data in GCA and PMR are similar. The principal findings are those associated with inflammation. Marked elevation of the erythrocyte sedimentation rate is characteristic of these two diseases. There are, however, typical and atypical cases with positive biopsy results and normal sedimentation rates (Wong and Korn, 1986). A recent report emphasized vasculitic involvement of the occipital artery in patients presenting with "occipital neuralgia" and normal sedimentation rates (Jundt and Mock, 1991). However, it is not unusual to confirm the diagnosis in patients with mild elevations, especially if the patient has been treated with nonsteroidal anti-inflammatory agents. Normal values for sedimentation rates are age dependent but, in general, rates above 35 to 40 mm/hour can be accepted as abnormal in patients of any age. Values of 100 mm/hour or greater are common in these diseases. When possible, the Westergren method should be used. Variations in results occur when blood is allowed to stand, and therefore the test should be set up within 1 hour of drawing the sample.

In addition to elevated sedimentation rates, a mild to moderate normochromic anemia is often seen along with mild leukocytosis. Nonspecific changes in plasma proteins are common, including elevation of plasma fibrinogen levels, α_2 globulins, complement, and γ globulins with slight depression of the serum albumin. Liver function tests are frequently abnormal; especially common are mild elevations of the alkaline phosphatases with elevations of serum transaminases. In several cases percutaneous liver biopsies were performed. Most often, fine bile ducts with intracellular deposition of bile pigment characteristic of cholestasis have been reported. In one personally observed case, in addition to cholestasis, a granuloma was present in the biopsy specimen. In spite of the prominent proximal muscle pain in patients with PMR, the tests for muscle inflammation are normal. An elevated creatine kinase or aldolase level suggests the diagnosis of an inflammatory myopathy of another sort.

Interest has been increasing in markers of vessel inflammation that might be helpful in distinguishing the subgroup of patients with PMR who also have cranial arteritis. Elevated levels of von Willebrand factor antigen have been found in the blood of patients with GCA and other forms of vasculitis. Nusinow et al. (1984), Persellin et al. (1985), and Clompi et al. (1988) found elevated levels of von Willebrand factor in PMR patients both with and without biopsy-proven GCA. It appears that, although von Willebrand factor antigen is elevated in GCA and PMR compared to controls, it does not predict biopsy results.

Should the temporal artery be biopsied when a diagnosis of GCA is suspected? In most cases, yes. In an emergency (e.g., when vision is threatened), the biopsy can be done after corticosteroid therapy has been started. When consigning patients to long-term therapy with corticosteroids, however, we prefer to have a tissue diagnosis whenever possible. In patients with a diagnosis of PMR in whom there is no clinical or historic evidence of GCA, we do not proceed to biopsy.

BIOPSY FINDINGS

In GCA the involved arteries are grossly seen as tortuous, swollen, nodular vessels with or without pulsation, with cellulitis of contiguous tissue. Biopsies of temporal arteries have been performed in more than half of the cases reported, and some patients have come to autopsy. Microscopic examination reveals a panarteritis. The typical section reveals hypertrophy of the intima, medial necrosis associated with the formation of granulomatous tissue and the presence of foreign body giant cells, periarterial cellular infiltration, and thrombus formation (Figures 11–1 and 11–2). Eosinophilic invasion of the artery in cranial arteritis is rare. The presence of giant cells has suggested a tuberculous etiology, but no tubercules have been seen and no acid-fast bacilli have been demonstrated.

Consecutive biopsies on three cranial arteritis patients were studied by electron microscopy by Kuwabara and Reinecke (1970). All biopsies showed a combination of pathologic changes of various stages of the disease with inflammation and smooth muscle cell involvement. Biopsies obtained in the clinically acute periods showed predominantly inflammatory elements. Later biopsies from the same patients showed granulomatous reactions and muscular regeneration.

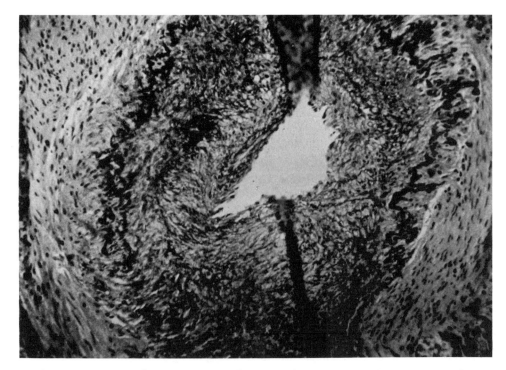

Figure 11–1. Cranial arteritis. Section of a biopsy of temporal artery showing acute inflammatory cells and giant cells (hematoxylin and eosin stain).

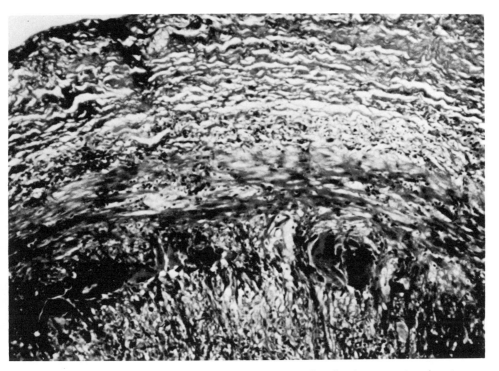

Figure 11–2. Higher power view of Figure 11–1, graphically demonstrating the giant cells.

Klein et al. (1976) called attention to the intermittency of pathologic changes (skip lesions) that may occur in cranial arteritis. They identified skip lesions in 17 of 60 patients with temporal arteritis, based on a retrospective and prospective examination of temporal artery biopsy specimens. Examining more than 6,000 serial sections of arteries from patients with skip lesions, they found foci of arteritis as short as 330 mm in length in an otherwise normal biopsy specimen. Their study suggests the need to biopsy long segments of the artery, to examine multiple histologic sections, and perhaps to consider performing a contralateral temporal artery biopsy when frozen section examination of the first side is normal.

Lie and colleagues (1970) studied 150 temporal arteries from cadavers and described senile changes in these arteries occurring with advancing age. Progressive intimal thickening and alteration of the internal elastic lamina occurred from infancy to senility without development of atheroma.

Senile changes in temporal arteries are not associated with giant cell reaction and should not be confused with the active phase of cranial arteritis. The residual changes of cranial arteritis that may persist for many years are sufficiently different from the ordinary changes of senescence to enable one to distinguish between senescent arteries and arteries previously involved with the inflammatory reaction characteristic of temporal arteritis.

Other forms of arteritis have been found in the temporal arteries, including polyarteritis nodosa and Wegener granulomatosis (Small and Brisson, 1991). Histopathologic classification criteria have been published by Lie (1990).

IMMUNOLOGIC STUDIES

Liang et al. (1974) performed immunofluorescent studies on 15 consecutive temporal artery biopsy specimens and on control specimens obtained from 10 patients with unrelated diseases. They found four different patterns of immunoglobulin deposition. Immunoglobulins (Igs) were prominent in nuclei outlined by cytoplasmic staining and also were found at the disrupted internal elastic membrane in 7 of 15 patients. These patterns were not present in the 10 control temporal artery specimens obtained at autopsy. The authors suggested that the cytoplasmic staining for IgG, IgM, IgA, and the third component of complement resulted from phagocytosis of antibodies, complexed with antigen and complement within the vessel wall. They further suggested that the elastic pattern is consistent with two mechanisms: (1) elastic tissues may bind antibody specific to the tissue or (2) immune complexes may penetrate the endothelium and then lodge passively against the internal elastic membrane. These findings parallel those for other forms of vasculitis and suggest that antibodies participate in the pathogenesis of cranial arteritis. The immunoglobulins in these vessels may be antibodies to a component of the arterial wall, presumably elastin, or they may result from the deposition of circulating immune complexes.

Reyes et al. (1976) described a 67-year-old woman with a 5-month history of progressive, multiple neurologic deficits; an autopsy revealed viruslike particles associated with granulomatous angiitis of the central nervous system. The small parenchymal and leptomeningeal blood vessels of the brain and spinal cord were particularly affected. Electron microscopic studies of formalin-fixed brain disclosed intranuclear particles resembling herpesvirus. Although definitive proof cannot be established, Reyes and his collaborators suggest that some cases of granulomatous angiitis of the central nervous system may result from virus infection.

Malmvall and associates (1976) studied immunoglobulin levels in the serum of 36 patients (25 women and 11 men) with a mean age of 70 years. Twenty-four (15 women and 9 men) had histologic findings of cranial arteritis in temporal biopsy specimens. Complement levels were determined in 30 of the patients. A control group consisted of 39 hospitalized patients with a mean age of 74 years, none of whom had fever or elevated sedimentation rate and in whom there was no evidence of immunologic, malignant, or infectious diseases. In the group with GCA, the mean values of IgE, total complement, and complement factors C_3 and C_4 were statistically significantly higher than those in the control group. There was no increase of IgM concentration. The concentration of IgA was higher in men with GCA than in men in the control group, but no difference was seen among the women.

We surveyed 36 temporal artery biopsies obtained from 1975 through 1978

Table 11–1   Hematoxylin/eosin and immunofluorescence findings in 9 patients with cranial arteritis

Age (years)	H/E stain diagnosis	Immunofluorescence findings					
		IgG	IgA	IgM	C1q	C3	Fib
74	Temporal arteritis	Luminal	—	Luminal	—	—	Luminal
68	Giant cell arteritis	Internal elastic membrane	—	—	—	—	Diffuse
71	Consistent with temporal arteritis	Linear in smooth muscle	Minimum amount in smooth muscle	Minimum amount in smooth muscle	Linear in smooth muscle	—	Linear in smooth muscle
74	Giant cell arteritis	—	—	—	—	—	—
68	Giant cell arteritis	—	—	—	—	—	Luminal
69	Giant cell arteritis	—	—	—	—	—	—
62	Giant cell arteritis	—	—	—	—	—	—
78	Arteritis with intact elastica "not temporal"	Scattered in intima/media	—	Fine granular deposits at elastica	—	—	Deposits in all parts
76	Temporal arteritis	In media and intima	—	—	In media	In media	In media

Key to abbreviations: H/E, hematoxylin and eosin; IgA, IgG, IgM, immunoglobulins A, G, M; C1q, C3, complement components; Fib, fibrinogen.

in 21 women and 15 men. All were examined with standard pathologic techniques, hematoxylin and eosin staining (H&E), and immunofluorescent methods. In some selected cases, elastin stains were done. Immunofluorescent studies included IgG, IgA, IgM, C_{1q}, C_3, and fibrinogen. The results from nine representative patients with GCA are presented in Table 11–1. In addition, only H&E and immunofluorescent studies were done in eight other cases. Of these, half showed fibrinogen within the lumen and IgG on the internal elastic membrane.

The initial cells infiltrating the blood vessel wall have been described by Cid et al. (1989) as interdigitating reticulum cells. These appear at an early stage prior to the arrival of lymphocytes (primarily T cells). These thymic-derived lymphocytes express human lymphocyte antigen DR on their surfaces, suggesting local activation (Andersson et al., 1988). Macrophages act as antigen-presenting cells. The nature of the inciting antigen is unknown, although some evidence favors an inert substance such as elastin in the vessel wall.

These data suggest two possible immunologic mechanisms for vascular damage. One would involve deposition in the arterial wall of immunoglobulin and complement, and the second a cellular attack directed against antigens in the vessel wall.

CLINICAL ASPECTS

The symptomatology of the disease may be divided into nonspecific complaints of a generalized, systemic nature and specific complaints directly attributable to inflammation and distention of the temporal and other arteries (Table 11–2) (Wilkinson and Russell, 1972).

Table 11–2 Numerical incidence of involvement of the various arteries

Artery	No. of arteries described (i.e., their state was definitely ascertained at the time of autopsy) in the 12 patients	No. of arteries severely involved in the 12 patients	No. of arteries mildly involved in the 12 patients	"Incidence" of severe involvement (%)	"Incidence" of mild involvement (%)
Superficial temporal	22	22		100	
Vertebral	13	13		100	
Ophthalmic	17	13		76	
Posterior ciliary	12	9		75	
External carotid	15	7	4	47	27
Petrous and cavernous segments of internal carotid	8	3	5	38	62
Proximal central retinal	10	6	3	60	30
Distal central retinal	11	3	4	26	36
Cervical segment of internal carotid	8		2		25
Common carotid	14		2		14
Large arteries at base of brain	10		2		20
Small intracranial	10		1		20

Reproduced with permission from Wilkinson, I. M. and R. W. Russell (1972). Arteries of the head and neck in giant-cell arteritis. *Arch. Neurol.* 27:378–391.

Not all patients with GCA have headache but, when present, the headache is of high intensity, of a deep aching quality, throbbing in nature, and persistent. In addition to the aching and throbbing, there is often a burning component, unlike most other vascular headaches. The headache is slightly worse when the patient lies flat in bed, and is diminished in intensity by the upright or half-upright position. It is somewhat reduced in intensity by digital pressure on the common carotid artery on the affected side and is made worse by stooping over. Hyperalgesia of the scalp is present; because the distended arteries are extremely tender, any pressure greatly increases the pain.

Some patients may suffer pain on mastication, and in some this may be the initial symptom. Facial swelling and redness of the skin overlying the temporal arteries, with the addition of the burning component of pain, are usually noted after the onset of headache. Immediate relief from burning pain and headache may follow biopsy of the inflamed temporal artery, and it is assumed that this follows the interruption of the afferents for pain about the vessel.

Before the onset of full-blown GCA, pain often occurs in the teeth, ear, jaw, zygoma and nuchal region, and occiput. The distribution of these symptoms suggests primary involvement of other branches of the external carotid artery, notably the external and internal maxillary arteries. In addition, peripheral arteries may be involved, and claudication of one or more extremity may be a sign of the disease or its relapse (Halpin et al., 1988).

Ocular Symptoms

The presenting complaint may be of ocular origin. It has become evident that more than a third of patients with GCA are threatened with partial or even complete loss of vision. Diplopia and photophobia have been noted, ophthalmoscopic evidence of occlusion of the central retinal artery has been apparent in some cases, and complete loss of vision may occur secondary to anterior ischemic optic neuropathy. In addition, a variety of neuro-ophthalmologic complications, including cortical blindness and visual hallucinations, have been described by Mehler and Rabinowich (1988).

Cerebral Symptoms

Some patients have presented signs suggestive of cerebral damage and encephalitis during the acute stage of the illness. Mental sluggishness, dizziness, vomiting, dysarthria, delirium, and even coma have been described. Cases of GCA with involvement of intracranial arteries may occur. In addition to the usual constitutional symptoms of weight loss, anorexia, low-grade fever, and headache, these patients also demonstrate lethargy, depression, and cranial nerve palsies. Dementia may be an initial complaint and has been described as a sign of disease recurrence by Pascuzzi et al. (1989). Major stroke may occur.

Other Symptoms

In every case, signs and symptoms have been present that cannot plausibly be related to the sterile inflammation of the temporal arteries alone and are more suggestive of systemic arteritis. Prevalent symptoms and signs are weight loss, anorexia, general malaise, fever, sweating, and weakness. The weight loss may be profound, and the patient may be emaciated. This condition is probably secondary to anorexia, which, although in certain cases is a concomitant of the excruciating pain and headache, may antedate the onset of pain. Sweating is a common symptom.

Inconstant low-grade fever not associated with shaking chills is recorded in 70% of the cases. The average temperature is 37.8°C, although recordings as high as 39.5°C have been made.

Other complaints of a nonspecific nature are weakness, lassitude, malaise and "grippy feelings," and fatigue (occasionally to the point of prostration) (see Table 11–3).

PAINFUL OPHTHALMOPLEGIA (TOLOSA-HUNT SYNDROME)

Six cases of retro-orbital pain and involvement of the structures lying within the cavernous sinus and its wall were studied by Hunt et al. (1961). Pain may precede the ophthalmoplegia by several days, or may not occur until some time

Table 11–3 Presenting symptoms in 50 patients with GCA

Symptoms[a]	Patients (No.)	Percentage
Headache	45	90
Jaw pain	20	40
Generalized aching, stiffness	19	38
Visual complaints	17	34
Cerebral symptoms	15	30
Tender aching temporal arteries	12	24
Fatigue, malaise, insomnia	14	28
Neck and back pain	10	20

[a] Not mutually exclusive.

later. It is not a throbbing hemicrania occurring in paroxysms, but a steady pain behind the eye that is often described as "gnawing" or "boring." The defects are not confined to the third cranial nerve; the fourth, sixth, and first divisions of the fifth cranial nerve are also implicated. Periarterial sympathetic fibers and the optic nerve may be involved. The symptoms last for days or weeks. Spontaneous remissions occur, sometimes with residual motor or sensory deficit. Attacks recur at intervals of months or years. No systemic reaction occurs. The syndrome is presumably caused by an inflammatory lesion of the cavernous sinus. However, this syndrome can be caused by tumor, aneurysm, or syphilis and requires a complete evaluation (see Chapter 17). Tolosa (1954), of the Neurological Institute of Barcelona, published the report of a single case that met the preceding criteria. His patient expired after an exploratory operation, and autopsy showed an inflammatory lesion of the cavernous sinus. The syndrome, also called pseudotumor of the orbit, has been carefully considered, reviewed, and discussed by Ingalls (1953) and, as a "syndrome of the superior orbital fissure," it has been studied by Lakke (1962), who supplied an additional bibliography.

Occasional cases of Tolosa-Hunt syndrome still appear in the medical literature. Smith and Taxdal (1966) have emphasized the dramatic response of the syndrome to systemic corticosteroid therapy. Takeoka et al. (1978) have described angiographic findings in a patient with the Tolosa-Hunt syndrome. During the acute episode, at a time when a right third nerve paresis was present, there was evidence of irregular narrowing in the carotid siphon and incomplete opacification of the anterior cerebral artery when angiography was repeated. Ten days later, after treatment with corticosteroids, a remarkable improvement in the prior stenosis had occurred.

A few observations on the Tolosa-Hunt syndrome deserve emphasis. There is a close relationship between the oculomotor paresis that occurs and the angiographic abnormalities. In most patients pupillary function remains normal, with only 20% showing some pupillary involvement. The onset of the third-nerve paresis is rather rapid, but recovery is almost always complete when appropriate therapy is provided.

POLYMYALGIA RHEUMATICA

PMR does not have an "official" set of criteria for its diagnosis. It may represent a group of related disorders; however, it is generally recognized as a clinical syndrome characterized by the following:

1. Marked stiffness and pain in the muscles of the shoulder and pelvic girdles at night and especially in the morning. Improvement occurs throughout the day with activity.
2. Patients generally over age 50.
3. Absence of prominent symmetric synovitis.
4. Negative latex fixation test for rheumatoid arthritis.
5. Elevation of the erythrocyte sedimentation rate to 50 mm/hour (Westergren).
6. Prompt (usually within 48 hours) response to 15 mg/day of prednisone.

The etiologies of GCA and PMR are unknown and, although they are often found together, their precise relationship is controversial. They may represent stages in a common inflammatory process, and the clinical picture may reflect certain host responses to an inciting agent. PMR is a more commonly recognized clinical entity, and although it may precede the development of GCA, it also exists as a stable clinical syndrome for long periods without the development of clinically recognized vessel inflammation. Whether or not all PMR patients are at risk for the development of vessel inflammation is not clear; however, if one biopsies the temporal arteries of patients with PMR in the absence of any signs or symptoms of vessel inflammation, evidence of arteritis will be found in 10 to 15%. The significance of determining the presence or absence of vessel inflammation—that is, PMR versus PMR with GCA—has great prognostic and risk significance in the untreated patient; however, in the patient who is about to be started on therapy, the difference is more a matter of levels of steroid use than choices between therapeutic agents. The inability to detect occult vessel inflammation in a certain subgroup of patients with a clinical diagnosis of PMR does raise questions regarding the use of nonsteroidal anti-inflammatory agents in this disease, because such agents do not eliminate the possibility of blindness or stroke.

TREATMENT OF GCA AND PMR

Short-Term and Long-Term Goals

GCA can be considered as a semiacute inflammatory disease that demands rapid treatment. On occasion, if vision is threatened, treatment should be considered as a medical emergency. In the short term, the goal is to relieve the patient's complaints. Longer term goals are to suppress the disease sufficiently using the least amount of medication, presuming that the illness will eventually prove self-limiting and will "burn out."

Indications for hospitalization include rapid progression of complaints, especially if vision is threatened. Usually patients with GCA are easily managed on an outpatient basis. The temporal artery biopsies are well suited to an outpatient surgical procedure. Long-term management is almost always in the outpatient department.

Nonpharmacologic Measures

A graduated physical therapy program should be instituted for patients with PMR, particularly emphasizing range of motion, exercise, heat, and hot packs. After the diagnosis has been made and corticosteroids have been begun, similar programs may be useful for patients with GCA.

Drug Therapy

Corticosteroids should be used promptly in the therapy of GCA and PMR. They should be begun as soon as the diagnosis is made—if necessary, before a temporal artery biopsy. The corticosteroids control the progress of the arteritis, reducing symptoms and preventing the development of ocular complications. Blindness or defects in vision do not always correlate with the severity of the cranial arteritis; thus, all patients should be treated promptly. In GCA the treatment is usually initiated with 40 to 60 mg of prednisone daily. Thereafter, this dose may be rapidly tapered to a maintenance level, depending on the relief of symptoms and the decline in the sedimentation rate toward normal. In PMR, prednisone may be started at a dosage of 15 mg given as a single dose in the morning. The duration of therapy is uncertain. It may be necessary to continue corticosteroids for months or even years, although eventually it is possible to discontinue treatment in almost all patients.

Absence of response to prednisone within 5 to 7 days is unusual and indicates the need for a more comprehensive evaluation of the presenting complaints. In PMR the response usually, but not invariably, occurs within the first 24 to 72 hours.

Alternate-day corticosteroid therapy is not advisable in GCA, at least initially, because systemic symptoms will not be controlled by the drug when used in this manner (Hunder et al., 1975). It is advisable to use a single morning dose of prednisone to minimize the additional side effects associated with split-dose regimens, although the latter may be useful in the initial treatment program when the maximum effect of the drug is desired.

If treatment is stopped in less than 2 years, about 20% of patients with GCA will relapse. As the dose of steroids is being tapered in patients with GCA, mild to moderate symptoms of PMR sometimes become evident. Generally, this does not constitute an indication to increase the prednisone levels unless there is significant elevation of the sedimentation rate. The sedimentation rate should be checked for several months after the cessation of therapy, and the physician should be aware of possible relapses at extended intervals. We recently observed a relapse of PMR after a 2-year asymptomatic, steroid-free interval and the development of a vasculitic lesion in another patient previously treated for PMR for 18 months, again with a 2-year drug-free interval. These examples illustrate the continued risk of patients with this disease and point out the problems in considering any individual patient as "cured."

In long-term treatment of PMR, it may be possible to manage the patient on a low maintenance steroid dose, in the range of 1 to 5 mg/day. If this is done, the clinician should be alert to the appearance of GCA despite the low-dose steroid therapy; involvement of the ophthalmic artery, producing blindness, is a particular concern in this situation.

It is known that other anti-inflammatory drugs, such as the nonsteroidals, are capable of lowering the sedimentation rate and relieving some of the constitutional symptoms of PMR. There are those who argue for their use in PMR patients without signs or symptoms of GCA. One of the authors had such a patient referred to him who developed sudden, irreversible monocular blindness while on nonsteroidal anti-inflammatory agents for PMR. Clearly, these agents do *not* protect patients from such serious complications and we do not advocate their use in the initial management of PMR or GCA. They may have a role in the later therapy of patients when corticosteroids have been tapered to a low level and the patient experiences symptoms of a musculoskeletal nature associated with the steroid discontinuation. In all cases the physician must be aware of the potential for relapse, and the use of the nonsteroidal anti-inflammatory agents in this group of patients may mask the sedimentation rate elevation that accompanies a relapse of either GCA or PMR.

Finally, it is important to realize that in every series of patients there are those who, in the process of tapering of corticosteroids, eventually develop a polyarthritis that develops into classic rheumatoid arthritis. Such patients may or may not have positive latex fixation tests. We have observed several patients who have had biopsy-proven GCA and subsequently developed seropositive rheumatoid disease.

Complications of Treatment

The complications are those of treatment with corticosteroids. In a personal series of patients with GCA, about 40% developed a moon face–Cushingoid appearance, 15% had symptomatic vertebral compression fractures, and 10% had demonstrable proximal muscle weakness.

Some diabetic patients will note increased insulin requirements. The physician must be alert to rapid development of cataracts, exacerbation of peptic ulcers, avascular necrosis of bone, and reappearance of pulmonary infection, especially tuberculosis, which may occur in treating patients with GCA with prednisone.

SUMMARY

Giant cell arteritis and polymyalgia rheumatica may represent different phases of the same disease. Most patients will present with signs and symptoms generally associated with inflammation (anorexia, prostration, fever, sweats, weight loss, and leukocytosis) and, in GCA, heat, swelling, tenderness, redness, and pain locally over the artery. GCA probably represents an example of immunologic vasculitis associated with the deposition of immune complexes within the walls of the affected blood vessels or a cell-mediated attack producing localized vascular injury and inflammation.

Prompt therapy with corticosteroids is indicated in all patients with GCA and, we believe, in PMR. Long-term follow-up is indicated in both diseases, and the possibility of relapse must be kept in mind, even several years after the discontinuation of corticosteroids.

REFERENCES

Andersson, R., G. Hansson, T. Söderström et al. (1988). HLA-DR expression in the vascular lesion and circulating and lymphocytes of patients with giant cell arteritis. *Clin. Exp. Immunol. 73*:82–87.

Cid, M.C., E. Campo, G. Ercilla et al. (1989). Immunohistochemical analysis of lymphoid and macrophage cell subsets and their immunologic activation markers in temporal arteritis. *Arthritis Rheum. 32*:884–893.

Clompi, M.L., G. Marotta, L. Puccetti et al. (1988). Behavior of von Willebrand factor antigen in follow-up of polymyalgia/giant cell arteritis. *Scand. J. Rheumatol. 17*: 491–495.

Halpin, D.P., K.T. Moran, and E.R. Jewell (1988). Arm ischemia secondary to giant cell arteritis. *J. Vasc. Surg. 4*:381–384.

Hunder, G.G., D.A. Bloch, B.A. Michel et al. (1990). The American College of Rheumatology 1990 criteria for the classification of giant cell arteritis. *Arthritis Rheum. 33*:1122–1128.

Hunder, G.G., S.G. Sheps, G.L. Allen et al. (1975). Daily and alternate-day corticosteroid regimens in the treatment of giant-cell arteritis: Comparison in a prospective study. *Ann. Intern. Med. 82*:613–618.

Hunt, W.E., J.N. Meagher, H.E. LeFever, and W. Zeman (1961). Painful ophthalmoplegia. Its relation to indolent inflammation of the cavernous sinus. *Neurology 11*:56.

Huston, K.A., G.G. Hunder, J.T. Lie et al. (1978). Temporal arteritis: A 25 year epidemiologic, clinical and pathologic study. *Ann. Intern. Med. 88*:162–167.

Ingalls, R.G. (1953). *Tumors of the Orbit.* Charles C. Thomas, Springfield, IL.

Jundt, J.W. and D. Mock (1991). Temporal arteritis with normal sedimentation rates presenting as occipital neuralgia. *Arthritis Rheum. 34*:217–219.

Klein, R.G., R.J. Campbell, G. Hunder, and J. Carney (1976). Skip lesions in temporal arteritis. *Proc. Mayo Clin. 51*:504–510.

Kuwabara, T. and R. Reinecke (1970). Temporal arteritis. *Arch. Ophthalmol. 83*: 692–697.

Lakke, J.P.W.F. (1962). The superior orbital fissure syndrome caused by local pachymeningitis, with a case report. *Arch. Neurol. 7*:289.

Liang, G.C., P. Simkin, and M. Mannik (1974). Immunoglobulins in temporal arteritis. *Ann. Intern. Med. 81*:19–23.

Lie, J.T. (1990). Illustrated histopathologic classification criteria for selected vasculitic syndromes. *Arthritis Rheum. 33*:1074–1087.

Lie, J.T., A.L. Brown, Jr., and E.T. Carter (1970). Spectrum of aging changes in temporal arteries. *Arch. Pathol. 90:*278–285.

Malmvall, B., B. Bengtsson, B. Kaijser et al. (1976). Serum levels of immunoglobulin and complement in giant cell arteritis. *JAMA 236:*1876–1878.

Mehler, M.F. and L. Rabinowich (1988). The clinical neurophthalmologic spectrum of temporal arteritis. *Am. J. Med. 85:*839–844.

Nusinow, S.R., A.B. Federici, T.S. Zimmerman, and J.G. Curd (1984). Increased von Willebrand factor antigen in the plasma of patients with vasculitis. *Arthritis Rheum. 27:*1405–1410.

Pascuzzi, R.M., K.L. Roos, and D.E. Thomas, Jr. (1989). Mental status abnormalities in temporal arteritis: A treatable cause of dementia in the elderly. *Arthritis Rheum. 32:*1308–1311.

Persellin, S.T., T.M. Daniels, L.J. Rings et al. (1985). Factor VIII-von Willebrand factor in giant cell arteritis and polymyalgia rheumatica. *Mayo Clin. Proc. 60:*457–462.

Reyes, M.G., R. Fresco, S. Chokroverty, and E. Salud (1976). Virus-like particles in granulomatous angitis of the central nervous system. *Neurology 26:*797–799.

Small, P. and M.L. Brisson (1991). Wegener's granulomatosis presenting as temporal arteritis. *Arthritis Rheum. 34:*220–223.

Smith, J.L. and D.J.R. Taxdal (1966). Painful ophthalmoplegia: The Tolosa-Hunt syndrome. *Am. J. Ophthalmol. 61:*1466–1472.

Takeoka, T., F. Gotoh, Y. Fukuuchi, and Y. Inagaki (1978). Tolosa-Hunt syndrome. *Arch. Neurol. 35:*219–223.

Tolosa, E. (1954). Periarteritic lesions of carotid siphon with clinical features of carotid infra-clinoidal aneurysm. *J. Neurol. Neurosurg. Psychiatry 17:*300.

Wilkinson, I.M. and R.W. Russell (1972). Arteries of the head and neck in giant-cell arteritis. *Arch. Neurol. 27:*378–391.

Wong, R.L. and J.H. Korn (1986). Temporal arteritis without an elevated sedimentation rate. *Am. J. Med. 80:*959–964.

SUGGESTED READINGS

Cooke, W.T., P.C.P. Cloake, A.D.T. Govan, and J.C. Colbeck (1946). Temporal arteritis: A generalized vascular disease. *Q. J. Med. 15:*47.

Crompton, M.R. (1959). The visual changes in temporal (giant-celled) arteritis. *Brain 82:*377–390.

Enzmann, D. and W.R. Scott (1977). Intracranial involvement of giant cell arteritis. *Neurology 27:*794–797.

Gocke, D.J., C. Morgan, M. Lockshin et al. (1970). Association between polyarteritis and Australia antigen. *Lancet 2:*1149–1153.

Heptinstall, R.H., K.A. Porter, and H. Barkely (1954). Giant cell (temporal) arteritis. *J. Pathol. Bacteriol. 67:*507–519.

Hollenhorst, R.W., J.R. Brown, H.P. Wagener, and R.M. Shick (1960). Neurologic aspects of temporal arteritis. *Neurology 10:*490.

Horton, B.T. and T.B. Magath (1937). Arteritis of temporal vessels; report of seven cases. *Proc. Mayo Clin. 12:*548.

Russell, R.W. (1959). Giant cell arteritis; a review of thirty-five cases. *Q. J. Med. 28:*471–489.

Scott, T. and E.S. Maxwell (1941). Temporal arteritis; a case report. *Int. Clin. 2:*220–222.

12

Major Vascular Diseases and Headache

DONALD J. DALESSIO

Headache is a common complaint of patients with cerebrovascular disease. It is consistently associated with acute events characterized by vessel rupture and bleeding. It may not be present when thrombosis is present; for example, even with a major cerebral infarction patients rarely complain of pain, another striking example of the insensitivity of the brain parenchyma to ischemia.

ANATOMIC CONSIDERATIONS

The cerebral arterial tree in humans, unlike that of many other organs, has no hilum from which the vessels plunge into the body of the structure. On the contrary, the internal carotid and vertebral arteries are united by the circle of Willis and its six large branches, which encircle the globoid hemispheres at the base of the brain. These six great trunks then divide into branches. A few enter the basal ganglia and choroid plexus, but for the most part they spread themselves like a net in finer and finer branches over the surface of the cortex. Smaller arteries at innumerable points dive deeply into the cortical and subcortical tissues where, through their capillaries, they anastomose with one another and with others coming through the brain substance from the opposite surface of the hemisphere.

The cerebral veins are divided into two groups, the internal and the external, with incomplete anastomoses between them. The internal group drains through the great cerebral vein of Galen, running back directly over the pineal body. The external veins emanate from the region of the insula. Because with growth there is anterior displacement of the frontal lobe and posterior development of the main mass of the hemispheres, the direction of the terminal portion of the great veins is altered; the anterior veins are thus directed posteriorly and the posterior veins course obliquely and anteriorly as they pass to the superior sagittal sinus. The large venous sinuses drain into channels at the base of the skull. The blood then flows from the cranial cavity like fluid from a flask with a gradually tapering neck.

SUBARACHNOID HEMORRHAGE

Genesis of Cerebral Aneurysm

The main cerebral blood supply derives from the basilar and internal carotid arteries, meeting in the polygonal arrangement known as the circle of Willis. The internal carotid arteries branch abruptly to give rise to the anterior cerebral and middle cerebral vessels, and a further abrupt branching, the anterior commissure, connects two of these, the anterior cerebrals. The paired vertebrals join to form the basilar, which forks at its anterior end into the posterior cerebrals, and these last are connected with the rest of the "circle" by still another abrupt bifurcation, the posterior commissures, which join the internal carotid. A rapidly moving volume of blood is thus forced through a highly angular system of arteries.

The vessels composing the circle of Willis are characterized by a high frequency of aneurysm, particularly at or near the points of bifurcation. A major factor in the occurrence of such aneurysm is congenital weakness of the artery walls, and this appears to be closely related to the angularity of the circle. The relation of the architecture of the circle of Willis to the incidence of aneurysm is shown in Figures 12–1 and 12–2.

Most saccular aneurysms are located on the anterior aspects of the circle of Willis. The most common sites include the following:

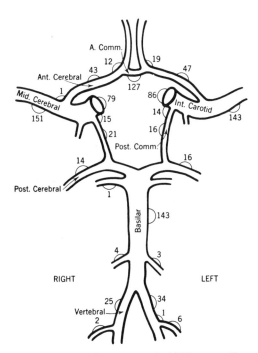

Figure 12–1. Location of intracranial aneurysms in 1023 cases. (Reproduced with permission from McDonald, C. and M. Korb (1939). Intracranial aneurysms. *Arch. Neurol. Psychiatry 42*: 289–307.)

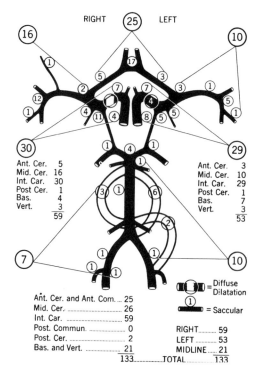

Figure 12–2. Arteries involved in 133 aneurysms. There were 108 patients, but in 16 of these the aneurysms were multiple. The total number of aneurysms for each main area is shown in each of the large circles near the outer borders. (Reproduced by permission from Dandy, W.E. (1944). *Intracranial Artery Aneurysms.* Comstock Publishing, Ithaca, NY.)

1. Adjacent to the anterior communicating artery
2. At the origin of the posterior communicating artery
3. At the bifurcation of the internal carotid into the middle and anterior cerebral arteries
4. At the first bifurcation of the middle cerebral artery

In 20 to 30% of cases, these may be multiple aneurysms.

Although most aneurysms are saccular, they vary greatly in form. Rarely, giant aneurysms are seen.

Qualities and Temporal Features of the Headache Associated with Subarachnoid Hemorrhage

Headache is the most common symptom of subarachnoid hemorrhage and occurs in almost every conscious patient. It is usually of very high intensity and of sudden onset. It is often described as "something snapping inside the head," followed by an intense throbbing ache. The ache at the start is commonly located in the occipital region and then radiates down the neck and back. Less commonly, it is located first in the frontal region, bilaterally or unilaterally, in the temporal region, at the vertex, or deep in the eye, but such headache soon radiates into the occipital region. When associated with neck rigidity, the headache is worsened by flexure of the neck.

In more than half of patients, the attack of sudden intense pain is accompanied by vomiting and drowsiness, neck rigidity, and loss of consciousness. Convulsions occur after the onset of headache in approximately 10 to 15% of patients. In 10% there are prodromes lasting a few hours to several days, such as low-intensity frontal or occipital headache, pain in the eye, pain in the back of the neck, backache, or pain in the hamstring muscles. Occasionally the severe headache is preceded by vertigo, photophobia, diplopia, and rarely vomiting.

The high-intensity headache following subarachnoid hemorrhage persists with little modification for approximately 1 week from its onset, with subsequent complete elimination of pain within 2 months. Sustained, chronic, or recurrent headache persisting longer than 2 months following rupture of intracranial aneurysm with subarachnoid hemorrhage is rare in patients who have not had headaches before the accident.

The initial severe headache associated with sudden hemorrhage into the subarachnoid space about the base of the brain is probably due to traction, displacement, distention, and rupture of pain-sensitive blood vessels and the pia arachnoid. The headache of several days' duration is probably secondary to a sterile inflammatory reaction about the blood vessels and meninges.

Other Presentations of Aneurysms

Full-blown subarachnoid hemorrhages are difficult to miss. Sometimes, however, there are "minibleeds" as only a few cubic centimeters of blood leak from an aneurysm whose point of rupture is partially sealed by thrombus. The occurrence of such aneurysmal leaks is uncommonly recognized. The headaches produced by such leaks may be abrupt and severe, although not as prostrating as those from larger hemorrhages. Often they are occipital and, like those from larger hemorrhages, are worsened by movement or jarring. They last a shorter time than the headaches of larger hemorrhages—sometimes for only hours, sometimes for a day or two. If such minibleeds occur in patients who are chronic headache sufferers, they may be dismissed as "an unusually severe migraine."

Some authors have referred to minibleeds as sentinel headaches. Day and Raskin (1986) have also described "thunderclap" headache in a patient whose computerized tomography (CT) scan and lumbar puncture were normal, but who was found to have an unruptured cerebral aneurysm by subsequent study. In a more recent prospective study of thunderclap headache, Harling et al. (1989) described 14 of 49 patients presenting to a Regional Neurosurgical Unit with sudden headache, suggestive of subarachnoid hemorrhage, who had normal cerebrospinal fluid and a normal CT scan. It did not prove possible, on clinical grounds alone, to distinguish these 14 patients from those who had bled. The patients were followed for a minimum of 18 months. Only one had no further headache, four had musculoskeletal pain, five psychogenic pain, and four migraine-type symptoms. None went on to have an unequivocal subarachnoid hemorrhage. The authors concluded that angiography cannot be justified in patients with thunderclap headache.

Fewer than 10% of aneurysms present in ways other than bleeding (Sahs et al., 1969). Most of these aneurysms are at the junction of the internal carotid and posterior communicating arteries. This location affords the aneurysm the opportunity of pressing either on the oculomotor nerve, producing diplopia, squint, ptosis, and/or pupillary dilation, or on the first division of the trigeminal nerve, producing ipsilateral orbitofrontal pain. Other "prerupture presentations" of aneurysms, even more uncommon, include visual disturbances from involvement of the ophthalmic circulation by aneurysms of the ophthalmic or anterior communicating arteries and hemiparesis or seizures due to pressure on the cerebral cortex from middle cerebral artery aneurysms.

Diagnosis of Aneurysms

If aneurysm rupture is suspected, a CT scan of the head should be done. In the majority of cases, the diagnosis of subarachnoid hemorrhage can be made with the unenhanced scan, which will demonstrate blood in the ventricles and/or basal cisterns. Acute hydrocephalus is often present as well. One may then decide whether or not to use lumbar puncture, which may not be necessary. If no lesions are seen, contrast medium may be given to complete the CT examination. If the CT scan is negative for intracranial blood and aneurysm is still suspected, lumbar puncture should be done.

Currently arteriography is usually done early in the course, to establish the anatomy and to help plan the surgery. All four vessels should be visualized; it is not enough to demonstrate the aneurysm responsible for the hemorrhage because multiple aneurysms may be present. Magnetic resonance imaging angiography (MRA) is becoming increasingly useful to diagnose aneurysm. The false-negative rate is still unknown.

Treatment

The modern treatment of subarachnoid hemorrhage is an unsettled and continuously changing issue, because rebleeding may occur throughout the life of the patient. The greatest risk to the patient is in the month after the initial bleeding episode.

Current therapy of the acute episode is aggressive, emphasizing early evaluation and operation, management of rebleeding, and amelioration of vasospasm. Intensive monitoring of the patient's status is essential, with special attention to relief of headache, anxiety, agitation, and straining. Hunt and Kosnik (1974) have developed a classification of patients with aneurysms based on extensive clinical experience (see Table 12–1). All authors agree that operation should be done rapidly on patients in Grades 0 through II. Many neurosurgeons now believe that the best management of aneurysmal rupture is one that emphasizes early operative intervention in almost all cases (Ljunggren et al., 1982).

In a recent randomized double-blind, placebo-controlled study, nimodipine treatment was associated with a significant reduction in delayed ischemic deteri-

Table 12-1 Classification of patients with intracranial aneurysms according to surgical risk

Grade	Criteria[a]
0	Unruptured aneurysm
I	Asymptomatic, or minimal headache and slight nuchal rigidity
IA	No acute meningeal or brain reaction, but with fixed neurologic deficit
II	Moderate to severe headache, nuchal rigidity, no neurologic deficit other than cranial nerve palsy
III	Drowsiness, confusion, or mild focal deficit
IV	Stupor, moderate to severe hemiparesis, possibly early decerebrate rigidity and vegetative disturbances
V	Deep coma, decerebrate rigidity, moribund appearance

[a] Serious systemic disease, such as hypertension, diabetes, severe artheroslerosis, chronic pulmonary disease, or severe intracranial arterial spasm seen on arterography, results in placement of the patient in the next less favorable grade.

oration (Pickard et al., 1989). Generally the drug is begun within 96 hours of the hemorrhage and continued for 21 days (Allen et al., 1983). The recommended dosage regimen is 60 mg every 4 hours in Hunt grade I through III patients (Table 12-1). The prevention of clot lysis using ε-aminocaproic acid remains a controversial issue.

Prognosis of Aneurysms

Jane et al. (1977) have studied the natural history of intracranial aneurysms with rebleeding rates during acute and long-term periods of observation. For a patient with an anterior communicating aneurysm seen on day 1, the chance that he or she will rebleed within the first day is approximately 50%. For posterior communicating aneurysms, the expected chance of rebleeding on the first day is 60%. Thereafter, the rate rapidly diminishes for both aneurysms. By day 30, the chance of rebleeding during the first 6 months has dropped to less than 10%. The authors have also followed a group of 213 patients for up to 21 years; of these, 54 had another bleeding episode during the first 10 years, and another 7 patients rebled between the 10th and 20th years. To summarize, the first decade following subarachnoid hemorrhage is characterized by rebleeding episodes at the rate of approximately 3% per year. Subsequent rebleeding occurs at the rate of 2% per year. In 67% of subsequent hemorrhages, death occurs. Jane and his colleagues made the point that subarachnoid hemorrhage secondary to aneurysms should be considered as a chronic disease with a "relentless rate of rebleeding."

Sahs and his colleagues (1984) have undertaken a long-term follow-up study of patients with subarachnoid hemorrhage seen between 1958 and 1965 and treated "conservatively," or without surgery. Of 568 cases, 378 were dead (66.5%) at the time of the survey in 1981-82. Of the deceased, 40% had expired within 6 months of hemorrhage. Those with multiple aneurysms did not differ significantly from those with a single lesion. Sahs estimates the rebleeding rates, after 6 months from the initial ictus, as 2.2%/year for the first 9.5 years and 0.86%/year for the second decade.

PARENCHYMATOUS CEREBRAL HEMORRHAGE

Although it is theoretically possible for hemorrhage in the brain parenchyma to occur without pain, this almost never happens. Cerebral (or cerebellar) hemispheric bleeding of any significant magnitude is accompanied by excruciating headache and, usually, by disturbance of consciousness. The venerable term "apoplexy," implying sudden paralysis with total or partial loss of consciousness and sensation, is most appropriate in this situation. Usually the intrahemispheric blood distends the brain, producing traction on pain-sensitive structures, and frequently it ruptures into the subarachnoid space, producing typical signs and symptoms associated with subarachnoid bleeding.

Certain signs and symptoms are common to all forms of intracranial bleeding. These include progressive headache, stiffness of the neck, disturbances of consciousness, nausea, and vomiting. Transient or progressive neurologic signs and/or seizures should be anticipated. Hypertension of any etiology is by far the most frequent cause of parenchymatous cerebral hemorrhage. The rupture may occur in an artery or cerebral vein, but the most common source of bleeding is from an arteriole that has degenerated in relation to the hypertensive atherosclerotic process. Persistent elevation of the blood pressure, particularly in acute situations of malignant hypertension, will produce necrosis of the smooth muscle and elastic laminae of the vessel wall, evoking Charcot–Bouchard aneurysms. These frequently rupture and are a common source of parenchymatous hemorrhage and brain destruction. These microaneurysms are distributed particularly in the lenticulostriate branches of the middle cerebral arteries that supply the internal capsule and the basal ganglia. They also occur in the brainstem, especially in the pons. Charcot–Bouchard aneurysms may be identified with arteriographic techniques or a magnified CT scan, or by MRI angiography.

Thus, parenchymatous cerebral hemorrhage usually occurs in the region of the internal capsule or the basal ganglia and pons. Approximately one fifth occur in the brainstem and cerebellum. The remainder are found in the frontal and occipital lobes.

Work-up of the patient with intracranial hemorrhage should proceed rapidly. A CT or MRI scan should be done as an emergency procedure, particularly if acute cerebellar hemorrhage is suspected, in which case surgery may be life saving. If there is suspicion of increased intracranial pressure, lumbar puncture should be delayed unless infection, such as bacterial meningitis, is a possibility. Spinal puncture may hasten herniation. At times, particularly if anticoagulants are to be used, a careful lumbar puncture is necessary.

Most of these patients have pre-existing hypertension, and many will have striking elevation of the blood pressure during the cerebral hemorrhage. Because there is evidence that elevated blood pressure will promote further hemorrhage and increasing cerebral edema, the hypertension should be treated.

HEADACHE AND ARTERIOVENOUS MALFORMATIONS

Arteriovenous malformations (AVMs) are uncommon. They account for only about 6% of subarachnoid hemorrhages. At least a third of all diagnosed AVMs do not bleed but present instead as focal or generalized epilepsy or with focal deficits such as hemiparesis. Walker (1956) has found that the incidence of chronic headaches in people with AVMs is not greater than that in the general population. Despite this study, which should de-emphasize any relationship between the two, a formidable mythology has grown up to connect AVMs with chronic headaches (Lees, 1962).

It has frequently been stated that the occurrence of migraine headaches persistently localized to the same side of the head should arouse suspicion of an underlying AVM. This has led to the infliction of angiography on many hapless patients who have lacked the versatility to have alternating hemicrania. In the definitive study by Blend and Bull (1967), however, it was found that no patient with migraine alone, even if persistently localized, had an abnormal angiogram; of those patients with migraine and abnormal angiograms, all were found to have persistently abnormal signs on neurologic examination, or bruits, seizures, or a history of subarachnoid hemorrhage. Thus, even the most persistently localized migraine does not warrant angiography unless there are clear-cut neurologic abnormalities.

AVMs may produce small leaks on multiple occasions, and headaches due to these leaks may occur; they are similar to those of leaking aneurysms. Rarely, blood from these multiple leaks organizes within the subarachnoid space of the basal cisterns, leading to a communicating hydrocephalus. The headache produced by the hydrocephalus is that of increased intracranial pressure—a dull, diffuse ache, more likely to be present in the morning, worse in the head-down position, and increasing over weeks and months.

HEADACHE AND OCCLUSIVE DISEASE, INCLUDING TRANSIENT ISCHEMIC ATTACKS

Medina and colleagues (1975) have observed that patients with transient ischemic attacks (TIAs) may describe headache in an incidence ranging from 25 to 40%. Often the head pain occurs in association with neurologic symptoms, or with their resolution. Sometimes headache is appreciated as a harbinger of the TIA. The pain is usually throbbing and brief, and may be accentuated by effort or position. The pain locale is variable, but headache associated with carotid TIAs is generally frontal, and that associated with vertebrobasilar TIAs is often occipital, as one would predict.

Edmeads (1979) has done studies of regional cerebral blood flow during TIAs in patients with and without headaches. No apparent differences that would explain the appearance of headache in some and not in others can be found in these subjects.

Leviton et al. (1975) have described a severe ipsilateral headache following closely on carotid endarterectomy. This complication may occur in those subject to migraine before surgery. This postendarterectomy hemicranial pain is indistinguishable from migraine. It often appears 36 to 72 hours after surgery and is typically described as intense and pounding. Generally, this is a benign and self-limiting phenomenon, perhaps related to a sudden increase in blood flow through a system disposed to low-pressure flow.

Portenoy et al. (1984) reported prospectively on 215 patients with cerebrovascular events. In their study, 34% of patients able to respond complained of headache. Typically the headache was throbbing and lateralized, usually to the side of the ischemia. Most headaches (60%) started prior to the event, beginning either gradually or abruptly. Headache was most frequently associated with parenchymal hemorrhage (57%), then TIA (36%), bland infarct (29%), and lacunar infarct (17%). Headache will usually not distinguish the lesion type or its location.

Nichols et al. (1990) described focal headache produced by balloon inflation of the internal carotid and middle cerebral arteries. The authors reported on 18 patients who underwent balloon inflation in the distal internal carotid artery and middle cerebral artery stem during embolization therapy for intracerebral arteriovenous malformations. Eleven patients had reproducible patterns of headache during balloon inflation. Inflation in the proximal middle cerebral artery stem produced pain primarily in the ipsilateral temple, that in the middle of the middle cerebral artery stem produced pain referred primarily retro-orbitally, and inflation in the distal middle cerebral artery stem produced pain referred primarily to the forehead. Experimental studies have demonstrated similar patterns of referred pain. The fact that these areas of referred pain are so reproducible is of potentially great clinical importance in the approach to management of patients with cerebrovascular disease and migraine.

HEADACHE AND VENOUS OCCLUSION

Thrombosis of the large intracranial venous sinuses, notably the lateral and sigmoid sinuses, may cause increased intracranial pressure with papilledema and no focal signs, mimicking the "pseudotumor cerebri" syndrome. The headache so produced is that of increased intracranial pressure. In the past the common causes were contiguous pyogenic infection, trauma, dehydration, cachexia, and the puerperium; recently, oral contraceptives have been recognized as an important cause.

Thrombosis of the superior sagittal sinus may produce headache from increased intracranial pressure, but this usually also produces hemorrhagic cerebral infarction with focal neurologic deficits, which give a clue to the diagnosis. Fronto-orbital pain may arise from involvement of the fifth nerve in cavernous sinus thrombosis, but the associated chemosis and oculomotor palsies usually make the diagnosis evident.

SPONTANEOUS INTERNAL CAROTID DISSECTION

Spontaneous internal carotid artery dissection is an uncommon but not altogether rare cause of headache and acute neurologic deficits in younger patients (Fisher, 1982; Mokri, 1990). Headache, the most common symptom, is often unilateral and located in the orbital, periorbital, and frontal regions. Often these patients have neck pain as well. The pain is usually moderate to severe and steady or throbbing in nature. A bruit or Horner syndrome is often seen. Focal cerebral symptoms (TIA or stroke) can precede the headache but frequently follow it by up to 2 weeks. These symptoms are seen in 60 to 75% of cases, and when present point to a vascular etiology for the headache. When absent, the presence of Horner syndrome, bruit, dysgeusia, and neck pain should suggest a diagnosis that can be confirmed by arteriography or MRI (Biousse et al., 1991; Cox et al., 1991; Fisher, 1982; Mokri, 1990). The physician should systematically look for internal carotid artery dissection in patients with any of the following: painful Horner syndrome, head pain preceding ischemic symptoms, or unilateral, severe, persistent neck pain of sudden onset, with or without headache. Biousse et al. (1991) have shown that cephalic pain is a frequent symptom of dissection (75%), is often inaugural (60%), and is usually located on the side of the dissection (76%).

TRANSIENT MIGRAINE ACCOMPANIMENTS—VASCULAR OR NOT?

We owe interest in this topic particularly to the efforts of Fisher (1968, 1980), whose observations deserve careful review and consideration. His patients presented with episodic transient visual and other neurologic symptoms, but when the conditions were investigated, embolic phenomena and occlusive vascular disease could not be demonstrated. Fisher believes, therefore, that these episodes are migrainous accompaniments of later adult life, occurring without headache—hence the term "transient migrainous accompaniments" (TMAs).

A reliable sign of migrainous paresthesias is the "march" of numbness as it gradually spreads over the face or fingers and hands and migrates from face to limb or vice versa, or crosses to the face and hand on the opposite side. This evolution may last for 30 minutes, commonly 15 to 25 minutes. This gradual spread is unusual in thrombotic or embolic cerebrovascular disease. Pure sensory stroke resulting from thalamic ischemia is the only stroke whose evolution may resemble the typical march of migraine paresthesias, but this occurs only rarely. Conversely, the march of sensory seizures is much more rapid, being measured in seconds.

The occurrence of two or more episodes, particularly if they closely resemble one another, is important in the diagnosis. This history helps to exclude cerebral embolism, which is a prime diagnostic possibility when there is only one attack. The history of a similar spell as long as 20 to 30 years before is also evidence for migraine. An identical vascular spell or series of spells, occurring years ago, also favors migraine over thrombotic vascular disease. The time between episodes varies widely. The duration of the episode may also be of importance in the diagnosis. Migrainous episodes classically last 15 to 20 minutes or longer, whereas most TIAs last less than 15 minutes.

Other points of value in the diagnosis of transient migraine equivalents are the benign nature of the spell in retrospect and the rarity of permanent sequelae. Repeated good recovery from what appears initially to be a threatening situation is evidence for migraine. In Fisher's series, there were no permanent deficits. Fisher further stressed the importance of a normal arteriogram and the absence of a source of emboli as prerequisites for establishing the diagnosis of TMA. Where atherosclerotic plaque and migraine coexist, the diagnosis becomes more difficult and the judgment depends on the experience and expertise of the clinician.

Murphey (1973) has described his own experiences with TIA. He noted that visual TIAs are usually unilateral and that they may be obliterated by closing the eye and presumably altering retinal arterial flow. This is in contrast with migrainous scotomata, which are often bilateral, sometimes homonymous, related to occipital cortical ischemia, and persist with eye closure.

MIGRAINE AND STROKE

Since the last edition of this book, episodic reports linking migraine and stroke have continued to appear in the literature, often as isolated cases (Bernsen et al., 1990; Lindboe et al., 1989). In Lindboe's case, for example, a 50-year-old woman with migraine was admitted to the hospital shortly after having abruptly developed hemiparesis. CT scan revealed infarction in the territory of the right middle cerebral artery. Death ensued after 3 days as a result of cerebral edema with herniation. Autopsy revealed no pathologic findings in the heart or in the extra- or intracranial arteries. The authors suggested that the fatal stroke may have resulted from arterial spasm caused by ergotamine overdosage and possibly complicated by thrombosis.

Sacquegna et al. (1989) reported on 61 consecutive patients, 40 years old or less, who were hospitalized for cerebral infarction between 1977 and 1985. Evaluation included CT brain scan, arteriography, echocardiography, and blood tests. A probably migrainous infarction was diagnosed in six patients (10%) (all women with a history of migraine) who survived the initial stroke and were followed up for an average of 4 years. In five patients the stroke occurred during an attack of migraine without aura and in one patient during an attack of migraine with aura. The site of infarction was invariably the occipital lobe. During the follow-up, no subject had a further stroke. All six women had a permanent hemianopic deficit.

Frequin et al. (1991) described a 25-year-old male with recurrent prolonged episodes of life-threatening coma varying from 3 to 10 days, with slow clinical recovery. They found evidence for ischemic dysfunction of the brainstem as a result of severe spasm of the basilar artery, demonstrated graphically by angiography, with recovery and disappearance of the spasm, again demonstrated angiographically, 2 weeks later.

Pope et al. (1991) described a group of young patients with cerebral ischemic events, endocardial lesions, and lupus anticoagulant. Fourteen consecutive patients (10 females, age range 17 to 53 years [mean 38 years]) who had evidence of the lupus anticoagulant syndrome at onset of symptoms of cerebral ischemia and were being followed prospectively were reviewed. All had abnormal phospholipid-dependent coagulation test results, and most had anticardiolipin antibody at the time of presentation. Three of 14 had four or more American Rheumatism Association criteria for definite systemic lupus erythematosus, and the remaining patients were considered to have primary lupus anticoagulant syndrome.

The common features among these patients included at least one cerebral ischemic event at presentation (stroke or TIA) or recurrent episodes suggesting cerebral ischemia (amaurosis fugax, recurrent severe migraine headaches); livedo reticularis; endocardial valvular lesions noted on echocardiography (11 mitral and 2 aortic valve) that were often associated with discrete vegetations; retinal vascular lesions; and CT/MRI scanning or angiographic evidence of multiple cerebral infarction. Venous thromboembolic events were uncommon (3 of 14). Common laboratory studies included thrombocytopenia (10 of 14), positive direct Coombs test result (11 of 14), and hypocomplementemia (11 of 14). Follow-up after initial treatment with either salicylates or anticoagulant therapy (warfarin) for up to 10 years indicated that, although many patients had recurrent symptoms suggesting cerebral ischemia, major stroke syndromes did not recur nor did new episodes emerge.

The authors concluded that the combination of multiple cerebral ischemic lesions and endocardial lesions, including valvular vegetations, suggests that these cerebral ischemic events represent cerebral emboli, and that these cerebral embolic events originate from vegetative lesions on the mitral or, less commonly, aortic valve, in association with lupus anticoagulant. Some cases may be due to undiagnosed spontaneous internal artery dissection.

SUMMARY

The headache of subarachnoid hemorrhage is of high intensity and sudden onset, is commonly located in the occipital region, and in almost all patients is associated with neck rigidity. It usually persists at a very high intensity for a few days, but seldom for as long as a week, and subsides thereafter, with complete elimination of pain within 2 months. The persistence of headache for longer periods following subarachnoid hemorrhage in patients who have had no previous headaches is rare. The initial headache of subarachnoid hemorrhage is probably due to traction, displacement, distention, and rupture of pain-sensitive blood vessels and the pia arachnoid. The headache of several days' duration is probably secondary to a sterile inflammatory reaction about the blood vessels and meninges.

Ruptured cerebral aneurysm based on a congenital defect with or without arteriosclerotic changes is responsible for the headache, stupor, coma, convulsions, and other disturbances in a high proportion of patients with subarachnoid hemorrhage. However, it is unlikely that periodic headaches of a few hours' duration, recurring over many years as they do in some patients, could stem from the slowly developing structural changes in an aneurysm. Ruptured subarachnoid hemorrhage is an extremely serious condition. Death occurs in approximately 45% of patients with each major bleeding episode and there is a significant risk of recurrence. Approximately one third of those who succumb will do so in the first 48 hours after bleeding, another third within the next month, and the remainder from recurrent bleeding episodes thereafter.

A precise regimen for every case of subarachnoid hemorrhage cannot be recommended with certainty. Early intervention is justified in many cases of aneurysmal hemorrhage characterized by prompt diagnosis, angiography showing no vasospasm, a favorable location, and the absence of serious neurologic signs.

Cerebral (or cerebellar) hemispheric bleeding that is of any significant magnitude is accompanied by excruciating headache and usually by disturbance of consciousness. Hypertension is the most frequent cause of parenchymatous cerebral hemorrhage. The hemorrhage usually occurs in the region of the internal capsule or the basal ganglia and pons, but one fifth of such hemorrhages occur in the brainstem and cerebellum.

Headache may be a manifestation of occlusive vascular disease. Transient migrainous accompaniments of later adult life may be confused with recurrent embolic episodes. With attention to the history, however, the former diagnosis can often be established, especially if arterial studies are normal. Headache, neck pain, and focal neurologic deficits may result from internal carotid artery dissection.

REFERENCES

Allen, G.S., H.S. Ahn, T.J. Preziosi et al. (1983). Cerebral arterial spasm: A controlled trial of nimodipine in patients with subarachnoid hemorrhage. *N. Engl. J. Med.* *308*:619–624.

Bernsen, H.J.J.A., C. Van de Vlasakker, W.I.M. Verhagen et al. (1990). Basilar artery migraine stroke. *Headache 30*:142–144.

Biousse, V., J.D. D'Angletan, P. Touboui et al. (1991). Headache in 67 patients with extracranial internal carotid artery dissection. *Cephalalgia 11*:232–233.

Blend, R. and J.W.D. Bull (1967). The radiological investigation of migraine. In *Background to Migraine: First Migraine Symposium*, pp. 1–10. Springer-Verlag, New York.

Cox, L.K., T. Bertorini, and R.E. Laster (1991). Headaches due to spontaneous carotid artery dissections: Magnetic resonance imaging evaluation and follow-up. *Headache 31*:12–16.

Dandy, W.E. (1944). *Intracranial Arterial Aneurysms*. Comstock Publishing, Ithaca, NY.

Day, J.W. and N.H. Raskin (1986). Thunderclap headache: Symptom of unruptured cerebral aneurysm. *Lancet 2*:124–128.

Edmeads, J.G. (1979). The headaches of ischemic cerebrovascular disease. *Headache 19*:345–349.

Fisher, C.M. (1968). Migraine accompaniments vs. arteriosclerotic ischemia. *Trans. Am. Neurol. Assoc. 93*:211–213.

Fisher, C.M. (1980). Late life migraine accompaniments as a cause of unexplained transient ischemic attacks. *Can. J. Neurol. Sci. 7*:9–17.

Fisher, C.M. (1982). The headache and pain of spontaneous carotid dissection. *Headache 22*:60–65.

Frequin, S.T.F.M., W.H.J.P. Linssen, J.W. Pasman et al. (1991). Recurrent prolonged coma due to basilar artery migraine. *Headache 31*:75–81.

Harling, D.W., R.C. Peatfield, P.T. VanHille et al. (1989). Thunderclap headache: Is it migraine? *Cephalalgia 9*:87–90.

Hunt, W.E. and E.J. Kosnik (1974). Timing and periorbital care in intracranial aneurysm surgery. *Clin. Neurosurg. 21*:79–89.

Jane, J.A., H.R. Winn, and A.E. Richardson (1977). The natural history of intracranial aneurysms: Rebleeding rates during the acute and long-term period and implication for surgical management. *Clin. Neurosurg. 24*:176–184.

Kassell, N.F., H.P. Adams, Jr., J.C. Torner, and A.L. Sahs (1981). Influence of timing on admission after aneurysmal subarachnoid hemorrhage on overall outcome: Report of the Cooperative Aneurysm Study. *Stroke 12*:620–631.

Lees, F. (1962). The migrainous symptoms of cerebral angiomata. *J. Neurol. Neurosurg. Psychiatry 25*:45–50.

Leviton, A., L. Caplan, and E. Salzman (1975). Severe headache after carotid endarterectomy. *Headache 15*:207–210.

Lindboe, C.F., T. Dahl, and B. Rostad (1989). Fatal stroke in migraine: A case report with autopsy findings. *Cephalalgia 9*:277–280.

Ljunggren, B., L. Brandt, G. Sunbay et al. (1982). Early management of aneurysmal subarachnoid hemorrhage. *Neurosurgery 11*:412–418.

McDonald, C. and M. Korb (1939). Intracranial aneurysms. *Arch. Neurol. Psychiatry 42*:289–307.

Medina, J.L., S. Diamond, and F.A. Rubino (1975). Headaches in patients with transient ischemic attacks. *Headache 15*:194–197.

Mokri, B. (1990). Traumatic and spontaneous extracranial internal carotid artery dissections. *J. Neurol. 237*:356–361.

Murphey, F. (1973). The scotoma of carotid artery disease as I remember them. *J. Neurosurg. 39*:390–393.

Nichols, F.T., M. Mawad, J.P. Mohr et al. (1990). Focal headache during balloon inflation in the internal carotid and middle cerebral arteries. *Stroke 21*:555–559.

Pickard, J.D., G.D. Murray, R. Illingworth et al. (1989). Effect of oral nimodipine on cerebral infarction and outcome after subarachnoid hemorrhage. *BMJ 298*: 636–642.

Pope, J.M., C.L.B. Canny, and D.A. Bell (1991). Cerebral ischemic events associated with endocarditis, retinal vascular disease, and lupus anticoagulant. *Am. J. Med. 90*:299–309.

Portenoy, R.K., T.J. Abisi, B.B. Lipton et al. (1984). Headache in cerebrovascular disease. *Stroke 15*:1009–1012.

Sacquegna, T., A. Andreoli, A. Baldrati et al. (1989). Ischemic stroke in young adults: The relevance of migrainous infarction. *Cephalalgia 9*:255–258.

Sahs, A.L., H. Nishioka, J.C. Torner et al. (1984). Cooperative study of intracranial aneurysms and subarachnoid hemorrhage: A long-term prognostic study. *Arch. Neurol. 41:*1140–1151.

Sahs, A.L., G.E. Perret, H.B. Locksley, and H. Nishioka (1969). *Intracranial Aneurysms and Subarachnoid Hemorrhage, A Cooperative Study.* J.B. Lippincott, Philadelphia.

Walker, A.E. (1956). Clinical localization of intracranial aneurysms and vascular anomalies. *Neurology 6:*79–90.

13

Allergy, Atopy, Nasal Disease, and Headache

DONALD D. STEVENSON

The term "allergy" was derived by von Pirquet (1906) from the Greek words *allos* (other) and *ergon* (action). von Pirquet used allergy to describe the "changed reactivity" that occurred in animals after immunization with antigens (allergens). A striking example of changed reactivity is anaphylaxis. An animal, after prior immunization with specific antigen, forms immunoglobulin (IgE) antibodies with combining sites directed at the same antigen. On re-exposure to the antigen a systemic reaction occurs. This reaction is the consequence of union between specific antigens and specific cell-fixed IgE antibodies, followed by release of chemical mediators and their rapid effects on smooth muscles, vascular beds, and mucous membranes.

Although an antigen-induced, IgE-mediated anaphylactic reaction is universally accepted as an "allergic event," physicians agree less frequently when the term "allergy" is used to describe other immunologic inflammatory reactions, and agreement is frequently replaced by confusion and acrimony when nonimmunologic untoward reactions are included in a classification of "allergic reactions." The classification of Gell and Coombs (1968) has been widely accepted as a reasonable description of directions in which the immune system can respond to introduction of specific antigens (Figure 13–1).

The "atopic state" refers to allergic reactions (such as asthma and hay fever) that are familial and for which intracutaneous injections of the offending allergens leads to immediate wheal and erythema in the cutaneous injection sites.

TYPE I REACTIONS

When IgE antibodies, fixed to tissue mast cells or circulating basophils, combine with specific antigens, a cascade of intracellular biochemical events occurs that culminates in the release of chemical mediators into surrounding tissue or fluid (Kaliner and Austen, 1973). These mediators produce the allergic inflam-

	TYPE I	TYPE II	TYPE III	TYPE IV
Immuno-chemical reaction	IgE-mediated chemical mediator release	cytotoxic or cytolytic Ab. (IgM or IgG)	circulating complexes of Ab. Ag and complement	sensitized lymphocytes
Time of reaction	Immediate (15 min)	Immediate to delayed (minutes to hours)	Intermediate (4-24 hr)	Delayed (24-72 hr)
Clinical state	Anaphylaxis Allergic rhinitis	Hemolytic anemia	Vasculitis	Contact dermatitis

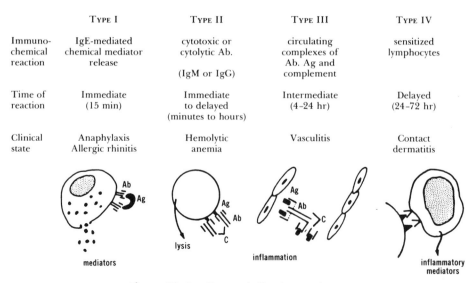

Figure 13–1. Types of allergic reactions.

matory response. Figure 13–2 depicts the interactions between primary effector cells, basophils (circulating in the bloodstream), and mast cells (tissue fixed), releasing primary mediators, and their targeted effects in directly stimulating and attracting eosinophils, platelets, and neutrophils. These secondary cells also release mediators and participate directly in the late allergic inflammatory reactions. Such events tend to amplify the original inciting stimulus (Austen, 1984).

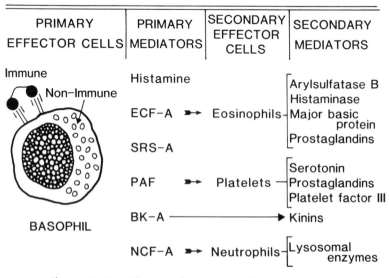

Figure 13–2. Allergic inflammatory cells and mediators.

Although the stimulus to the allergic cascade is frequently an interaction between antigen and IgE antibodies, mast cells and basophils can be activated by nonimmunologic stimuli, such as physical stimuli (trauma, heat, cold, vibration, solar radiation); complement products (C_{3a}, C_{5a}); enzymes (phospholipase A_2, chymotrypsin); polysaccharides (dextran); polypeptides (bradykinin, polymyxin B, eosinophil major basic protein); neuropeptides and hormones (substance P, neurotensin, somatostatin, gastrin, endorphins, enkephalins, acetylcholine); lymphokines from T cells; and drugs (morphine, tubocurarine, radiocontrast media, codeine) (Plaut and Lichtenstein, 1983).

Primary Mediators of Allergic Reaction

Histamine
Histamine combines with receptors in certain tissue cells to produce a variety of special events, depending on the response of the tissue where the receptors reside. For pharmacologic convenience, these receptors are called H_1 and H_2 (Goth, 1978). Important countermechanisms exist for degrading histamine rapidly. Radiolabeled histamine, injected intravenously, disappears from the circulation in about 1 minute (Beall and Van Arsdel, 1960).

Eosinophilic Chemotactic Factor of Anaphylaxis
Eosinophilic chemotactic factor of anaphylaxis (ECF-A) is a glycopeptide with a molecular weight between 500 and 1,000. After release from mast cells, ECF-A attracts eosinophils to this site of anaphylactic reaction, through a countergradient mechanism (Kay and Austen, 1971). Eosinophils have profound inflammatory effects, releasing major basic protein, leukotrienes, and other enzyme products (Altman and Gleich, 1990).

Prostaglandins
Prostaglandins (PGs) are a group of closely related chemicals that are derived from a common essential fatty acid, arachidonic acid, contained in the wall of many mammalian cells and released by the enzyme phospholipase A_2. Prostaglandin synthetase (cyclo-oxygenase) converts arachidonic acid to hydroperoxide, then into PGH and eventually into the PGF and PGE series. For the most part, these mediators appear as a consequence of any inflammation and tend to modulate or amplify other systems. For instance, PGF_2 directly stimulates bronchoconstriction and decreases cyclic adenosine monophosphate (AMP) levels in mast cells and basophils. PGE_1, on the other hand, stimulates bronchodilation and increases cyclic AMP levels in mast cells, diminishing or interrupting mediator release from storage cells (Vane, 1976).

The role of prostaglandins in neurovascular biology is incompletely defined. Some prostaglandins, particularly thromboxanes, aggregate platelets with disruption and release of stored serotonin, a potent vasodilator. Bergstrom et al. (1959) showed that intravenous injection of PGE_1 in susceptible individuals was associated with the onset of vascular headaches, whereas all patients in whom PGE_1 was infused experienced burning pain along the injected vein.

Leukotrienes

Leukotrienes C_4, D_4, and E_4 (slow-reacting substances of anaphylaxis) are also newly synthesized molecules derived from arachidonate in the cell wall. Leukotrienes are formed when membrane lipid is hydrolyzed by phospholipases to form free arachidonic acid, the fatty acid substrate for all additional derived molecules in the synthetic pathways. These powerful lipoxygenase products induce smooth muscle contraction, mucus secretion, and increased vascular permeability (Lewis et al., 1990). Also formed through the 5-lipoxygenase pathway is leukotriene B_4, which is chemotactic for neutrophils and eosinophils.

Platelet-Activating Factor

Platelet-activating factor (PAF) was initially discovered when shown to be generated from guinea pig lung mast cells after antigen challenge (Benveniste, 1974). PAF is also formed by human alveolar macrophages, platelets, neutrophils, and eosinophils (Mencia-Huerta et al., 1990). PAF combines with platelet receptors, stimulating release of serotonin and histamine from rabbit platelets. The role of PAF in humans is only partly clarified. Aggregation of platelets has profound effects on the coagulation and kinin systems. Induction of neutropenia and basopenia, release of platelet amines, and generation of thromboxanes are other effects that have been recently demonstrated.

Kinin-Activating Factor

Kinin-activating factor is released from IgE-sensitized basophils after antigen challenge, with a time course similar to that of histamine release (Newball et al., 1975). More recently it has been demonstrated that three different proteins are released from basophils after immune or nonimmune challenge. These are basophil kallikrein (molecular weight 400,000), basophil Hageman factor activator (molecular weight 13,000), and basophil prekallikrein activator (molecular weight 80,000) (Wasserman, 1983).

Kinins

A circulating globulin, kininogen is the protein substrate for bradykinin. Kininogen is cleaved by the enzyme kallikrein to produce the active peptide bradykinin (Proud et al., 1986). Kallikrein is generated from prekallikrein after interaction with activated Hageman factor (from the coagulation cascade) or released from basophils or mast cells during type I reactions. The generation of the nonapeptide, bradykinin, produces a potent mediator that increases vascular permeability, contracts smooth muscles, and interacts with sensory nerve endings to produce a painful stimulus (Kaplan and Austen, 1975).

For the most part, kinin activation appears to be a secondary system, resulting from release of mediators from basophils, activation of the complement system, or intravascular coagulation. Bradykinin is a potent vasodilator but is rapidly cleaved in normal plasma to an inactive octapeptide, limiting its systemic effects in normal humans and animals. Because of the lability of bradykinin in normal mammalian circulations, it has been extremely difficult to study its in vivo effects and to assign a clear role for the kinin system in disorders such as vascular shock, asthma, pain syndromes, or vascular dilation of the cerebral circulation (Cochrane and Griffin, 1982; Proud et al., 1986).

Neutrophil Chemotactic Factor

Neutrophil chemotactic factor was identified by Wasserman et al. (1977) in the sera of patients with cold urticaria. Partial purification of this material indicates it has a high molecular weight (750,000) and shows a preferential chemotactic activity toward neutrophilic polymorphonuclear leukocytes. Its release into the venous effluent follows a time course identical to that of histamine and low-molecular-weight ECF-A, suggesting that these mediators are released together during anaphylactic cellular discharge.

T-Lymphocyte Chemotactic Factors

T-lymphocyte chemotactic factor, a 1,400-molecular-weight protein, is released from mast cells and attracts T lymphocytes. B-lymphocyte chemotactic factor, a 500-molecular-weight protein, is released from mast cells and attracts B lymphocytes (Wasserman, 1983).

Comments

Although type I reactions can produce rapid and profound changes in the caliber of circular smooth muscles, vasodilation, increased vascular permeability, infiltration of eosinophils and neutrophils, aggregation of platelets, and activation of the kinin and coagulation systems, the compensatory and counterregulatory systems that either destroy the circulating mediators or block their effects by activating the sympathomimetic autonomic responses are also developed. These balances serve to either localize IgE-mediated (type I) reactions to the site of antigen–antibody interaction or shorten the time of their systemic effects (Austen, 1984).

TYPE II REACTIONS

Cytolytic or cytotoxic reactions occur when antigens are part of the cell wall, as in autoimmune hemolytic anemia or transfusion reactions, or when the antigens firmly adhere to cell walls. When penicillin or quinidine, for example, adhere to red blood cell membranes, type II reactions can be initiated if circulating antibodies of the IgG or IgM classes, which have been synthesized in response to penicillin or quinidine, combine with these strategically bound antigens. The combination of antibody and adherent antigen or cell wall antigen does not damage the cells. However, antibodies from both the IgG and IgM classes activate the complement system through the classic pathway, beginning with the C_1 trimolecular complex, through C_4, C_2, C_3, and $C_{5,6,7}$, C_8, and C_9. With the addition of the terminal complement components, spaces are formed in the lipid membrane of the cell wall, the cellular contents extrude into the extracellular space, and cytolysis occurs (Ruddy et al., 1972). To our knowledge, type II hypersensitivity reactions are not involved in the pathogenesis of headache.

TYPE III REACTIONS

Immune complex reactions occur within blood vessels when circulating soluble antigens (drugs, nuclear antigens, virus particles) combine with IgG or IgM antibodies, which fix complement components. These active immune complexes of antigen, antibody, and complement adhere to endothelial surfaces of blood vessels. Activated complement releases C_{3a} and C_{5a} anaphylatoxins, which stimulate nonimmunologic release of stored mediators from circulating basophils, activation of the kinin system through C_2, and release of chemotactic complexes of complement cleavage proteins that attract neutrophils to the site of complement activation (Kohler, 1978).

In type III reactions, inflammation occurs in the walls of blood vessels where immune complexes are deposited. The renal endothelial surfaces are common sites of immune complex deposition, presumably because immune complexes adhere more easily to endothelium when the rate of blood flow diminishes. Biopsy and immunofluorescent staining for antibody or complement show a lumpy, bumpy arrangement of complexes in the subendothelial cell walls, with infiltration of inflammatory cells, particularly polymorphonuclear leukocytes. Type III reactions can produce headache through the pathophysiologic mechanism of arteritis, when immune complexes are deposited in those arteries that carry blood to both intracranial and extracranial structures.

TYPE IV REACTIONS

Cellular immune reactions occur when thymus-derived T lymphocytes, previously sensitized to specific antigens, arrive at the site of antigen introduction. When the original antigen is either introduced through the skin or arrives with certain lipids (as in *Mycobacterium tuberculosis*), lymphocytes are preferentially sensitized or stimulated. Reintroduction of specific antigens stimulates sensitized lymphocytes to migrate toward the site of antigen entry or concentration. Activated lymphocytes secrete bioactive chemicals or factors (David and David, 1972), which produce inflammation in the area of their release. The tuberculin cutaneous reaction, occurring 24 to 72 hours after introduction of killed *M. tuberculosis* antigens, is the classic example of a delayed cellular reaction. With the exception of certain infectious diseases, such as tuberculosis and fungal meningitis, cellular immune reactions probably do not produce headaches.

EXPERIMENTAL STUDY OF PAIN FROM NASAL AND PARANASAL STRUCTURES

Harold Wolff and his associates studied the distribution of intensity of pain originating from the nasal and paranasal structures. Using a probe, faradic electrical current, and cotton pledgets soaked in epinephrine (1:1,000), they stimulated various sites in the nose and surrounding structures. These classic experiments are presented in this section in their original descriptive form as published in the earliest editions of this textbook.

* * * * *

Volunteers consisted of 5 normal subjects, 10 subjects who had undergone complete extirpation of a left acoustic neuroma with section of the left facial nerve, 5 with chronic sinusitis, 4 with acute sinusitis, and 1 with a fistulous opening into the left maxillary sinus. Subjects covered the tips of their index fingers with red wax and were instructed to press the pigment-covered finger against the skin at the place where painful sensation was experienced. Pain was subjectively classified as 1 (least intense) through 10 (most intense). The degree of electrical (faradic) current used in these experiments was determined as follows: the level of current that could elicit a 1 + reaction when the tip of the stimulator was applied to the tongue was the threshold of electrical current used for that experimental subject.

Sensation from Stimulation of the Pharynx, Nasopharynx, and Eustachian Tube

A 1 + to 2 + aching pain was elicited by pressing against the mucous membrane of the pharynx and posterior nasopharynx. The pain was described as being deep within the throat and was marked on the skin as being approximately along the thyroid cartilage of the larynx and at the edge of the hyoid bone, extending to the border of the trachea. Stimulation of the tonsils with faradic current was felt as an uncomfortable tickle at the site of stimulation, but pain was occasionally referred to an area in back of the ear.

Contact of the nasal catheter with the rim of the soft palate and fossa of Rosenmüller was felt as touch, which was described as unpleasant but not painful. Inflation of the eustachian tube was felt as "air blowing through and striking the eardrum." Subjects with prior section of the fifth or seventh cranial nerve continued to feel the same sensations with inflation of the eustachian tube. In one subject, in whom the fifth and ninth cranial nerves had previously been severed, the pharynx and fossa of Rosenmüller were reported to be insensitive, but blowing air through the eustachian tube produced the usual sensation.

Sensation from Stimulation of the Nasal Floor and the Septum

In all subjects with an intact cranial nerve supply, touch and pressure stimuli were recognized as such on stimulation of the nasal floor, and local unpleasant sensations were elicited by passage of a nasal catheter. In subjects with complete section of the fifth cranial nerve root, the insertion of a catheter through

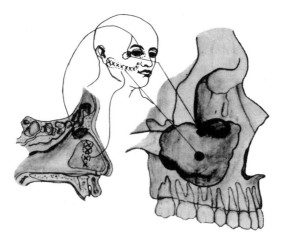

Figure 13–3. The points stimulated on the septum are shown by crosses and on the lateral wall of the maxillary sinus by cross-hatched circles. The areas in which pain of 1 + to 2 + intensity was felt are indicated by crosses within an outline on the small head above. Note that widely separated stimuli cause pain to be felt in the same areas.

the nose was not felt until it impinged on the soft palate and the fossa of Rosenmüller. These patients, however, stated that they felt "a pressure from the posterior portion of the nasal floor."

The nasal septum in normal subjects was sensitive throughout to light touch. Faradic current stimulation and pressure with a probe elicited moderate pain (1 + to 2 +), which was felt locally and sometimes referred as follows. Stimulation of the middle part of the the septum caused pain to be felt along the zygoma and toward the ear. On stimulation of the ethmoid portion of the septum, pain was felt in both the outer and inner canthus of the eye on the homolateral side (Figure 13–3).

Sensation from Stimulation of the Nasal Turbinates

The lower, middle, and upper turbinates, whether stimulated mechanically with a probe or by faradic current, were considerably more sensitive than the nasal floor or the septum. A sharp, burning pain was felt at the site of stimulation and along the lateral wall of the inside of the nose. A duller, aching pain was referred into the upper teeth when faradic current or pressure was applied to the anterior portion of the inferior turbinate. When the middle and posterior portions of the inferior turbinate were stimulated, pain was also felt under the eye, along the zygoma, and toward the ear. On stimulation of the middle turbinate, pain was felt along the zygoma, extending back toward the ear and into the temple and occasionally deep into the ear. On stimulation of the anterior tip of the superior turbinate, pain was felt in the inner canthus of the eye and spread to the forehead and along the lateral wall of the nose (Figure 13–4).

Pain elicited by inserting a cotton pledget soaked with epinephrine along the turbinates usually reached an intensity of 4 + to 5 +. The intensity of pain

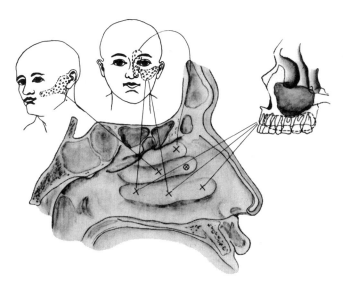

Figure 13–4. The points stimulated on the turbinates are indicated by crosses, from which lines lead to the indicated areas in which pain of 4 + to 6 + intensity was felt.

elicited by stimulation of these structures, and its extent of spread, varied from subject to subject. It was observed in subjects with engorged mucous membranes of the nose, specially of the turbinates, that experimentally induced pain was more intense, was referred to a large area, and was longer lasting than when mucous membranes were normal.

In patients with complete section of the fifth cranial nerve root, stimulation of the turbinates by pressure, faradic current, or epinephrine pledgets did not elicit sensation at the site of stimulation, except for a feeling of pressure "deep in." Two such patients also said they felt a pain deep in the ear when the middle turbinate was pressed with a probe, but they could feel nothing at the site of stimulation, and referred pain was not recorded.

Sensation from Stimulation of the Ostium of the Maxillary Sinus

In three subjects the normal ostium was stimulated by a probe or faradic electrode. As soon as the probe touched the walls of the ostium, there was a sharp, burning pain of 6 + intensity at the site of stimulation, accompanied by profuse lacrimation and injection of the eye on the stimulated side. When attempts were made to push the probe or electrode through the ostium into the antrum, a 5 + to 8 + sharp, burning pain was felt at the site of stimulation and an intense 4 + aching pain was felt in the posterior nasopharynx, in the back teeth, along the zygoma, and back into and well above the temple on the side stimulated. There was a deep aching pain in the pharynx. The skin over the zygoma was flushed and hyperalgesic (Figure 13–5). The skin over the zygoma and the temple remained hyperalgesic and the upper teeth were "sore" for approximately 24 hours following this procedure.

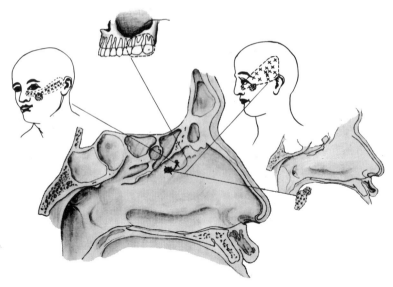

Figure 13–5. Large crosses indicate stimulation of the ostium of the maxillary sinus. Lines lead to the areas indicated by small crosses in which pain of 6 + to 9 + intensity was felt. A dotted circle over the zygoma indicates the area of erythema and hyperalgesia that long outlasted stimulation of the ostium.

Sensation from Stimulation of the Nasofrontal Duct

The nasofrontal duct and the lower part of the channel leading to the frontal sinus were likewise found to be exceedingly pain sensitive. Figure 13–6 illustrates the areas in which pain was felt when the duct of the frontal sinus was stimulated with faradic current, or merely with the passing of the electrode or a metal probe into the frontal sinus. Pain was felt at the inner canthus of the eye and in a wide band under the eye, along the zygoma, and into the temple on the stimulated side. Pain was also felt at the angle of the jaw and in the last two or three upper teeth. Profuse lacrimation and injection in the eye, as well as photophobia, also were present.

Sensation from Stimulation of the Sinuses

Frontal Sinus
When the walls and roof of the frontal sinus were stimulated by pressure with a probe, or by faradic current, minimal pain of no more than a ½ + intensity was felt directly over the site of stimulation.

Ethmoid Sinuses
In two of the normal subjects it was possible to investigate the pain sensitivity and sites of pain reference from stimulation in the superior nasal cavity, near the ethmoid sinuses. The sinuses themselves could not be explored. By pressing a probe against the wall of the superior nasal cavity in the general region of the

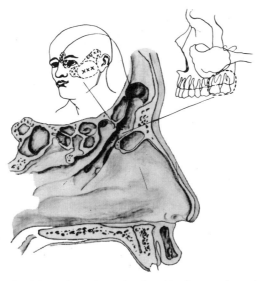

Figure 13–6.   Lines lead from the points stimulated in the nasofrontal duct to the areas in which pain of 5 + to 7 + intensity was felt. On stimulation of the inner wall of the frontal sinus, minimal pain of no more than ½ + intensity was felt only in the area indicated directly over the sinus.

anterior cells of the ethmoid sinuses, pain of 6 + intensity was felt directly over the eye and deep in the eye at its inner canthus. Pain was also felt in the upper jaw just above the superior nasal cavity over the posterior cells of the ethmoid; the conjunctiva adjacent to the nose became injected and profuse lacrimation and photophobia were present.

Pressing this region of the superior nasal cavity over the posterior ethmoid cells with a probe produced an intense aching pain of 5 + to 6 + intensity in the upper teeth, including the canine, the cuspids, and the first molar; profuse lacrimation in both eyes, and photophobia. The pupils were observed to be dilated. Moderate aching pain occurred just under and over the outer canthus of the homolateral eye. Also, pain extended from the teeth up the side of the nose (Figure 13–7).

Sphenoid Sinus

When the wall of the superior nasal cavity in the region of the sphenoid sinus was pressed by a probe, pain of 5 + to 6 + intensity was felt immediately, and most intensely, deep in the pharynx, which was described by the subject as "seeming to be deep in the head." Pain of a lesser intensity was referred over the eye and into the upper teeth on the stimulated side (Figure 13–7).

During an operation on the head for removal of a pituitary tumor, Dr. Bronson Ray stimulated the mucosal lining of the interior of the sphenoid sinus. In this patient, slight pain (1 + to 2 +) was felt at the vertex of the skull (Figure 13–8).

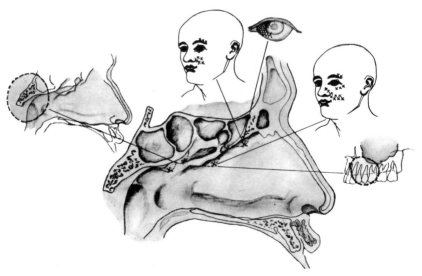

Figure 13–7. Crosses indicate the points of pressure against the walls of the superior nasal cavity in the region of the sphenoid and ethmoid sinuses, with the indicated areas in which pain of 5 + to 6 + intensity was felt.

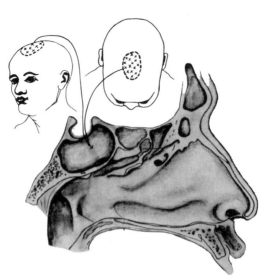

Figure 13–8. The area is indicated in which pain of 1 + to 2 + intensity was felt on faradic stimulation of the mucosal lining of a sphenoid sinus by Dr. Bronson Ray.

Maxillary Sinus

The maxillary sinuses in normal subjects could not be entered through the ostia. However, in three patients who had operative procedures performed on the nose and paranasal sinuses, the ostia were accessible and so large that a faradic stimulator could be introduced into the antrum with ease, and the walls of the latter could be stimulated by faradic current and by pressure. It was doubtful the mucous membrane linings of these antra were free of inflammation, because all the patients had been operated on because of inflammatory sinus diseases. Stimulation of the upper wall was felt up into the eye. Stimulation of the lower lateral wall was felt in the jaw and the back teeth. The sensation elicited from the walls of the sinus was of the same intensity and quality as that elicited by the same amount of faradic current applied to the tip of the tongue and to the mucous membrane of the septum (see Figure 13–3). When this threshold current was applied to the lower and middle turbinates in the same patient, however, a pain of 3 + to 4 + intensity was elicited. These three patients felt a sensation with a probe against the walls of the maxillary sinus as "pressure" but did not report it as painful.

In two of the patients with complete fifth cranial nerve root section, pressure on the posterior wall of the maxillary sinus was felt as "pressure deep in." Faradic stimuli were not felt on the walls of the sinus, nor was any sensation experienced in the teeth of these patients when faradic current was applied to the lateral wall. The ostia on the side of the fifth cranial nerve root section in these patients were also insensitive.

It was possible to explore a normal maxillary sinus in a unique way. A 28-year-old woman who had a sinus tract into the left maxillary sinus following extraction of the first left molar in the upper jaw was studied. This fistulous tract was large enough to allow the entrance of a Holmes laryngoscope for direct visualization of the mucous membrane lining the maxillary sinus cavity.

Experiment 1. The mucous membranes of the sinus were seen to be smooth and glistening throughout and were free of inflammation or atrophy. The normal ostium could also be observed as open and without surrounding inflammatory reaction or scar tissue.

When the wall of the maxillary sinus in this subject was stimulated with faradic current just under the orbital plate, a vibrating sensation was felt at the site of stimulation, and a ½ + pain up through the eye and over the eye along the supraorbital ridge was reported. On the lateral wall and the posterior wall, faradic stimulation was felt as an electric shock along the upper jaw and in the teeth, but the subject stated that the sensation was not painful. When faradic current was applied to the mucous membrane close to the ostium, however, 2 + pain was experienced, and pain was felt in the upper teeth, in and over the eye, and along the zygoma toward the left temple.

Experiment 2. This experiment explored the effect of prolonged positive pressure within the maxillary sinus. A thin rubber balloon was attached with adhesive tape binding over the end of a small perforated rubber catheter. This was inserted into the maxillary sinus through the fistulous opening after injection of

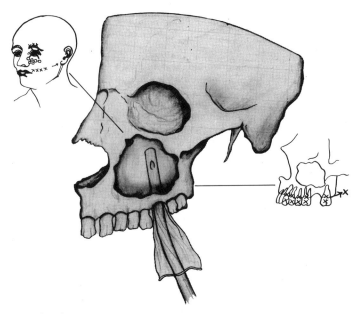

Figure 13–9. The thin rubber balloon is shown in the maxillary sinus. The areas are indicated in which pain was felt when positive pressure was applied to the walls of the sinus for prolonged periods.

procaine local anesthesia into the gum around the opening. The catheter was attached to a manometer so that pressure applied inside the sinus could be measured in millimeters of mercury (Figure 13–9). A positive pressure of 15 to 25 mm Hg elicited a sensation of pressure and fullness in the side of the face, but was maintained for 3.5 hours without eliciting pain. The pressure in the sinus could be gradually raised to 200 mm Hg before pain was experienced.

Pressure was maintained between 50 and 80 mm Hg for a period of 2.25 hours before the subject experienced a 1 + pain in and just below the area of the zygoma and in the upper teeth, radiating back toward the ear. However, quick, forced inhalations of air though the left naris increased the intensity of the pain to 3 + and 4 + and enlarged the area in which it was felt. Reducing the pressure to 0 mm Hg did not immediately abolish the pain, but its intensity gradually diminished during a 10-minute period.

The state of the turbinates was noted at fixed intervals throughout a 6-hour period of balloon inflation. The left turbinate gradually became swollen during this time, but it was not until this engorgement had occluded the left nasal passage that pain was experienced. Moreover, at the beginning of this period, balloon pressure could be raised to 200 mm Hg before pain was experienced, whereas when the turbinates had become swollen and engorged, balloon pressures over 50 mm Hg caused pain.

The pain associated with pressure in the maxillary sinus and swollen, engorged turbinates could be materially reduced in intensity, or almost entirely abolished, by topical application of procaine onto the engorged turbinates, in spite of continued pressure and a feeling of fullness in the side of the face.

Comment: One might infer from the preceding experiment that sustained, increased intramural pressure within the antrum might be associated with pain. However, such sustained stimulation of the walls of the sinus also evoked engorgement of the homolateral turbinates. It appeared from a temporal basis that reflex engorgement of nasal turbinates was responsible for the majority of the pain, since procainization of the inferior and middle turbinates markedly reduced pain intensity, even at a time when the pressure within the sinus was maintained and perceived as pressure in the side of the face.

Experiment 3. This experiment investigated the effect of negative pressure within the maxillary sinus. The nasal side of the ostium was occluded by inserting a cotton and petroleum jelly tampon over the middle turbinate. Negative air pressure was then applied to the sinus by inserting a tube through the fistulous opening. A "drawing" sensation was felt in the face, which the subject described as the feeling that "my face will collapse." This sensation was elicited with a negative pressure of 100 to 150 mm Hg. The experience was accompanied by considerable apprehension on the part of the subject, but in spite of this she maintained that she did not feel pain. However, after the negative pressure was increased to 250 mm Hg, an immediate 4 + pain was felt in the side of the nose and in the teeth.

Comment: When the cotton pledget occluding the ostium was removed at the termination of the experiment, a portion of its surface presented the appearance of having been drawn into the ostium. It is quite likely that the pain experienced with high negative pressures resulted from mechanical stimulation of the ostium by the moving cotton pledget. Thus, although the effects of negative pressures were not explored as extensively as were those of positive pressures, the available evidence makes it seem likely that most of the resulting pain was secondary to stimulation of the ostium and nasal structures.

Experiment 4. A thin rubber balloon was inserted into the sinus and filled with hot (45°C) and cold (19°C) water. Of these stimuli, the cold was not distinguished immediately and the hot not at all. After 10 minutes, the cold water was recognized as "a slight feeling of coolness." While the balloon was in the antrum, filled (under pressure with a syringe) with either hot or cold water, the teeth in the upper jaw felt sore when pressed, but these procedures did not elicit any aching pain anywhere in the side of the face.

When the maxillary sinus was irrigated through the fistulous opening with saline, no pain was elicited other than irritation of the fistulous opening itself. When the sinus was irrigated with saline through the nose and the ostium, however, a 4 + to 5 + pain was felt in the nasal wall, along the zygoma into the temple, over the eye, and all through the upper teeth. Similar pain was induced by inserting a cotton tampon soaked with epinephrine under the middle turbinate and over the ostium.

Comment: The feeling of cold after 10 minutes of exposure to cold within the sinus could have resulted from cooling of neighboring structures. The soreness of the teeth probably resulted from direct stimulation of the dental nerve.

"Sinusitis," Headache, and Anesthetization of the Turbinates

The following experiments are from a series of investigations that illustrate the effects of local anesthesia on nasal mucous membranes in patients with headache associated with disease of the nasal and paranasal structures.

Experiment 1. This patient had pain in the jaws and teeth and on both sides of the face along the zygomas and into the temples. Pain in the frontal region, increased lacrimation, and photophobia were also experienced. The pain was described as a steady ache of a 3 + intensity except in the forehead, where it was 4 +.

Roentgenograms showed both maxillary and frontal sinuses to be opaque. The nasal mucous membrane was bright red, and the turbinates were swollen. The inferior turbinate was in contact with the septum. Purulent secretions were present beneath both middle turbinates in the region of the ostia.

Cotton tampons soaked with 1% procaine hydrochloride were inserted along the inferior turbinates. At the end of 10 minutes the tampons were removed. The subject then stated that the pain in the teeth and jaw was nearly gone. Similar tampons were inserted under the middle turbinates approximately 5 mm beneath the ostia for 10 minutes. Within 8 minutes all pain in the jaw, teeth, and face was gone but a 1 + pain remained in the frontal region. In another 10 minutes the subject stated that all of the pain in the head was gone, and shaking the head vigorously did not produce pain.

Experiment 2. On the eighth day of an upper respiratory infection, the patient had pain over the right side of the face, from the side of the nose, under the eye, along the zygoma, into the temple and ear, and in the upper teeth and jaw. The pain was of 1 + intensity and of a dull, aching quality. The nasal mucous membranes were injected throughout. The turbinates were swollen and in contact with the septum. The middle turbinate was bright red and extremely pain sensitive. When the middle turbinate was touched with a probe, pain in the right side of the face was described as 3 +. There were purulent secretions beneath the middle turbinate in the region of the maxillary ostium. A procaine-soaked cotton tampon was inserted along the medial surface of the inferior turbinate and left in place for 10 minutes. The pain decreased slightly, especially along the side of the nose. Another tampon was inserted under the middle turbinate in the region of the maxillary ostium for 10 minutes, and when it was removed all pain in the side of the face, temple, ear, and teeth was gone, and only a sense of fullness and stiffness remained. All discomfort was gone within an hour and did not return.

Comment: The effect of placing procaine under the middle turbinate and about 5 mm beneath the ostium cannot be explained as a direct procaine effect on nerves entering the ostium to innervate the walls of the sinus. Such nerves, which penetrate the ostium through the nose, enter mostly posteriorly and along the upper margin of the maxillary bone. Therefore, the effect of local anesthesia on the sinus ostia appears to be the reason for disappearance of pain.

Experiment 3. This experiment involved pressure symptoms associated with a cyst in the left antrum. The patient, with a history of pain for 3 days in the left side of the face and head, was observed to have engorged turbinates that were in contact with the nasal septum, causing complete occlusion of the nasal passage. A local anesthetic was placed on the mucous membranes of the inferior and middle turbinates. Within 15 minutes the patient stated that he had a sense of fullness in the left side of the face and beneath the eye, but almost complete alleviation of the pain. The left antrum was entered with a trocar, and straw-colored fluid escaped from the needle under a pressure sufficient to send a stream in a straight line for 10 to 12 inches. Thereafter, the subject had no sensation of head fullness or pain.

Comment: This experiment provided further evidence that increased pressure in the maxillary sinus per se produces sensations of head fullness, and that the pain that the subject experienced had its origin in the inflammation of the adjacent turbinates. This experiment further illustrated that increased pressure in the antrum may exist for a long time without inducing any symptoms. Only with the onset of an upper respiratory infection and the associated inflammation of the turbinates was pain experienced by this subject.

Variations in Venous Pressure and the Size and Appearance of the Turbinates

Experiment 1. This subject had no gross infection of the nose. The jugular outflow on the left side of the neck was occluded for 3 minutes, which caused a gradually increasing engorgement of the turbinates on the left side. Ultimately, swelling of the inferior turbinate placed it in contact with an anterior deviation of the septum, so that the air passage was occluded on the left side. Toward the end of the 3-minute period there was an increase of watery secretion from the left naris.

Experiment 2. When the appearance of the nose was again normal, the experiment was repeated so that venous occlusion was produced on the opposite side. The same engorgement occurred, but nasal airway obstruction was not completed because the septum was not deviated on that side.

Experiment 3. The head was tilted to the horizontal in such a way as to avoid pressure on the neck and to minimize venous stasis. No change in the appearance of the turbinates was noted within 3 minutes, although over a 45-minute period some swelling gradually occurred on the dependent side.

Experiment 4. In addition to tilting the head as in Experiment 3, the face and neck were firmly pressed with a pillow or the supporting hand. The turbinates on the dependent side were noted to become swollen to the point of occluding the air passage within 1 to 3 minutes.

Effect of Vigorously Shaking the Head on Subjects with Engorged Turbinates

The intensity of headache associated with disease of the nasal and paranasal sinuses is increased by shaking the head. The following experiments showed that this increased pain results from the sudden displacement of swollen, inflamed structures.

The subject, about 12 days after the onset of an upper respiratory infection, and during a headache-free period when the turbinates in the right nasal passage were moderately engorged, induced further engorgement by occluding venous return in the right jugular vein with pressure of the hand and by lying on the right side for 5 minutes. The air passage in the right side of the nose was completely occluded and there was a sense of fullness in the right side of the head, but no pain was noted. The turbinates were observed to be swollen, the middle turbinate being especially engorged and in septal contact. At this time, shaking the head vigorously induced pain over the right side of the face from the side of the nose, along the zygoma, into the temple, and into the right upper teeth and jaw. The pain was of a dull, aching quality, was of a 1+ intensity, and persisted for 2 hours. A cotton tampon soaked with a vasoconstrictor (Neo-Synephrine HCl) was then inserted along the inferior turbinate and in contact with the middle turbinate, and was left in place for 10 minutes. When the pack was removed, the turbinates were observed to be pale and shrunken and all pain in the side of the face was gone. Vigorously shaking the head at this point did not elicit pain.

Site of Origin of Headache from Disease of the Nasal and Paranasal Structures

It is evident from these studies that the linings of the sinuses are relatively insensitive when compared with their extremely sensitive ducts and ostia and the nasal turbinates. Although the term "sinus headache" is commonly assigned to those headaches associated with nasosinus disease, proof that the pain has its origin in the mucous lining of the paranasal sinuses is lacking. The issue has been confused by the fact that sinus inflammation rarely if ever occurs without concomitant inflammation of the ostia and other nasal structures. The rare exception is sinus infection secondary to periapical abscess. It is interesting and significant that this type of sinus infection causes minor or no discomfort until the infection spreads into the ostia or nasal structures such that they are directly or indirectly inflamed as well.

It is inferred, therefore, that the site of paranasal headache is related chiefly to the region of the nose that is most inflamed and engorged. Disease of the superior nasal structures causes headaches primarily in the front and top of the head, and in and between the eyes. Disease of the middle and inferior nasal structures causes headaches primarily over the zygomas and temples and in the teeth and jaws.

PATHOPHYSIOLOGY OF HEADACHE FROM DISEASE OF NASAL AND PARANASAL STRUCTURES

Variations in Venous Pressure

Variations in venous pressure modify the intensity of the paranasal headache. Unilateral pressure on the jugular vein, both internal and external, increases the turgescence of the turbinates on the homolateral side. When the turbinates were previously inflamed and engorged, this effect is more striking than when they were normal at the time of this experiment. When the turbinates are already moderately painful, the pain is augmented by further turgescence, and still further augmented by shaking the head or lowering the head between the knees. When a subject with turgescent turbinates rests in a lying-down position on his or her side, there is a momentary slight increase in pain as the swollen turbinates are displaced. Gradually the uppermost turbinates shrink slightly, whereas the dependent turbinates become more engorged and occlude the air passage completely.

However, venous pressure is not a factor of primary importance in sinus headache, because intensity of pain is usually greatest when the subject is in the erect position and the cranial venous pressure is at its lowest.

Negative and Positive Air Pressure

The fact that the headache is usually worse in the upright position and better when the patient is lying down has been used as evidence that pain is due to negative or positive air pressure in the sinuses, resulting from the drainage out of the sinuses of, or their filling up with, purulent secretion. However, because changes in pressure have been demonstrated to be inadequate stimuli for producing serious discomfort in sinus cavities, other factors must be more important as causes of pain.

Irritants on the Nasal Mucosa

Toxic or noxious chemicals, in either the liquid or gaseous phase, can produce inflammation in the nasal mucosa by direct interaction with the mucous membranes. This is not immunologically mediated, although variations in the degree of sensitivity of dose–effect relationships in certain patients have been observed by careful clinicians. Some individuals with exquisite sensitivity to inhaled cigarette smoke, smog, and chemical fumes are already suffering from other forms of nasal mucosal inflammation (allergic or vasomotor rhinitis). The superimposition of chemical molecules on already inflamed surfaces increased the inflammation and swelling, and this may be enough to exceed pain thresholds and produce paranasal pain. In the absence of underlying rhinitis, chemical fumes would not be an adequate stimulus to produce paranasal pain in this subgroup of patients.

Vasomotor Changes in the Nasal Membranes

Local vasomotor changes in the erectile tissue of the nose as accompaniments of stress, exhaustion, anxiety, hormonal stimulation, sexual excitement, and various emotional states have been observed. Ordinarily such variations are not associated with nasal symptoms, but sometimes the effects of these changes produce enough congestion of the turbinates to induce obstruction of the nasal passages with or without associated paranasal head pain.

NASAL DYSFUNCTION AND HEADACHE IN PATIENTS HAVING ADAPTIVE DIFFICULTIES

Functional alterations in the structures of the human nose have been studied and correlated with a wide variety of circumstances, including noxious stimulation inside the nose by chemical agents, noxious stimulation of other portions of the head, variations in environmental temperature, interruption of afferent nerve pathways, weeping, and numerous life-threatening situations with their accompanying affective states.

In general, two patterns of disturbance of nasal function were recognized. The first involved vasoconstriction in the nose with shrinkage of the membranes and increase in the size of the air passages. Such changes in reaction to threats accompanied feelings of fear, sadness, and other emotions that, although strong, involved minimal conflict (Figure 13–10).

The second type of disturbance in the nose appeared to have greater significance in relation to disease. It was characterized by the initial hyperemia associated with turgescence of the erectile tissues in the turbinates and nasal septum, engorgement of the nasal mucosa, and increased secretion. These changes were accompanied by obstruction to breathing and often by paranasal pain. After hyperemia subsided, secondary pallor ensued, with the mucous membranes of the nose remaining boggy and edematous. This second type of nasal disturbance, characterized by hyperfunction, occurred in response to a variety of environmental threats against the individual and appeared to constitute part of a defense mechanism for shutting out and washing away a noxious environment at the head of the organism. Such a pattern was found to occur in response to local stimulation by the noxious fumes of ammonium carbonate (Figure 13–11) or by grass pollen to which the subject was immunologically sensitive (Figure 13–12). It also occurred following noxious stimulation not directed specifically at the nose or respiratory passages—for example, the painful tightening of a metal headband. In fact, this defensive pattern of shutting out occurred even in response to noxious environmental stimuli that did not involve physical contact with the organism, such as situational threats occurring during interpersonal adjustment. Weeping, which followed frustrating or humiliating experiences,

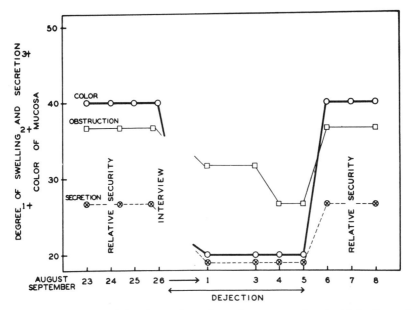

Figure 13–10. Pallor and shrinkage of nasal membranes associated with feelings of sadness, fear, and dejection.

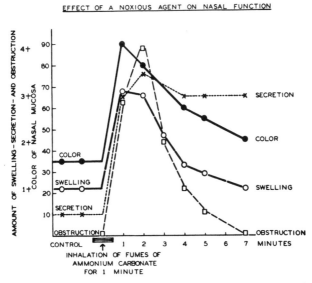

Figure 13–11. Nasal hyperfunction following inhalation of the noxious fumes of ammonium carbonate.

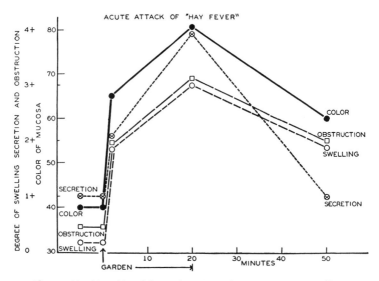

Figure 13–12. Nasal hyperfunction after exposure to pollens.

was accompanied by swelling, hyperemia, hypersecretion, and obstruction in the nose (Figure 13–13). Such changes also accompanied anger and feelings of frustration without weeping.

One subject, a 25-year-old physician, was studied in detail over 8 months. He exhibited alterations in nasal function that were observed during naturally occurring day-to-day life stresses. Pallor of nasal membranes with an increase in size of the air channels occurred in a setting of abject fear and dejection

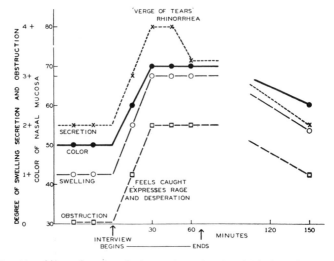

Figure 13–13. Nasal hyperfunction during an interview in which the subject experienced rage and desperation.

following his wife's hemoptysis. In situations of conflict, however, when decisions were required regarding threats to his career or to his position as head of his household, nasal hyperemia with swelling, hypersecretion, and obstruction to breathing occurred. At such times he also experienced frequent colds with sneezing and coughing, postnasal discharge, and sinus headache.

He approached his problems in an energetic, aggressive, outgoing, and self-confident fashion. Situations within his realm of responsibility were rarely out of his control. His system of security relied on three props: (1) the approval of his superiors; (2) his ability to be assertively independent in the economic and social spheres; and (3) his achievement of a recognized position in a competitive society—that is, "success in his career."

At the time when the subject's wife was 5 months pregnant, a decision had to be made to relinquish their own apartment and go to live with the wife's aunt in a suburb of the city. During this period, in which the subject was exposed to serious threats to his independence, he was also subjected to threats to his career and to the danger of losing the approval of his superiors. Working with him under his supervision was an intern about 4 years his senior, who found it difficult to perform the menial but essential chores customarily assigned to an intern and who was unwilling to accept the responsibility for his patients. The subject hesitated, because of his subordinate's experience and age, to reprimand him openly and frankly. He first tried to cope with the situation by suggesting a plan to maintain the ward's efficiency. When this failed, the subject began, in addition to his own work, to perform the intern's neglected duties himself. He finally confronted the intern frankly with the issue, but the latter refused to accept criticism from a younger, less-experienced man.

In this setting of threat to his career, with feelings of anger and resentment and the fear of loss of the approval of his senior colleagues, as well as the conflict arising from his being forced to sacrifice those symbols of independence his own home represented, the subject was aware of an increase in postnasal accumulations of secretions and the need to "clear his throat" frequently. His nose felt occluded, and there was burning pain in both nostrils. Figure 13–14 demonstrates the increase in redness of the nasal mucosa associated with a significant increase in the amount of secretion, swelling, and obstruction sustained throughout this 12-day period.

During weeping, not only the eyes but also the nose were found to participate in this reaction. (In two other individuals in this study, deeper structures, including the bronchi, constricted during threatening situations, thus participating in the bodily reaction of exclusion. Against local intrusion by dust, for example, or noxious fumes, the reaction of shutting out and washing away proved highly effective.) Against situational threats involving interpersonal relations, the nasal changes afforded incomplete relief and were often counterproductive.

When the nasal changes in the bodily pattern of shutting out and washing away were unduly sustained, they gave rise to troublesome symptoms, including burning pain of low intensity. This was increased by forced inspiration, and a dull, aching pain spread from the bridge of the nose into the orbit and along the zygoma to the ear on each side of the swollen nasal structure. When the

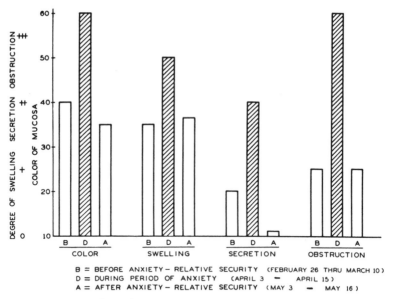

Figure 13–14. Sustained nasal hyperfunction during 12 days of anxiety and resentment compared with control periods before and after.

swelling shifted to the opposite nostril, the pain correspondingly changed position. The pain, which also involved the teeth, especially those of the upper jaw, alternated with a feeling of fullness that was worse during the working hours of the day, especially during periods of stress, and was minimal in the early morning and late evening. When pain was relatively intense, local deep tenderness was also noted. Photophobia occurred, especially on the painful side, with injection of the sclerae and the skin of the cheek. Distribution of headache is shown schematically in Figure 13–15.

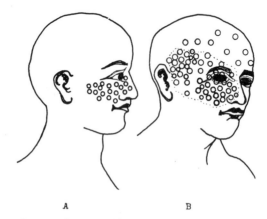

Figure 13–15. Distribution of pain and hyperalgesia during nasal hyperfunction associated with emotional conflict. A., baseline pain distribution. B., spreading pain distribution after emotional conflict.

These observations indicate that, during sustained conflict, prolonged nasal hyperfunction may occur, accompanied by obstruction, facial pain, and tenderness. Such symptoms are often attributed to acute sinusitis. In this case no infection of the sinuses was demonstrated, however, and the disturbance with accompanying symptoms subsided completely when the subject's conflicts were resolved.

* * * * *

PARANASAL HEAD PAIN AND ALLERGY

It is clear that any stimulus that causes engorgement or inflammation of the nasal turbinates can produce nasal or paranasal head pain. Therefore, the proper perspective in which to view allergy and headache is within the context of the causes of swelling and inflammation of the nasal membranes (rhinitis). Because allergic reactions are one of many provoking mechanisms leading to rhinitis, they are included in the list. However IgE-mediated reactions do not hold exclusive rights to induction of swelling of turbinates and their associated paranasal head pain.

Allergic Rhinitis

Paranasal head pain develops in some patients when IgE-mediated inflammation occurs in nasal mucous membranes. Thus, allergic rhinitis can be responsible for paranasal headache, with or without associated inflammation in the paranasal sinuses. The percentage of patients with allergic rhinitis who also report paranasal head pain is unknown. Many individuals with allergic rhinitis experience mild "pressure" in the paranasal structures, but their individualized definition of "pain" in large part determines whether or not they report paranasal "pain" during allergic rhinitis episodes. In our allergy clinic, only 20% of patients with proven IgE-mediated rhinitis reported any paranasal discomfort, including pain, as a significant complaint. Thus, most patients with allergic rhinitis rarely seek medical attention because of their paranasal head pain, but instead volunteer symptoms such as rhinorrhea, nasal congestion, sleep disturbance, or sneezing as their complaints.

Other Types of Rhinitis

The term "rhinitis" is nonspecific. A number of inflammatory mechanisms can induce swelling and congestion of the nasal membranes, and all can lead to paranasal pain. Important variables in the production of paranasal pain include (1) the anatomic arrangements between the nasal septum, turbinates, and sinus ostia; (2) the relative size of the nasal passages; and (3) the presence or absence of nasal polyps and their location with respect to the sinus ostia. All of these variables in concert determine whether or not turbinates are sufficiently enlarged within a confined nasal space to induce pressure on other turbinates and sinus ostia.

Table 13-1 Characteristics of the major forms of rhinitis

	Allergic rhinitis	Infectious rhinitis	Vasomotor rhinitis	Irritant rhinitis
Seasonal incidence	Frequent	Increased in winter	None	Smog
Itching and sneezing	Usual	Rare	Unusual	Unusual
Collateral allergy	Common	Occasional	Occasional	Occasional
Family history allergy	Common	Occasional	Occasional	Occasional
Sore throat	Rare	Common	Rare	Rare
Fever	Rare	Common	Rare	Rare
Conjunctivitis	Itching common	Occasional	Rare	Burning common
Nasal pallor	Usual	Rare	Common	Occasional
Nasal polyps	Occasional	Occasional	Occasional	Occasional
Injection of pharynx	Rare	Common	Rare	Rare
Eosinophil nasal secretions	Usual	Absent	Absent	Absent
Purulent nasal secretions	Rare	Usual	Occasional	Occasional
Positive allergy skin tests	Usual	Rare (coincidental)	Rare	Rare (coincidental)
Paranasal pain	Occasional	Common	Occasional	Occasional

The characteristics of all forms of rhinitis are compared with those of allergic rhinitis in Table 13–1. *Allergic rhinitis* is the only type that is initiated by IgE and antigen interaction. *Infectious rhinitis* is usually the consequence of a viral agent infecting the nasal membranes and inciting an inflammatory response. A viral infection frequently extends to the sinus ostia, eustachian tubes, pharynx, larynx, and trachea. Primary or secondary bacterial infections, usually *Staphylococcus aureus, Haemophilus influenzae, Pneumococcus pneumonia,* or *Streptococcus hemolyticus,* also occur in the nasal and sinus membranes. Paranasal head pain is more prominent during infectious rhinitis than in any other form of rhinitis (Solomon, 1967).

Vasomotor rhinitis mimics allergic rhinitis, but antigens and antibodies do not produce this type of nasal congestion. Instead, a variety of stimuli, including temperature changes, exercise, change in position, change in barometric pressure or humidity, anger and frustration, and certain odors, precede the onset of nasal congestion. How these nonallergic stimuli induce nasal congestion is not entirely clear, but most evidence favors dysfunctional control of nasal vascular beds by the autonomic nervous system. Interruption of the cervical sympathetic nerves is followed by unilateral nasal obstruction and hypersecretion. Disruption of the parasympathetic fibers produces dry, crusted, small atrophic nasal membranes (Millonig et al., 1950). If a cold stimulus is applied to the nasal membranes or to skin of the extremity, there is prompt homolateral engorgement of the nasal turbinates in patients suffering from vasomotor rhinitis (Ralston and Kerr, 1945). Thus parasympathetic discharge, relative to opposing sympathetic nervous system discharge, appears to be important in the pathogenesis of vasomotor rhinitis.

Irritant rhinitis is sometimes subclassified as a form of vasomotor rhinitis. As implied by its name, irritant chemicals activate congestion and inflammation of the nasal membranes through direct contact with these structures. The precise role of the vasomotor autonomic reflexes in the resulting nasal congestion is unclear. Normal individuals who inhale volatile acidic fumes, smoke, or smog invariably develop mild to moderate nasal congestion. At the other end of the spectrum, selected "sensitive" individuals experience severe conjunctival or nasal congestion on contact with minimal atmospheric concentrations of smog, cigarette smoke, perfumes, or cocaine. Although many of these patients also have vasomotor rhinitis, others experience nasal congestion only when their nasal membranes are in contact with irritant fumes.

Rhinitis medicamentosa is the rebound response of the nasal vascular beds to topical application of sympathomimetic drops or sprays. Neo-Synephrine and oxymetazoline HCl are the preparations usually applied to the nasal membranes. Rhinitis medicamentosa almost never occurs by itself, and attention to the underlying rhinitis mechanism is necessary both in order to wean the patient away from sympathomimetic nasal sprays and to initiate a treatment plan that will prevent the need for using topical sympathomimetic sprays in the future. By the time these individuals seek medical attention, the syndrome of underlying rhinitis with superimposed rhinitis medicamentosa is frequently associated with paranasal head pain. However, despite their discomfort and desire to receive medical assistance, some patients are reluctant to disclose their use of sympathomimetic sprays because of their complete dependence on the sprays and fear that the physician will take away their topical decongestant without providing alternative treatment. Close questioning and even observation may be necessary to obtain this essential information.

Finally, although the features of rhinitis are presented in Table 13–1 as separate entities, few individuals experience only one type of rhinitis during their lifetimes. An individual who develops IgE-mediated rhinitis from inhaling grass pollen in the spring may experience irritant rhinitis in the fall on exposure to smog, vasomotor rhinitis while skiing in the winter, and a viral upper respiratory infection in March. This chronology can be further complicated by the simultaneous appearance of two or even more rhinitis mechanisms. Diagnostic and treatment ingenuity can be severely strained when several types of rhinitis occur simultaneously (Tennenbaum, 1972). In addition, because nasal obstruction leads to sleep deprivation, the disease of rhinitis can cause fatigue from sleep disruption and psychosocial distress that, through the autonomic nervous system, directly causes further congestion of the nasal turbinates, with paranasal pain or head pain of either muscle contraction or vascular origin.

Clinical Features of Paranasal Head Pain

The headache associated with frontal sinus disease and the usual inflammation around the sinus ostia are localized over the frontal region. Antral disease produces headache over the maxillary region and into the zygoma or temporal areas. The headache associated with sphenoid and ethmoid sinus disease is experienced between and behind the eyes and over the vertex of the skull.

Commonly, when sinus disease is of sufficient duration, pain also occurs in the back of the head, neck, and shoulders, suggesting a muscle contraction type of head pain resulting from sleep deprivation or stress of a prolonged disease. Headaches are less frequent when the patient has been in the supine position and are less prominent at night than during the day. Moreover, the pain associated with maxillary sinus disease gradually diminishes over about 30 minutes when the patient lies down with the diseased sinus uppermost.

The headache associated with frontal sinus disease commonly begins about 9 A.M., gradually becomes worse, and terminates toward evening or on retiring. The pain associated with maxillary sinus disease frequently has its onset in the early afternoon.

In all instances, the pain is of a deep, dull, aching, nonpulsatile quality. It is seldom, if ever, associated with nausea. Chronic sinus disease produces headache pain of lower intensity than that associated with acute sinus disease, depending on the association of nasal membrane congestion. In both instances, the intensity of pain is increased by shaking the head or assuming the head-down position. The headache is intensified by procedures that increase the venous pressure, such as "straining," coughing, or wearing a tight collar.

The headache associated with disease of the nasal and paranasal structures is commonly reduced in intensity or abolished by nasal decongestant sprays or pills. Aspirin may reduce the intensity of the pain but usually does not abolish it. Patients frequently report the simultaneous disappearance of nasal congestion and paranasal head pain after appropriate decongestant therapy has been initiated.

NASAL SEPTAL CONTACT HEADACHE

Deviation of the nasal septum can occur in many forms and degrees of obstruction. Because the septum itself is relatively insensitive to pain, the mechanism of pain induction is through pressure of the septum on pain-sensitive structures, such as the nasal turbinates (Ryan and Ryan, 1979). Using topical decongestants, this type of pain should disappear after shrinking the adjacent turbinates.

ANGIOEDEMA AND HEAD PAIN

After release of vasodilating mediators, soft tissue swelling can occur in tissues of the face, tongue, or larynx. Antigens such as penicillin, sulfa, horse serum, or insulin can combine with specific IgE antibodies to initiate type I hypersensitivity reactions, manifested by either urticaria, angioedema, or both. Urticaria (crops of wheals frequently surrounded by erythema and associated with pruritus) occurs either in specific locations or over most of the body's surface. Angioedema, by contrast, is a condition characterized by nonpitting localized edema without associated pruritus (Mathews, 1974). These two forms of abnormal cutaneous or subcutaneous vasodilation can appear separately or at the same time. Both urticaria and angioedema are associated with vasodilation and increased permeability of small venules and capillaries; vascular congestion occurs in the upper corium vessles in urticaria and in the subcutaneous vessels in angioedema (Lever, 1961).

Intradermal injection of histamine produces local wheal-and-flare urticarial lesions that are indistinguishable from spontaneous urticaria (Lewis, 1961). However, many patients who have urticaria do not respond to antihistamines (H_1 blockers), and the pathogenic mechanisms that produce urticaria and angioedema are now recognized to be heterogeneous with immunologic, nonimmunologic, emotional, neural, and physical inciting events triggering a complicated chain of mechanisms culminating in vasodilation and increased permeability of cutaneous vessels (Kaplan, 1978; Soter, 1990).

Although most angioedema is painless, in certain forms and/or locations it causes head pain. For the most part, these instances are obvious; pain is directly adjacent to soft tissue swelling on the scalp or face. Angioedema of the tongue, pharynx, and larynx is manifested by other symptoms, such as obstruction, sensation of a mass, or difficulty with swallowing or speaking. Pain is rarely a manifestation of these latter angioedema locations, and referred pain is even more unusual. Generalized, severe angioedema has been reported in at least one patient with associated headaches, epilepsy, hemiplegia, and coma (Fowler, 1962). We have observed a patient who reacted to parabens (stabilizer chemicals in injectable medications) by developing generalized erythrodermia with tissue edema, including cerebral edema, headache, and semicoma. She was treated with systemic corticosteroids and recovered completely.

CEREBRAL ARTERITIS SYNDROMES

Systemic lupus erythematosus (SLE) is a disease manifested by deposition of complexes of DNA, antibody, and complement in arterial walls (type III reactions). The resulting inflammation or arteritis can produce systemic symptoms such as fever, malaise, myalgias, and arthralgias, or localized symptoms that are the consequences of occlusion and perinflammation of specific arteries. Cerebral head pain can be caused by inflamed superficial arteries, as a consequence of arterial obstruction with ischemic pain, or may be due to a generalized cerebritis with dull, pressure-type pain (Atkins et al., 1972).

Giant cell arteritis may occur in the cerebral arteries. Because the superficial temporal arteries are accessible and can be sacrificed for biopsy, the term "temporal arteritis" has gained popular acceptance. Actually, in this disease, giant cell arteritis is present in large arteries to the brain or those that supply the skeletal muscles (polymyalgia rheumatica syndrome) (Healey and Wilske, 1977) and viscera (O'Neil et al., 1976), as well as the axillary, brachial, femoral, and coronary arteries (Stanson et al., 1976).

Evolving evidence supports the hypothesis that giant cell arteritis, temporal arteritis, cranial arteritis, and polymyalgia rheumatica are all manifestations of a type III immunologic reaction, appearing in a number of large and medium-sized arteries. Immunofluorescent studies of biopsied arteries (particularly the superficial temporal) show deposits of IgG, IgA, sometimes IgM, fibrin, and complement components (Waaler et al., 1976) in a number of biopsy specimens, depending on the stage of disease and the biopsy site (Klein et al., 1976). Hazelman et al. (1975) reported lymphocyte stimulation by arterial wall antigen extracts in polymyalgia rheumatica, suggesting that cellular immune hypersensitivity or type IV reactions may also occur in this disease. The main deterrent in categorizing giant cell arteritis as an immune disease, however, has been failure to identify the inciting antigen(s). By contrast, in SLE, a variety of nuclear antigens have been separated and studied (Nutman et al., 1975).

The relationship between the arteritis syndromes and headaches is described in greater detail in Chapter 11.

HEADACHE REACTIONS TO DRUGS USED TO TREAT ALLERGIC DISEASES

Common and frequently overlooked causes of head pain in patients with allergic diseases are reactions to the drugs used to treat these patients. Individuals with allergic rhinitis receive antihistamine and sympathomimetic decongestants; asthmatics receive theophylline, sympathomimetic bronchodilators, and corticosteroids; and patients suffering from systemic arteritis syndromes frequently receive high dosages of corticosteroids. Therefore, when evaluating a patient who has one or more of these diseases and also complains of head pain, physicians are encouraged to assess the consequences of those drugs used to treat the disease rather than assuming that the disease is responsible for the head pain syndrome.

Table 13-2 lists the major drugs used to treat allergic diseases, along with their side effects.

RELATIONSHIP BETWEEN ALLERGY AND MIGRAINE HEADACHE

Migraine is a common disorder that occurs in 15% of the adult population, twice as frequently in women as in men (Dalsgaard-Nielsen, 1974). Because migraine headaches tend to occur intermittently, it has been tempting to identify provoking factors responsible for each migraine attack. Infrequent exposure to allergens constitutes a hypothetical provoking event for each or some migraine headaches. However, proving that antigens, combining with IgE antibodies, actually cause migraine or vascular headaches has been difficult. Most of the controversy regarding allergy and migraine headaches is the result of differing interpretations of incomplete data and failure to define descriptive terms in a mutually agreeable manner.

Table 13–2 Side effects of drugs used to treat allergic diseases

	Consequences of drugs	
	---	---
Drugs	Head-pain type	Other side effects and manifestations

Decongestants
  Antihistamines and
    sympathomimetics
	Vascular, pounding
	  headaches
		Somnolence, or excitation

Sympathomimetics
  Epinephrine
  Ephedrine
  Isoproterenol
  Metaproterenol
  Albuterol
	Vascular, pounding
	  headaches
		Tremor, palpitations,
		  tachyarrythmias

Aminophylline or
  theophylline
	Toxic, sick headache,
	  generalized
		Nausea, emesis, tremor,
		  excitation, convulsions,
		  tachyarrhythmias

Corticosteroids
  Prednisone
  Methylprednisolone
	Cervico-occipital headaches
	Vascular headaches
		Hypertension, Cushing
		  syndrome, osteoporosis

History of Allergy and Migraine Headaches

One of the earliest relationships between migraine and allergy was based on definitions. In 1873, Trousseau stated that migraine was one of the "allergic manifestations of the atopic state." He declared, without evidence, that periodic headache, along with hay fever, urticaria, and eczema, were all features of an "asthmatic state." He failed to provide any data to support his statement. Other physicians have attempted to link migraine headache to allergy by identifying common associations. For example, Neusser (1892) reported eosinophilia during a migraine attack. Van Leeuwen and Zeydner (1922) described an activity in the blood of patients with asthma, urticaria, epilepsy, and migraine that induced smooth muscle contraction in vitro but was absent from the blood of normal control subjects.

Pagniex et al. (1919), DeGowin (1932), Rinkel (1933), Balyeat and Brittain (1930), Hahn (1930), Hamburger (1935), Gonzales (1953), Ogden (1951), and others followed with reports of allergy and migraines appearing in the same individuals. Vaughan's work (1934) is representative of these publications. On the basis of a clinical history of migraine attacks after ingesting certain foods and the presence of positive skin tests in response to these foods, he concluded that allergic reactions were a causative factor in 70% of patients with migraine headache. In half of his patients, a reduction in migraine headaches occurred after the diet was modified. The chief food offenders have varied from study to study: wheat, milk, chocolate, and eggs in the opinion of Balyeat and Brittain (1930); celery, peas, and onions in DeGowin's report (1932).

The position that allergy causes migraine headaches was championed in the United States by Vaughan and others (Rowe, 1932; Unger and Unger, 1952). By defining migraine as an allergy, Rinkel, in 1933, was able to show that migraine patients had a family history of "allergy." Although some migraine patients came from families in which true atopic diseases, such as allergic rhinitis, asthma, urticaria, and eczema existed, in the majority of family members interviewed by Rinkel the so-called family history of allergy turned out to be migraine headaches. Another interpretation of the same data is that the majority of migraine patients came from families in which other members also had migraine headaches. Despite the passage of time, the controversy continues. More recent publications by Unger and colleagues (1970, 1974) and Speer (1975) continue to report that allergy causes migraine headaches.

Dietary Migraine

The major arena of controversy with respect to a cause-and-effect relationship between allergic reactions and migraine has been that of food allergy. From the outset, those who favored the allergic migraine hypothesis observed migraine headache attacks after food ingestion in many of their patients. Wolf and Unger (1944) recorded migraine headache attacks in one patient after he consumed food extracts that had induced positive wheal-and-flare skin test responses. They then failed to produce headache in the patient after administering harmless extracts presented to the known offending allergen. Hyslop (1934) reported a patient who suffered migraine after ingesting pork only when the patient was under emotional stress.

However, in most of the studies, a critical experimental control was omitted. If the alleged offending food had been administered without the patient's awareness, and headache had always occurred, a direct cause-and-effect relationship between food and headache would be more convincing. When this step was carried out at the New York Hospital, with the administration of chocolate, disguised in capsules for those allegedly sensitive to chocolate, or milk given through a stomach tube to those who were said to be sensitive to milk, the results did not confirm the earlier work. No headache ensued. Moreover, in 1950 Loveless gave milk, corn, arrowroot, and tapioca, as well as placebo preparations, in disguised form, to persons alleged to have had headache attacks precipitated by the ingestion of these foods. She noted, in her well-controlled study, no predictable relationship between the administration of these substances and the occurrence of headache.

In another well-controlled, double-blind food challenge and elimination study, Walker (1960) showed that there was no predictable relationship between disguised offending foods and the occurrence of migraine headache attacks. Many have concluded that the effect of the doctor's and patient's belief that the allergen offered would produce a migraine headache could have triggered migraine attacks through fear and psychic anticipation of stress in the earlier, uncontrolled feeding experiments.

The presence of positive wheal-and-flare skin test responses to certain foods has been used as evidence for food allergy in migraine patients (Vaughan, 1934). Unfortunately, positive skin tests occur in up to 25% of asymptomatic, nonallergic control populations (Smith, 1978). A variation on food skin testing was provided by Monro et al. (1980), who used radioallergosorbent testing (RAST) to measure serum-specific IgE antibodies. In 47 patients, the authors believed they could predict food allergy from RAST results and, after challenge with forbidden foods, demonstrated an increase in the serum levels of food-specific IgE antibodies. They could "provoke" headaches with open challenges with food and "block" headaches with open ingestion of chromolyn sodium.

Not only are positive food skin tests and elevated titers of serum-specific IgE (on RAST) found in asymptomatic individuals, but a cause-and-effect relationship between addition and elimination of foods in known atopic conditions has been difficult to prove. The difficulties of establishing a diagnosis of food hypersensitivity have been outlined by May and Bock (1978). In migraine, the problem is further compounded by a significant psychological factor—that a positive skin test for a food can induce fear of that food in the susceptible patient, which, in turn, can precipitate a migraine headache when that forbidden food is reintroduced.

The many problems in the interpretation of skin tests make it difficult to establish their relevance to migraine. It is noteworthy that, although the gastrointestinal tract is more permeable to food allergens in the very young, Vahlquist (1955) has shown that the incidence of migraine in children is at most one third to one half that found in adults. If food allergy, which has a high incidence in children when compared with adults, were important in the pathogenesis of migraine, the opposite relationship should exist, with migraine headaches being two to three times more common in children than in adults.

Despite the above controversies, in recent years it has been convincingly demonstrated that, in a few selected patients, milk, wheat, corn, egg, soybean, and peanut can induce IgE-mediated migraine headaches (Mansfield et al., 1985). Out of a large population of patients who reported food-associated migraine headaches, a few patients were identified as having the following experimental findings: history of migraine each time after eating a specific food, positive wheal-and-flare skin test responses to that food, and migraine headache appearing within 30 minutes of ingesting the suspect food during double-blind ingestive challenges (using freeze-dried foods and placebos). Finally, in three patients who developed headaches after ingesting suspect foods, simultaneous sampling of their venous blood revealed elevated levels of histamine just prior to the onset of the vascular headache. Control challenges with placebos were not associated with migraine headaches or the appearance of histamine in the plasma (Mansfield et al., 1988). Although these studies convincingly demonstrate that, after food ingestion, histamine was released into the vascular space at the same time that a vascular headache occurred, several observations and questions remain unanswered. First, in both studies a substantial number of patients thought they were allergic to foods but had negative skin tests, or positive skin tests to that food followed by negative oral challenges. Unfortunately, the incidence of true food allergy inducing headaches in a migraine population continues to be unknown but could be quite low; such headaches may even be unusual. Second, although appearance of histamine suggests that an IgE-mediated reaction has occurred, plasma histamine determinations are difficult to perform, histamine can be found in certain foods themselves, and nonspecific stimuli can induce release of histamine from either mast cells or basophils. Therefore, until serum tryptase levels (specific for mast cell discharge) have been measured after ingestive challenges with specific foods, the cell source of histamine cannot be stated.

Another approach to the question of food inducing migraine headaches was to eliminate all foods (except lamb, pears, and spring water) for 5 days in a group of 60 migraine patients (Grant, 1979). All patients had previously been told to avoid cheese, chocolate, citrus fruits, alcohol, cigarette smoke (active or passive), hunger, and excessive stress and yet were still having frequent headaches. At the end of the first 5 days, new foods were tested as follows: Pulse rate and all symptoms were recorded before, 20 minutes after, and 1.5 hours after ingestion of each new food. All the patients experienced "reactions" to between 1 and 30 foods per patient, averaging 10 foods for each patient. Patients then eliminated the offending foods from their diet, with dramatic improvement in the frequency of migraine headaches. For the group of 60 patients, the number of headaches declined from 402 per month (prediet) to 6 per month (after starting the diet). The author concluded that the elimination of offending food allergens was the reason for the declining numbers of migraine headaches.

The reduction in frequency and intensity of migraine attacks by the ingestion of elimination diets is difficult to evaluate when attempting to use these data to support a cause-and-effect relationship between specific foods and migraine headaches. This is particularly the case during a "study" in which the investigator must be involved in recording the "results." The investigator's desire to help achieve a positive effect and the patients' motivation to help the results or at least not disappoint the investigator are variables that confound the result. Wolff (1955) put forth the thesis that the interest and good will of the physician and the expectation of improvement on the part of the patient may effect relief in many patients through neural rather than allergic avoidance mechanisms.

The term "dietary migraine" has been used by Dalessio (1972) to describe the relationship between eating certain foods and the onset of migraine headaches. Despite the controversy as to the existence of food-induced, IgE-mediated reactions, the observation that certain patients develop headaches after ingesting selected foods remains valid. It is now clear that many of those foods that appear to produce migraine have one thing in common. In addition to their food antigens, these ingestants also contain vasoactive chemicals or substrates for enzyme systems that synthesize vasoconstrictors. These chemicals and substrates have direct or indirect effects on cerebral blood vessel receptors, stimulating vasoconstriction of the susceptible migraine arteries. (See Chapter 5 for a list of vasoactive chemicals that all migraine patients should avoid.)

Epidemiologic Investigations of Migraine and Atopic Populations

Lance and Anthony (1966), in their headache clinic, studied 500 patients with migraine headaches and 100 patients with tension-type headaches. Of the migraine patients, 17% were found to have allergic disorders, including asthma, hay fever, hives, and eczema; 13% of the patients with tension-type headaches had similar allergies. There were no statistical differences between the populations, which strongly implied that migraine sufferers had no greater propensity toward allergies than did a control group of patients with tension-type headaches. Furthermore, an epidemiologic study of an entire Michigan community (population 11,305) showed that the incidence of asthma and allergic rhinitis was 21.8% for males and 25.3% for females (Broder et al., 1974). Urticaria is extremely common, occurring at least once during the lifetime of at least 20% of the general population (Smith, 1978). Our best available information leads to the conclusion that 20% of the adult population suffers from one or more manifestations of allergy or atopy, an incidence exceeding that found in Lance and Anthony's headache populations.

In a neurology clinic in Chicago, Bassoe (1933) found that only 3% of 270 migraine patients had any historic manifestations of allergy. Ziegler and colleagues (1972) studied 289 migraine patients and also found a very low incidence of associated allergic rhinitis and asthma.

In looking at the allergic population for the incidence of migraine, Schwartz (1952) examined 241 asthmatics and 200 nonallergic controls as well as their 3,815 relatives. He found an incidence of approximately 5% for migraine headaches among the asthmatics, normal controls, and their relatives. This figure is actually lower than the 15% incidence of migraine in the general population reported by Dalsgaard-Nielsen (1974). In another study by Kallos and Kallos-Deffner (1955), the incidence of migraine in their allergic population was 15%. Therefore, because migraine and allergy are frequently found in the general population, it is not surprising that nonrandom studies identified some patients with both conditions. It appears that approximately 20% of migraine patients have allergy and 15% of allergy patients have migraine headaches. Figure 13–16 illustrates this point.

Because of the difficulty in identifying some patients with allergic disease, even by allergy specialists, a potential criticism of studies that attempted to identify allergies in a migraine population has been that the nonallergist investigators failed to identify allergic patients accurately. Therefore, Medina and

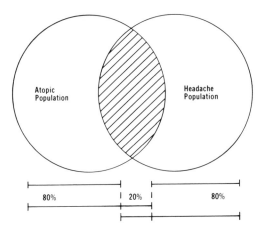

Figure 13–16. Schematic representation of the overlap between the atopic and migraine populations. The hash-marked area between the circles represents those atopic patients who also have migraine headaches.

Diamond (1976) measured total serum IgE levels in 89 unselected patients with migraine headaches and 27 control patients with tension-type headaches. Elevated levels of serum IgE were found in 6% of patients with migraine and 4% of patients with tension-type headaches, incidences not significantly different from each other or from those in the general population. By contrast, elevated levels of serum IgE were found in 41% of patients with respiratory allergy and in 79% of patients with atopic dermatitis and respiratory allergy (Smith, 1978).

Although there is no universal test to identify atopy and one must rely on the history to identify migraine patients, data linking these two conditions into a monogenetic or even polygenetic defect have been difficult to obtain or interpret. In a large study of babies born to women who enrolled in the Collaborative Perinatal Project, these children were followed through age 7. There were 2,510 pairs of mothers and babies who were divided into combinations of mothers without migraine headaches or asthma and allergies (1,765), those mothers without migraine headaches but who did have asthma and allergies (404), those mothers who did have migraine headaches but did not have asthma or allergies (238), and those mothers who had both migraine headaches and asthma and allergies (103). The follow-up of the children from these mothers indicated that asthma was slightly more frequent in the children if the mothers had either asthma and allergies or migraine headaches. Asthma appeared in 3.2% of children from headache- and asthma/allergy-free mothers, as contrasted with 6.3% from mothers with migraine and no asthma/allergies, 6.8% from mothers who were headache free but with asthma/allergies, and 11.6% from mothers with both migraine headaches and asthma/allergies. Interpretation of these epidemiologic observations was further confounded by variables such as race, environment, and smoking history. Even if one could bypass such variables, the differences among groups were not striking, although statistical differences were observed (Chen and Leviton, 1990). Because both allergy and migraine are common conditions, they will segregate in epidemiologic studies with some frequency. Whether or not they are linked genetically cannot be proven or discarded. However, the presence of one does not appear to protect against the other. Some patients have both and, in these individuals, it is important to deal realistically with both disorders.

Migraine Headaches in Allergic Patients

Patients who have allergic disease may also have other disease processes that are not caused by their allergy but under certain circumstances may be worsened by the allergy itself, drugs used to treat the allergy, or the psychological consequences of having a chronic disease. Allergic patients may develop paranasal sinus headaches, tension-type headaches from tension and worry over their diseases, and (in susceptible individuals) migraine headache with aura. Is there any evidence that type I IgE-mediated reactions precipitate migraine headaches in the allergic subgroup of migraine patients?

Kallos and Kallos-Deffner's (1955) experiments are particularly interesting. They selected a small group of 28 patients who had both migraine headaches and urticaria, rhinitis, or asthma. They injected extracts of specific allergens into these patients, using concentrations great enough to produce typical IgE-mediated reactions of rhinitis, asthma, or urticaria. In most patients, a vascular headache followed the parenteral injections of large dosages of allergenic extracts. However, two important clarifying observations were made. Headache always appeared in association with rhinitis, asthma, or urticaria and never as the only manifestation of an allergen-induced systemic reaction. Second, the migraine aura was universally absent. The nasopulmonary reaction could then be prevented by pretreating the patient with antihistamine (H_1 blockers), but the vascular headache continued to occur unless the patient was pretreated with ergotamine, which blocked the headache but had no effect on the respiratory tract reactions. These very interesting observations suggest that mediators released during IgE-mediated anaphylaxis can produce vascular headaches. If this mediator is histamine, it would also require H_2 cerebral arterial receptors, since H_1 antihistamines do not block vascular headache.

The role of histamine in vascular headaches was first reported by Pickering (1933), who injected 0.1 mg of histamine intravenously, producing vascular headaches in all subjects. Keeney (1946) systematically reviewed this topic and studied 37 patients with periodic vascular headache. Twenty-four developed typical vascular headaches after subcutaneous injections of 0.1 mg histamine. In 7 of 10 patients, 0.6 mg of nitroglycerine sublingually also produced vascular headache, suggesting that vasodilation, rather than a specific susceptibility to histamine, represented the pathogenic event in vascular head pain.

Although it is clear that subcutaneous or intravenous injections of large dosages of histamine or other vasodilators will produce headaches in susceptible individuals, it is not clear if these observations have any relevance to spontaneous migraine occurring as a consequence of IgE-mediated rhinitis, asthma, or urticaria.

In an important study by Kaliner et al. (1982), plasma and histamine levels were measured during continuous infusions of histamine into eight normal volunteers and four asthmatics not taking any medications. Resting or baseline plasma histamine levels were 0.62 ± 0.12 ng/ml and rose progressively in direct proportion to the concentration of infused histamine. Plasma levels of histamine required to elicit symptoms were as follows: 1.61 ± 0.30 ng/ml produced a 30% increase in heart rate, and 2.39 ± 0.52 ng/ml produced significant flush and headache. Pretreatment with hydroxyzine (H_1 blocker) or cimetidine (H_2 blocker) failed to influence the amount (level) of histamine associated with flush and headache. However, pretreatment with both an H_1 and an H_2 blocker raised the threshold whereby histamine produced the same symptoms (5.76 ± 0.78 ng/ml) when compared with the lower levels of histamine previously associated with headache and flush (2.39 ng/ml) when pretreatment was not carried out.

Another interesting study of intravenous histamine infusion (Krabbe and Olesen, 1980) was conducted in three patient groups: 13 normal, non–headache-prone volunteers, 10 patients who suffered from tension-type headaches, and 25 patients with recurrent migraine headaches. Histamine infusion of 0.16, 0.33, and 0.66 µg/kg/minute were used. The results showed that normal volunteers did not develop headache, although flushing and other systemic symptoms prevented maximum infusion of histamine in 4 out of 13 subjects. In the 10 tension-type headache patients, 5 had mild throbbing headache and 4 experienced a pressing type of head pain during the histamine infusion; 1 patient did not experience head pain despite maximum histamine infusion. In the 25 migraine patients, all but one developed severe pounding head pain during histamine infusions that were often less than 0.66 μ/kg. In 15 out of 18 migraine patients, simultaneous infusion of the H_1 blocker mepyramine diminished or blocked the headache. Cimetidine (H_2 blocker) also decreased headache significantly. Pretreatment with H_1 and H_2 blockers was not attempted.

The relevance of these artificial laboratory experiments to naturally occurring migraine headaches is not clear. For instance, Anthony et al. (1978) conducted a clinical trial using both chlorpheniramine (H_1 blocker) and cimetidine (H_2 blocker) in the chronic prophylaxis for prevention of migraine headaches. They found no benefit over the placebo treatment regimen.

In patients with allergic diseases such as asthma, neither spontaneous exacerbations of asthma with elevated histamine, 1 to 5 ng/ml (Simon et al., 1977), nor antigen inhalation–induced asthma with plasma histamine of 1 to 6 ng/ml (Bhat et al., 1976) was associated with any headaches despite other systemic symptoms of histaminemia, including significant asthma and flushing.

In spontaneous rhinitis, asthma, or urticaria, it seems unlikely that enough histamine molecules spill into the vascular space, escape active degradation, and become available to vascular receptors in the cerebral arteries to effect significant vasodilation in most normal subjects. However, in patients with vascular headaches and significant target organ susceptibility to any vasodilators, such mechanisms may play an occasional role in producing head pain.

There are several artificial systems wherein a large intravascular discharge of mediators can occur. In systemic anaphylaxis, antigen is circulating in the vascular space and interacting with IgE fixed to circulating basophils. This leads to the release of mediators from these storage cells that are within the vascular spaces. Under such circumstances, 100 ng/ml of histamine may be measured in the plasma and patients frequently develop generalized peripheral vasodilation and hypotensive shock. Selected patients also develop vascular headaches. These have been recorded in the absence of treatment with epinephrine, another pharmacologic cause of head pain. Systemic anaphylaxis occurs in the following instances: after a bee sting, after injection of drugs (penicillin) or proteins (horse serum), with food anaphylaxis, and as a side effect of desensitization injections for the treatment of hay fever and asthma.

In 1950 Loveless studied the occurrence of headache, as well as other effects of overdosage of allergens, in 177 pollen-sensitive persons. Headache, when it occurred in these subjects after allergen injection overdosage, was generalized and not hemicranial. It occurred in both those with and those without histories of frequent headache attacks. Of the 177 subjects, there were 925 overdosage reactions. Twelve of the 177 subjects experienced headaches as part of such overdosage reactions on one or more occasions. Indeed, these 12 persons experienced 26 headaches during 121 overdosage reactions, or 21% of the time. For the entire group, the incidence of headache as an aspect of allergen overdosage effects was 2.8%, and headache always occurred as part of a widespread allergen overdosage syndrome, including urticaria, rhinitis, asthma, and/

or hypotension. In the Loveless study, headache never occurred as an isolated phenomenon during IgE-mediated reactions.

Because most allergy practices have an incidence of systemic reactions to injected allergy extracts on the order of 1:500 injections, this artificial or iatrogenic event cannot begin to account for spontaneous vascular or migraine headaches, even in the small portion of atopic population receiving immunotherapy.

Walker (1960) again emphasized the insignificance of the effects of food allergens in the migraine headache attack. She was not able to demonstrate a significant therapeutic effect from elimination diets but was convinced that for some patients the occurrence of allergic phenomena is so disturbing and exhausting it is sufficient to precipitate migraine attack by psychoneural pathways. Sleep deprivation is a major problem in chronic allergic disease.

SUMMARY

Allergic reactions can be categorized into four types, according to Gell and Coombs (1968). Any type of rhinitis can be associated with paranasal head pain. The headache is dull, deep, aching, and nonpulsatile. It is associated with nasal congestion. One type of rhinitis is IgE mediated and a legitimate cause of paranasal head pain. The mucosa covering the approaches to the paranasal sinuses was found to be the most pain sensitive of the nasal and paranasal structures and cavities, whereas the mucosa lining the sinuses was of relatively low sensitivity.

Inflammation and engorgement of the turbinates, ostia, nasofrontal ducts, and superior nasal spaces are responsible for most of the pain emanating from the nasal and paranasal structures. Most of the pain arising from faradic, mechanical, and chemical stimulation of the mucosa of the nasal and paranasal cavities was referred pain—that is, it was felt at a site other than that stimulated. It was referred chiefly to those areas supplied by the first division of the fifth cranial nerve.

The phenomena of migraine headaches and certain allergic responses are similar in many respects. In both, attacks are paroxysmal, with associated edema and hyperemia, presumably mediated by protein breakdown products and terminated by vasoconstrictor drugs. However, there is evidence that histamine infusion or ingestion of allergens with release of histamine is implicated in the etiology of some migraine headache attacks. It is very unlikely that allergic mechanisms account for most migraine headaches. Stress induced by chronic, sleep-depriving allergic diseases and medications used to treat allergy seems to be an important linkage between allergic disease of the respiratory tract and headaches.

REFERENCES

Altman, L.C. and G.J. Gleich (1990). Eosinophils. *Immunol. Allergy Clin. North Am.* *10*:263–271.

Anthony, M., G.D.A. Lord, and J.W. Lance (1978). Controlled trials of cimetidine in migraine and cluster headache. *Headache 18*:261–264.

Atkins, C.J., J.J. Kondon, and F.P. Quismorio (1972). The choroid plexis in systemic lupus erythematosus. *Ann. Intern. Med. 76:*165–172.

Austen, K.F. (1984). The heterogeneity of mast cell populations and products. *Hosp. Pract. 19:*135–146.

Balyeat, R.M. and F.L. Brittain (1930). Allegic migraine—based on a study of 55 cases. *Am. J. Med. Sci. 180:*212–220.

Bassoe, P. (1933). Migraine. *JAMA 101:*599–605.

Beall, G.N. and P.P. Van Arsdel (1960). Histamine metabolism in human disease. *J. Clin. Invest. 39:*676–684.

Benveniste, J. (1974). Platelet-activating factor, a new mediator of anaphylaxis and immune complex desposition from rabbit and human basophils. *Nature 249:* 581–582.

Bergstrom, S.H., H. Duner, U.S. Von Euler et al. (1959). Observations on the effects of infusions of prostaglandin E in man. *Acta Physiol. Scand. 45:*144–153.

Bhat, K.N., C.M. Arroyave, S.R. Marney et al. (1976). Plasma histamine changes during provoked bronchospasm in asthmatic patients. *J. Allergy Clin. Immunol. 58:* 647–656.

Broder, E., M.W. Higgins, K.P. Mathews, and J.B. Keller (1974). The epidemiology of asthma and hay fever in a total community: Tecumseh, Michigan. *J. Allergy Clin. Immunol. 54:*100–112.

Chen, T.C. and A. Leviton (1990). Asthma and eczema in children born to women with migraine. *Arch. Neurol. 47:*1227–1230.

Cochrane, C.G. and J.H. Griffin (1982). The biochemistry and pathophysiology of the contact system of plasma. *Adv. Immunol. 33:*241–305.

Dalessio, D.J. (1972). Dietary migraine. *Am. Fam. Physician 6:*60–65.

Dalsgaard-Nielsen, T. (1974). The nature of migraine. *Headache 14:*13–18.

David, J.R. and R.R. David (1972). Cellular hypersensitivity and immunity: Inhibition of macrophage migration and lymphocyte mediators. *Prog. Allergy 16:*300–332.

DeGowin, E.L. (1932). Allergic migraine: Review of sixty cases. *J. Allergy 3:*557–564.

Fowler, P.B.S. (1962). Epilepsy due to angioneurotic edema. *Proc. R. Soc. Med. 55:* 13–15.

Gell, P.G.H. and R.R.A. Coombs (1968). The allergic response and immunity. In *Clinical Aspects of Immunology,* pp. 423–456. F.A. Davis, Philadelphia.

Gonzales, S. (1953). Association of asthma and headache of allergic origin. *Med. Ibera 2:*747–753.

Goth, A. (1978). Antihistamines. In *Allergy: Principles and Practice* (E. Middleton, C. Reed, and E. Ellis, eds.), pp. 454–463. C.V. Mosby, St. Louis.

Grant, E.C.G. (1979). Food allergies and migraine. *Lancet 1:*966–968.

Hahn, L. (1930). Relation between migraine and allergy. *Med. Klin. 26:*1219–1226.

Hamburger, J. (1935). Migraine: Role of food allergy. *Rev. Immunol. (Paris) 1:*102–109.

Hazelman, B.L., I.C.M. MacLennan, and R.G. Earler (1975). Lymphocyte proliferation to artery antigen as a positive diagnostic test in polymyalgia rheumatica. *Ann. Rheum. Dis. 34:*122–128.

Healey, L.A. and K.R. Wilske (1977). Manifestations of giant cell arteritis. *Med. Clin. North Am. 61:*261–270.

Hyslop, G.H. (1934). Migraine: Suggestions for its treatment. *Med. Clin. North Am 17:* 827–842.

Kaliner, M. and K.F. Austen (1973). A sequence of biochemical events in the antigen-induced release of chemical mediators from sensitized human lung tissue. *J. Exp. Med. 138:*1094–1102.

Kaliner, M., J.H. Shelhamer, and E.A. Ottesen (1982). Effects of infused histamine:

Correlation of plasma histamine levels and symptoms. *J. Allergy Clin. Immunol.* 69:283–289.

Kallos, P., and L. Kallos-Deffner (1955). Allergy and migraine. *Int. Arch. Allergy Appl. Immunol.* 7:367–392.

Kaplan, A. (1978). Urticaria and angioedema. In *Allergy: Principles and Practice* (E. Middleton, C. Reed, and E. Ellis, eds.), pp. 1080–1099. C.V. Mosby, St. Louis.

Kaplan, A.P. and K.F. Austen (1975). Activation and control mechanisms of Hagemen factor–dependent pathways of coagulation, fibrinolysis and kinin generation and their contribution to the inflammatory process. *J. Allergy Clin. Immunol. 5b:* 491–503.

Kay, A.B. and K.F. Austen (1971). The IgE-mediated release of an eosinophil leukocyte chemotactic factor from human lung. *J. Immunol.* 107:899–906.

Keeney, E.L. (1946). Periodic vascular head pain. *Immunology and Allergy Clinics N. America 5:*550–567.

Klein, R.G., R.J. Campbell, G.G. Hunder, and J.A. Carney (1976). Skip lesions in temporal arteritis. *Mayo Clin. Proc. 51:*504–510.

Kohler, P.F. (1978). Immune complexes and allergic disease. In *Allergy: Principles and Practice* (E. Middleton, C. Reed, and E. Ellis, eds.), pp. 155–176. C.V. Mosby, St. Louis.

Krabbe, A.E. and J. Olesen (1980). Headache provoked by continuous intravenous infusion of histamine. *Pain 8:*253–259.

Lance, J.W. and M. Anthony (1966). Some clinical aspects of migraine. *Arch. Neurol.* 15:356–361.

Lever, W.F. (1961). Urticaria and angioedema. In *Histopathology of the Skin,* pp. 114–120. J.B. Lippincott, Philadelphia.

Lewis, G.P. (1961). Bradykinin. *Nature 192:*596–600.

Lewis, R.A., K.F. Austen and R.J. Soberman (1990). Leukotrienes and other products of the 5-lipoxygenase pathway. *N. Engl. J. Med. 323:*645–655.

Loveless, M.H. (1950). Milk allergy. A survey of its incidence: Experiments with a masked ingestion test. *J. Allergy 21:*489–501.

Mansfield, L.E., T.R. Vaughan and S.F. Waller (1985). Food allergy and migraine: Double blind and mediator confirmation of an allergic etiology. *Ann. Allergy 55:* 126–129.

Mansfield, L.E., T.R. Vaughan and S.F. Waller (1988). Food allergy in headaches: Whom to evaluate and how to treat. *Postgrad. Med. 83:*46–55.

Mathews, K.P. (1974). A current view of urticaria. *Med. Clin. North Am. 58:*185–196.

May, C.D. and S.A. Bock (1978). Adverse reactions to food due to hypersensitivity. In *Allergy: Principles and Practice* (E. Middleton, C. Reed, and E. Ellis, eds.), pp. 1159–1171. C.V. Mosby, St. Louis.

Medina, J.L. and S. Diamond (1976). Migraine and atopy. *Headache 15:*271–274.

Mencia-Huerta, J.M., B. Dugas and P. Braquet (1990). Immunologic reactions in asthma. *Immunol. Allergy Clin. North Am. 10:*337–353.

Millonig, A.G., H.E. Harris, and W.J. Gardner (1950). Effect of autonomic denervation on the nasal mucosa. *Arch. Otolaryngol. 52:*359–365.

Monro, J., J. Brostoff, C. Carini, and K. Zilkha (1980). Food allergy in migraine. *Lancet 1:*1–4.

Neusser, E. (1892). Klinisch-hamatologische Mittheilungen. *Wein. Klin. Wocherschr 5:* 41–45.

Newball, H.H., R.C. Talamo, and L.M. Lichtenstein (1975). Release of leukocyte kallikrein mediated by IgE. *Nature 254:*635–637.

Nutman, D.D., N. Kurata, and E.M. Tan (1975). Profiles of antinuclear antibodies in systemic rheumatic diseases. *Ann. Intern. Med. 83:*464–469.

Ogden, H.D. (1951). The treatment of allergic headache. *Ann. Allergy* 9:611–619.

O'Neil, W.N., Jr., S.P. Hammar, and H.A. Bloomer (1976). Giant cell arteritis with visceral angiitis. *Arch. Intern. Med.* 136:1157–1160.

Pagniez, P., P. Vallery-Radot and A. Nast (1919). Therapeutique preventive de certaines migraines. *Presse Med.* 27:172–176.

Pickering, G.W. (1933). Histamine headache. *Clin. Sci.* 1:77–101.

Plaut, M. and L.M. Lichtenstein (1983). Cellular and chemical basis of the allergic inflammatory response. In *Allergy: Principles and Practice* (E. Middleton, C. Reed, and E. Ellis, eds.), pp. 119–146. C.V. Mosby, St. Louis.

Proud, D., C.R. Baumgarten, R.M. Naclerio, and L.M. Lichtenstein (1986). The role of kinins in human disease. *NER Allergy Proc.* 7:213–218.

Ralston, H.J. and W.J. Kerr (1945). Vascular responses of the nasal mucosa to thermal stimuli with some observations on skin temperature. *Am. J. Physiol.* 144:305–312.

Rinkel, H.J. (1933). Considerations of allergy as a factor in familial recurrent headache. *J. Allergy* 4:303–312.

Rowe, A.H. (1932). Allergic migraine. *JAMA* 99:912–917.

Ruddy, S., I. Gigli, and K.F. Austen (1972). The complement system in man. *N. Engl. J. Med.* 287:489–495.

Ryan, R.E., Sr., and R.E. Ryan, Jr. (1979). Headache of nasal origin. *Headache* 19: 173–177.

Schwartz, M. (1952). Is migraine an allergic disease? *Acta Allerg.* 5(Suppl. II):426–432.

Simon, R.A., D.D. Stevenson, D.M. Arroyave, and E.M. Tan (1977). The relationship of plasma histamine to the activity of bronchial asthma. *J. Allergy Clin. Immunol.* 60:312–316.

Smith, J.M. (1978). Epidemiology and natural history of asthma, allergic rhinitis and atopic dermatitis (eczema). In *Allergy: Principles and Practice* (E. Middleton, C. Reed, and E. Ellis, eds.), p. 637. C.V. Mosby, St. Louis.

Solomon, W.R. (1967). Hay fever, allergic rhinitis and asthma. In *A Manual of Clinical Allergy* (J.M. Sheldon, ed.), pp. 78–88. W.B. Saunders, Philadelphia.

Soter, N.A. (1990). Urticaria: Current therapy. *J. Allergy Clin. Immunol.* 86:1009–1014.

Speer, F. (1975). The many facets of migraine. *Ann. Allergy* 34:273–285.

Stanson, A.W., R.G. Klein, and G.G. Hunder (1976). Extracranial angiographic findings in giant cell arteritis. *Am. J. Roentgenol.* 137:957–963.

Tennenbaum, J.I. (1972). Allergic rhinitis. In *Allergic Diseases* (R. Patterson, ed.), p. 172. J.B. Lippincott, Philadelphia.

Trousseau, A. (1873). *Clinique Medical de L'Hotel-Dieu de Paris*, 4th ed., Vol. 2, p. 460. Bailliere, Paris.

Unger, A.H., and L. Unger (1952). Migraine is an allergic disease. *J. Allergy* 23:429–436.

Unger, L. and J.L. Cristol (1970). Allergic migraine. *Ann. Allergy* 28:106–112.

Unger, L. and M.C. Harris (1974). Stepping-stones in allergy. *Ann. Allergy* 33:353–363.

Vahlquist, B. (1955). Migraine in children. *Int. Arch. Allergy* 7:348–360.

Vane, J.R. (1976). The mode of action of aspirin and similar compounds. *J. Allergy Clin. Immunol.* 58:691–712.

Van Leeuwen, W. and Z. Zeydner (1922). Occurrence of toxic substance in blood in cases of broncial asthma, urticaria, epilepsy and migraine. *Br. J. Exp. Pathol.* 3: 282–287.

Vaughan, W.T. (1934). Analysis of allergic factor in recurrent paroxysmal headache. *Trans. Assoc. Am. Physicians* 49:348–358.

von Pirquet, C. (1906). Allergie. *Munchen. Med. Wochenschr.* 53:1457–1465.

Waaler, E., O. Tonder, and E.J. Milde (1976). Immunological and histological studies of temporal arteries from patients with temporal arteritis and/or polymyalgia rheumatica. *Acta Pathol. Microbiol. Scand.* 84:55–63.

Walker, V.B. (1960). *Report to the Ciba Foundation Conference on Migraine*. CIBA Foundation, London.

Wasserman, S.I. (1983). Mediators of immediate hypersensitivity. *J. Allergy Clin. Immunol.* 72:101–115.

Wasserman, S.I., N.A. Soter, D.M. Center, and K.F. Austen (1977). Cold urticaria: Recognition and characteristics of a neutrophil chemotactic factor which appears in serum during experimental and cold challenge. *J. Clin. Invest.* 60:189–196.

Wolf, A.A. and L. Unger (1944). Migraine due to milk; Feeding tests. *Ann. Intern. Med.* 20:831–843.

Wolff, H.G. (1955). Headache mechanisms. *Int. Arch. Allergy* 7:210–225.

Ziegler, D.K., R. Hassanein, and K. Hassanein (1972). Headache syndromes suggested by factor analysis of symptom variables in a headache prone population. *J. Chron. Dis.* 25:353–362.

14

The Teeth and Jaws as Sources of Headache and Facial Pain

FRANCIS V. HOWELL

Both odontalgia and the broad area of myofascial pain, sometimes referred to as temporomandibular joint (TMJ) syndrome, are of considerable interest to the physician and the dentist. The fifth cranial nerve (trigeminal nerve) has wide distribution in the anterior portion of the head, and disturbances over this distribution may produce variable responses that are often difficult to evaluate. Trigeminal neuralgia may mimic toothache, and many teeth have been removed or pulps extirpated for root canal therapy by the uninitiated clinician. Conversely, odontalgia can, in certain instances, produce many of the symptoms of trigeminal neuralgia.

Ruling out dental disease and TMJ dysfunction is mandatory in evaluating headache and other facial pain, particularly when it is unilateral. Bilateral pain is frequently associated with emotional disturbances. Pilling (1968) and Clark (1987) have written good reviews of the relationship of structural disharmony and psychological stress, and McCreary et al. (1991) examined the psychological differences among diagnostic subgroups of TMJ dysfunction patients and found that "somatic overconcern" was a significant factor in pain and its control, but anxiety or depression was not.

Pain due to inflammatory and retrograde pulpal disease and to independent or concomitant periodontal disease is relatively common. It is not difficult to eliminate, particularly if the specific lesion can be demonstrated clinically or radiologically. However, in some atypical manifestations of pulpal disease and the TMJ syndrome, direct etiology may not always be obvious.

The dental profession is well aware that apprehension regarding impending dental procedures constitutes a real barrier to adequate diagnosis, and that pain perception may be altered by affecting the threshold of response to painful stimulation like that during nerve testing, digital palpation, percussion, or some other painful procedure. In the TMJ syndrome, emotional factors are often of extreme importance.

ANATOMIC AND PHYSIOLOGIC CONSIDERATIONS

Impulses from the teeth and TMJ area are carried by branches of the second and third divisions of the fifth cranial nerve. Nerves enter the pulp through the apex and accompany the larger vessels to form an almost complete mantle around the arteries (Berkelback van der Sprenkle, 1935–36). These nerve fibers form a complicated network between the odontoblasts and extend partially into the calcified portion of the dentinal tubule, permitting the dentin, wherever exposed, to transmit pain (Lewinsky and Stewart, 1935–36). Brashear (1936) found that more than half of the unmyelinated and small myelinated nerve fibers were less than 6 μ, with the remainder varying in size up to 10 μ. Thermal, mechanical, and chemical stimulation of dentin in a normal tooth results only in pain, with the patient unable to differentiate its exact cause.

Therefore, a tooth that is "alive" can be stimulated by numerous irritants, and the resultant pain can be described by the patient only as "pain." In contrast, sensations such as touch and pressure appear to be transmitted primarily to the nerve endings in the periodontal ligament and the alveolar bone. These sensations are often easily described by the patient.

A classic study by Robertson et al. (1947) demonstrated the distribution and pathophysiology of headache and other pain in the face and head resulting from afferent impulses originating in the teeth. Comparisons were made between experimental stimulation of the teeth and clinical situations in which morbid processes were present. In the study, two different electrical methods were employed: one for inducing toothache well above the pain threshold, and the other for inducing pain only at the threshold. Pain was estimated on an arbitrary basis of 1 to 10, with 10 + being extremely high intensity or the point at which the patient experienced the "worst" pain. Toothache was held at the 4 to 6 intensity for a period of 10 minutes. In the lower ranges of intensity, initial current inducing toothaches had to be increased to continue to induce pain.

The second method used to induce pain at its threshold employed a "vitalometer," as described by Ziskin and Wald (1938). This is a method similar to the pulp-testing procedures performed clinically by most dentists. The pain threshold in this phase of the experiment was expressed as the smallest voltage that would elicit a painful sensation.

DEGENERATIVE AND INFLAMMATORY ODONTALGIA

Description of Headache Resulting from Noxious Stimulation of Teeth

In a study conducted at the New York Hospital, headache that occurred after experimental induction of toothache in the manner described above was divided into series 1 (noxious stimulation of teeth in the upper jaw) and series 2 (noxious stimulation of teeth in the lower jaw). In series 1, with stimulation to a premolar or first molar tooth in the maxilla, pain of 4 + to 8 + intensity was manifested by pain in the tooth. However, following a break in the stimulating current, a jab of more intense pain was experienced as a "narrow column of pain which spread vertically into the eye, the orbital ridge, and the temple." With extremely intense toothache (10 +), pain spread into adjacent teeth and along the maxilla.

During the period of toothache, intense apprehension, profuse salivation, lacrimation, and flushing of the face on the side of stimulation were noted, with generalized sweating. On termination of stimulation, pain decreased quickly to 1 + intensity, with only a sensation of pressure between the teeth. After toothache completely diminished, there was a continuing sensation of tightness, slight numbness, and fullness over the cheek, and a tight, stiff sensation in the skin and deep tissues in the temporal region, the forehead, and scalp on the same side. Some stiffness in the TMJ and fullness in the ear were described. Within 5 to 10 minutes after all pain in the tooth was terminated, a steady aching and diffuse pain of 1 + intensity was experienced in the temporal region, along the zygomatic ridge, and for a short distance over the eye. Figure 14–1 presents a graphic demonstration of the pattern of head pain 5 minutes (A) and 20 minutes (B) after stimulation. Most headache persisted from 1 to 8 hours, and in one instance for up to 24 hours, with gradually diminishing intensity. Although the sensation of tightness, fullness, and numbness was rather short lived, during the period of diminishing intensity there was photophobia and injection of the conjunctiva, with tenderness to the temporal muscle and overlying tissues on palpation. Sensation to a pinprick was sharper.

In series 2, a lower premolar or first molar tooth was stimulated in the same

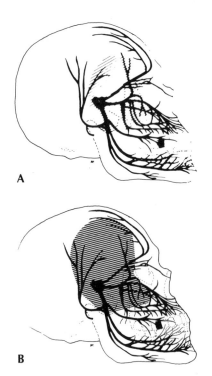

A

B

Figure 14–1. (A), The distribution of sensations of fullness, numbness, and stiffness 5 minutes after noxious stimulation of the upper right second bicuspid (4). (B), The distribution of headache 20 minutes after noxious stimulation of the upper right second bicuspid (4).

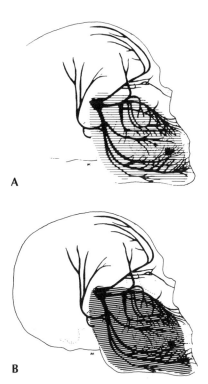

Figure 14–2. (*A*), The distribution of fullness, numbness, and stiffness 5 minutes after noxious stimulation of the lower right second bicuspid (29). (*B*), The distribution of headache 20 minutes after noxious stimulation of the lower right second bicuspid (29).

manner as in series 1, maintaining the 4+ to 8+ toothache for a period of 10 minutes. During the stimulation, there was intense aching pain in the tooth with a less intense pain throughout the lower jaw extending into the anterior wall of the ear canal. At the end of the stimulation, the high-intensity pain was quickly terminated but a persistent sensation of pressure in the tooth was noted, often accompanied by a dull, diffuse, aching pain of low intensity throughout the lower jaw on the same side. Subsequently, a sensation of fullness and heaviness developed, and a 2+ to 3+ intensity of pain extended throughout the upper and lower jaws into the zygoma and temporal area and over the top of the ear. There was also fullness and aching in the ear. This "lower-half" headache was increased in intensity by biting and bending over. The pattern is well demonstrated in Figure 14–2. Many of the same effects were noted as in series 1: apprehension, lacrimation, salivation, flushing of the face, photophobia, and generalized sweating as well as stiffness of the masseter muscle. The amount of pain in response to aspirin was the same in series 1 and series 2. In each series, the effects of noxious stimulation were completely reversible and no sequelae were noted. Results of this classic and extensive study are well documented by the clinical pattern of pain resulting from retrograde and inflammatory odontalgia.

In the same experiment, the effect of application of local anesthetic to the source of noxious stimulation adjacent to the tooth was investigated in two phases. In the first, there was direct injection of procaine into the area of headache. Pain persisted in a scattered fashion, with the greatest area of pain diminished. However, there was complete absence of pain following local anesthetic injection by an infiltrative procedure (tuberosity injection). Some pain returned following the cessation of anesthesia to the area; in some cases, the area remained pain-free when normal sensation returned to the tooth.

The elimination of headache after blocking the path of afferent impulses from the tooth and adjacent tissues allows one to assume that the painful experience was caused by afferent impulses arising from the stimulated tooth. These afferent impulses gave rise to excitatory processes in the brainstem, which spread to exert effects on many trigeminal structures.

Practical Clinical Considerations

Although it can be demonstrated by the described experiments of toothache-induced headache and by clinical manifestation of odontalgia that the headache follows certain prescribed patterns, there is a practical clinical consideration. Only under unusual circumstances can this type of headache be seen without accompanying odontalgia from a diseased pulp or an inflamed periodontium. A relatively easy elimination of this pain by nerve blockage or infiltrative local anesthesia produces a fairly clear-cut cause-and-effect relationship. Unfortunately, the observation made experimentally that the headache can return when the local anesthetic effect dissipates often leads, in a clinical situation, to discomfort for the patient. The present practice of using short-acting, local anesthetics for all dental operative procedures should possibly be modified by the clinician. Certainly, the patient who is undergoing routine filling procedures on the teeth does not want local anesthetic effects for a long period of time. However, when the clinician is aware that nerve tissue has been subjected to considerable agitation, the use of long-acting local anesthetics such as bupivacaine hydrochloride should be considered.

Odontalgia from the usual degenerative and inflammatory etiologies produces fairly predictable patterns of pain, which become obvious when local anesthesia is used and the pain dissipates. Occasionally, the localization of the tooth involved in the odontalgia may be difficult because in early pulpal degenerative stages the tooth may not be sensitive to percussion or show other evidence of pressure building within. All dentists are aware that analgesics may be required for the patient until the exact source of the problem can be determined in a few hours or even a few days.

CRACKED TOOTH SYNDROME

Another type of pain, termed the "cracked tooth syndrome" (incomplete tooth fracture, greenstick fracture, etc.) is of considerable clinical significance to the physician as well as to the dentist in evaluating pain because the pain does not follow the "usual" patterns of directly induced and referred pain. Frequently, the patient is seen by the dentist, who can find no organic evidence of dental disease and then seeks referral to a physician, often a neurologist. In my experience, almost half of the patients who are seen with this syndrome are referred by physicians.

The condition has been recognized in the dental literature for a number of years. Gibbs (1954) termed the condition "cuspal fracture odontalgia." Sutton (1962) described the condition as greenstick fracture, and Cameron (1964) coined the term "cracked tooth syndrome," which appears to predominate in the current dental literature. The term "incomplete tooth fracture," suggested by Maxwell and Braly in 1977, indicated that the syndrome itself resulted because the tooth did not fracture completely; rather, only dentinal tubules were involved. In the most comprehensive study to date, Cameron (1964) presented a series of significant cases (Table 14–1) that indicated that more than half of all cracked teeth are mandibular molars, with the second molar being the most commonly involved. There has been considerable speculation as to the preponderance of involvement of the lower molar teeth. Possibly the motion of the mandible and the position of the lingual cusps of the maxillary molars produce a cleavage action.

Unlike ordinary odontalgia caused by retrograde pulpal disease, most of the teeth involved in this syndrome have few, if any, restorations. The cusps are usually normal in appearance. Examination of prehistoric skulls does not reveal significant incidence of cracked teeth, and it has been speculated that the popularity of hot liquids, such as coffee and soup, and the ready availability of cold and frozen foods, such as ice cream, combine to produce extensive expansion and contraction of the enamel and dentin, thus making the coronal structure susceptible to fracture. In my experience, many of these patients are ice chewers, and it is believed that the melting of the ice cube into the fossae between the cusps can produce considerable lateral pressure against the cusps as the ice crystal fractures under pressure. Ice chewing appears to be a definite hazard to all patients who have small fillings within the central grooves between the cusps as well as to those who have no restorations.

In Figure 14–3 (a dental radiogram from a patient who is an ice chewer), the second molar tooth (to the right) contains an anteroposterior (mesiodistal)

Table 14–1 Locations of cracked teeth

Tooth	No.	Percentage
Mandibular		
Second molars	17	34
First molars	9	18
Third molars	1	2
Bicuspids	1	2
Maxillary		
First molars	12	24
Second molars	2	4
First bicuspids	6	12
Second bicuspids	2	4
Totals	50	100

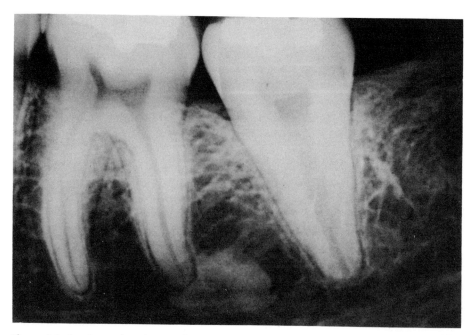

Figure 14–3. Second molar (single-rooted tooth) exhibits thickening of periodontal ligament on sides near apex. This is an indication of a split tooth.

crack beneath the small occlusal restoration. The pulp tests were "normal." In this particular case, the patient presented with pain to cold and pressure, particularly compression of tough foods. Pain was present only at certain times, and the patient could be free of pain for weeks. As the crack was subjected to more occlusal pressure, particularly from ice chewing, the pain became more intense until finally the crack was discovered and a crown was placed on the tooth. This completely eliminated the symptoms, and, after 5 years, the tooth is completely normal.

The symptomatology of a cracked tooth is summarized in Table 14–2. Typically, a patient will complain of pain radiating to the side of the head after biting on compressible food, such as nuts, meat, or bread crusts. The pain is often sudden, and after the initial impulse cannot be localized to a specific tooth

Table 14–2 Symptoms of cracked teeth

Pain	No. of patients
Pressure	27
Cold	16
Heat	14
Ache	9
Cellulitis	5
Sweet	1
None reported	6

by the patient. Following such an incident, there is extreme sensitivity to cold. This sensation will continue to be an important diagnostic consideration because the electric pulp tester often does not differentiate between a normal tooth and the cracked tooth. Cold applied to a tooth can be a distinguishing feature if the tooth is hypersensitive.

As the cracked tooth syndrome proceeds, if not discovered, the traumatization to the dental tubules will allow direct penetration of the dental pulp and actual pulpal death, with the usual sequelae. It is extremely important for the dentist as well as the physician to realize that, when the condition is first discovered, coronal protection is indicated to preserve the vitality of the pulp tissue. Without preserving the pulp, no repair can take place. Many dentists, on finding such a tooth, often resort to root canal therapy. Because oral fluid will continue to seep into the cracked areas, endodontic treatments are unsuccessful. In addition, Campbell et al. (1990) have recently shown that about 5% of patients who had had endodontic treatment by open surgical procedures had continual pain. Half of these cases were due to post-traumatic dysesthesia and half to phantom tooth pain.

TEMPOROMANDIBULAR JOINT SYNDROME (MYOFASCIAL PAIN DYSFUNCTION SYNDROME)

Costen's (1934) concept of occlusal disharmony with resultant damage to the TMJ was attributed to a wide variety of signs and symptoms; this has now been totally discarded and replaced by concepts probably first delineated by Schwartz in 1955. The term "temporomandibular joint pain dysfunction syndrome" appears to some investigators to be descriptive of both muscular and articular disturbances. The more popular term, myofascial pain dysfunction (MPD) syndrome, was introduced by Laskin (1969). Most clinicians now believe that the etiology of TMJ dysfunction and/or MPD is multifactorial, involving a variety of factors that include dental occlusion, articular abnormalities, and muscular dysfunction (Hall, 1987; Jankelson, 1979; Reeh and El Deeb, 1991).

Bell (1982), responding to the rather confusing numbers of TMJ disturbances and disorders, developed a useful classification (Table 14–3). It is interesting to note that not all the conditions have pain that involves large areas of the distribution of the fifth nerve. The acute muscle disorder has a definite

Table 14–3 Classification of TMJ disorders

Class	Disorder
A	Acute muscle disorders
B	Disk—interference disorders of the joint
C	Inflammatory disorders of the joint
D	Chronic mandibular hypomobilities
E	Growth disorders of the joint

symptom complex. A review of all TMJ disorders is not necessary here. Only the masticatory muscle spasm disorder (MPD) need be discussed because of its complexity and wide spectrum of symptoms. MPD is unique because it is frequently associated with the type of pain seen in headache or confused with disturbances of the fifth nerve. Pain in this syndrome is due to spasm of the masticatory muscles and not to disease of the joint itself. This is often precipitated by an overextension of the jaw, which stretches the muscle and then produces spasm on contraction. Although muscle overextension can be produced by encroachment by prosthetic appliances of dental restorations or may result from decreased space between the mandible and the maxilla, resulting in overclosure, these features are not as important as oral habits coupled with psychophysiologic characteristics of the patients. The median age of patients with this syndrome is 32, and nearly 85% are women. Brooke et al. (1980) noted that patients often exhibit features of emotional stress.

There are varying clinical features, but four signs and symptoms must be present for the diagnosis: (1) muscle tenderness, (2) clicking or popping noise in the joint, (3) limitation of jaw motion, and (4) pain. Two negative findings must be present to differentiate this syndrome from organic disease of the joint: (1) no clinical, radiographic, or laboratory evidence of joint disease; and (2) lack of tenderness in the joint on palpation though the external auditory meatus, thus demonstrating the muscular nature of the condition.

Specific muscles are involved. In a study by Greene et al. (1969), the following were involved:

Lateral pterygoid: 84%
Masseter: 70%
Temporalis: 49%
Medial pterygoid: 35%
Cervical, scalp, and facial: 43%

Tenderness in these muscles usually produces a high degree of limitation of movement. Vertigo and subluxation occur infrequently.

Sudden onset is often described by patients, but this may be due to threshold effects. Intensification of pain often occurs as a distinctive feature because of the contralateral nature of the masticatory apparatus. For this reason, a patient who has pain on the right side of the face favors that side by chewing on the left, thereby increasing the luxation of the apparatus on that side and, naturally, increasing the muscle spasm. Because of the distribution of the fifth nerve, patients often describe the resulting pain as toothache, earache, sore neck, headache, sinus, and neuralgia. The clinician, utilizing the pressure points of muscle attachment, should have little difficulty in diagnosing the condition.

Treatment is controversial, because the symptoms of MPD mimic so many conditions. Most treatments are usually symptom oriented and empiric, without criteria for either diagnosis or treatment. Despite numerous studies, two schools of thought regarding etiology still exist, which lead to two types of treatment. One group still believes the primary cause of MPD is emotional stress. This group relies on biofeedback, psychiatric and/or psychologic counseling, and associated medications. The other group, led by Cooper and Rabuzzi (1984), believes that "the physical course is muscle fatigue and resultant spasm due to the misuse of mandibular muscles that occurs with the mandibular movement required to produce occlusion of the teeth." They believe the use of electromyography and mandibular kinesiography is necessary to make an appropriate diagnosis.

Most clinicians today believe that, in the absence of organic disease of the joint itself, conditions that fit this category should be treated conservatively, and the patient is instructed concerning contralateral aspects of muscle function and the pattern of pain in these muscles. Pain can often be brought under control rapidly. Establishing a hinge relationship, banning forward movement of the jaw, will often eliminate muscle spasm. Pointing out that favoring the more painful side can intensify the problem by leading to more extensive muscle spasm and aggravating already overextended muscles helps the patient understand the difficulty. The judicious use of muscle relaxants for patients who have severe spasm and anxieties has proven effective as well. Utilization of a physical therapist to provide instruction on balanced muscular motion has proved to be helpful. Biofeedback techniques have also been of value. Of considerable importance to the physician is the recognition that these patients are often under stress or have emotional disturbances that must be given appropriate therapeutic consideration.

SUMMARY

With appropriate stimulation of healthy and diseased teeth, it is possible to analyze a variety of face and head pains that stem from the teeth. Use of locally acting anesthetics to interfere with toothache-induced headache allows one to assume that the painful experience was caused by afferent impulses arising from the stimulated tooth.

The cracked tooth syndrome (incomplete tooth fracture) may produce pain radiating to the head following mastication. Appropriate therapy will help resolve the matter.

The TMJ syndrome represents a dysfunction of the entire masticatory apparatus. It is associated with muscle tenderness, clicking or popping noises in the joint, limitation of joint movement, and pain. Much of the pain is related to muscle spasm. Treatment should invariably be conservative.

REFERENCES

Bell, W.E. (1982). *Clinical Management of Temporomandibular Disorders*. Year Book Medical Publishers, Chicago.

Berkelbach van der Sprenkle, S. (1935–36). Microscopical investigation of the tooth and its surroundings. *J. Anat. 70*:233.

Brashear, A.D. (1936). Innervation of the teeth. *J. Am. Dent. Assoc. 23*:662.

Brooke, R., I. Stern, P. Gould, and M.A. Mothersill (1980). The diagnosis and conservative treatment of myofascial pain dysfunction syndrome. *J. Prosthet. Dent. 44:* 844–852.

Cameron, C.E. (1964). Cracked tooth syndrome. *J. Am. Dent. Assoc. 68:*405.

Campbell, R.L., K.W. Parks, and R.N. Dodds (1990). Chronic facial pain associated with endodontic therapy. *Oral Surg. Oral Med. Oral Pathol. 69:*287–290.

Clark, G.T. (1991). Diagnosis and treatment of painful temporomandibular disorder patients. *Pain 44:*29–34.

Cooper, B.C. and D.D. Rabuzzi (1984). Myofascial pain dysfunction syndrome: A clinical study of asymptomatic subjects. *Laryngoscope 94:*68.

Costen, J.B. (1934). A syndrome of ear and sinus symptoms dependent upon disturbed function of the temporomandibular joint. *Ann. Otol. Rhinol. Laryngol. 43:*1.

Gibbs, J.W. (1954). Cuspal fracture odontalgia. *Dental Dig. 60:*158.

Greene, C.S., M.D. Lerman, H.D. Sutcher, and D.M. Laskin (1969). The TMJ pain-dysfunction syndrome: Heterogeneity of the patient population. *J. Am. Dent. Assoc. 79:*1168.

Hall, E.H. (1982). Organic abnormalities of the TMJ. *Ear Nose Throat J. 61:*84–89.

Jankelson, B. (1979). Neuromuscular aspects of occlusion: Effects of occlusal position on the physiology and dysfunction of the mandibular musculature. *Dent. Clin. North Am.* 123.

Laskin, D.M. (1969). Etiology of the pain-dysfunction syndrome. *J. Am. Dent. Assoc. 79:*147.

Lewinsky, W. and D. Stewart (1935–36). The innervation of the dentine. *J. Anat. 70:* 349.

Maxwell, E.H. and B.V. Braly (1977). Incomplete tooth fracture. *J. Calif. Dental Assoc. October:*51–55.

McCreary, C.P., B.T. Clark, R.L. Merril et al. (1991). Psychological distress and diagnostic subgroups of temporomandibular disorder patients. *Pain 44:*29–34.

Pilling, L.F. (1968). Psychosomatic aspects of facial pain. In *Facial Pain* (L.F. Pilling, ed.), pp. 107–119. Lea & Febiger, Philadelphia.

Reeh, E.S. and M.E. El Deeb (1991). Referred pain of muscular origin resembling endodontic involvement. *Oral Surg. Oral Med. Oral Pathol. 71:*223–227.

Robertson, H.S., H. Goodell, and H.G. Wolff (1947). Studies on headache: The teeth as a source of headache and other pain. *Arch. Neurol. Psychiatry 57:*277.

Schwarz, L. (1955). Pain associated with the temporomandibular joint. *J. Am. Dent. Assoc. 51:*394.

Sivestri, A.R. (1976). The undiagnosed split-root syndrome. *J. Am. Dent. Assoc. 92:* 930.

Sutton, P.R.N. (1962). Greenstick fracture of the tooth crown. *Br. Dent. J. 112:*362.

Ziskin, D.E. and A. Wald (1938). Observations on electrical pulp testing. *J. Dent. Res. 17:*79.

15

The Major Neuralgias, Postinfectious Neuritis, and Atypical Facial Pain

DONALD J. DALESSIO

Perhaps no subject in medicine is as confusing to patient and physician alike as that of recurrent chronic facial pain. Often unilateral, frequently unresponsive to therapy, long lasting, and discomforting, some chronic facial pains have resisted even simple nosologic classification. Some patients with severe protracted facial pain will develop complications related to attempts at pain relief as significant as the original cause of their problem. Drug addiction or dependence, serious (even suicidal) depression, disability, and invalidism are among the most frequently encountered complications of long-term intense facial pain. This knowledge notwithstanding, a physician who understands how to deal with patients with chronic facial pain and who understands the mechanisms behind their pain-centered behavior may be able to effect a significant improvement for many of these patients by using a judicious combination of drug therapy, surgery, and other modalities.

TRIGEMINAL NEURALGIA

Clinical Features of Trigeminal Neuralgia Pain

Trigeminal neuralgia (tic douloureux) almost always begins after the age of 30 years unless the patient has concomitant multiple sclerosis. The pain is of high intensity and tends to occur in association with trigger zones (which are areas of increased sensitivity on the face), especially about the nares and mouth, that set off the attack when they are stimulated—often by trivial sensations (Figure 15–1). Thus, the behavioral characteristics of patients with trigeminal neuralgia are to avoid touching the face, washing, shaving, biting or chewing, or any other maneuvers that stimulate the trigger zones and produce the pain. This avoidance technique is an invaluable clue to the diagnosis. In almost every other facial pain syndrome patients will be found massaging the painful area,

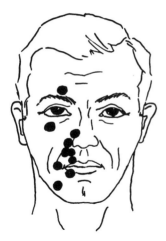

Figure 15–1. Trigger zones in trigeminal neuralgia.

abrading it, or applying heat or cold, but in trigeminal neuralgia exactly the opposite occurs; the patient goes to great lengths to avoid any stimulation of the face or mouth whatsoever.

The pain paroxysm is usually a high-intensity jab lasting less than 20 to 30 seconds, followed at times by a period of relief lasting a few seconds to a minute, again followed by another jab of pain. Repeated episodes of pain may occur, but the pain is not usually long lived compared with other chronic facial pains.

Fromm and his colleagues (1990) described 18 patients whose initial trigeminal pain was not characteristic of neuralgia, but suggested a toothache or sinus pain, often lasting several hours. Often this pain was set off by drinking hot or cold liquids or by jaw movements. Then, at some later time ranging from several days to 12 years, more typical trigeminal neuralgia developed in the same general area as the initial pain. Six of these patients became pain free while taking carbamazepine or baclofen. The authors noted that pretrigeminal neuralgia must be differentiated from trigeminal tumors, atypical facial pain, atypical odontalgia, and facial migraine, among other entities. They recommended a magnetic resonance imaging (MRI) scan of the middle and posterior fossa as a diagnostic study in this situation.

Pathologic Anatomy and Function of the Trigeminal (Gasserian) Ganglion

Alterations in the anatomy of the gasserian ganglion and sensory root have been reported for years. In 1934 Dandy found aberrant arteries and other vascular anomalies in 40% of patients with trigeminal neuralgia as he exposed the fifth nerve root through the posterior fossa. Subsequently, Jannetta (1967) and Janetta and Rand (1967) demonstrated small arterial loops impinging on nerve fibers during subtentorial microdissection of the trigeminal root in patients with trigeminal neuralgia. Separation of these vessels from the root, combined with partial rhizotomy, relieved the neuralgia without producing a major sensory abnormality.

Following an anatomic study, Kerr (1963) proposed that contact between the internal carotid artery and the undersurface of the gasserian ganglion may be a significant factor in the development of trigeminal neuralgia. He based this proposal on sections of the petrous tip that demonstrated that a lacuna in the bony root of the carotid canal may be frequently present in normal patients. He found considerable variability in the fascial reinforcements of this lacuna, with a tendency for it to become reduced in thickness with age. Kerr believed that this structural variant was compatible with features peculiar to trigeminal neuralgia. In addition, electron microscopic abnormalities in the gasserian ganglion itself have been described. Tashiro et al. (1991) have reported "transfixings" of the trigeminal nerve by the compressing artery.

Pathophysiology

Kugelberg and Lindblom (1959) have studied the neuropathophysiology of trigeminal neuralgia. Their results indicate that the excitatory state necessary to fire an attack may be built up over a considerable time by temporal summation of afferent impulses. Antiepileptic drugs, when effective, raise an attack threshold and shorten the duration of attacks by diminishing the self-maintenance of the excitation. Kugelberg and Lindblom postulated that periodic discharges in the brainstem, in structures related to the spinal nucleus of the fifth cranial nerve, may explain the suddenness, intensity, and brevity of the attack.

Fromm et al. (1984) suggested that trigeminal neuralgia has a peripheral cause and a central pathogenesis. In other words, both peripheral and central factors are operative in this disease. For example, chronic "irritation" of the peripheral trigeminal nerve, from whatever cause, leads to failure of segmental inhibition in the trigeminal nucleus, and to the production of ectopic action potentials in the trigeminal nerve. This consideration of increased neuronal discharges and reduced inhibitory mechanisms produces a hyperactive sensory circuit, leading eventually to paroxysmal discharges in the trigeminal nucleus. These "antidromic jolts" are perceived by the patient as painful attacks of trigeminal neuralgia.

Medical Treatment

The medical treatment of trigeminal and other cranial neuralgias is based on the capacity of the drugs employed to interrupt the temporal summation of afferent impulses that set off the painful attack. If the trigger zones are touched repeatedly, a curve can be developed demonstrating a spatial and temporal relationship of repetitive stimuli to pain (Figure 15–2). If carbamazepine is then given for 24 hours, the shape of this curve will be altered, and as the responsiveness of the trigger zones becomes less evident, the condition is gradually relieved.

Most authorities agree that medical treatment is indicated first, if for no other reason than that its use constitutes a therapeutic challenge to the diagnosis. For example, if a patient presumed to have trigeminal neuralgia does not rapidly respond to carbamazepine in 24 to 48 hours, the diagnosis is seriously in doubt. After all, the diagnosis is made on the basis of history alone, and, in general, patients are not good observers of their own pains or sensations.

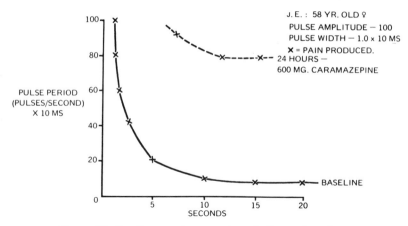

Figure 15–2. Temporal summation of afferent impulses.

If the patient does respond to carbamazepine, then clearly this is the treatment of choice. Those clinicians who have followed patients with trigeminal neuralgia for more than a decade realize that the disease is often remitting, and it may be possible, using drugs, to nudge the patient into another remission, following which medication can sometimes be stopped. If this is not the case, and the response to carbamazepine is only partial, other drugs may also be useful in the treatment of this condition, including phenytoin, baclofen, and chlorphenesin. Some neurosurgeons suggest that unpleasant side effects occur frequently with carbamazepine and that up to 20 to 30% of patients taking this drug need to stop it, which is surprising because the drug seems better tolerated when used in epilepsy.

Nonetheless, one cannot deny that carbamazepine may produce undesirable sedation or idiosyncratic reactions, including blood dyscrasias (rarely). Thus, caution must be employed when using it.

Specifics of Medical Treatment

To inhibit or reduce synaptic transmission and relieve pain, one naturally turns to the anticonvulsants. These drugs reduce the sensitivity of the trigger zones and relieve the pain within 4 to 24 hours, often dramatically. Generally, treatment is begun with carbamazepine, 100 to 200 mg two or three times daily. If this dose is well tolerated and if the pain is rapidly relieved, it may be continued for several weeks or months, depending on the course of the disease. One should attempt to titrate the medication to the severity of the patient's pain. It may be necessary to continue the carbamazepine at a maintenance level, such as 200 mg/day, in order to keep the patient pain free.

If symptoms persist on carbamazepine, another drug can be added to the regimen, such as baclofen, in doses ranging from 10 to 80 mg/day. Rarely, three drugs are employed (Table 15–1). By the time the three-drug treatment level is reached, one should be considering referring the patient for appropriate surgery. Generally, parenteral doses are not used.

Table 15-1 Drugs commonly used in medical therapy of trigeminal neuralgia

Drug	Route of administration	Dosage (mg/day)	Side effects/precautions
Carbamazepine	Oral	200–600	Drowsiness, ataxia, confusion Monitor for blood disorders weekly at first, then monthly
Phenytoin	Oral	200–400	CNS, hematopoietic, oral
Chlorphenesin	Oral	800–2400	Drowsiness
Baclofen	Oral	30–80	Drowsiness, weakness, nausea, vomiting

New developments in drug therapy. Lechin et al. (1989) used pimozide for trigeminal neuralgia in a double-blind crossover trial. In 48 patients described as "refractory to medical therapy," pimozide was superior to carbamazepine for relief of pain. Pimozide is given in a dose of 4 to 12 mg daily. The drug is described as an antipsychotic of the piperidine series, which blocks dopaminergic receptors in the brain. Multiple side effects occur with this medication, which the physician must review carefully before considering its use in trigeminal neuralgia.

A keto derivative of carbamazepine, oxcarbazepine, has also been tested in patients with trigeminal neuralgia who are refractory to medical treatment (Zakrzewska and Patsalos, 1988). Six patients were treated over 6 months and had an "excellent therapeutic response." The authors suggested that oxcarbazepine has potent antineuralgic properties in the absence of significant side effects and, therefore, may be useful in intractable trigeminal neuralgia. This drug is not available in the United States.

Monitoring serum levels. Serum levels of anticonvulsants are a useful way of monitoring treatment. For carbamazepine, at least initially, levels of 6 to 12 μg/ml (25 to 50 μmol/liter) are usually required to relieve the pain. For phenytoin, therapeutic levels are 10 to 20 μg/ml (40 to 80 μmol/liter).

Use of baclofen. Fromm et al. (1984) have reported on the use of baclofen in refractory trigeminal neuralgia. These authors treated 14 patients who were refractory to or unable to take carbamazepine, starting with 10 mg three times a day, and achieved pain relief in 10 patients. At two subsequent visits a week apart, baclofen was increased to 60 to 80 mg/day, or a mean dose of 1.03 mg/kg. Concomitant drugs were carbamazepine in five patients, phenytoin in one, and carbamazepine and phenytoin in two. Although side effects occurred (especially including drowsiness), some patients did achieve satisfactory control.

Pharmacologic Activity of Drugs Used in Medical Treatment

The pharmacologic effects of the four drugs most commonly used to treat trigeminal neuralgia are similar (see Table 15-2). Note that all four drugs have anticonvulsant, muscle relaxant, and sedative properties, which could be predicted from the evidence reviewed below. None is anesthetic or analgesic.

Table 15–2 Pharmacologic activity of baclofen, chlorphenesin, phenytoin, and carbamazepine

Effect	Baclofen	Chlorphenesin	Phenytoin	Carbamazepine
Anticonvulsant activity	+	+	+ + +	+ +
Muscle relaxant effect	+ + +	+ + +	+	+ +
Sedative effect	+ +	+ +	+	+ +
Anesthetic activity	0	0	0	0
Analgesic effect	0	±	0	±

Despite this paradox, pain relief is achieved by interrupting the neurophysiologic state that produces the pain.

Carbamazepine and phenytoin. Phenytoin reduces post-tetanic potentiation of synaptic transmission within the spinal cord as well as the stellate ganglion of animals. Post-tetanic potentiation can be considered an enhancement of synaptic transmission following rapid, repetitive, presynaptic stimulation. Carbamazepine also depresses post-tetanic potentiation at the spinal cord level in animals, and significantly inhibits polysynaptic reflex activity in the spinal cord (Fromm, 1969). Both drugs depress synaptic transmission in the spinal trigeminal nucleus. Laboratory studies have shown that these anticonvulsants depress synaptic transmission in the trigeminal system, as evidenced by decreasing amplitude and increasing latency of evoked potentials (Fromm and Landgren, 1963).

Chlorphenesin. Chlorphenesin depresses transmission to a number of spinal and supraspinal polysynaptic pathways. It also depresses polysynaptic potentials in spinal cords of animals and inhibits convulsions induced by strychnine (Matthews et al., 1963). Our laboratory studies have demonstrated depression of synaptic transmissions by chlorphenesin in the trigeminal system of the cat.

Baclofen. Baclofen depresses excitatory synaptic transmission in the spinal trigeminal nucleus, and resembles the other drugs in this respect. It increases the latency of response and decreases the number of spikes in trigeminal nucleus neurons elicited by maxillary nerve stimulation (Fromm et al., 1984).

Side Effects of Medical Treatment
Carbamazepine. The side effects of carbamazepine that most frequently limit therapy include ataxia, drowsiness, and fatigue. Older patients may note confusion while taking the drug. Idiosyncratic side effects include leukopenia, agranulocytosis, and, rarely, aplastic anemia. It is therefore advisable to obtain pretreatment baseline values of blood and platelets, and to repeat these tests at regular intervals (e.g., monthly) during treatment.

Phenytoin. The most common side effects of this drug are drowsiness, dizziness and diplopia, which can be reduced by appropriate dosage modification. More severe central nervous system effects, such as ataxia, nystagmus, and slurred speech, are an indication for immediate reduction of the dosage. Idiosyncratic side effects of phenytoin include gum hypertrophy and occasionally megaloblastic anemia.

Chlorphenesin and baclofen. The most common side effect noted with chlorphenesin is drowsiness. Similarly, drowsiness, weakness, nausea, and vomiting may occur with baclofen.

Surgical Treatment of Major Trigeminal Neuralgia

A number of patients with trigeminal neuralgia, between 25 and 50%, will eventually fail on medical therapy and will need some form of neurosurgical treatment. The type of operation performed varies widely from place to place. Patients must be completely and clearly apprised of the nature of the operations proposed, the procedures to be undertaken, possible side effects, costs, and morbidity and mortality. Informed consent regarding these neurosurgical procedures, given their many differences, is mandatory (Table 15–3). Two operations, including local ablation of peripheral nerves and wide section of the sensory roots of the trigeminal nerve (Dandy, 1925), are rarely done because better methods are usually available for surgical pain relief.

Radiofrequency Rhizotomy

Selective lesioning of the trigeminal root using a radiofrequency electrode placed in the root under radiographic control (radiofrequency rhizotomy) is an operative procedure that has gained wide acceptance (Sweet and Wepsic, 1974; Tew and Keller, 1977). It has the advantages of safety and simplicity. The anesthesia used is light, and the patient is awake during some of the procedure, recovers rapidly, and is often found eating supper a few hours after the operation has been completed. Almost always the patient can be discharged the next day.

However, there is a recurrence rate of about 25%, occasional corneal anesthesia occurs, and rarely uncomfortable dyesthesias or jaw weakness result. Altered sensation in the face is reported by many patients, but only a few are

Table 15–3 Comparison of operative techniques for trigeminal neuralgia[a]

Technique	Description	Complications
Radiofrequency rhizotomy	90% effective minor percutaneous needle procedure, brief hospital stay	Facial sensory loss is frequently quite severe; corneal hypesthesia (10–15%), occasional masseter weakness
Glycerol injection	85% effective minor percutaneous needle procedure, brief hospital stay	Facial sensitivity loss is slight; persistent corneal hypesthesia and masseter weakness is rare
Microvascular decompression	90% effective major craniotomy, 4–10-day hospital stay	+4% serious postoperative complications, 1% mortality

[a] Each of the procedures is associated with a modest recurrence rate. The recurrence rate is least with microvascular decompression and modestly greater with radiofrequency rhizotomy and glycerol injection.

bothered by it. To the present, there has been no mortality associated with this operation.

Glycerol Rhizolysis

A variation on the radiofrequency rhizotomy procedure has been proposed by Hakanson (1981). He injects 0.3 to 0.4 ml of glycerol by the anterior percutaneous route into the trigeminal cistern (Meckel's cave). Hakanson reported excellent response to this procedure, with only minimal disturbance of facial sensitivity. Sweet and his colleagues (1981) have also reported their experience with this procedure. They described greater pain on injection and more sensory loss than Hakanson. The presumption is made that glycerol is neurotoxic, acts on partially demyelinated nerve fibers, and eliminates the compound action potential in the trigeminal rootlets that are associated with pain.

Although some neurosurgeons continue to favor percutaneous radiofrequency rhizotomy, the trend is to glycerol rhizolysis of the trigeminal ganglion (Young, 1988). That has also been our experience, and we now routinely suggest the glycerol procedure in our patients who wish to avoid craniotomy (Waltz et al., 1989). Linderoth and Hakanson (1989) also reported success using glycerol injection in treating trigeminal neuralgia caused by multiple sclerosis.

Microvascular Decompression

An alternative procedure is microvascular decompression of the trigeminal root (Bederson and Wilson, 1989; Jannetta, 1977b). The rationale for decompression is the assumption that the neurosurgeon will find a lesion (usually an arterial loop) compressing the trigeminal root close by the brainstem. Tash et al. (1989) have used MRI to evaluate the relationship of vascular structures to the trigeminal nerve root in six patients with trigeminal neuralgia and in 85 asymptomatic individuals. In all patients with trigeminal neuralgia, a vascular structure at the root entry zone of the fifth nerve was identified. Of the 85 asymptomatic people, contact between a vascular structure and the trigeminal nerve root was noted in 30% but only 2% had deformities of the nerve root. If and when it is found, the offending compressing lesion is lifted from the trigeminal root, often by interposing a sponge; by deduction, then, it is suggested that in most cases trigeminal neuralgia is a compressive cranial mononeuropathy.

Meglio and Cioni (1989) have described a new percutaneous microcompression of the trigeminal ganglion as a variation on the usual surgical technique. They employ a small balloon, with a filling capacity of about 1 ml, introduced by percutaneous means through the foramen ovale, which is inflated against the ganglion for periods ranging from 1 to 10 minutes. The results reported were in the range of 90% improvement in pain and compare favorably with other standard neurosurgical procedures. In effect, this is a variation on older concepts of compressing the trigeminal ganglion to achieve pain relief.

Factors in Selection of Surgical Procedure

There are, of course, significant differences in costs between these various operations. Radiofrequency lesions and glycerol injections are done rapidly and almost always the patient is quickly discharged. With microsurgical decompression of the trigeminal root, a formal craniotomy is required, and the patient frequently spends 4 to 10 days in the hospital and a similar period of time in convalescence.

Trigeminal Evoked Potentials

A major difficulty in treating trigeminal neuralgia is an objective method for assessing therapy. One approach to this dilemma is to try to establish a reliable and practical method for obtaining trigeminal somatosensory evoked potentials (TEPs).

We have devised a noninvasive method, involving a mild electric shock to the lower lip, to elicit reliable evoked potentials from the trigeminal nerve in 20 normal young adults (Dalessio et al., 1990). The wave forms were morphologically similar to those observed with invasive procedures. No substantial differences for stimulation of the right or left side, recording electrode, or subject sex were obtained for any of the individual potential amplitudes or latencies. The same procedures were applied to 10 patients who had been treated with retrogasserian glycerol injections for trigeminal neuralgia. TEPs were elicited in all patients, although the quality of the individual waveforms was more variable than that observed for the normal subjects. Comparison of the treated with the unaffected sides of the face in the patients demonstrated significantly smaller N2–P2 amplitudes and longer N2 latencies for the affected face side. The results suggest that these procedures produce reliable evoked potential measures of trigeminal nerve function noninvasively, which can provide an objective index of treatment efficacy.

Trigeminal Neuralgia and Multiple Sclerosis

Sensory disturbances in the distribution of the trigeminal nerve are relatively common in multiple sclerosis and may even involve the inside of the mouth. The usual descriptions of facial hypesthesia are nonspecific. Often patients speak of numbness or deadness of the face, or of a feeling that part of the face has been anesthetized by novocaine. Pain may or may not be associated with these sensations, which may be quite transient, last for a day or two or more, or sometimes become permanent. Objective signs of sensory loss are difficult to elicit, but there may be associated impairment of pain and temperature sensitivity and loss of touch in the region involved. The corneal reflex may be diminished or absent when the loss of sensation affects the first division of the trigeminal nerve.

Intermittent trigeminal neuralgia, as opposed to the condition described above (which might be termed trigeminal neuritis), is uncommon in multiple sclerosis, and varies between a 1 and 2% incidence (Garcin et al., 1960; Harris, 1950). Conversely, the incidence of multiple sclerosis among patients with trigeminal neuralgia is approximately 3%. Typically, the classic history of trigeminal neuralgia (Parker, 1978) will be obtained in patients with multiple sclerosis except that it may appear at a younger age than when the disease occurs in its idiopathic form. Some patients with multiple sclerosis manifest recurrent episodes of face pain, generally long lasting and not stabbing or lancinating, without associated trigger zones. These patients are assumed to have a form of atypical facial pain and not true trigeminal neuralgia.

In my experience, trigeminal neuralgia almost never occurs as the first manifestation of the disease, and all of the patients seen with trigeminal neuralgia in association with multiple sclerosis have had very significant physical signs of multiple sclerosis before the facial pain began. Most, for example, have paraparesis or paraplegia, disorders of sensory function including posterior column signs, and the like. Single cases of trigeminal neuralgia appearing as the first manifestation of multiple sclerosis are rare.

With regard to the pathogenesis of trigeminal pain in multiple sclerosis, it can be stated that in this situation demyelinating plaques may be found at the point of entry of the fifth root, or involving the main sensory nucleus or the descending root of the trigeminal nerve. Demyelinating plaques may also be found in the gasserian ganglion. If this is the case, plaques are often found in adjacent structures also involving the facial nucleus, sometimes producing facial weakness and continuous rhythmic fascicular contractions, termed "facial myokymia." Presumably the plaques occurring either in the ganglion or in the main sensory nucleus alter the electrophysiology of facial sensation, allowing hyperactive sensory circuits to appear, producing trigger zones and the characteristic manifestations of trigeminal neuralgia, as we have come to know them.

The treatment of trigeminal neuralgia occurring in association with multiple sclerosis is the same as that given previously for the idiopathic variety.

GLOSSOPHARYNGEAL NEURALGIA

Glossopharyngeal neuralgia (tic) is characterized by severe pain in the region of the tonsil and ear. It has timing features like those of trigeminal neuralgia, and may be initiated by yawning and swallowing or contact of food with the tonsillar region. Rarely the patient may become unconscious during a paroxysm of pain (probably as a result of asystole). Examination reveals no evidence of reduction in perception of pinprick or touch, or of motility function in the nasopharynx.

Some authors use the term "glossopharyngeal and vagal neuralgia" or "vagoglossopharyngeal neuralgia" instead of glossopharyngeal neuralgia, implying that the pain can radiate into the distribution of the vagus nerve as well as that of the glossopharyngeal nerve. The original term, "glossopharyngeal neuralgia," is recognized by most neurologists and is more commonly used.

Often the pain of glossopharyngeal neuralgia can be relieved by temporary cocainization of the involved side of the throat. Extracranial block of the glossopharyngeal nerve with alcohol is not recommended because the injection of alcohol in the region of the jugular foramen might well cause paralysis of the 10th, 11th, and 12th cranial nerves and could conceivably also involve the sympathetic trunk.

If the patient does not respond to carbamazepine, the treatment of choice for glossopharyngeal neuralgia is intracranial section of the nerve. Usually the exposure is through a unilateral suboccipital craniectomy. The nerve can be identified as it passes along the floor of the posterior fossa to emerge through the jugular foramen.

TICLIKE NEURITIDES OF THE FIFTH CRANIAL NERVE ASSOCIATED WITH BRAIN TUMORS AND OTHER PATHOLOGIC PROCESSES

These relatively uncommon painful states resemble trigeminal neuralgia but can usually be differentiated, because each painful paroxysm is commonly a sustained, high-intensity ache of several minutes' duration, whereas true neuralgia is characterized by recurrent, brief, painful jabs of approximately 30 seconds' duration. Cushing (1920), in describing these neuralgias resulting from tumor involvement of the sensory root, the trigeminal ganglion, or the fifth nerve, has divided them into four groups on the basis of the site of the precipitating cause.

Tumors of the Cerebellopontine Recess

Tumors of the cerebellopontine recess on the trigeminal root may rarely be accompanied by paroxysms of pain that resemble trigeminal neuralgia. The pain is not eliminated by trigeminal ganglion operation. Sometimes there is a low-intensity, steady, dull ache, but usually little or no pain is produced by such tumors, and there is a gradual hypesthesia in the distribution of the fifth cranial nerve.

Tumors of the Middle Fossa

Tumors of the middle fossa that involve the trigeminal ganglion by direct pressure from above, mainly on the dura overlying the ganglion, are growths with a meningeal attachment, such as endothelial tumors, granulomas, and occasional gliomas. The pain, again, rarely resembles trigeminal neuralgia in its temporal features. Furthermore, it is an inconspicuous symptom of the underlying disorder. Usually when pain occurs, it is of a sustained aching and burning character and is associated with hypesthesia of an appropriate area of the skin. Paroxysms of high-intensity pain of 10 to 15 minutes' duration may occur.

Tumors of the Cranium or Extracranial Tissues

Tumors that arise in the cranium or in the extracranial tissues beneath the ganglion, often metastatic, are almost certain to involve the ganglion in the course of time. Occasionally the nerve may be completely destroyed, resulting in total anesthesia in its territory without production of pain. More often the process is accompanied by aching and burning pain of high intensity occurring in paroxysms of 10 to 15 minutes' duration.

Endothelial Tumors

Endothelial tumors originating from the envelopes of the trigeminal ganglion give rise to pain in the region supplied by one or more branches of the fifth nerve. The character of the pain, a more or less sustained, steady ache, readily distinguishes it from true trigeminal neuralgia. It is also inevitably accompanied by a hypesthesia, if not anesthesia, and motor paralysis. Also, the third, sixth, and eighth nerves may be involved by the tumor. Avulsion of the sensory root on the side affected, resulting in total anesthesia, eliminates the pain.

GENICULATE NEURALGIA OF HERPETIC ORIGIN

Generally, geniculate neuralgia is related to herpes zoster infection of the geniculate ganglion and is characterized by severe pain in the tympanic membrane, the walls of the auditory canal, the external auditory meatus, and the external structures of the ear. The pain is typically deep and may be associated with a herpetic rash in the auricle, or the rash may be present in the external auditory canal. The disease may be associated with facial palsy, difficulty with hearing, vertigo, and tinnitus. Treatment is symptomatic.

HEMIFACIAL SPASM

Maroon (1978) has reviewed the literature on hemifacial spasm and described his therapy of this syndrome. Recent surgical observations indicate that hemifacial spasm is most likely caused by normal or pathologic vascular structures that cross-compress the facial nerve. The critical area of compression is found at the brainstem exit zone of the seventh nerve. In this area, the central glial investment of the facial nerve changes to peripheral or schwannian myelin. It is suspected that this anatomic junction zone may be of pathophysiologic significance when directly compressed or irritated. Maroon recommended a retromastoid craniectomy and vascular decompression operation to relieve hemifacial spasm while preserving facial nerve function. This is in contrast to commonly used destructive operations for hemifacial spasm. He emphasized, however, that microsurgical techniques must be employed or high morbidity and mortality may occur using the retromastoid approach. Interestingly, in Maroon's series of cases, facial pain or headache associated with clonic facial spasm was extremely rare. He emphasized that the problem is primarily a muscular one related to predominant contraction of the orbicularis and zygomatic muscles.

Hemifacial spasm should be differentiated from blepharospasm and the synkinesis that may occur following a Bell palsy. In my experience, blepharospasm is always bilateral, and it affects primarily the periorbital muscles but may spread to the upper facial muscles as well. In a small number of patients with Bell palsy, hemifacial synkinetic movements may develop as the patient recovers from the episode but is left with persisting weakness. This history is clearly different from that of hemifacial spasm. Also, facial myokymia may appear as a form of fascicular twitching of the facial muscles, especially the orbicularis oculi. In none of these conditions is facial pain common.

HEADACHE AND DIABETIC NEUROPATHY

Isolated cranial nerve palsies, especially of the third and sixth nerves, are known to occur in diabetics. Neuralgia of the fifth nerve with diabetic ocular paresis may occur. No suitable explanation for the pain is available. It appears likely that the third, fourth, and sixth cranial nerve defects stem from vascular occlusive disease of the vasa nervorum, and that the fifth cranial nerve may rarely become similarly involved.

HERPETIC AND POSTHERPETIC NEURITIS

Herpes Zoster Involvement of the Gasserian Ganglion and Trigeminal Nucleus

The pain of herpes zoster, in contrast to that of trigeminal neuralgia as regards timing features, is steady and sustained. Although the pain often spontaneously regresses within 2 or 3 weeks, it may persist for several months, and when it occurs in persons past age 70, as it frequently does, its duration may be a year or more. Rarely, it may persist indefinitely. The pain is unilateral, and the quality of the pain is both burning and aching. It may be experienced in any part of the distribution of the fifth cranial nerve, although involvement of the forehead is most common. The pain is nonthrobbing and relatively uniform, and usually diminishes gradually in intensity. Examination soon after onset reveals erythema and the typical herpetiform lesion of the skin associated with hyperalgesia and paresthesia. Examination later reveals hypesthesia and paresthesia of the involved areas, and sometimes scarring and pigmentation of the skin. There may be weakness of the masseter muscle and pterygoid muscle on the homolateral side. The judicious use of codeine and salicylates, with reassurance of better days to come, makes the period of spontaneous regression tolerable. Sensory root section does not usually give complete relief. Often it has no effect.

Herpes Zoster and Involvement of Other Dorsal Root Ganglions and Nerve Tissues

Steady pain in the face and ear, back of the head, and neck, associated with vertigo and palsy of the homolateral side of the face, results from widespread inflammation involving the gasserian and glossopharyngeal and the first two or three dorsal root ganglions and the dorsal horns of the cervical portion of the cord. The pain has the qualities and duration previously described. As with all cases of herpes, there may be a slight or moderate palsy. Herpetiform lesions may or may not be present.

Occipital Neuritis Due to Herpes, Other Infections, and Cervical Cord Tumors

Occipital headache due to inflammation, injury, or pressure on the occipital nerves, upper cervical spinal roots, dorsal horn, or root ganglions is a long-lasting, sustained, nonthrobbing ache of moderate intensity. It is difficult to separate from tension-type headache because it also is always associated with muscle tenderness. The characteristic feature is paresthesia or algesia of the tissues of the scalp and the skin of the neck. Discoloration or scarring of the skin, such as follows herpes, may also occur. When the headache is postherpetic, section of nerves or roots will probably not eliminate the pain, although it may be somewhat reduced. Procaine injections about the sensory roots have a similar slight effect in reducing the intensity of pain.

Occipital headache due to tumors of the upper cervical cord, especially to those masses attached or adjacent to the first two or three roots, closely resembles that already described. In most instances, in addition to the pain there is disturbance in sensory perception within the dermatomes involved. Enhanced computerized tomography is the diagnostic procedure of choice, after plain cervical spine films are done. Removal of the tumor or rhizotomy, when removal is possible, eliminates or reduces the intensity of headache.

Sustained contraction of the neck with a radiographic picture of a straight cervical spine may also be associated with a variety of cervical defects, including displaced cervical intervertebral disk nuclei. Unilateral neck ache extending to the occiput, and sometimes also including the temple and forehead, may appear in patients with mid and upper cervical joint disorders. Cautious extension of the neck by manual or other traction may have a therapeutic effect.

Patients who survive after rupture of the odontoid ligament have severe headache in the neck and the suboccipital region.

HEADACHE AND DISEASES OF THE CERVICAL SPINE

Brain et al. (1952) called attention to the headache and other clinical manifestations of cervical spondylosis (see also Chapter 8). Pain is commonly referred to the deep structures about the neck and back of the head, as well as into the arms and digits, which is likely to be worsened by moving the neck and pulling on the arms. Hyperalgesia, wasting, and fasciculations may be present. In addition, symptoms may arise from the impairment of function of the cervical spinal cord. Brain and his colleagues defined cervical spondylosis as a degenerative disorder of the cervical spine leading to narrowing of the intravertebral spaces and protrusion of the intravertebral disks. These changes can cause pressure on the spinal nerves in their foramina as well as pressure on the spinal cord.

Because the disorder is degenerative rather than inflammatory, Brain et al. selected the term "spondylosis" rather than "spondylitis." They considered trauma and the degeneration of the intravertebral disks with age to be the main precipitating factors. It is more common in men than in women and produces symptoms chiefly in the fifth and sixth decades. As a result of the morbid process, the nerve roots are compressed in the foramina, now the site of a secondary formation of fibrous tissue. Thus, nerve fibers undergo degeneration. The cord is directly compressed and tethered by the adhesions around the nerve roots, and normal neck movement causes continual mild injury. Blood supply may be affected by compression of the spinal veins and the anterior spinal artery. Spinal fluid may show a slight rise in protein, and when the neck is extended there may be a demonstrable obstruction on manometric tests. Brain et al. found that rest by immobilization with a plastic collar for 3 months usually eliminates the pain, rendering operative intervention unnecessary. When the spinal cord is compressed, however, surgical procedures are sometimes helpful if the operation takes place early in the course of the disorder.

A number of other workers have called attention to the occurrence of headache with pathologic changes of the cervical spine, and especially to the possibility of painful implication of the frontal part of the head. Headache is said to be a common accompaniment of cervical disk lesions. High cervical bony defects or root damage do indeed become linked with headache, which may become frontal. Conspicuous in this category is the headache that accompanies the development of Paget's disease, involving the bones of the base of the skull and the upper cervical spine. The distortions and the displacements that occur under these circumstances may also be linked with occipital headache.

PAINFUL TIC CONVULSIF

Painful tic convulsif is characterized by periodic contractions of one side of the face, accompanied by great pain. It may be confused with the facial contortions and masticatory movements on the involved side that rarely accompany the paroxysms of true trigeminal neuralgia. Cushing (1920) has reported five cases of the disorder, which is rare.

Painful tic convulsif is reported to be more severe in women than in men. It may begin in or about the orbicularis oculi as a fine intermittent myokymia, with some spread thereafter into the muscles of the lower part of the face. Occasionally strong spasms may involve all of the facial muscles on one side almost continuously. Rarely, the face may become weak and some of the facial muscles may atrophy.

A recent report of tic convulsif by Harsh and colleagues (1991) is of interest. A 54-year-old patient is described with a 5-year history of left hemifacial spasm and a 2-month history of left trigeminal neuralgia. MRI imaging with enhancement showed massively ectatic vertebral and basilar arteries, distorting the brainstem and the trigeminal and facial nerves. Surgical therapy included selective trigeminal rhizotomy (the patient had not responded to carbamazepine), decompression of the seventh nerve, and "cushioning" of the residual trigeminal nerve at the point of maximum distortion by the underlying basilar artery. Postoperatively the patient did well, with neither facial pain nor abnormal movement.

ATYPICAL FACIAL PAINS

The head and face pains included for consideration in this section differ from the typical or major facial neuralgias chiefly as follows:

1. In the atypical neuralgias the pain is seldom limited to the distribution of the fifth or ninth cranial nerves, but usually spreads over the area supplied by the cervical roots.
2. The pain is not significantly reduced or eliminated by division of the fifth or ninth cranial nerves.
3. The pain is of a steady, diffuse, aching quality of hours' or days' duration; it does not occur in paroxysms of short duration (1 to 30 seconds) followed by freedom from pain, as in trigeminal neuralgia.
4. The atypical facial neuralgia syndromes do not present trigger zones.
5. These disorders occur in a younger age group than the major neuralgias, and far more commonly in women.
6. Attacks are not precipitated by cold, drafts, cold water in the mouth, swallowing, talking, chewing, shaving, or washing the face, as in typical neuralgias considered in the previous sections.

Many factors may be responsible for this complaint. A careful search should be made for local pathology of the eyes, nose, teeth, sinuses, and pharynx. In particular, nasopharyngeal cancer should be excluded by MRI.

Some patients with atypical facial pains may be suffering from a form of migraine involving the face. This is particularly the case if the pain is throbbing in nature, and a trial of ergotamine or dihydroergotamine (DHE-45) may be helpful. If autonomic symptoms, including cutaneous pallor, sweating, flushing, and rhinitis, occur, attempts to alter responses to autonomic stimuli using β-adrenergic blockers such as propranolol (Inderal) can be employed.

Many patients with chronic long-standing atypical facial pains require intensive inpatient evaluation. A pain center approach to the problem is indicated to identify, if possible, the origins of the pain, medical or otherwise; to isolate factors contributing to the pain problem; and to quantify or measure the severity of the pain the patient is experiencing. In this situation, psychological testing and pain measurements should be included in the evaluation. Treatment can include pain-relieving or analgesic medications, attitude-influencing or psychotropic medications, nerve blocks, electrical neurostimulation, biofeedback techniques for reduction of muscle spasm, activity management, and family counseling.

Carotidynia

Fay (1932) introduced the word "carotidynia" to describe a variety of pain that arises in the neck. He suggested that the pain originated in the common carotid and external carotid arteries and its maxillary branches, and that the course of afferent impulses to the central nervous system was indirect, involving in part the vagus nerve. Carotidynia is a syndrome that features tenderness, swelling, and sometimes conspicuous pulsation of the common carotid artery on the affected side. If the thumbs are placed on the common carotid arteries just below the bifurcation and the structures are pressed back against the transverse cervical processes with a rolling movement, a severe pain is produced. Patients who already have a dull aching pain referred to the eye, deep in the malar region, and spreading back to the ear, behind the ear, and down the neck have the pain accentuated. The attacks are usually periodic, are more likely to occur on the same side, and are not associated with visual disturbances.

Roseman (1967) has reviewed the literature on carotidynia and reported his observations in young and middle-aged adults. He described a unilateral or bilateral neck pain of high intensity but relatively short duration, lasting 11 days on average. In 90% of cases the disease was self-limited. Systemic signs of illness were absent. Treatment of carotidynia is usually supportive. Simple analgesics such as aspirin may be helpful; corticosteroids are rarely necessary.

Lovshin (1977) has reported a series of 100 cases of carotidynia from the Cleveland Clinic. All of the patients were examined, treated, and followed by the author. There were 82 females and 18 males, and 67 patients had a history of vascular headache. Forty-five patients volunteered the information that the glands in the neck had been swollen. Lovshin found that the most common form of carotidynia is related to overdistention, relaxation, and increased pulsation in the carotid artery. This syndrome of vascular neck pain is closely associated with various forms of migraine. It is more common in women than in men, the ratio being about 4:1. The syndrome occurs at almost any age but is more prevalent during the fourth and fifth decades, and there is often a history of migraine. The only significant abnormality on physical examination is the presence of a tender, throbbing, often dilated carotid artery. The condition is frequently misdiagnosed and therefore not properly treated. Lovshin stated that the preferred treatment is similar to that of migraine and other painful vasodilating conditions of the head. In particular, he suggested various oral preparations of ergotamine tartrate, or methysergide, 2 mg three or four times daily in a short course. Apparently carotidynia is not characterized by an inflammatory arteritis. The condition is not related to cranial arteritis.

Raeder Syndrome and the Pericarotid Syndrome

Raeder paratrigeminal syndrome is a rare illness characterized by oculosympathetic paralysis, the sudden onset of severe frontotemporal burning, aching pain of rapid onset with associated ptosis and meiosis, often in a periorbital distribution, no previous history of headache, and normal sweating in the supraorbital area of the ipsilateral forehead. Raeder (1924) based his conclusions on five cases in which there were cranial nerve dysfunctions, usually involving the optic, oculomotor, trochlear, trigeminal, and abducens nerves.

Raeder's first patient had a tumor arising from the region of the trigeminal ganglion infiltrating all of these cranial nerves. Two of his cases had multiple cranial nerve lesions and sympathetic paralysis related to head injury. In two cases, no particular cause could be identified. In essence then, Raeder's patients had multiple cranial nerve involvements, primarily parasellar, associated with oculosympathetic paralysis and intact facial sweating. Others have since described almost any lesion in which there is oculosympathetic paralysis associated with head pain as Raeder syndrome. Given this confusion, it would probably be best to abandon the eponym and more precisely classify patients with oculosympathetic paralysis and headache, who may or may not have disturbances of sweating as well. Many patients with cluster headaches have an associated oculosympathetic paralysis, but in this situation the tempo of the cluster headache establishes the diagnosis, rather than the autonomic dysfunction.

Vijayan and Watson (1978) have described a pericarotid syndrome characterized by oculosympathetic paralysis, ipsilateral head pain, and anhidrosis over the forehead with otherwise intact facial sweating. They suggest that the site of the lesion involving the oculosympathetic fibers in their patients is pericarotid. Their patients had no previous history of headache. They were able to establish a pathogenesis in only one of their six patients in whom a left internal carotid artery occlusion had occurred. In the other five patients, the etiology was unknown.

SUMMARY

Both medical and surgical therapies may be used in the individual patient with trigeminal neuralgia. Ordinarily, the treatment is medical. However, if a response to drugs is not forthcoming, or if the patient becomes toxic while taking medications or refuses to abide by an appropriate medical program, then surgical consultation should be obtained and the appropriate operation performed. The form and type of the neurosurgical procedure will probably depend to a considerable extent on the expertise of the neurosurgeon and his or her training. Generally, in the elderly the simplest procedures should be attempted first. It may be necessary to employ both medical and surgical procedures in the individual patient. The medical drug of first choice is carbamazepine.

Atypical facial neuralgia is a general term used to cover a variety of head and face pains, some of which are poorly defined. The pathogenesis of the atypical facial neuralgias is uncertain, and multiple causation seems likely. A search for neoplasms, local inflammatory pathology, vasomotor phenomena, and depressive symptoms is indicated, with treatment guided by the findings.

REFERENCES

Bederson, J.B. and C.B. Wilson (1989). Evaluation of microvascular decompression and partial sensory rhizotomy in 252 cases of trigeminal neuralgia. *J. Neurosurg. 71:* 359–367.

Brain, W.R., D.W.C. Northfield, and M. Wilkinson (1952). The neurological manifestations of cervical spondylosis. *Brain 75:*187.

Cushing, H. (1920). The major trigeminal neuralgias and their surgical treatment, based on experiences with 332 Gasserian operations. The varieties of facial neuralgia. *Am. J. Med. Sci. 160:*157.

Dalessio, D.J. (1977). Medical treatment of trigeminal neuralgia. *Clin. Neurosurg. 24:* 579–583.

Dalessio, D.J. (1982). Trigeminal neuralgia. A practical approach to treatment. *Drugs 24:*248–255.

Dalessio, D.J., H. McIsaac, M. Aung, and J. Polich (1990). Noninvasive trigeminal evoked potentials: Normative data and application to neuralgia patients. *Headache 30:*696–700.

Dandy, W.E. (1925). Section of the sensory root of the trigeminal nerve at the pons. *Bull. Johns Hopkins Hosp. 36:*105.

Dandy, W.E. (1934). Concerning the cause of trigeminal neuralgia. *Am. J. Surg. 24:*447.

Fay, T. (1932). Atypical facial neuralgia, a syndrome of vascular pain. *Ann. Otol. 41:* 1030.

Fromm, G.H. (1969). Pharmacological consideration of anticonvulsants. *Headache 9:* 35.

Fromm, G.H. and S. Landgren (1963). Effect of diphenylhydantoin on single cells in the spinal trigeminal nucleus. *Neurology 13:*34.

Fromm, G.H., S.B. Graff-Radford, C.F. Terrence, and W.H. Sweet (1990). Pre-trigeminal neuralgia. *Neurology 40:*1493–1495.

Fromm, G.H., C.F. Terrence, and J.C. Maroon (1984). Trigeminal neuralgia. Current concepts regarding etiology and pathogenesis. *Arch. Neurol. 41:*1204–1207.

Garcin, R., S. Godlewski, and J. leLapresle (1960). Neuralgie du trijumeau et sclerose en plaques. *Rev. Neurol. 102:*441.

Hakanson, S. (1981). Trigeminal neuralgia treated by injection of glycerol into the trigeminal cistern. *Neurosurgery 9:*638–646.

Harris, W. (1950). Rare forms of paroxysmal trigeminal neuralgia and the relation to disseminated sclerosis. *BMJ 1:*831.

Harsh, G.R., C.B. Wilson, G.B. Hieshima, and W.P. Dillon (1991). Magnetic resonance imaging of vertebrobasilar ectasia in tic convulsif. *J. Neurosurg. 74:*999–1003.

Jannetta, P.J. (1967). Structural mechanisms of trigeminal neuralgia. *J. Neurosurg. 26:* 159.

Jannetta, P.J. (1977a). Observations on the etiology of trigeminal neuralgia, hemifacial spasm, acoustic nerve dysfunction and glossopharyngeal neuralgia. Definitive microsurgical treatment and results in 117 patients. *Neurochirurgia 20:*145–154.

Jannetta, P.J. (1977b). Treatment of trigeminal neuralgia by suboccipital and transtentorial cranial operations. *Clin. Neurosurg. 24:*538–549.

Jannetta, P.J., and R.W. Rand (1967). Gross (mesoscopic) description of the human trigeminal nerve and ganglion. *J. Neurosurg. 26:*109.

Kerr, F.W.L. (1963). The etiology of trigeminal neuralgia. *Arch. Neurol. 8:*15.

Kugelberg, E., and U. Lindblom (1959). The mechanism of the pain in trigeminal neuralgia. *J. Neurol. Neurosurg. Psychiatry 22:*36.

Lechin, F., B. van der Dijs, M.E. Lechin et al. (1989). Pimozide therapy for trigeminal neuralgia. *Arch. Neurol. 46:*960–963.

Linderoth, B. and S. Hakanson (1989). Paroxysmal facial pain in disseminated sclerosis treated by retrogasserian glycerol injection. *Acta Neurol. Scand. 80:*341–346.

Lovshin, L. (1977). Carotidynia. *Headache 17:*192–195.

Maroon, J.C. (1978). Hemifacial spasm. *Arch. Neurol. 35:*481–483.

Matthews, R.J., J.P. DaVanzo, and R.J. Collins (1963). The pharmacology of chlorphenesin carbamate. *Arch. Int. Pharmacodyn. 143:*574.

Meglio, M. and B. Cioni (1989). Percutaneous procedures for trigeminal neuralgia: Microcompression versus radiofrequency thermocoagulation. *Pain 38:*9–16.

Parker, H.L. (1978). Trigeminal neuralgia associated with multiple sclerosis. *Brain 51:* 46.

Raeder, J.G. (1924). Paratrigeminal paralysis of oculopupillary sympathetic. *Brain 47:* 149–158.

Raskin, N.H. and S.P. Prusiner (1977). Carotidynia. *Neurology 27:*43–46.

Roseman, D.M. (1967). Carotidynia. A distinct syndrome. *Arch. Otolaryngol. 85:*81.

Rushton, N., P. Goldstein, and J.A. Gibilisco (1969). A psychiatric study of atypical facial pain. *Can. Med. Assoc. J. 100:*26.

Sternbach, R.A., R.J. Ignelzi, L.M. Deems, and G. Timmermens (1976). Transcutaneous electrical analgesia: A follow-up analysis. *Pain 2:*35–41.

Sweet, W.H., C.E. Poletti, and J.B. Macon (1981). Treatment of trigeminal neuralgia and other facial pains by retrogasserian injection of glycerol. *Neurosurg. 9:*647–653.

Sweet, W.H. and J.G. Wepsic (1974). Controlled thermocoagulation of trigeminal ganglion and rootlets for differential destruction of pain fibers. Part 1: Trigeminal neuralgia. *J. Neurosurg. 40:*143–156.

Tash, R.R., G. Sze, and D.R. Leslie (1989). Trigeminal neuralgia: MR imaging features. *Radiology 172:*767–770.

Tashiro, H., A. Kondo, I. Aoyama et al. (1991). Trigeminal neuralgia caused by compression from arteries transfixing the nerve. *J. Neurosurg. 75:*783–786.

Tew, J.M. and J.R. Keller (1977). The treatment of trigeminal neuralgia by percutaneous radio frequency technique. *Clin. Neurosurg. 24:*557–575.

Vijayan, N. and C. Watson (1978). The pericarotid syndrome. *Headache 18:*244.

Waltz, T., D.J. Dalessio, B. Copeland, and G. Abbott (1989). Percutaneous injection of glycerol for the treatment of trigeminal neuralgia. *Clin. J. Pain 5:*195–198.

Young, R.F. (1988). Glycerol rhizolysis for treatment of trigeminal neuralgia. *J. Neurosurg. 69:*39–45.

Zakrzewska, J.M. and P.N. Patsalos (1988). Oxcarbazepine: A new drug in the management of intractable trigeminal neuralgia. *J. Neurol. Neurosurg. Psychiatry 52:* 472–476.

16

Post-Traumatic Headaches

OTTO APPENZELLER

Nowhere is scientific medicine less evident than in the treatment and management of post-traumatic headaches. Great difficulties arise in interpreting and assessing subjective symptoms that usually become overwhelmingly important in the subject's life only some variable time after head injury is sustained. This has led to a proliferation of anecdotal reports that often are contradictory and inconclusive and, despite their extent, leave a fuzzy clinical picture, the description of which causes problems for practitioners who wish to fit their patients into recognizable categories. Many neurologists and neurosurgeons favor their individual pathogenic mechanisms for post-traumatic headache; however, it should be stressed that probably no one factor is responsible for the ubiquitous occurrence of this vexing symptom, and only a minority of patients can be clearly helped by specific pharmacotherapy. Only carefully organized prospective studies of this ever-increasing problem, with adequate follow-up and large enough numbers of patients and assessment of the extent of injury and its relation to subsequent symptoms, might clarify the picture.

HISTORIC ASPECTS

Medical records from the earliest times, although limited, describe damage to the head with visible fractures of the skull. In such individuals, the cause of headache was obvious. However, the idea that damage to the brain can occur without obvious external trauma first appeared in a description of a criminal who committed suicide by hitting his head against a wall. At autopsy, the skull was intact and no visible brain damage was seen. In the 19th century, persistent and intractable symptoms after head injury were noted when Rigler (1879) ascribed the increasing incidence of post-traumatic disability to the acceptance of financial compensation for accidental injuries on the Prussian railways. He was skeptical about symptoms in railway workers who demanded compensation and suggested that they may not have a "molecular derangement within the nervous system."

A clear distinction between symptoms due to damage of the brain and those associated with compensation claims was drawn by Strumpell in 1888. He thought that symptoms not obviously due to cerebral damage were widespread and exaggerated. In 1892, Friedmann described a triad of headache, dizziness, and alcohol intolerance. Later, irritability and difficulty in concentration were added, and this quincade was labeled the postconcussion syndrome, headache being the most troublesome and prominent symptom.

This constellation of complaints is common after head injury, but its pathogenesis and management continue to arouse controversy. Many war-injured patients were extensively studied and considerable knowledge about post-traumatic syndromes has accrued, but this has come mainly from severe and penetrating injuries, typical of casualties. However, more and more seemingly superficial or minor closed injuries to the head are even more troublesome to the physician. Even in patients who initially had no obvious evidence of cranial or cerebral trauma, subsequent verifiable atrophic areas in the brain may be demonstrable. Although the headache may not be causally related to the radiographic findings, litigiousness necessitates the admission that "*certo pronunciare non possumus; certum tamen est graves contusiones capitis plerumque molesta sui monumenta post se relinquere*" (I cannot judge; the only certainty is the head injury that continues to trouble)—the opinion of a judge given in 1694 in relation to a patient of Wepfer (1727). This patient, a 26-year-old servant, was hit on the head by a staff, with consequent well-described retrograde amnesia, and 6 months later had a continuing headache, dizziness, ringing in the ear, and lassitude.

PATHOGENESIS

A brain concussion imposed on delicate neurotransmitter, neuromodulator, and electrical brain activity interferes with the regulatory capacity of the central, and subsequently the peripheral, autonomic and vasomotor systems. The abnormalities in cerebral blood flow following concussion may lead to very serious consequences. From this alteration in vasomotion arises primary traumatic brain damage and more diffuse secondary disorders of the brain. It is sometimes possible to observe a remarkably rapid post-traumatic atrophy of cerebral tissue attributed to vasomotor disturbances leading to serious impediment of blood flow to the damaged and other parts of the brain (Tonnis, 1956). Courville (1950) and others (de Morsier, 1943) found diffuse ischemic parenchymatous damage after blunt head trauma, and Strich (1956) demonstrated pathological areas of demyelination years after apparently mild blunt head injuries.

Nevertheless, secondary changes in the brain after trauma and atrophic or demyelinated areas do not seem to be pathogenetically related to post-traumatic headaches, because brain tissue itself is insensitive. These pathologic findings instead demonstrate the relationship between brain concussion and vascular disorders and the serious circulatory disturbance occurring in the peritraumatic period. These derangements of the circulation are characterized by a fall in diastolic blood pressure with orthostasis predisposing to changes in blood flow and changes in blood vessel diameter, including pulsatility of major blood vessels sensitive to pain that are related to the symptomatology of vascular headaches of the migrainous type.

Thus, the immediate postconcussion headache is clinically very similar to migraine. This pulsatile headache increases with Valsalva's maneuver, bending forward, or exertion. The pain, however, is more or less continuous or occurs phasically or in attacks that are diffuse, sometimes frontal. However, pain of this nature, if it persists for years after a head injury, can only with difficulty be attributed to the original impact. True post-traumatic migraine is said to be rare.

Cluster headache after a postinjury interval of several months, as reported by Nick and Sicard-Nick (1969), must be unusual because no such case has been observed by Heyck (1975) or others. Recently, however, cluster-like headache ipisilateral to a post-traumatic subdural hematoma has been reported in another patient (Formisano et al., 1990). The pain appeared 45 days after the injury.

After reviewing hundreds of head-injured patients with headache, Heyck found post-traumatic migraine to be uncommon in adults, but not in children (Heyck, 1975). Ophthalmic post-traumatic migraine in younger subjects, with flashes of light, scotomata, unilateral headache, vomiting, sonophobia, and photophobia after head trauma, is perhaps related to the excessive reactivity of the autonomic nervous system in children, in whom the head injury may also unmask a latent migrainous diathesis. Self-limited cortical blindness was reported in six children (Kaye and Herskowitz, 1986). In five of these, normal visual function returned within 24 hours. These children had relatively minor trauma. In the one child with demonstrated parieto-occipital contusion, a striking visual recovery (with a remaining altitudinal defect) was evident 1 week after trauma.

In older individuals, often those with brain atrophy, continuous nonmigrainous post-traumatic headaches are more frequent. These are attributed to the age-related changes in the cerebral vasculature and impairment of vascular adaption with age. In addition, predisposition to bleeding and numerous microhemorrhages in the meninges and dura after even minor head trauma, with consequent scars and adhesions, play a role in the genesis of the headaches.

INCIDENCE

In assessing incidence, it is necessary to exclude headache resulting from complications of the injury itself, such as subarachnoid hemorrhage, bacterial meningitis, or subdural hematoma. The incidence of headaches without obvious recognizable structural injury varies with the selection of the clinical material and the duration of follow-up. In a number of patients, moreover, analysis of post-traumatic headache is complicated by their development of recurring headaches after a symptom-free interval. The reported incidence varies from 28% (Penfield and Norcross, 1936) to nearly double that in a review of 200 cases of non–war-related head injuries, in which 46% of the patients complained of headache when consciousness returned. The proportion remained the same at the time of discharge; 3 months later, however, only 21% had returned to work, and a further decrease in the number working was found in subsequent months (Guttman, 1943). Surprisingly, headache was a more troublesome symptom in those who were thought to have a less severe injury, but no such relationship was found in patients who had headaches for longer periods of time after the injury. Age was not important in determining the incidence of headache, but those who had an antecedent history of recurrent headache were more prone to develop post-traumatic headache.

After very severe blunt head trauma, the risk of behavioral and emotional sequelae is greater in younger than in older patients (Thomsen, 1989). All patients in this study had at least 1 month or more of post-traumatic amnesia, and were first seen about 4.5 months after injury and followed for a period ranging from 2.5 to 10 to 15 years later. There was, however, no correlation between age when injured and post-traumatic amnesia. In another series (Russell, 1933–34) post-traumatic headache lasting longer than 2 months was found in 100% of patients over the age of 50, which contrasted with an overall incidence of 60% in this series. No relationship was found between the severity of the headache, the duration of residual disabilities, and the severity of injury, but a clear relationship to possible financial compensation was evident. A different experience was reported by Guttman (1943) and Brenner et al. (1944), who were unable to relate the severity and duration of headache to age, neurologic disablement, sex, occupation, circumstances of injury, or intelligence of the subjects. The conclusion that 30 to 50% of patients develop headache after head injury seems to be adequately supported by a variety of authors (Miller, 1968).

The estimated incidence of head injuries ranges from 75,000 to 3 million annually in this country (Caveness, 1979; Jennett and Teasdale, 1981). Injuries sufficiently severe to cause residual disability occur in about 60,000 people annually, and although neurologic sequelae are often overemphasized, those without obvious clinical deficits but with persistent headache and mental symptoms form the bulk of post-traumatic handicaps and seem to be generally forgotten.

Careful reviews to assess the connection between severity of the injury as evidenced by coma or amnesias or the presence of focal brain damage, subarachnoid bleeding, increased cerebrospinal fluid pressure, or electroencephalographic (EEG) abnormalities and the severity and duration of post-traumatic headache have failed (Brenner et al., 1944; Friedman and Merritt, 1945). Some have even suggested that post-traumatic headache is singularly less troublesome after major cerebral injury and more disabling after minor concussion (Miller, 1961). Nevertheless, scalp lacerations promote headache; whether this is because of neuroma formation resulting from injury to cutaneous scalp nerves or other factors remains unclear. Extensive experience (Gurdjian and Webster, 1958) has shown that patients with major cerebral damage and serious parenchymal brain atrophy usually have little in the way of post-traumatic headache. The troublesomeness of headache in those with head injuries without loss of consciousness and those with only momentary impairment of awareness suggests that personality traits play a role in promoting such headaches.

CLINICAL FEATURES

There is no uniform description of the character of the headaches. Russell (1933–34) thought they were continuous, but others believed they were mostly intermittent (Simons and Wolff, 1946). The varied and nonspecific nature of post-traumatic headaches was best characterized by Symonds (1960), who showed the variation in the nature of the pain, its location, and the importance of the behavior of the sufferer. The headaches may be throbbing or hammering and occasionally bursting or stabbing in nature. The descriptions given by patients emphasize the distress and are often exaggerated in those with litigation pending.

Symptoms of Post-traumatic Headache

The best-defined and probably most easily understood post-traumatic headache is associated with injury to the scalp. The origin is visible, and the pain is often associated with a sharp, well-localized area of tenderness in the scar or nearby. Percussion may cause a spreading sharp stab of pain. Sometimes head gear cannot be tolerated, or exposure to cold or emotional stress may trigger pain. Compression of a neuroma by contraction of scalp muscles or through release of neurotransmitters and neurohormones might trigger painful afferent stimuli. Sometimes the local pain spreads to cause generalized intermittent headache. Usually, the pain subsides spontaneously within a few months after injury, but repeated injections of local anesthetic in and around painful trigger points often speeds recovery. An associated spreading paresthesia from the injury site is often exaggerated by percussion but usually fades with the disappearance of the pain or after the use of local anesthetic.

Injury to the ligamentous structures of the cervical spine or more serious injury to the spine itself often complicates injury to the head, and this is sometimes overshadowed by extensive head trauma. For variable periods thereafter, such patients may complain of symptoms referable to the cervical spine long after those due to the head injury have disappeared. The injuries to the bony skeleton, disks, or ligaments, and sometimes pressure on spinal nerves, often contribute to the post-traumatic syndrome, including the headache. The cause of the pain may be actual skeletal damage; more often, however, pressure, irritation, or traction on cervical roots is largely responsible for occipital and posterior cervical neck pain and headache. Many patients are relieved by manipulation. However, this is risky, particularly in elderly individuals. Disastrous occlusions of vertebral arteries have been well documented following such maneuvers. The injection of local anesthetic into tender points in the neck repeated at 2- or 3-day intervals often helps break the vicious pain cycle. This is usually accompanied by the administration of tricyclics. Physical therapy and traction have advocates, but their effects are unpredictable (Simons and Wolff, 1946).

Generalized post-traumatic headache is difficult to account for and categorize. It is described often not as a pain, but as a fuzziness or dizzy sensation or a feeling of fullness in the head. Such patients are usually able to clearly distinguish between post-traumatic sensations and headache of a different kind, to which they may have been prone before their injury. Similar categorizations are often made by patients whose headache may be a symptom of depression, in whom, again, inadequate descriptions of abnormal head sensations often distinguish depressive manifestations from headaches due to migraine, increased intracranial pressure, or a hangover.

Generalized headache, which is clearly pain rather than an amorphous head sensation, usually makes its onset with some delay after the injury. This lag has been attributed to post-traumatic amnesia (Symonds, 1942), but it may also appear without an intervening amnestic period. Whether this delay results from a gradual change in neurotransmitters in the perivascular nerve plexus or in the brain itself, which only reaches its pain-promoting patterns sometime after injury, is not certain. This type of headache is often unilateral at the onset and may spread from the site of injury. It may be related to exertion or to posture, especially bending forward. When the headache is severe, vomiting may also occur. Stress, fatigue, excitement, bright lights, noise, concentration, or consumption of alcohol often exacerbates the headaches. Rest, quiet, and lying down in a darkened room bring improvement. Analgesics are not universally successful in alleviating the pain, and many patients pass from mild use of over-the-counter medication to serious polypharmacy dependence.

Patterns of Post-traumatic Headache

Within this wide spectrum of post-traumatic headache symptoms, certain patterns are discernible. One pattern is characterized by the features of tension-type headache, usually the sense of a tight band around the head or bilateral temple nonthrobbing pain, sometimes occipital. This is often accompanied by tenderness of extracranial structures. It is occasionally relieved by local anesthetic injection, local massage, heat or ice, sedatives, voluntary relaxation, and tricyclic antidepressants. This pattern is very similar to an ordinary tension-type headache but without antecedent trauma.

The second variety of post-traumatic headache is often generalized, occasionally unilateral, and paroxysmal. It may be throbbing and has all the features of migraine, accompanied occasionally by nausea and vomiting, photophobia, and sonophobia. This post-traumatic migraine, although much less common than the tension-type headache, responds to treatment with ergotamine and other standard migraine therapy. Because of its association with trauma, resolution of litigation is occasionally helpful in decreasing the frequency of attacks. Nevertheless, many patients become regular migraineurs, with exacerbation and improvement in the frequency and severity of attacks most often related to the usual situational factors.

A third variety, termed "post-traumatic disautonomic cephalalgia" (Vijayan and Dreyfus, 1975), is distinct but rare, and follows injury to the neck. The cause is thought to be trauma to the perivascular sympathetic fibers in the carotid artery sheath. Pain and tenderness of the neck remain for weeks after the injury. Later, severe unilateral episodic pulsatile headache occurs ipsilateral to the injury, in the temporal and frontal areas, associated with ipsilateral sweating and dilation of the pupil, blurred vision, photophobia, and nausea. The headaches may last for hours to days and recur at frequent intervals. Sympathetic overactivity (perhaps as a result of partial injury of sympathetic fibers) with excessive firing, and later sympathetic denervation confirmed by response of the pupil to a weak solution of epinephrine, were found in these patients. Ergotamine is not effective, but propranolol may be useful.

Postconcussion Syndrome

The postconcussion syndrome remains a mystery, and the clinical spectrum is broad. Symptoms include headache, dizziness, impairment of memory, difficulty in concentrating, fatigue, anxiety, irritability, personality changes, and depression (Lindvall, 1974). The occurrence of this syndrome is perhaps even more common after mild head trauma (Kay et al., 1971; Merrett and McDonald, 1977). Immediately after head injury and for a few days thereafter, the headache and dizziness dominate the symptomatology; the cause is probably multifactorial, including pain at the injury site and diffuse, dull pressure thought in the past to be a result of muscular contraction (Simons and Wolff, 1946). It may be associated with a "whiplash" phenomenon arising from the cervical spine, from musculoskeletal structures or pressure or tension on nerve roots, or it could be post-traumatic migraine. Dizziness is common early in the post-traumatic period; abnormal electronystagmographic, audiologic, and vestibular–caloric findings have been reported in such patients (Toglia et al., 1970), but these investigations remain controversial (Lindvall, 1974). Many neuropsychological abnormalities, including slowed information processing and difficulty with memory, inability to concentrate, fatigability, irritability, and anxiety, are common features (Gronwall and Wrightson, 1974; Rimel et al., 1982).

Evidence for brain damage after even minor head injury has been repeatedly presented (Oppenheimer, 1968; Strich, 1956), and the delayed onset of symptoms may be due to difficulties and stressful situations encountered on return to work because of inability to perform previously easy tasks (Gronwall and Wrightson, 1974). Although symptoms continue for months or years after the accident, the perpetuation of disability is the result not only of putative brain damage, usually undetected by present methods of investigation, but also of psychological responses to the accident. Litigation and compensation, although not entirely to blame for persistent disability, certainly promote its continuation (Brooks, 1972). Continued disability after head injury is associated with middle age, married status, social class IV (U.K. classification by Hollingshead), industrial accidents, relatively unskilled occupations, and previous behavioral abnormalities (Kay et al., 1971).

Neuropsychiatric Disorders following Head Injury

Symptoms persisting for some time after head injury almost invariably involve the development of secondary psychiatric problems. An explanation of the basis of the symptoms, if available, and exploration of life situations, stresses, the occurrence of reactive depression, and alcoholism all may be appropriately addressed by psychotherapy, including the use of pharmacologic intervention. Good responses to tricyclics have been reported (Adeloye, 1971; Tyler et al.,

1980). More recent studies are at variance with this conclusion. Saran (1988) compared the responses to amitriptyline in patients with headache associated with depression and depression after minor closed head injury. The former group responded to the drug, but the post-traumatic patients did not improve, showing neither reduction in headache nor a decrease in depression. Although many patients eventually recover, this is in large part because of the support of relatives and family, who realize that patients may not be exactly the same after the injury and may react differently to stresses and emotional stimuli and have difficulty achieving adaptive responses and behaviors.

The relationship of head injury to psychiatric illness is not easily defined by modern techniques, which do not provide an understanding of neuropsychiatric disorders after injury.

EEG and sleep EEG may be useful in those with closed head injury and the post-traumatic syndrome. Abnormal sleep patterns have been found 5 years after head injury (Prigatano et al., 1982), and a correlation has been reported between the percentage of rapid eye movement (REM) sleep and sleep fragmentation and the development of behavior problems and symptoms of psychopathology after head injury. During the acute recovery period after head injury, a correlation between REM sleep percentage time and cognitive function has also been found. In addition, a post-traumatic hypersomnia is recognized. This is sometimes prominent 6 months or more after head injury (Association of Sleep Disorders Centers, 1979). The use of EEG for prognostic purposes, however, is not as yet possible.

Schizophrenia-like symptoms may follow head injury (Davison and Bagley, 1969; Lishman, 1978). Conversely, 15% of schizophrenics have had head injuries preceding their first psychotic episodes (Lishman, 1978). A variable number ranging from 0.07 to 9.8% of injured patients develop schizophrenialike psychosis (Davison and Bagley, 1969), and there is less genetic predisposition to schizophrenia in those with the disease and antecedent brain injury. Although focal brain lesions have not been clearly related to the subsequent development of schizophrenia, some have suggested that temporal lobe damage or diffuse brain damage is more likely to result in schizophrenia (Davison and Bagley, 1969).

A group of schizophrenics with brain atrophy and computerized tomographic evidence of ventricular enlargement, together with intellectual deterioration, has been identified. These patients also show intellectual impairment on neuropsychological tests (Johnstone et al., 1976). However, the distinction between chronic schizophrenics and those who have brain atrophy from other causes is difficult by these methods, and only 54% can be correctly assigned to one or the other group. Chronic schizophrenics also have flattening of affect, retardation, and poverty of speech (Johnstone et al., 1978). Enlargement of ventricles, sometimes a sequela of head trauma, has been correlated with eventual clinical outcome, and the intellectual and memory deficits and social and vocational disabilities seem related to these radiographic findings (Levin et al., 1981). It is tempting to also relate ventricular enlargement to development of schizophrenialike post-traumatic symptoms. In addition, gliosis in the brain of chronic schizophrenics is found in the midbrain, diencephalon, and limbic system, areas that may show significant damage after head trauma and that are linked to behavioral changes resembling chronic schizophrenia or post-traumatic symptoms (Stevens, 1982).

The post–head-injury depression is frequently associated with headache and is often expressed as discouragement, loss, and demoralization (Rimel et al., 1982). The severity of the injury, the time after injury of onset of symptoms, and the location of focal neurologic deficits might be related to the development of this post-traumatic affective disturbance. The frontal and temporal lobes are often implicated in those with post-traumatic depression (Robinson and Szetela, 1981). The role of nonrepinephrine projections to the frontal lobe from the locus ceruleus in the genesis of these depressive disorders remains to be further assessed, but adrenergic agonists have been used in treatment of cognitive deficits (Arnsten and Goldman-Rakic, 1985).

Few neurochemical studies are available to determine the changes in neurotransmitters and neuromodulators that occur after head trauma. An increase in homovanillic acid and 5-hyroxyindoleacetic acid immediately following head injury has, however, been found (Van Woerkom et al., 1977). Moreover, the release of acetylcholine occurring simultaneously with trauma to the brain may be an additional trigger for postconcussive affective disorders (Ward, 1966).

The frequent personality changes after head injury and the accompanying post-traumatic headache have been attributed to diffuse brain damage. Emotional lability, a decrease in control of impulsive actions, apathy, and sometimes indifference associated with intellectual impairment are common (Levin et al., 1982). It is thought that, in a number of such cases, damage to localized brain areas or to neurotransmitter systems responsible for the integration of the personality is the cause of the syndrome, and frontal and temporal lobe personality disorders are frequently found because of the propensity of these areas of the brain to suffer damage. Such patients, particularly those with frontal lobe lesions, may have minimal or no detectable intellectual deficits on testing and show profound personality disorders, but special psychological tests such as the Wisconsin Card Sort and the Stylus Maze tests may reveal an inability to change behavior in response to verbal signals, a lack of the capacity to follow instructions, and frequent impulsive mistakes (Milner, 1964).

In temporal lobe damage, personality disorders are common and often associated with complex partial seizures. Impulsivity, hyperorality, hypersexuality, visual agnosia, and impairment of memory are the features of more severely brain-injured patients and this, together with somatic complaints of headache and dizziness and the need to treat seizures, leads to polypharmacy and sometimes complicated personality changes resulting more from therapy than from the brain lesions. Sudden violent outbursts with minimal or no provocation in frontal and temporal lobe–damaged patients are often part of the syndrome. These outbursts are facilitated by excessive or immoderate alcohol intake and continued depression, which may perpetuate the aggressive outbursts and persistent psychosocial maladjustments. This, together with the somatization of complaints to the head and persistent headache, makes the management of such patients very difficult (Kwentus et al., 1985).

General Considerations

After head injury, the patient is an expert in this field, and an examination of the patient's complaints may give a more complete description of post-traumatic states and generate hypotheses to explain the deficits found in such patients. An endless list of symptoms, including headache with varying degrees of post-traumatic amnesia, emerges from numerous inquiries; nevertheless, no stable constellation of complaints to satisfy the criteria for a "post-traumatic syndrome" has been found. In a review of 57 patients who sustained a severe closed head injury and who were followed up for 2 years, 84% reported some residual deficits in psychological function, with forgetfulness heading the list. In seeking a relationship between post-traumatic amnesia and return to preinjury work, forgetfulness, slowness, inability to concentrate, and inability to divide attention between two simultaneous activities were found to be positively related to the severity of the injury. Numerous other complaints were not related to severity. A similar pattern emerged when analyses were based on deficits as reported by patients' relatives, but the severity of injury was not related to the number of complaints. In addition, the longer the post-traumatic amnesia persisted, the less likely it was that a patient could resume work at preinjury levels (Van Zomeren and van den Burg, 1985).

Whiplash Injury Headaches

Whiplash injury has multiple pathogenetic origins. It results from strain or rupture of paraspinous muscles or ligaments. Cartilage end plates or intervertebral disks may be avulsed, and a traumatic arthropathy of the zygapophyseal joints may appear. Cervical spondylosis may predispose to whiplash injury and consequent post-traumatic headache arising from osteoarthritis of the cervical zygapophyseal joints or contraction of muscles resulting from splinting of the cervical spine reflexly and tension myalgia (Edmeads, 1978).

Treatment of these headaches is by heat, neck immobilization, sometimes manipulation and traction, or injection with local anesthetic and steroids. Several injections and the use of anti-inflammatory drugs or tricyclic antidepressants and analgesics are often successful. Some refractory patients may require anterior body fusion of a segment identified as the cause of headache by using distention and analgesic diskography (Pawl, 1977). This should rarely be necessary and should be preceded by a trial of neck immobilization in a collar.

INNERVATION OF CEREBRAL VESSELS—A PATHOGENETIC ROLE?

Patients with head injuries and a definite site of impact often complain of ipsilateral headaches during the post-traumatic period. There is no universally accepted explanation relating ipsilateral headache to symptomatic cerebral hemispheres in migraine, but a trigeminal innervation of the pia and arachnoidal vessels arising from ipsilateral trigeminal structures in the cat has been found. These nerve fibers release substance P, a vasodilator associated with pain per-

ception. Ipsilateral trigeminal sensory responses to cortical stimulation by subdural electrodes in humans have also been reported (Lesser et al., 1985). These
responses have been attributed to nerve fibers that accompany pial vessels,
which are presumably related to the trigeminal vascular system (Moskowitz,
1984). These findings support the existence of such a perivascular plexus system
in the human cerebrovasculature also. It is therefore conceivable that pain
perception in patients with unilateral head injuries may be ipsilateral to the
injury and may even be accompanied by visual phenomena sometimes found in
patients with post-traumatic headache (Lesser et al., 1985).

The cerebral vessels, like other blood vessels, were until recently thought
to be innervated only by sympathetic norepinephrine-containing nerve fibers
that mediate constriction and parasympathetic acetylcholine-containing fibers
thought to act in a dilatory fashion. This is clearly an incomplete view, because
it has become obvious, using selective and sensitive immunohistochemical
methods, that neuropeptides are also present in perivascular nerve fibers. Cerebral autoregulation of the vasculature depends in part on sympathetic nerves
that modulate cerebral capacitance vessels (Edvinsson, 1982). It is possible,
however, that the increasingly larger number of transmitter candidates found
in walls of cerebral vessels of animals and humans may play a role as well. It
has been suggested that they act by rapidly modifying vessel tone. They are
thought to maintain homeostasis in the cerebral circulation, ensuring oxygen
and glucose supplies adequate for brain function. The neuropeptides now demonstrated in perivascular nerve plexuses of cerebral vessels include neuropeptide Y, substance P, calcitonin gene-related peptide (CGRP), and vasoactive
intestinal polypeptide (VIP), all of which probably act as neurotransmitters. In
addition, gastrin-releasing peptide (GRP), cholecystokinin, neurotensin, and
somatostatin have also been found, but their role in the control of cerebral
vessel tone is less well defined (Edvinsson, 1985).

Physiologic evidence shows that, apart from norepinephrine, vasoconstrictor activity results from cotransmitter-released neuropeptide Y from sympathetic nerves, and fibers containing this peptide are abundant around major
arteries supplying blood to the brain. The additional observation that neuropeptide Y disappears after superior cervical sympathectomy or after the administration of 6-hydroxydopamine, a sympathetic ganglion poison, supports the coexistence of norepinephrine and neuropeptide Y in sympathetic fibers (Edvinsson,
1985).

Direct neurogenic mechanisms mediating rapid dilation of cerebral vessels
have also been found. Metabolic factors that are released during normal and
pathologic states (e.g., epilepsy or head injury) are important in maintaining
blood flow to the brain, but cholinergic mechanisms arising in central cholinergic neurons are also involved (Bartus et al., 1982). In addition, transmitters
distinct from acetylcholine have been shown to cause dilation of brain vessels.
These transmitters are VIP and substance P, stored in perivascular nerves in
the cerebral vessels (Edvinsson et al., 1981; Larsson et al., 1976). Moreover,
nerve fibers showing VIP immunoreactivity are found to a variable extent in
the walls of cerebral arteries of laboratory animals and of humans. These fibers
are found in the adventitia or at the adventitial–medial border of the arteries

and are most densely distributed in the rostral part of the circle of Willis. The origin of VIP-containing nerve fibers is not clear, but it has been suggested that they arise from local ganglia or in the brain itself. VIP causes relaxation of isolated cerebral arteries from all animals examined (Edvinsson and Ekman, 1984). Microapplication or superfusion of VIP causes cerebral vasodilation and an increase in flow, and the experimental injection of VIP into the striatum or the cortex causes metabolic activation with increases in local glucose consumption in both ipsilateral and contralateral homologous regions (McCulloch and Kelly, 1983). These and many other experimental findings suggest an important role for VIP in cerebral blood flow regulation.

The evidence for sensory nerve endings on intracranial vasculature has recently been strengthened. These endings are of particular importance in the mechanism of vascular head pain. In animals and humans, it is clear that the central portions of intracranial blood vessels are pain sensitive. In addition, meningeal manipulation and distention of dural arteries are associated with pain. Stimulation of various parts of the vasculature in humans is associated with different types of pain; for example, the pial arteries at the base of the brain, when stimulated, cause a dull and intense ache. Substance P has been demonstrated around these blood vessels and might be a transmitter in some sensory fibers surrounding them. Substance P is thought to be important in transmission of nociceptor stimuli to the central nervous system through primary sensory neurons (Pernow, 1983). Substance P–containing fibers around cerebral arteries and veins in various mammals, including humans, are not affected by removal of the superior cervical ganglion or chemical sympathectomy with 6-hydroxydopamine, but capsaicin treatment causes a significant loss of these fibers. The major effect of capsaicin is on the sensory system, which implies that substance P–containing fibers may be part of the sensory trigeminal system but not part of the sympathetic ganglia (Hokfelt et al., 1980). Substance P is released from perivascular plexuses by a variety of stimuli, including electrical field stimulation; this suggests a neurotransmitter role for this peptide also.

CGRP may also be involved in nociception and affects the autonomic and endocrine systems. Nerve fibers containing CGRP have been demonstrated by immunohistochemical techniques around cerebral arteries, and this peptide is thought to coexist with substance P fibers in perivascular nerve plexuses. CGRP is potentially of great importance in regulating cerebral blood flow. GRP is strikingly homologous with the amphibian peptide bombesin. Its presence has been demonstrated around cerebral vessels, but neither GRP nor bombesin are of physiologic importance in experimental cerebral blood flow studies. Low levels of somatostatin have also been found around some cerebral vessels in experimental animals, but the importance of this peptide in the cerebral circulatory regulation is problematic.

Peptides affect cerebral blood flow and, in turn, are influenced by the electrical activity of brain structures, which is clearly deranged at some point in association with cerebral trauma. The effect of trauma on peptides, and consequently on cerebral blood flow and pain, has not been investigated in animals or humans. It is tempting to speculate, however, that the intimate morphologic association of peptide-containing perivascular nerve plexuses, and their partial origin in sympathetic extracranial systems or in the brain itself and effect on the blood–brain barrier subsequent to changes in vasomotor function, may profoundly influence the post-traumatic course of individual patients and their eventual symptomatology.

POST-TRAUMATIC HEADACHE—A REFLEX SYMPATHETIC DYSTROPHY?

The cause of reflex sympathetic dystrophy (RSD), like that of post-traumatic headache, remains unknown. Nevertheless, the sympathetic nervous system and vasoregulation are important components of the pathologic mechanisms in both conditions. RSD usually involves a limb and consists of a triad of pain, edema, and sympathetic dysfunction occurring after trauma to the limb, injury to nerves, or central nervous system dysfunction. This triad is also present in post-traumatic headache.

Endothelia—Role in Post-traumatic Headache and RSD

A recent observation is that vascular endothelium is heterogeneous; that is, not only are there endothelial cells of arteries and veins, but these cells differ in their function in various organs and express different phenotypes (Goerdt et al., 1989). This clearly shows that endothelia serve different organs in adapative and specialized ways and are not just a sheath of cells that function as a semi-permeable membrane. It is therefore to be expected that endothelial cell products such as endothelin, a powerful vasoconstrictor (Lerman et al., 1990), participate in the responses to injuries because vascular responses to injury are not uniform. Thus, during head injury, vasodilation occurs in the cerebral vasculature and vasoconstriction in the skin and other vascular beds. Endothelial cells interact with perivascular nerves, which modulate vessel diameter and in turn change the paracrine function of endothelial cells (Appenzeller, 1991). At the time of injury to the head, the vasoreactivity of cerebral vessels may profoundly affect endothelial cell function.

Changing levels of catecholamines occurring during injury may cause the release of endothelin and in turn affect vasoconstrictor responses induced by endothelin release (Yang et al., 1990). Moreover, vasodilation and consequent decrease in shear stress also tend to increase endothelin release (Yoshizumi et al., 1989).

In RSD and after head trauma, local factors have assumed an increasing importance, particularly in sympathetic disregulation (Janig, 1989). It is likely that such factors at the injury site or within the brain contribute to the pathogenesis and perpetuation of the post-traumatic syndrome. For example, hypoxia has profound effects on endothelial cell paracrine function, including the induction of endothelin (VanHoutte, 1989). The accumulation of inflammatory cells at the site of injury has similar effects, and the release of vasoactive substances from these cells compounds and alters neurogenic vasoregulation and in turn the function of endothelial cells (Springer, 1990). Thus, one proposal worthy of further exploration is to regard post-traumatic headache as a RSD affecting the head and to apply to the head the methods used for the study of the pathogenesis of RSD affecting a limb. Thus, blood flow studies not only in the intracranial arteries but in brain coverings should be revealing, and the manipulation of the sympathetic supply to the head might, just as in some cases of RSD, be useful.

The use of calcitonin, found effective in RSD (Gobelet et al., 1986), might also be tried in post-traumatic headache. Epidemiologic studies have established a statistical link between cigarette smoking and RSD (An et al., 1988). Because the consumption of nicotine causes vasospasm, and this is a feature of RSD and the post-traumatic syndrome some time after injury, such an association has been sought in a study of long-term effects of head injuries (Carlsson et al., 1987). It was found that smoking and alcohol were powerful factors confounding the postinjury picture. Thus, both RSD and the post-traumatic injury syndrome share the link with smoking.

The use of barbiturates in RSD has been linked to the syndrome, and withdrawal of the drug seemed to be a precondition for recovery (Horton and Gerster, 1984). Barbiturates are often part of the treatment of post-traumatic headache. A review of their effectiveness or role in prolongation of headache after head trauma should be revealing.

EFFECTS OF HEAD INJURY IN CHILDREN

Prominent symptoms are sometimes seen in children after relatively minor head trauma. Temporary neurologic deficits including post-traumatic blindness (Griffith and Dodge, 1968), hemiparesis (Pickles, 1949), somnolence, irritability, and vomiting (Mealy, 1968) have been reported and associated with the syndrome of post-traumatic migraine. In children, post-traumatic attacks associated with focal neurologic deficits resulting from head trauma are transient in nature and have a tendency to recur. They resemble those described in British soccer players who develop classic migraine after heading the ball or receiving other minor blows to the head (Matthews, 1972).

A study of 25 children with transient post-traumatic neurologic focal deficits produced a constellation of clinical findings. Hemiparetic blindness and somnolent irritable states were attributed to involvement of the cerebral vasculature. This syndrome resembles migraine with aura and presumably has a similar pathogenesis. Head trauma may affect perivascular peptide-containing nerve plexuses and may lead to release of neurotransmitters and neuromodulators, with subsequent migrainous symptoms. In general, patients with this syndrome sustain a blow to the head that is sufficient to daze momentarily and rarely causes transient unconsciousness. A latent interval between the trauma and the onset of neurologic symptoms is usual, and this varies from seconds to hours, but in the majority the focal neurologic deficits appear within minutes. Many such post-traumatic attacks in children are mistaken for cerebral concussion or contusion or acute epidural or subdural hematomas, but it is more likely that they are migrainous in nature.

Some patients with this syndrome studied by angiography showed occlusion of branches of the middle cerebral arteries after transient focal neurologic deficits. Such attacks might therefore reliably be attributed to vascular spasms (Haas et al., 1975). Neurogenic mechanisms are primarily responsible for vascular phenomena and consequent focal neurologic deficits superimposed on, and complicated by, dysfunction of the brain and of the nerve supply to its blood vessels.

LATE EFFECTS OF HEAD INJURY

Good recovery after closed head injury is not always assurance that deficits may not appear and be measurable at a later date. Twenty patients with good recovery from closed head injury, according to the Glasgow Head Injury Scale, matched with a group of similar intelligence, language capacity, age, sex, and handedness, underwent intensive neuropsychological examination. The results showed that, despite good immediate recovery, poorly defined symptoms including difficulties in concentration, irritability and fatigue, and problems with tasks comparable to those carried out prior to injury persisted. The previous history of these patients was unremarkable and did not include psychiatric, neurologic, medical, or other behavioral disorders or alcoholism. Results of the head injury patients on verbal or performance vigilance tests, the Wechsler Memory Quotient, the trailmaking test, Wisconsin Card Sorting, and the Stroop Test, including word list generating or indexes of aphasia and apraxia, were no different from those of controls. Patients were, however, significantly worse on consonant trigram tests, which require the recall of three consonants after varying intervals of counting backward by threes, and on the Wechsler Memory scale. The speed of tapping of the dominant finger was difficult for patients to assess, and the Stroop color time story delay reproduction, results on the Wechsler Memory scale, and perseverative errors were all abnormal.

The two groups were best distinguished from each other by the trigram consonant test and the delay in the Wechsler Memory scale. Both of these could correctly classify 85% of participants in this study. Subtle deficiencies may remain even after good recovery, and the most important impairment involves the amount of information that can simultaneously be handled by postinjury patients (Stuss et al., 1985).

REFERENCES

Adeloye, A. (1971). Clinic trial of fluphenazine in the post-concussional syndrome. *Practitioner* 206:517–518.

An, H.S., K.B. Hawthorne, and W.T. Jackson (1988). Reflex sympathetic dystrophy and cigarette smoking. *J. Hand Surg.* 13:458–460.

Appenzeller, O. (1991). Pathogenesis of migraine. *Med. Clin. North Am.* 75:763–789.

Arnsten, A.F.T. and P.S. Goldman-Rakic (1985). α_2-adrenergic mechanisms in prefrontal cortex associated with cognitive decline in aged non-human primates. *Science* 230:1273–1276.

Association of Sleep Disorders Centers (1979). Diagnostic classification of sleep-wake disorders. *Sleep 2:*5–119.

Bartus, R.T., R.L. Dean III, B. Beer, and A.S. Lippa (1982). The cholinergic hypothesis of geriatric memory dysfunction. *Science 217:*408–417.

Brenner, C., A.P. Friedman, H.H. Merritt, and D.E. Denny-Brown (1944). Post-traumatic headache. *J. Neurosurg. 1:*379–391.

Brooks, D.N. (1972). Memory and head injury. *J. Nerv. Ment. Dis. 155:*350–355.

Carlsson, G.S., K. Svardsudd, and L. Welin (1987). Long-term effects of head injuries sustained during life in three male populations. *J. Neurosurg. 67:*197–205.

Caveness, W.F. (1979). Incidence of craniocerebral trauma in the United States in 1976 and trends from 1970–1975. *Adv. Neurol. 22:*1–3.

Courville, C.B. (1950). Contributions to the study of cerebral anoxia. *Bull. Los Angeles Neurol. Soc. 15:*99–103.

Davison, K. and C.R. Bagley (1969). Schizophrenia-like psychosis associated with organic disorders of the central nervous system. *Br. J. Psychiatry 4* (Suppl.): 113–184.

de Morsier, G. (1943). Les encéphalopathies traumatiques. Étude neurologique. *Schweiz. Arch. Neurol. Neurochir. Psychiatr. 50:*161–169.

Edmeads, J. (1978). Headaches and head pains associated with diseases of the cervical spine. *Med. Clin. North Am. 62:*533–544.

Edvinsson, L. (1982). Sympathetic control of cerebral circulation. *Trends Neurosci. 5:* 425–429.

Edvinsson, L. (1985). Functional role of perivascular peptides in the control of cerebral circulation. *Trends Neurosci. 8:*126–131.

Edvinsson, L. and R. Ekman (1984). Distribution and dilatory effect of vasoactive intestinal polypeptide (VIP) in human cerebral arteries. *Peptides 5:*329–331.

Edvinsson, L., J. McCulloch, and R. Uddman (1981). Substance P: Immunohistochemical localization and effect upon cat pial arteries in vitro and in situ. *J. Physiol. (Lond.) 318:*251–258.

Friedman, A.P. and H.H. Merritt (1945). Relationship of intracranial pressure and presence of blood in the cerebrospinal fluid to the occurrence of headaches in patients with injuries to the head. *J. Nerv. Ment. Dis. 102:*1–7.

Friedmann, M. (1892). Über eine besondere schwere From von Folgezustanden nach Gehirnerschutterung und über den vasomotorischen Symptomenkomplex bei der selben in Allgemeinen. *Arch. Psychiatr. 23:*230–267.

Formisano, R., A. Angelini, G. DeVuono et al. (1990). Cluster-like headache and head injury: Case report. *Ital. J. Neurol. Sci. 11:*303–305.

Gobelet, C., J.L. Meier, W. Schaffner et al. (1986). Calcitonin and reflex sympathetic dystrophy syndrome. *Clin. Rheumatol. 5:*382–388.

Goerdt, S., F. Steckel, K. Schulze-Osthoff et al. (1989). Characterization and differential expression of an endothelial cell-specific surface antigen in continuous and sinusoidal endothelia in skin vascular lesions and in vitro. *Exp. Cell. Biol. 57:*185–192.

Griffith, D.F. and P.R. Dodge (1968). Transient blindness following head injury in children. *N. Engl. J. Med. 278:*648–651.

Gronwall, D. and P. Wrightson (1974). Delayed recovery of intellectual function after minor head injury. *Lancet 2:*605–609.

Gurdjian, E.S. and J.E. Webster (1958). *Head Injuries, Mechanisms, Diagnosis and Management.* Little, Brown, Boston.

Guttman, L. (1943). Post-contusional headache. *Lancet 1*:10–12.

Haas, D.C., G.S. Pineda, and H. Lourie (1975). Juvenile head trauma syndromes and their relationship to migraine. *Arch. Neurol. 32*:727–730.

Heyck, H. (1975). *Der Kopfschmerz*, 4th ed., p. 218. Georg Thieme Verlag, Stuttgart.

Hokfelt, T., O. Johansson, A. Ljungdahl et al. (1980). Peptidergic neurones. *Nature 284*: 515–521.

Horton, P. and J.C. Gerster (1984). Reflex sympathetic dystrophy syndrome and barbiturates. A study of 25 cases with barbiturates compared with 124 cases treated without barbiturates. *Clin. Rheumatol. 3*:493–499.

Janig, W. (1989). Mechanisms of pain associated with abnormalities in the sympathetic nervous system. *New Issues Neurosci. 1*:369–387.

Jennett, B. and G. Teasdale (1981). *Management of Head Injuries*. F.A. Davis, Philadelphia.

Johnstone, E.C., T.J. Crow, C.D. Frith et al. (1976). Cerebral ventricular size and cognitive impairment in chronic schizophrenia. *Lancet 2*:924–926.

Johnstone, E.C., T.J. Crow, C.D. Frith et al. (1978). The dementia of dementia praecox. *Acta Psychiatr. Scand. 57*:305–324.

Kay, D.W.K., T.A. Derr, and L.P. Lassman (1971). Brain trauma and the postconcussion syndrome. *Lancet 2*:1052–1055.

Kaye, E.M. and J. Herskowitz (1986). Transient post-traumatic cortical blindness: Brief versus prolonged syndromes in childhood. *J. Child Neurol. 1*:206–210.

Kwentus, J.A., R.P. Hart, E.T. Peck et al. (1985). Psychiatric complications of closed head trauma. *Psychosomatics 26*:8–17.

Larsson, L.I., L. Edvinsson, J. Fahrenkrug et al. (1976). Immunohistochemical localization of a vasodilatory polypeptide (VIP) in cerebrovascular nerves. *Brain Res. 113*:400–404.

Lerman, A., F.L. Hildebrand Jr., K.B. Margulies et al. (1990). Endothelin: A new cardiovascular regulatory peptide. *Mayo Clin. Proc. 65*:1441–1455.

Lesser, R.P., H. Luders, G. Klem et al. (1985). Ipsilateral trigeminal sensory responses to cortical stimulation by subdural electrodes. *Neurology 35*:1760–1763.

Levin, H.S., A.L. Benton, and R.G. Grossman (1982). *Neurobehavioral Consequences of Closed Head Injury*. Oxford University Press, New York.

Levin, H.S., C.A. Meyers, R.C. Crossman et al. (1981). Ventricular enlargement after closed head injury. *Arch. Neurol. 38*:623–629.

Lindvall, F. (1974). Causes of postconcussional syndrome. *Acta Neurol. Scand. 56* (Suppl.):1–145.

Lishman, W.A. (1978). *Organic Psychiatry*. Blackwell Scientific Publications, London.

Matthews, W.B. (1972). Footballer's migraine. *BMJ 2*:326–327.

McCulloch, J. and P.A.T. Kelly (1983). A functional role for vasoactive intestinal polypeptide in anterior cingulate cortex. *Nature 304*:438–440.

Mealy, J., Jr. (1968). *Pediatric Head Injuries*, pp. 56–57. Charles C. Thomas, Springfield, IL.

Merrett, J.D. and J.R. McDonald (1977). Sequellae of concussion caused by minor head injury. *Lancet 1*:1–4.

Miller, H. (1961). Accident neurosis. *BMJ 1*:919–925, 992–998.

Miller, H. (1968). Post-traumatic headache. In *Handbook of Clinical Neurology*, Vol. 5 (P.J. Vinken and G.W. Bruyn, eds.), pp. 178–184. North-Holland Publishing, Amsterdam.

Milner, B. (1964). Some effects of frontal lobectomy in man. In *The Frontal Granular Cortex and Behavior* (J.M. Warren and K. Akert, eds.), pp. 313–334. McGraw-Hill, New York.

Moskowitz, M.A. (1984). The neurology of vascular head pain. *Ann. Neurol. 16:* 157–168.

Nick, J. and C. Sicard-Nick (1969). Chronic post-tramatic headache. In *Research and Clinical Studies in Headache,* Vol. II (A.P. Friedman, ed.), pp. 115–168. Karger, Basel.

Oppenheimer, D.R. (1968). Microscopic lesions in the brain following head injury. *J. Neurol. Neurosurg. Psychiatry 31:*299–306.

Pawl, R.P. (1977). Headache, cervical spondylosis and anterior cervical fusion. *Surg. Annu. 9:*391–408.

Penfield, W. and N. Norcross (1936). Subdural traction and post-traumatic headache. Study of pathology and therapeusis. *Arch. Neurol. Psychiatry 36:*75–94.

Pernow, B. (1983). Substance P. *Pharmacol. Rev. 35:*85–141.

Pickles, W. (1949). Acute focal edema of the brain in children with head injuries. *N. Engl. J. Med. 240:*92–95.

Prigatano, G., M. Stahl, W. Orr et al. (1982). Sleep and dreaming disturbances in closed head injury patients. *J. Neurol. Neurosurg. Psychiatry 45:*78–80.

Rigler, J. (1879). *Über die Folgen der Verletzungen auf Eisenbahnen, insbesondere der Verletzungen des Ruckenmarks.* G. Reimer, Berlin.

Rimel, R., B. Giordani, J. Barth et al. (1982). Moderate head injury: Completing the clinical spectrum of brain trauma. *Neurosurgery 11:*344–351.

Robinson, R.C. and B. Szetela (1981). Mood change following left hemisphere brain injury. *Ann. Neurol. 9:*447–453.

Russell, W.R. (1933–34). The after-effects of head injury. *Trans. Med. Chir. Soc. Edinb. 113:*129–141.

Saran, A. (1988). Antidepressants not effective in headache associated with minor closed head injury. *Int. J. Psychiatry Med. 18:*75–83.

Simons, D.J. and H.G. Wolff (1946). Studies on headache; mechanisms of chronic post-traumatic headache. *Psychosom. Med. 8:*227–242.

Springer, T.A. (1990). Adhesion receptors of the immune system. *Nature 346:*425–434.

Stevens, J.R. (1982). Neuropathology of schizophrenia. *Arch. Gen. Psychiatry 39:* 1121–1129.

Strich, S.J. (1956). Diffuse degeneration of the cerebral white matter in severe dementia following head injury. *J. Neurol. Neurosurg Psychiatry 19:*163–185.

Strumpell, A. (1888). *Über die traumatische Neurosen.* Gustav Fischer, Berlin.

Stuss, D.T., P. Ely, H. Hugenholtz et al. (1985). Subtle neuropsychological deficits in patients with good recovery after closed head injury. *Neurosurgery 17:*41–47.

Symonds, C.P. (1942). Discussion on differential diagnosis and treatment of post-contusional states. *Proc. Roy. Soc. Med. 35:*601–607.

Symonds, C.P. (1960). Post-traumatic headache. In *Injuries to the Brain and Spinal Cord* (S. Brock, ed.). Cassell, London.

Thomsen, I.V. (1989). Do young patients have worse outcomes after severe blunt head trauma? *Brain Inj. 3:*157–162.

Toglia, J.V., E. Rozenberg, and M. Ronis (1970). Post-traumatic dizziness. *Arch. Otolaryngol. 92:*485–492.

Tonnis, W. (1956). Beobachtungen an frischen gedeckten Hirnschadigungen. In *Das Hirntrauma* (R. Rehwald, ed.), pp. 77–111. Thieme, Stuttgart.

Tyler, S., H. McNelly, and L. Dick (1980). Treatment of post-traumatic headache with amitriptyline. *Headache 20:*213–216.

VanHoutte, P.M. (1989). Endothelin and control of vascular function. *Hypertension 13:* 658–667.

Van Woerkom, T.C.A.M., A.W. Teelken, and J.M. Minderhound (1977). Difference in neurotransmitter metabolism in frontotemporal-lobe contusion and diffuse cerebral contusion. *Lancet 1:*812–813.

Van Zomeren, A.H. and W. van den Burg (1985). Residual complaints of patients two years after severe head injury. *J. Neurol. Neurosurg. Psychiatry 48:*21–28.

Vijayan, N. and P.M. Dreyfus (1975). Post-traumatic dysautonomic cephalalgia. *Arch. Neurol. 32:*649–652.

Ward, A.A. (1966). The physiology of concussion. In *Head Injury Conference Proceedings* (W.F. Caveness and A.E. Walker, eds.), pp. 203–208. J.B. Lippincott, Philadelphia.

Wepfer, J.J. (1727). Observationes medicopracticae de affectibus capitis internis et externis. Observation 10, Schaffhausen.

Yang, Z., Z.H. Yang, V. Richard et al. (1990). Threshold concentrations of endothelin-1 potentiate contractions to norepinephrine and serotonin in human arteries. *Circulation 82:*188–195.

Yoshizumi, M., H. Kurhara, T. Sugiyama et al. (1989). Hemodynamic shear stress stimulates endothelin production by cultured endothelial cells. *Biochem. Biophys. Res. Commun. 161:*859–864.

17

Headache and the Eye

THOMAS J. CARLOW

Headache is commonly localized to the eye and periorbital region. Without obvious ocular pathology, the eye itself is rarely responsible for the pain and discomfort (Berhens, 1978; Cameron, 1976; Carlow and Appenzeller, 1976; Chamlin, 1962; Friedman, 1964; Harris, 1934; Lance, 1973; Newman and Burde, 1979; Worthen, 1980). The main topics discussed in this chapter are the neuroanatomy of eye pain, refractive and muscle imbalance headache, disease of the eye and orbit, referred eye pain, photophobia, and retinal migraine.

NEUROANATOMY OF EYE PAIN

The ophthalmic division of the trigeminal nerve carries afferent pain fibers from the orbit and periorbital region. Painful sensation is carried in this division from the cornea, ciliary body, iris, lacrimal gland, conjunctiva, nasal mucous membrane, eyelid, eyebrow, forehead, and scalp anterior to a coronal plane bisecting the head at the ears. In the cavernous sinus (Feindel et al., 1960; Penfield and McNaughton, 1940; Ray and Wolff, 1940; Whitnall, 1932) the trigeminal nerve branches to innervate the major vessels at the base of the brain, cerebellar tentorium, falx cerebri, and cranial nerves III, IV, and VI. The anterior fossa and sphenoid wing (McNaughton, 1937) are sparsely supplied by a few small ophthalmic nerve branches. The nasociliary nerve separates from the ophthalmic division at the level of the anterior cavernous sinus. After entering the orbit, it divides into multiple long ciliary nerves that course with the optic nerve to the base of the globe, then traverse the eye between the sclera and choroid to supply the ciliary body, iris, and cornea. Two other major ophthalmic branches enter the orbit at the superior orbital fissure. The frontal nerve hugs the orbit roof, then splits into the supratrochlear and supraorbital nerve supplying the forehead near the midline, the upper eyelid, and the superior lateral nose. The lacrimal nerve passes laterally in the orbit to innervate the lacrimal gland and a small area of upper outer eyelid.

REFRACTIVE AND MUSCLE IMBALANCE HEADACHE

Refractive disorders and muscle imbalance have been overemphasized as a source of ocular headache. Despite symptomatic relief achieved with correction of a refractive error or ocular motor imbalance, the etiologic site for "eye strain" (Mitchell, 1876) headache may be quite distant from the eye. Excessive accommodation and/or prolonged sustained extraocular muscle contraction have been formulated as explanations for this headache (Worthen, 1980). Bilateral orbital heaviness with a steady, dull, frontal, bitemporal headache typically manifests when schoolwork or other activity requires prolonged close work. Sleep or simply eye closure commonly relieves this afternoon or evening headache, which is temporally related to sustained eye use. It is never associated with other systemic symptomatology (e.g., nausea or vomiting).

Refractive Disorders

Myopia, hypermetropia, astigmatism, and presbyopia are common refractive errors. Myopia is the only refractive disorder unrelated to "ocular" headache. Hypertropia, astigmatism, and presbyopia can be partially corrected by either excessive accommodation or sustained extraocular muscle contraction, supporting the theories explaining refractive headache. Eckardt et al. (1943) experimentally induced refractive errors, resulting in bilateral periorbital heaviness and occasional frontal and bitemporal or even occipital headache in hyperopia and astigmatism, but not in myopia.

When two retinal images fail to fuse, a marked difference in image size, or aniseikonia, may be responsible, secondary to a pronounced asymmetry in ocular refractive power, or anisometropia. Eye strain headaches have been attributed to aniseikonia and anisometropia, and have been alleviated with refractive lenses designed to equalize the retinal image size disparity. This form of "ocular" headache may be primarily psychogenic.

Strabismus

Strabismus, or muscle imbalance, very rarely produces headache following a prolonged, sustained extraocular muscle effort to maintain monocular vision. Simultaneous contraction of neck and scalp muscles may contribute to the cephalalgia; however, cervical electromyography in tension headache and migraine has not shown a difference between the headache and headache-free states (Pozniak-Patewicz, 1976). Hyperphoria is the only statistically significant muscle imbalance related to ocular headache (Waters, 1970). A full medical and neurologic examination should be performed before prescribing prisms for muscle imbalance headache, particularly for a vertical dissociation, to obviate missing a posterior fossa or orbital lesion.

Convergence Insufficiency

Convergence insufficiency, in contradistinction to other heterophorias, can be responsible for "ocular" headache and is frequently overlooked. Generalized headache maximal in the periorbital region, blurred near vision, and horizontal diplopia with prolonged close work are common complaints. Reading will typically be unimpaired for a short period followed by the preceding symptomatology; complaints resolve with nonconvergent tasks and recur with repeated attempts at close work. Occasionally, an initial presbyopic correction can uncover convergence insufficiency when accommodation relaxes, resulting in an increased need for convergence with any near activity.

Two simple bedside tests are useful (Burian and Van Noorden, 1974). First, determine the point where a fixation target moving toward the nasion blurs or appears double and/or one eye breaks fixation and drifts outward. The distance from this point to the outer orbital rim is the objective near point of convergence (NPC); the normal value is 5 to 10 cm. If the NPC is 20 to 30 cm from the orbital rim, convergence insufficiency can be diagnosed. A second method utilizes a red glass placed before one eye and determines the point where a white fixation light, again moving toward the nasion, splits or is perceived as a red and white light. The distance from this break point to the outer orbital rim is the subjective NPC. The subjective and objective NPC have the same significance.

Orthoptic exercises to strengthen convergence can be beneficial. A fixation target held at arm's length is followed in to the tip of the nose as the arm is flexed and then out again as the arm is extended. This can be combined with jump exercises, in which a near point is fixated alternately with a distant target. These orthoptic exercises should be performed for 5 to 10 minutes, two to three times daily. Base-in prisms in a bilateral bifocal distribution can relieve the ocular symptomatology in patients refractory to orthoptic exercises (e.g., those with Parkinson disease). This subjective discomfort can be ameliorated during periods of extensive near work (e.g., preparation for a college examination) by occluding one eye.

Ocular Neurosis

Headache and "eye strain" beginning abruptly and coincident with any attempt to read or use the eyes, in the presence of a normal ophthalmologic examination, should be considered an ocular neurosis (Derby, 1930). Despite reassurance, these patients are frequently convinced that their symptoms are secondary to their glasses or an ocular muscle weakness. Simple psychotherapy should be instituted; recalcitrant cases may require psychiatric consultation.

DISEASE OF THE EYE AND ORBIT

Conjunctival and Corneal Diseases

Conjunctivitis causes minimal orbital discomfort with diffuse vascular injection and mild photophobia. The conjunctiva contains relatively few pain fibers, which accounts for the marked inflammatory response without severe pain

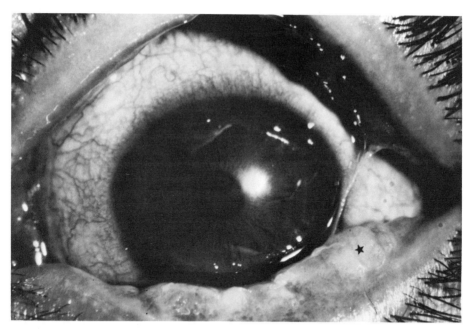

Figure 17–1. Chronic vernal conjunctivitis with an edematous, boggy palpebral conjunctiva (*star*) and diffusely injected bulbar conjunctiva.

(Figure 17–1). Tearing and itching are evident; conjunctivitis can be separated from other causes of a red or injected eye by a normal visual acuity, pupil, and cornea exam. Treatment depends on the underlying etiology.

Severe pain and tenderness will result from either trauma to or a foreign body on or in the cornea. Intense photophobia is combined with diffuse conjunctival injection, lacrimation, and blepharospasm. Corneal edema may cause minimally impaired visual acuity but the pupillary examination will be normal. If untreated, a mild iritis may result, with miosis and anterior chamber inflammation. Once the offending agent has been removed, pain can be relieved with a cycloplegic drug and a pressure patch. Antibiotics should be added under the direction of an ophthalmologist.

Recurrent corneal erosion syndrome can resemble cluster or other forms of episodic headache. It can follow corneal injury or infection, is unilateral involving the forehead and periorbital region, and is associated with marked blepharospasm and photophobia. The pain frequently occurs on awakening or after sustained eye closure. Slit-lamp examination will document a corneal epithelial break. Pressure patching during the period of re-epithelialization can give substantial pain relief.

Iris and Ciliary Body Diseases

Uveitis includes inflammation of the iris, ciliary body and/or choroid. It can be subdivided into anterior uveitis involving the iris (iritis) or ciliary body (cyclitis) or both (iridocyclitis), and posterior uveitis involving the choroid (choroiditis) or retina and choroid (chorioretinitis). Two major types of uveitis, nongranulo-matous and granulomatous, may be distinguished both clinically and pathologi-cally. Anterior uveitis is typically nongranulomatous, can be an autoimmune or collagen vascular disorder, and in the majority of cases has no clear etiology. Granulomatous uveitis is more diffuse, with pathologic signs in the posterior and anterior uvea. Both a slit-lamp examination and indirect ophthalmoscopy are required to identify and localize uveitis. Anterior uveitis or iritis is an impor-tant source of orbital pain. Eye discomfort is moderately severe in the distribu-tion of the trigeminal ophthalmic division. Vision is blurred, with marked photo-phobia, lacrimation, a clear cornea, and a miotic pupil. Marked limbal injection at the corneal and scleral junction is a hallmark of anterior uveitis. The eye is tender, with the periorbital discomfort worse at night and in the early morning hours. Pain may be referred to the ear, teeth, or sinuses. Marked reduction of headache intensity and orbital discomfort can follow the instillation of a mydri-atic. A definitive diagnosis can be elusive, and treatment can include topical or systemic antibiotics and/or steroids.

Glaucoma

Glaucoma is responsible for 15% of all blindness in the United States (Scheie and Albert, 1969). It is clinically useful to classify glaucoma as angle closure, open angle, a combination of angle closure and open angle, and congenital (Kolker and Hetherington, 1970).

Severe ocular pain that spreads to involve the entire head characterizes acute angle-closure glaucoma. Blurred vision and marked photophobia with nausea and vomiting can occasionally be intense enough to suggest laparotomy. Examination reveals a mid-dilated pupil, a steamy edematous cornea (Figure 17–2), and an exquisitely tender eye. Minimal ocular pressure demonstrates a hard, rigid globe and intensifies the ocular and periocular pain. The normal flow of aqueous fluid from the posterior chamber into the anterior chamber, to be absorbed by the trabecular meshwork and canal of Schlemm, is blocked at the angle formed by the iris and the cornea by a forward iris displacement. Intensive miotic therapy, carbonic anhydrase inhibitors, glycerol, and intravenous urea or mannitol can lower intraocular pressure and relieve the headache and eye discomfort. Angle-closure glaucoma can be a surgical emergency and should be referred to an ophthalmic surgeon.

A low-grade, diffuse headache can be present for years before open-angle glaucoma is diagnosed and decreased visual acuity noted. Examination docu-ments a pale optic nerve head, a large, vertically aligned optic cup (Figure 17–3), retinal nerve fiber layer dropout, and a corresponding visual field defect. Intraocular pressures range between 30 and 45 mm Hg, presumably from de-creased trabecular meshwork porosity. Open-angle glaucoma is an urgent oph-thalmologic problem, and should be referred to an ophthalmologist.

Optic Neuritis

Pain with eye movement is encountered in demyelinative optic neuritis, influ-enza, orbital cellulitis, orbital periostitis, and myositis (Roy, 1975). Retro-or-bital pain has been reported in 92% of patients with demyelinative optic neuritis;

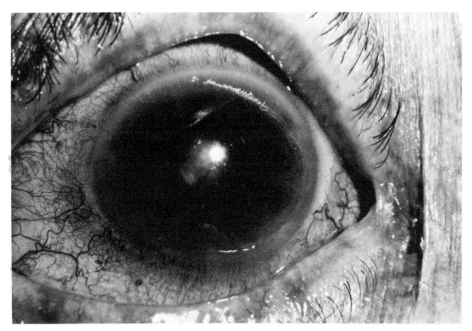

Figure 17–2. Acute angle-closure glaucoma with a mid-dilated fixed pupil, steamy cornea, and diffusely injected bulbar conjunctiva.

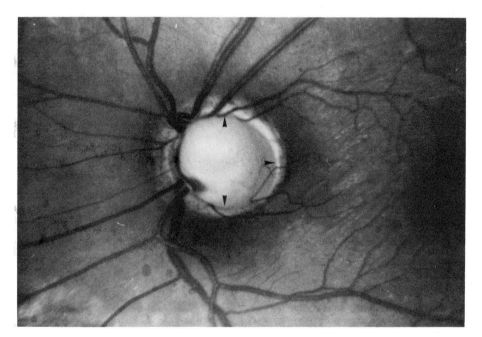

Figure 17–3. Severely cupped (*arrowheads*) glaucomatous optic nerve.

one third will have ocular pain with eye movement (Optic Neuritis Study Group, 1991). Pain commonly commences when the eyes are moved in one direction, and may proceed or follow the onset of visual dysfunction. The eye and periorbital region may be minimally tender to mild pressure. Long ciliary nerve irritation, coursing adjacent to the swollen optic nerve sheath, is one theoretical source for the ocular discomfort. Pain on eye movement has been ascribed to traction of the superior and medial recti origins on the optic nerve sheath, at the orbital apex (Lepore, 1991). Visual loss deteriorates over days to weeks, plateaus for several weeks, and then slowly improves to normal or near-normal visual acuity in 85 to 90% of cases within 6 months (Nikoskelainen and Riekkinen, 1973). The majority of patients with acute demyelinative optic neuritis will have a normal-appearing optic nerve head; 35% will have a papillitis or swollen optic nerve head (Figure 17–4). This entity is clinically indistinguishable from unilateral papilledema without an assessment of visual function. Color vision and brightness comparison will be depressed, and an afferent pupillary defect (Marcus Gunn pupil) will be observed on the involved side. If the ocular discomfort and eye pain are intense, prompt relief can be achieved with a burst of corticosteroids.

A randomized controlled trial comparing intravenous methylprednisolone (1 g/day intravenously for 3 days) followed by oral prednisone (1 mg/kg/day for 11 days) to oral prednisone (1 mg/kg/day for 14 days) and to placebo showed more rapid recovery of visual function in the intravenous methylprednisolone

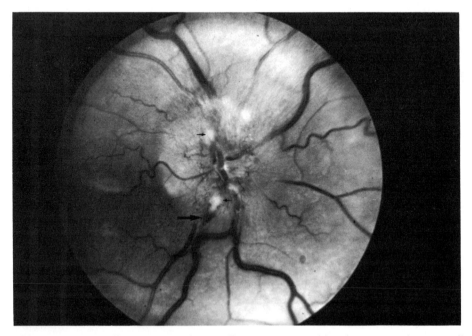

Figure 17–4. Papillitis is seen with a swollen optic nerve, dilated veins, exudates (*small arrows*), and a hemorrhage off the nerve head (*large arrow*).

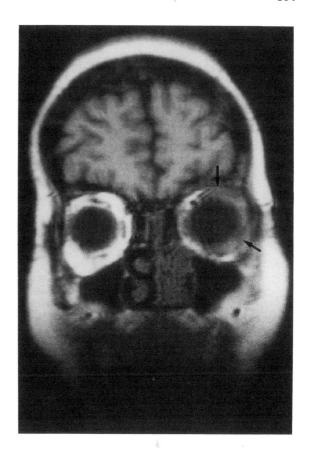

Figure 17–5. Metastatic breast carcinoma encases the left orbit (*arrows*) in a T_1-weighted coronal MRI.

group but no difference between the oral prednisone group and placebo. Vision was slightly better in the intravenous methylprednisolone group after 6 months. Oral prednisone alone was found to be an ineffective treatment and increased the risk of new episodes of optic neuritis (Beck et al., 1992). Optic neuritis secondary to a collagen vascular disorder may require large doses of intravenous methylprednisolone (Dutton et al., 1982).

Orbital Tumor

Primary orbital neoplasms usually are not associated with headache and eye pain. Metastatic orbital tumors (Figure 17–5) and neoplasms (Figure 17–6) that erode or irritate the orbital bony vault (e.g., nasopharyngeal carcinoma) can cause severe frontal head pain when the trigeminal ophthalmic division is compromised.

Orbital Pseudotumor

Orbital pseudotumor is responsible for approximately 10% of all exophthalmos (Henderson and Farrow, 1973; Ingalls, 1953), and is the only orbital lesion that consistently demonstrates both proptosis and orbital pain. This nonspecific

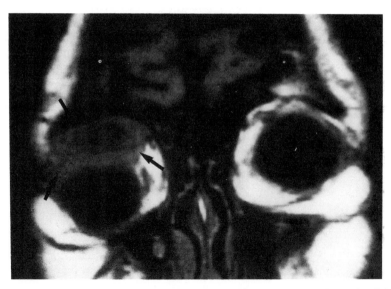

Figure 17–6. Carcinoma of the lacrimal gland (*arrows*) compresses the right globe in a T$_1$-weighted coronal MRI.

inflammatory process will cause abrupt orbital pain, unilateral and sometimes bilateral proptosis, conjunctival chemosis, and ophthalmoplegia with diplopia. Idiopathic orbital pseudotumor may have an elevated erythrocyte sedimentation rate, while all other laboratory studies are normal. A computerized tomography (CT) scan or magnetic resonance imaging (MRI) with contrast can help to separate this orbital process from disorders that mimic it clinically (Figure 17–7). A reactive adjacent sinus inflammation and a swollen, enlarged optic nerve may complicate radiologic interpretation. Dramatic resolution of proptosis, ophthalmoplegia, orbital pain, and visual loss can be seen 24 to 48 hours after initiating high-dose oral corticosteroids. The ophthalmoplegia and resultant diplopia may take weeks to months to finally become asymptomatic. Orbital cellulitis with lid and conjunctival edema, proptosis, and tenderness of the globe on retropulsion can give a similar clinical picture. Fever, prostration, an elevated white blood cell count with an abnormal differential, tenderness over the sinuses, radiographic studies, and an otolaryngologic consultation can help to separate these two entities.

Thyroid Orbitopathy

Thyroid orbitopathy does not cause severe orbital pain; however, patients may complain of relatively intolerable discomfort with eye movement, particularly with upgaze. High-dose corticosteroids can give remarkable pain relief; unfortunately, the pain frequently returns with any attempt to taper or discontinue treatment. Low-dose orbital irradiation, 1,500 to 2,000 rads, can also be beneficial (Palmer et al., 1987). Dysthyroid orbitopathy must always be considered

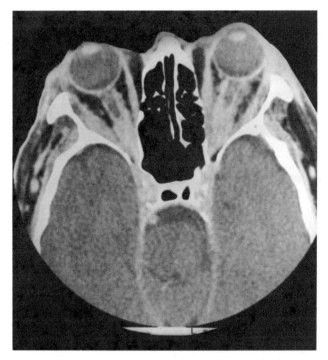

Figure 17–7. Bilateral orbital pseudotumor with enlarged extraocular muscles and swollen optic nerve sheaths.

an urgent medical problem, because optic neuropathy resulting from optic nerve compression at the orbit apex may complicate the clinical course (Figure 17–8).

Orbital Trauma

Orbital pain may follow significant orbital trauma (Sutula and Weiter, 1980) or surgery. Removal of a neuroma formed from the end of a severed nerve can occasionally resolve the ocular discomfort (Folberg et al., 1981; Wolter and Benz, 1964).

Superior Orbital Fissuritis—Tolosa-Hunt Syndrome

Multiple cranial nerves and blood vessels enter the orbit through the superior orbital fissure. Nongranulomatous or granulomatous disease of this bony aperture can result in a severe, boring, retro-orbital pain, with involvement of cranial nerves II through VI. This clinical constellation characterizes a superior orbital fissuritis, or Tolosa-Hunt syndrome (Kline, 1982; Smith and Taxdal, 1966). Retro-orbital pain commonly precedes a third nerve paresis with subsequent involvement of the fourth, fifth, sixth, and second cranial nerves. Pupil sparing is seen in approximately 50% of cases, and 10% show signs of impaired vision (Schatz and Farmer, 1972). Because this syndrome can be produced with tumor, aneurysm, inflammatory disease (e.g., systemic lupus erythematosus), and

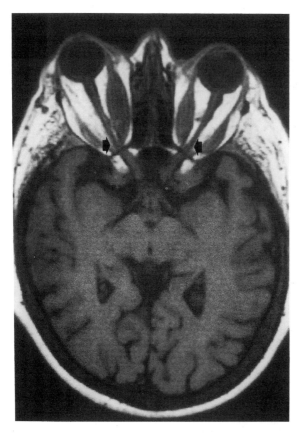

Figure 17–8. Bilateral thyroid orbitopathy can cause visual loss secondary to optic nerve compression from enlarged extraocular muscles (*arrows*) at the orbital apex.

syphilis, a complete laboratory and neuroradiologic evaluation is mandatory. MRI with gadolinium and MRI angiography may prove to be the only studies needed to permit a therapeutic trial of corticosteroids. This boring retro-orbital pain can be totally relieved within 24 hours after starting relatively high-dose oral corticosteroids (e.g., 100 to 120 mg of prednisone). As in orbital pseudotumor, the ophthalmoplegia can require weeks or months to resolve. Without treatment the symptoms can persist for months, only to spontaneously remit and then recur at irregular intervals. The superior orbital fissure syndrome and pseudotumor of the orbit may be a pathologic continuum delineated only by locale.

Herpetic and Postherpetic Trigeminal Neuralgia

Herpetic and postherpetic involvement of the trigeminal ophthalmic division results in a steady, uncomfortable, irritating, temporal and periorbital pain that can precede the herpetic rash by several days. Rash regression requires 2 to 3 weeks, with either total resolution or a postherpetic neuralgia. Corneal infiltrates and an iritis are frequently observed when the rash involves the nose, because the nasociliary nerve supplies both areas. Herpetic trigeminal neuralgia can be differentiated from the nonherpetic form by its steady, sustained, burning, nonstaccatic character. Treatment of the acute and postherpetic rash phases can be extremely discouraging. Levodopa (Kernbaum and Hauchecorne, 1981) begun during the acute phase has decreased pain intensity and the frequency of postherpetic neuralgia. Oral prednisone has been recommended for patients over 60 years of age (Keczkes & Basheer 1980) to reduce the incidence of postherpetic neuralgia. Acyclovir, begun within 72 hours of vesicle development, significantly reduces the incidence and severity of the most common herpes zoster ophthalmicus complications: keratopathy, keratitis, and uveitis. It has no effect on the incidence, duration, or severity of postherpetic neuralgia (Cobo et al., 1986). Postherpetic neuralgia, unfortunately, can be intractable to all current treatments; however, high-dose amitriptyline (Taub, 1973), baclofen (Fromm et al., 1984), narcotics, and a transcutaneous stimulator may be tried.

REFERRED EYE PAIN

Pathologic involvement of structures innervated by the trigeminal ophthalmic nerve in the cavernous sinus (Thomas and Yoss, 1970) and meningeal ophthalmic division branches that supply the cerebellar tentorium, falx cerebri, cribriform plate, and sphenoid wing can cause pain referable to the eye and periorbital region. Detailed discussions of these disorders can be found in the appropriate chapters (e.g., aneurysm, temporal arteritis, cluster headache, ophthalmoplegic migraine, temporomandibular joint syndrome and nasopharyngeal carcinoma).

Isolated Painful Oculomotor Palsy

A supraclinoid aneurysm (Green et al., 1964; Rucker, 1966; Rush and Younge, 1981) is the most common cause of an isolated third nerve palsy or paralysis. Thirty percent of all intracranial aneurysms lie at the junction of the internal carotid and posterior communicating arteries. Fifty percent of these will develop a third nerve paresis, predominantly in women. Retro-orbital pain (Soni, 1974) can precede the third nerve paresis by up to 2 weeks in the trigeminal ophthalmic nerve distribution. When the pupil is dilated and fixed to a *bright* light, a supraclinoid aneurysm at the junction of the internal carotid and posterior communicating artery compressing the third nerve as it enters the posterior aspect of the cavernous sinus must be a primary consideration.

The second most frequent etiology for an isolated third nerve paresis is vascular disease (hypertension or diabetes mellitus). As with a supraclinoid aneurysm, eye pain may antedate the onset of diplopia and the third nerve paresis by days to weeks; however, the pupil is spared (Goldstein and Cogan, 1960; Nadeau and Trobe, 1983). This oculomotor paresis is not dependent on the degree of diabetic or hypertensive control. The diplopia may disappear within weeks or persist for several months. Without definite subjective and objective signs of improvement at 3 months, other etiologies should be considered.

The diagnostic evaluation of an isolated painful oculomotor paresis or paralysis is somewhat controversial, but primarily depends on pupillary involvement. If the pupil is fixed to a *bright* light, a cerebral angiogram (possibly only an MRI or MRI angiogram) is mandatory (Figure 17–9), particularly with evidence of subarachnoid hemorrhage (SAH). If the pupil responds to light, a minimum of two fasting blood sugar determinations, a hypertension work-up and a complete neurologic examination are suggested. Rarely, an internal carotid–posterior communicating artery aneurysm may present without pupillary involvement or SAH, with pupillary dysfunction delayed for a week (Kissel et al., 1983). Close observation with a re-evaluation at 7 days is required. If the oculomotor paresis is not resolved by the third month, or if no evidence for diabetes or hypertension can be documented, a complete clinical and laboratory evaluation should be considered, including complete blood count, sedimentation rate, fluorescent titer antibody test, antinuclear antibody test, thyroid screen, Tensilon test, forced ductions, possible lumbar puncture, CT scan, MRI and/or MRI angiography, and cerebral angiography.

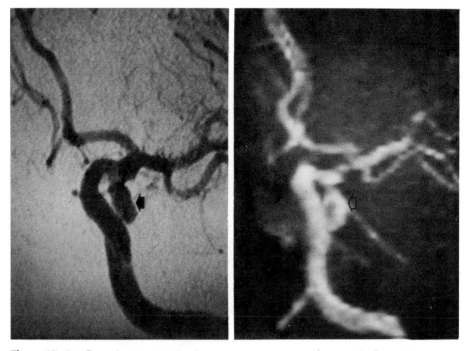

Figure 17–9. Posterior communicating artery aneurysm can be seen in the angiogram on the left (*solid arrow*) and in the MRI angiogram on the right (*open arrow*).

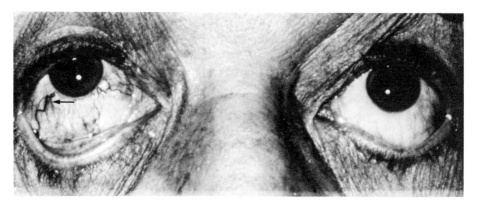

Figure 17–10. Carotid–cavernous fistula can present with dilated bulbar conjunctival vessels (*arrow*).

Carotid–Cavernous Fistula

Carotid–cavernous fistulas may be congenital, atherosclerotic, or traumatic and become manifest when a carotid artery or one of its branches ruptures into the cavernous sinus (Figure 17–10). Ocular bruit, pulsating proptosis, conjunctival chemosis and injection, diplopia, blurred vision, and periorbital pain and headache are all secondary to raised orbital venous pressure. The pain can be moderately severe, constant, boring, and retro-orbital in character. Preservation of visual function and periorbital pain relief may require either a direct surgical or invasive neuroradiologic procedure.

Pituitary Apoplexy

Rarely, spontaneous hemorrhage into a pituitary adenoma (Figure 17–11) can cause severe headache (Friedman et al., 1982), partial or complete ophthalmoplegia, and sudden bilateral blindness. Craniotomy or transsphenoidal decompression combined with corticosteroid replacement can be lifesaving.

Nasopharyngeal Carcinoma

Godtfredsen (1965) found that 25% of nasopharyngeal carcinoma patients present with ocular signs alone, primarily pain or numbness in the first or second trigeminal nerve division. Seventy percent of his entire series had first and second trigeminal division neuralgias, 65% had ophthalmoplegia, 17% had exophthalmos, and 16% had a Horner's syndrome. Otolaryngologic evaluation combined with CT or MRI are mandatory, particularly in a male in his seventh or eighth decade with unexplained chronic periorbital pain.

Vascular Disease

Ocular pain and headache (Andrell, 1943; Currier et al., 1961; Fisher, 1951, 1968) have been documented with internal carotid, middle cerebral, posterior cerebral, and vertebrobasilar artery disease. The pain can be excruciating, pre-

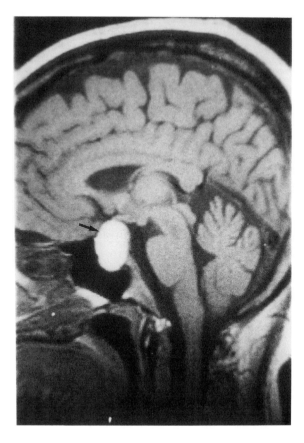

Figure 17–11. Pituitary apoplexy can result from acute hemorrhage into a pituitary adenoma (*arrow*).

cede the stroke, and resolve or persist after stroke completion. Acute or chronic carotid artery obstruction with insufficient collateralization can produce an injected painful globe, corneal edema, cells in the anterior chamber, a mid-dilated pupil, cataract, rubeosis, abnormal intraocular pressure, retinal microaneurysms, neovascularization, and nerve fiber infarcts (Knox, 1969). Acute eye pain has resolved following endarterectomy for high-grade internal carotid artery stenosis (Cohen and McNamara, 1980).

Spontaneous internal carotid artery dissection (Mokri et al., 1979) can result in ipsilateral periorbital head pain at the angle of the jaw and an ipsilateral Horner's syndrome (Figure 17–12). Anticoagulants can prevent further cerebral embarrassment from a subsequent distal thrombosis, and corticosteroids in high doses (Fisher, 1981) can dramatically relieve pain.

Severe orbital and supraorbital pain can occur ipsilateral to infarction in the vertebrobasilar artery distribution. It is usually described as a burning or soreness and can be transient or permanent. Currier et al. (1961) postulated that this orbital pain manifests when the trigeminal descending and the brainstem reticular pathways are simultaneously involved.

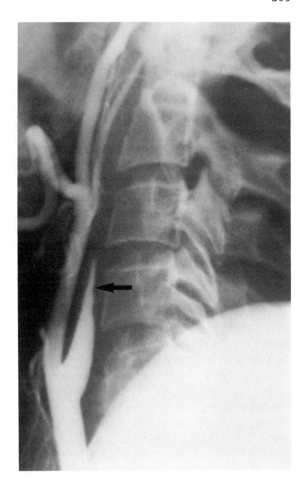

Figure 17–12. Internal carotid artery dissection is seen with a tapered (*arrow*) occluded internal carotid artery.

GREATER OCCIPITAL NEURALGIA

A frequently overlooked cause of isolated periorbital pain is referred pain from an inflammation or compression of the greater occipital nerve as it exits between the occiput and the first cervical vertebra to pierce the large cervical muscle tendinous insertions (Knox and Mustonene, 1975). Pain can begin in the occipital region, radiate over the scalp to the eye, or simply be isolated to the orbit (Bode, 1979; Lieppman, 1980). This periorbital referred pain is believed to be secondary to dysfunction in the descending brainstem trigeminal pathways and greater occipital nerve fiber interconnections. A soft cervical collar worn during sleep to prevent neck extension, hot packs applied at bedtime and on awakening, analgesics, extensive physical therapy, local anesthetic injection at a point halfway between the mastoid and greater occipital protuberance, and surgical avulsion of the nerve have all found advocates.

PHOTOPHOBIA

Photophobia, or intense painful intolerance to light exposure, has not been fully explained, especially without obvious ocular disease (Lebensohn, 1951). With iris irritation or inflammation, a light reflex inducing miosis and iris traction can partially explain local or orbital photophobia. Severe photophobia can be evident in the absence of ocular pathology (e.g., meningitis, SAH, migraine, and retrobulbar optic neuritis), suggesting a combined disturbance at brainstem and cortical levels (Worthen, 1980).

RETINAL MIGRAINE

Migraine is well covered in other chapters in this volume; however, a few comments relative to retinal migraine are made here. It typically implies a rapid, transient loss of vision, usually for less than 30 minutes, accompanied by an ipsilateral headache in a migraineur (Corbett, 1983). Rarely, the visual loss may be permanent. Anterior visual pathway migraine may be a more descriptive definition, because both the ciliary and retinal circulations can be involved. Ischemic optic neuropathy (Katz and Bamford, 1985), central retinal artery occlusion (Katz, 1985), retinal hemorrhage, vitreous hemorrhage, and central serous retinopathy have all been associated with this entity (Hupp et al., 1989). Retinal vascular ischemia has been documented during attacks of anterior visual pathway migraine (Coppeto et al., 1986; Gronvall, 1938; Wolter and Burchfield, 1971). Treatment has not been well defined because a well-controlled study has not been published. Vasoconstrictors should be avoided, excluding ergot-containing drugs. Amyl nitrite, aspirin, calcium channel blockers, isoproterenol, naproxen, nitroglycerin, pentoxifylline, and propranolol have all found advocates (Hupp et al., 1989). Sustained release calcium channel blockers have been particularly effective in my practice. It may be impossible to separate retinal migraine from an embolic source of amaurosis fugax by history alone, because headache may not accompany the visual loss.

SUMMARY

The eye is rarely responsible for headache and periorbital discomfort, if ophthalmic signs are not obvious. Correction of refractive and strabismus disorders seldom relieves headache. Convergency insufficiency is an exception. "Eyestrain" headache, commencing abruptly with any eye use, is commonly an ocular neurosis.

Conjunctivitis and corneal lesions are treatable causes of headache. The recurrent corneal erosion syndrome can mimic cluster and other episodic headache disorders. Anterior uveitis and angle-closure glaucoma are important causes of headache that are best treated by an ophthalmologist. Periorbital pain and tenderness seen with demyelinating optic neuritis is usually transient.

Metastatic orbital tumors can cause ocular pain, whereas primary orbital tumors rarely cause headache. Orbital pseudotumor and the Tolosa-Hunt syndrome are a continuum of the same pathologic process. Both respond to corticosteroids, recur at irregular intervals, and simulate other pathologic processes.

Any structure innervated by the ophthalmic division of the trigeminal nerve can be a source for referred pain. Oculomotor nerve palsy can be preceded by severe orbital and periorbital eye pain, commonly secondary to aneurysm or vascular disease. The pupillary exam usually separates these two entities. Cavernous sinus lesions are frequently responsible for referred eye pain (pituitary apoplexy, carotid–cavernous fistula, and nasopharyngeal carcinoma). Disease of the anterior and posterior cerebral circulation can present with eye pain. Spontaneous internal carotid artery dissection pain can be treated with corticosteroids.

Greater occipital neuralgia (referred cervical pain) is a common treatable cause of ocular and posterior head pain that is not well recognized. Photophobia may have an obvious orbital etiology or be unexplained and have both a central trigeminal and cortical substrate. Retinal migraine implies a rapid monocular loss followed by an ipsilateral headache in a known migraineur and may be confused with other similarly presenting disorders.

REFERENCES

Andrell, P. (1943). Thrombosis of the internal carotid artery: A clinical study of nine cases diagnosed by arteriography. *Acta Med. Scand. 114:*336–372.

Beck, R.W., P.A. Cleary, M.M. Anderson et al. (1992). A randomized controlled trial of corticosteroids in the treatment of acute optic neuritis. *N. Engl. J. Med. 326:* 581–588.

Behrens, M.M. (1978). Headaches associated with disorders of the eye. *Med. Clin. North Am. 62:*507.

Bode, D.D., Jr. (1979). Ocular pain secondary to occipital neuritis. *Ann. Ophthalmol. 11:*589–594.

Burian, H.M. and G.K. Van Noorden (1974). *Binocular Vision and Ocular Motility.* C.V. Mosby, St. Louis.

Cameron, M.E. (1976). Headaches in relation to the eyes. *Med. J. Aust. 1:*292–294.

Carlow, T.J. and O. Appenzeller (1976). Ophthalmic causes of headache. In *Pathogenesis and Treatment of Headache* (O. Appenzeller, ed.), pp. 187–195. Spectrum Publications, New York.

Chamlin, M. (1962). Headache of ocular origin. *Int. J. Neurol. 31:*360–367.

Cobo, L.M., G.N. Foulks, T. Liesegang et al. (1986). Oral acyclovir in the treatment of acute herpes zoster ophthalmicus. *Ophthalmology 93:*763–770.

Cohen, M.M. and M.F. McNamara (1980). Eye pain due to carotid stenosis. *Ann. Ophthalmol. 12:*1056–1057.

Coppeto, R.J., S. Lessell, R. Sciana et al. (1986). Vascular retinopathy in migraine. *Neurology 36:*267–270.

Corbett, J.J. (1983). Neuro-ophthalmic complications of migraine and cluster headaches. *Neurol. Clin. 1(4):*973–995.

Currier, R.D., C.L. Giles, and R.N. DeJong (1961). Some comments on Wallenberg's lateral medullary sydrome. *Neurology 11:*778–791.

Derby, G.S. (1930). Ocular neuroses: An important cause of so-called eyestrain. *JAMA 95:*913–917.

Dutton, J.J., R.N. Burde, and T.G. Klingle (1982). Autoimmune retrobulbar optic neuritis. *Am. J. Ophthalmol. 94:*11–17.

Eckardt, L.B., J.M. McLean, and H. Goodell (1943). Experimental studies on headache: The genesis of pain from the eye. *Proc. Assoc. Res. Nerv. Ment. Dis. 23:*209–227.

Feindel, W., W. Penfield, and F. McNaughton (1960). The tentorial nerves and localization of intracranial pain in man. *Neurology 14:*555–563.

Fisher, C.M. (1951). Occlusion of the internal carotid artery. *Arch. Neurol. Psychiatry 65:*346–377.

Fisher, C.M. (1968). Headache in cerebrovascular disease. In *Handbook of Clinical Neurology,* Vol. 5, (P.J. Vinken and G.W. Bruyn, eds.), pp. 124–156. North-Holland Publishing, Amsterdam.

Fisher, C.M. (1981). The headache and pain of spontaneous carotid dissection. *Headache 22:*60–65.

Folberg, R., V.B. Bernardino, G.L. Aguilar, and G.M. Shannon (1981). Amputation neuroma mistaken for recurrent melanoma in the orbit. *Ophthalmic Surg. 12:*275–278.

Friedman, A.H., R.H. Wilkins, P.D. Kenan et al. (1982). Pituitary adenoma presenting as facial pain: Report of two cases and review of the literature. *Neurosurgery 10:*742–745.

Freidman, A.P. (1964). Reflection on the problem of headache. *JAMA 190:*445–447.

Fromm, G.H., C.F. Terrence, and A.S. Chattha (1984). Baclofen in the treatment of trigeminal neuralgia: Double-blind study and long-term follow-up. *Ann. Neurol. 15:*240–244.

Godtfredsen, E. (1965). Diagnostic and prognostic roles of ophthalmoneurologic signs and symptoms in malignant nasopharyngeal tumors. *Am. J. Ophthalmol. 59:*1063–1069.

Goldstein, J.E. and D.G. Cogan (1960). Diabetic ophthalmoplegia with special reference to the pupil. *Arch. Ophthalmol. 64:*592–600.

Green, W.R., E.R. Hackett, and N.E. Schlezinger (1964). Neuro-ophthalmologic evaluation of oculomotor nerve paralysis. *Arch. Ophthalmol. 72:*154–167.

Gronvall, A. (1938). On changes in the fundus oculi and persistent injuries to the eye in migraine. *Arch. Ophthalmol. 16:*602–611.

Harris, W. (1934). Headaches in relation to ocular conditions. *BMJ 2:*298–299.

Henderson, J.W. and G.M. Farrow (1973). *Orbital Tumors.* W.B. Saunders, Philadelphia.

Hupp, S.L., L.B. Kline, and J.J. Corbett (1989). Visual disturbances of migraine. *Surv. Ophthalmol. 33:*221–236.

Ingalls, R.G. (1953). *Tumors of the Orbit and Allied Pseudotumors.* Charles C Thomas, Springfield, IL.

Katz, B. (1985). Migrainous central retinal artery occlusion. *J. Clin. Neuro-Ophthalmol. 6:*69–71.

Katz, B. and C.R. Bamford (1985). Migrainous ischemic optic neuropathy. *Neurology 35:*112–114.

Keczkes, K. and A.M. Basheer (1980). Do corticosteroids prevent post-herpetic neuralgia? *Br. J. Dermatol. 102:*551–555.

Kernbaum, S. and J. Hauchecorne (1981). Administration of levodopa for relief of herpes zoster pain. *JAMA 246:*132–134.

Kissel, J.T., R.M. Burde, T.G. Klingele, and H.E. Zieger (1983). Pupil-sparing oculomotor palsies with internal carotid posterior communicating artery aneurysms. *Ann. Neurol. 13:*149–154.

Kline, L.B. (1982). The Tolosa-Hunt syndrome. *Surv. Ophthalmol. 27:*79–95.

Knox, D.L. (1969). Ocular aspects of cervical vascular disease. *Surv. Ophthal. 13:* 245–262.

Knox, D.L. and E. Mustonene (1975). Greater occipital neuralgia: An ocular pain syndrome with multiple etiologies. *Trans. Am. Acad. Ophthalmol. Otolaryngol. 79:* 513–519.

Kolker, A.E. and J. Hetherington (1970). *Diagnosis and Therapy of the Glaucomas,* 3rd ed. C.V. Mosby, St. Louis.

Lance, J.W. (1973). *The Mechanism and Management of Headache,* 2nd ed. Butterworth, London.

Lebensohn, J.E. (1951). Photophobia: Mechanism and implications. *Am. J. Ophthalmol. 34:*1294–1300.

Lepore, F.E. (1991). The origin of pain in optic neuritis. *Arch. Neurol. 48:*748–749.

Lieppman, M.E. (1980). Occipital neuralgia: The ophthalmic entity and its treatment. *Ophthalmology 87:*94.

McNaughton, F.L. (1937). The innervation of the intracranial blood vessels and dural sinuses. *Arch. Res. Neuv. Ment. Dis. 8:*178.

Mitchell, S.W. (1876). Headaches from eye strain. *Am. J. Med. Sci. 71:*363–375.

Mokri, B., T. Sundt, and O. Houser (1979). Spontaneous internal carotid dissection, hermicrania, and Horner's syndrome. *Arch. Neurol. 36:*677–680.

Nadeau, S.E. and J.D. Trobe (1983). Pupil-sparing in oculomotor palsy: A brief review. *Ann. Neurol. 13:*143–148.

Newman, S. and R.M. Burde (1979). Headache and the ophthalmologist. *Sight Sav. Rev. 49*(3):99.

Nikoskelainen, E. and P. Riekkinen (1973). Retrospective study of 117 patients with optic neuritis. *Acta Ophthalmol. Scand. 50:*690–718.

Optic Neuritis Study Group (1991). The clinical profile of optic neuritis: Experience of the optic neuritis treatment trial. *Arch. Ophthalmol. 109:*1673–1678.

Palmer, D., P. Greenberg, P. Cornell et al. (1987). Radiation therapy for Graves ophthalmopathy: A retrospective analysis. *Int. J. Radiat. Oncol. Biol. Phys. 13:* 1815–1820.

Penfield, W. and F. McNaughton (1940). Dural headache and innervation of the dura mater. *Arch. Neurol. Psychiatry 44:*43–75.

Pozniak-Patewicz, E. (1976). "Cephalic" spasm of head and neck muscles. *Headache 15:*261–267.

Ray, B.S. and H.G. Wolff (1940). Experimental studies on headache: Pain-sensitive structures in the head and their significance in headache. *Arch. Surg. 41:*813–856.

Roy, F.H. (1975). *Practical Management of Eye Problems: Glaucoma, Strabismus, Visual Fields.* Lea & Febiger, Philadelphia.

Rucker, C.W. (1966). The causes of paralysis of the third, fourth, and sixth cranial nerves. *Am. J. Ophthalmol. 61:*1293–1298.

Rush, J.A. and B.R. Younge (1981). Paralysis of cranial nerves III, IV, and VI. *Arch. Ophthalmol. 99:*76–79.

Schatz, N.J. and P. Farmer (1972). Tolosa-Hunt syndrome. The pathology of painful ophthalmoplegia. In *Neuro-ophthalmology,* Vol. 6 (J.L. Smith, ed.), pp. 102–112. C.V. Mosby, St. Louis.

Scheie, H.G. and D.M. Albert (1969). *Adler's Textbook of Ophthalmology,* 8th ed. W.B. Saunders, Philadelphia.

Smith, J.L. and D.S.R. Taxdal (1966). Painful ophthalmoplegia: The Tolosa-Hunt syndrome. *Am. J. Ophthalmol. 61:*146–147.

Soni, S.R. (1974). Aneurysms of the posterior communicating artery and oculomotor paresis. *J. Neurol. Neurosurg. Psychiatry 37:*475–484.

Sutula, F.C. and J.J. Weiter (1980). Orbital socket pain after injury. *Am. J. Ophthalmol. 90:*692–696.

Taub, A. (1973). Relief of post-herpetic neuralgia with psychotrophic drugs. *J. Neurosurg. 39:*235–239.

Thomas, J.E. and R.E. Yoss (1970). The parasellar syndrome: Problems in determining etiology. *Mayo Clin. Proc. 45:*617–623.

Waters, W.E. (1970). Headache and the eye. *Lancet 2:*1–12.

Whitnall, S.E. (1932). *The Anatomy of the Human Orbit and Accessory Organs of Vision,* 2nd ed. Oxford University Press, New York.

Wolter, J.R. and C.A. Benz (1964). Bilateral amputation neuromas of eye muscles. *Am. J. Ophthalmol. 57:*287–289.

Wolter, J.R. and W.J. Burchfield (1971). Ocular migraine in a young man resulting in unilateral transient blindness and retinal edema. *J. Pediatr. Ophthalmol. 8:* 173–176.

Worthen, D. (1980). The eyes as a source of headache. In *Wolff's Headache and Other Head Pain,* 4th ed. (D.J. Dalessio, ed.), pp. 388–402. Oxford University Press, New York.

18

Radiologic Investigation of Headache

JACK ZYROFF
STANLEY G. SEAT

Because headache may be a symptom of many different diseases, its radiographic investigation traditionally involved all of the neuroradiologic procedures. Such investigations, however, were dramatically altered by computerized tomography (CT), introduced to the medical community by Godfrey N.
Hounsfield in 1973. CT revolutionized neurologic diagnosis through its sensitivity, specificity, and simplicity. Except for the intravenous injection of iodinated
contrast material, with its occasional adverse reactions, CT is a noninvasive
procedure that can be performed on outpatients. Magnetic resonance (MR)
imaging was the next major technical innovation in the practice of neuroradiology. Introduced as a clinical tool in the early 1980s, MR surpassed CT in its
exquisite demonstration of anatomic detail and its superior sensitivity to pathologic alterations. MR is based on the effects of radiofrequency waves on protons
in a magnetic field. Because it is a low-energy technique, it has none of the
biohazards known to be associated with x-rays. Although nuclear magnetic
resonance had been used by chemists for in vitro analysis since 1947, its application to imaging was made possible by computer advances that were a direct by-
product of CT technology.

Skull radiography and conventional tomography, although noninvasive and
low in cost, provide only limited information about the calvarial vault or intracranial calcifications and no direct information about the brain itself. They are
therefore poor screening tools and are relegated to an occasional supplementary
role.

Arteriography, however, continues to play a central role in neurovascular
diagnosis and therapy. Selective arteriography, enhanced by improved cathe-
ters and digital imaging techniques, is essential in confirming and mapping cerebral aneurysms, vascular malformations, and occlusive vascular diseases.
These vascular diseases are often suspected from noninvasive screening tests
such as Doppler sonography, CT, MR, and, more recently, MR angiography.
Arteriography is mandatory for treatment planning, particularly when demonstration of vascular anatomy is of utmost importance. The recent development

of innovative embolization and balloon catheter techniques has made endovascular treatment of these disorders possible, and, in some cases, the treatment of choice (Vinuela et al., 1989).

Other imaging modalities, such as positron emission tomography (PET), magnetic resonance spectroscopy (MRS), and single-photon emission computerized tomography (SPECT), may occasionally contribute to headache evaluation. However, these tools are limited by lack of widespread availability to clinical practitioners.

TUMORS

In patients with intracranial tumors, headache may be an early and prominent symptom. The frequency of headaches appears to be similar in rapidly growing and slowly growing neoplasms. A review of various neoplasms indicates the following incidence of headaches: meningioma (46%), pituitary adenoma (51%), glioblastoma (57%), and metastases (65%) (Heyk, 1968). In patients with nonlocalizing intracranial pressure, 20% had lateralizing supratentorial neoplasms and 10% had midline and intraventricular neoplasms (Huckman et al., 1976).

The chief goals of imaging in brain neoplasia include tumor detection, characterization of tissue type, and specific localization for treatment planning. MR satisfies all of these requirements more completely and accurately than does any other imaging technique. In the cooperative patient without contraindications, MR has become the imaging procedure of choice in those centers where it is available. Because of superior contrast resolution and multiplanar imaging capability, MR is superior to CT in tumor detection. MR demonstrates infiltrative gliomas not apparent or less confidently visualized by CT (Figure 18–1). Tumors of the posterior fossa, which may be concealed by bone artifacts on CT, are clearly displayed by MR (Figure 18–2).

The introduction in recent years of the intravenous paramagnetic contrast agent gadolinium–diethylenetriaminepentaacetic acid (Gd-DTPA) (Magnevist; Berlex Laboratories, Wayne, NJ) has significantly improved MR's sensitivity in tumor detection. This improvement was particularly helpful in extra-axial benign tumors, such as meningiomas and neuromas (Breger et al., 1987; Haughton et al., 1988). Tiny pituitary microadenomas and intracanalicular acoustic neuromas, some as small as 3 mm in diameter, have been visualized with the use of contrast (Stack et al., 1988). Gadolinium has also improved detection of intracranial metastases. Parenchymal metastases only a few millimeters in size are consistently seen (Healy et al., 1987; Sze et al., 1988). Their detection has had a significant impact on patient management (Figure 18–3).

One of the most important contributions of intravenous contrast has been the ability to visualize the meninges. MR with gadolinium is the first imaging technique to reliably demonstrate meningeal pathology. Numerous cases of meningeal involvement from metastases and lymphoma have been described, many of which presented with headache as a primary or sole symptom (Figure 18–4) (Rodesch et al., 1990).

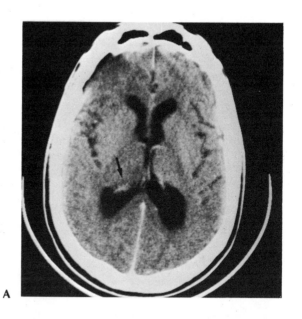

A

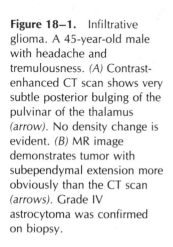

Figure 18–1. Infiltrative glioma. A 45-year-old male with headache and tremulousness. *(A)* Contrast-enhanced CT scan shows very subtle posterior bulging of the pulvinar of the thalamus *(arrow)*. No density change is evident. *(B)* MR image demonstrates tumor with subependymal extension more obviously than the CT scan *(arrows)*. Grade IV astrocytoma was confirmed on biopsy.

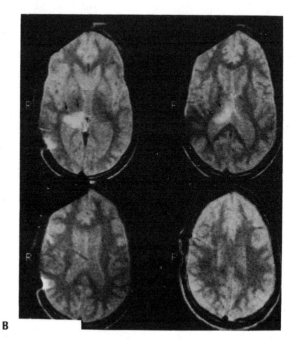

B

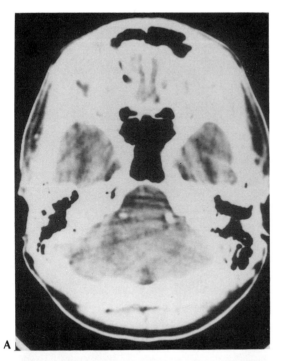

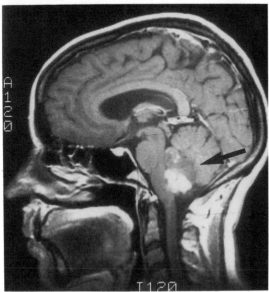

Figure 18–2. Ependymoma of the fourth ventricle in a 36-year-old female with chronic intermittent headaches. *(A)* Contrast-enhanced CT scan shows no abnormality in posterior fossa. Bone artifact limits evaluation of fourth ventricular region. *(B)* Sagittal MR image with intravenous contrast clearly shows a 3-cm mass in the inferior fourth ventricle *(arrow)*. An empendymoblastoma was surgically removed.

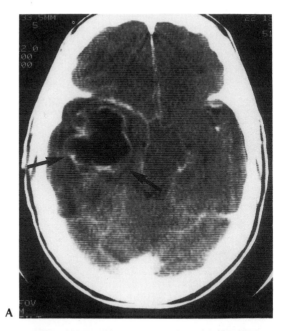

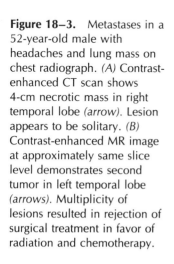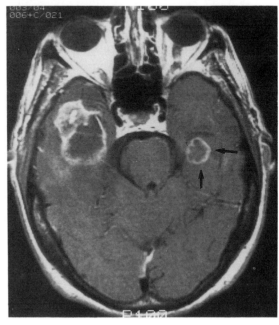

Figure 18–3. Metastases in a 52-year-old male with headaches and lung mass on chest radiograph. *(A)* Contrast-enhanced CT scan shows 4-cm necrotic mass in right temporal lobe *(arrow)*. Lesion appears to be solitary. *(B)* Contrast-enhanced MR image at approximately same slice level demonstrates second tumor in left temporal lobe *(arrows)*. Multiplicity of lesions resulted in rejection of surgical treatment in favor of radiation and chemotherapy.

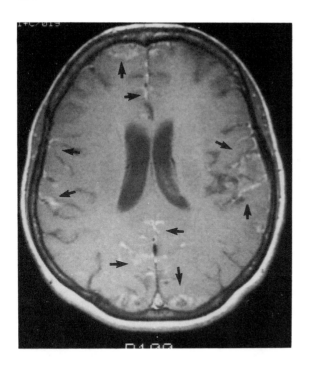

Figure 18–4. Carcinomatous meningitis in a 59-year-old female with known breast carcinoma, headaches, and mental status changes. Contrast-enhanced MR image reveals diffuse enhancement of pia and arachnoid *(arrows)*, compatible with carcinomatosis. Findings confirmed by cerebrospinal fluid cytology.

Contrast has been successful in separating tumor tissue from surrounding edema, a problem in earlier MR imaging. This has been especially important in planning surgery or radiation treatment and in assessing the efficacy of therapy. A close correlation between tumor margins defined on MR and postmortem pathology has been shown (Johnson et al., 1989). Contrast has aided in specificity of diagnosis, especially in separating benign from malignant tumors. However, MR continues to be limited in separating histologic types of malignancy. Location seems to be more important than appearance or signal characteristics in differentiating malignant lesions (Just and Thelen, 1988; Komiyama et al., 1987). Because of sampling errors in biopsy specimens, some believe that MR may be superior to histology in staging gliomas (Dean et al., 1990).

MRS and PET have been used to characterize brain neoplasms. Both techniques are predicated on depiction of metabolic differences between tissue types and have achieved early but limited success in staging neoplasms and predicting survival. PET has been successful in differentiating tumors from radiation necrosis (Patronas et al., 1985). At this time these techniques are confined to large investigational centers and may play a significant role in management of brain tumor patients in the future (Alavi et al., 1988; Glickson, 1989; Heindel et al., 1988).

CT has been reported to have an accuracy rate of over 90% in detecting brain tumors, especially with the use of iodinated contrast material (Christie et al., 1976; Salazar et al., 1981) (Figure 18–5). This makes CT an excellent alternative in situations in which MR is unavailable, contraindicated, or uneconomical.

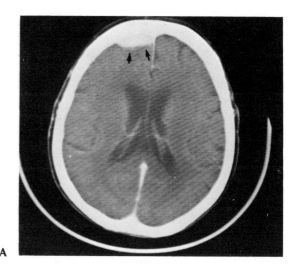

A

Figure 18–5. Meningioma. *(A)* Precontrast CT scan shows no abnormalities. *(B)* Postcontrast CT scan shows homogeneously enhancing mass that has a broad base of attachment to the frontal dura *(arrows)*. Typical appearance of meningioma. The importance of intravenous contrast material in tumor visualization is illustrated.

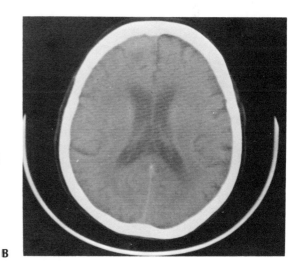

B

INTRACEREBRAL HEMORRHAGE

Subarachnoid and intracerebral hemorrhages are well-known causes of sudden headaches that represent neurologic emergencies. Although the diagnosis is often made by clinical examination or lumbar puncture, the etiology is usually established by radiologic investigation. The potential causes of intracerebral bleeding are numerous, including aneurysm, vascular malformation, tumors, infarction, and bleeding disorders (Figure 18–6).

CT is the preferred imaging procedure in acute hemorrhage because of its high specificity in imaging blood and its rapid imaging time in evaluating acutely ill patients. Although a *localized* intracerebral hematoma or large subarachnoid

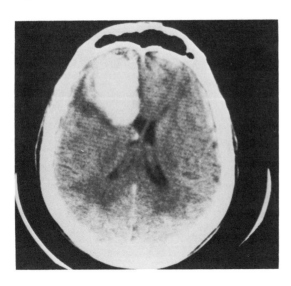

Figure 18–6. Intracerebral hemorrhage in an elderly male with sudden onset of frontal headache. Noncontrast CT scan shows high-density characteristics of acute hemorrhage in the right frontal lobe. Biopsy documented amyloid angiopathy.

hemorrhage is clearly seen by CT, a small bleed in the subarachnoid space may dissipate quickly and not be readily identified. The demonstration of intracranial aneurysms by CT is directly related to the size and location of the aneurysms. Because most aneurysms tend to be located near the skull base and are less than 1 cm in diameter, they may simply be too small to see. The larger aneurysms are usually identified, but may be confused with tumors unless they are clotted, calcified around the rim, or clearly associated with a hematoma. None of these limitations, however, minimizes the role of CT in aneurysm evaluation. The presence of a local intracerebral hematoma is extremely important in localizing the potential bleeding site and in aiding the arteriographer in the search for a bleeding source (Figure 18–7). Areas of ischemia may be identified that suggest severe arterial spasm, a fact that has prognostic implications and may alter angiographic and surgical timing (Davis et al., 1982).

Vascular malformations can often be suspected from their CT or MR appearance alone. A collection of serpentine or linear structures is usually specific enough for diagnosis (Figure 18–8). However, a small arteriovenous malformation (AVM) may be atypical in its CT presentation and simulate a small neoplasm. MR is more specific in these circumstances. Because of their proximity to bone, dural AVMs are infrequently identified by CT or MR unless large or hemorrhagic; angiography is required instead for demonstration (Figure 18–9). Conversely, some "cryptic AVMs," more accurately termed cavernous angiomas, may be seen with CT or MR and not with angiography.

MR has been particularly valuable in vascular disease. Because blood flow produces signal alterations relative to stationary tissue, arterial and venous anatomy can be visualized. AVMs and aneurysms can often be clearly identified and specifically diagnosed. MR angiography is a new methodology that is predicated on MR flow principles. This noninvasive technique is now able to demon-

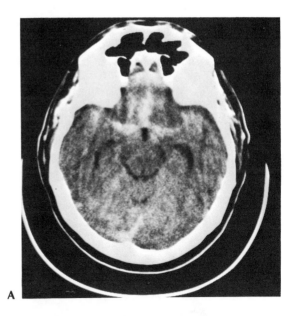

A

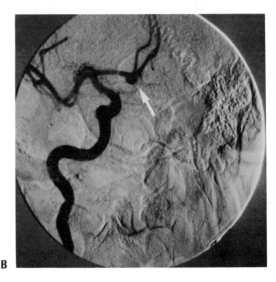

Figure 18–7. Subarachnoid hemorrhage and aneurysm in a 47-year-old male with abrupt onset of headache and photophobia. *(A)* Noncontrast CT scan shows high-density acute bleeding in basal cisterns and interhemispheric fissure. *(B)* Angiogram documents aneurysm of anterior communicating artery on an oblique view of the right **B** carotid artery injection *(arrow)*.

strate aneurysms as small as 3 mm (Masaryk et al., 1989). In the future it is hoped that MR angiography will supersede more conventional invasive angiography (Figure 18–10).

Any candidate for interventional therapy of aneurysms or AVMs requires selective multivessel arteriography for diagnosis and evaluation. No other procedure provides the vascular detail necessary for determining and planning operative or endovascular therapy.

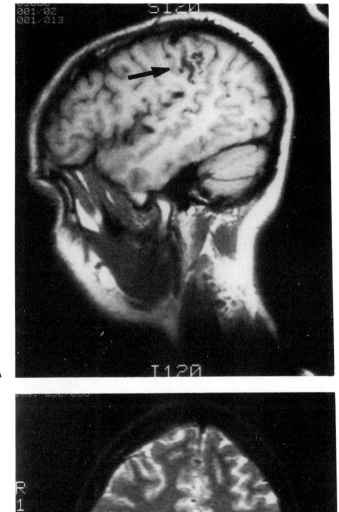

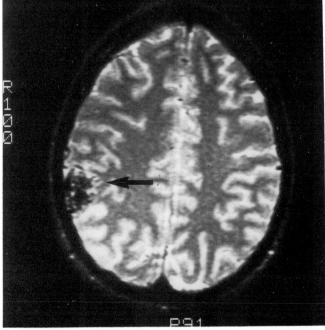

Figure 18–8. Parietal AVM in a 24-year-old female with parietal headaches and seizures. *(A)* Sagittal MR image shows serpentine dilated vessels in right parietal lobe *(arrow)*. *(B)* Axial MR image dramatically demonstrates signal void associated with rapidly flowing blood in AVM vessels *(arrow)*.

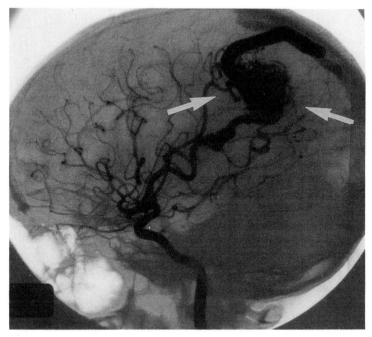

C

Figure 18–8. (C) Arteriography confirms AVM and better demonstrates arterial feeders and large draining veins *(arrows)*, information needed to plan therapy.

Figure 18–9. Carotid–cavernous fistula in a 50-year-old female with headaches and chemosis of right eye. Arteriography shows direct communication between the cavernous carotid artery and the cavernous venous sinus, subsequently treated by balloon occlusion. The cortical venous system fills extensively under arterial pressure. No history of trauma was present. Conventional head CT scan was unrevealing.

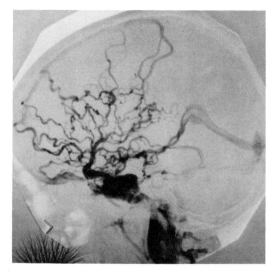

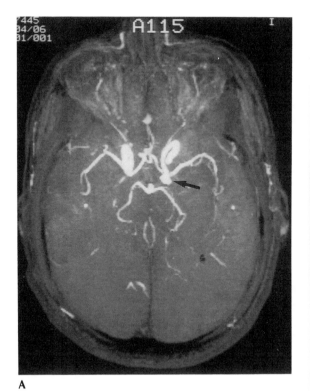

A

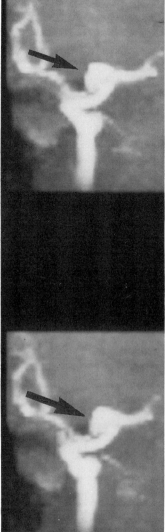

B

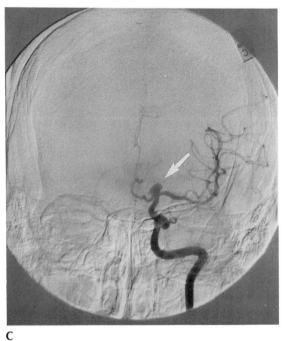

C

Figure 18–10. Carotid artery aneurysm. *(A)* MR angiogram in axial projection demonstrates 8-mm aneurysm at intracranial carotid artery bifurcation on the left *(arrow).* *(B)* Reprojected MR angiogram in sagittal oblique view again demonstrates aneurysm *(arrows).* *(C)* Conventional angiogram findings *(arrow).*

EXTRACEREBRAL HEMORRHAGE

Extracerebral hemorrhage may occur as a sequel to trauma, bleeding disorders, or cerebrospinal fluid hypotension and is often an occult cause for headache, sometimes presenting in the absence of other compelling neurologic findings. Both CT and MR are sensitive and specific in the diagnosis of subdural or epidural hematoma. Because blood composition changes with age, the appearance of hematomas on CT and MR also changes, creating pitfalls and the potential for missed diagnoses. In acute hemorrhage, the CT density of blood is almost always greater than that of normal brain tissue, probably secondary to the high protein concentration of red cells. As clot lysis takes place, the CT density diminishes with time. Careful examination of the ventricular system and white matter for mass effect is mandatory in situations in which the hematoma is isodense to brain on CT (Figure 18–11). In MR, the signal characteristics of clot will vary depending on its age and the imaging sequence utilized. At different times the paramagnetic effects of either deoxyhemoglobin, methemoglobin, or hemosiderin will predominate (Gomori et al., 1985). This can often create a complex and confusing MR picture, particularly when rebleeding results in the simultaneous appearance of all three stages (Figure 18–12).

Because of its coronal imaging capabilities, MR is more sensitive in detecting hematomas in the subtemporal and subfrontal regions. MR is also more sensitive than CT in uncovering parenchymal lacerations from shear injuries (Hesselink et al., 1988). When the content of an extracerebral fluid collection is uncertain by CT, MR can be useful in separating chronic hematoma from hygroma or cysts (Fobben et al., 1989).

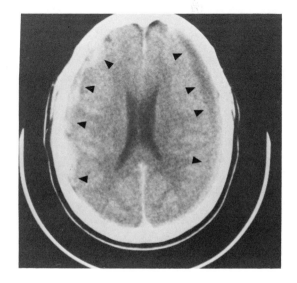

Figure 18–11. Bilateral subdural hematomas. Noncontrast CT scan demonstrates ventricular compression without midline shift. Extracerebral collections are evident bilaterally (*arrowheads*). The density of the hematomas ranges from white to black, depending on their age and stage of clot lysis.

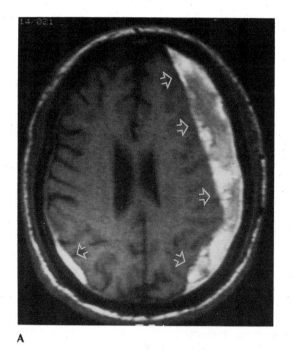

A

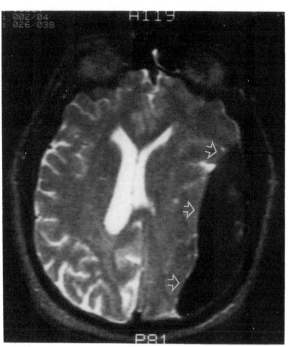

B

Figure 18–12. Subdural hematomas. *(A)* MR axial image with T_1 weighting demonstrates bilateral subdural hematomas that appear white because of methemoglobin *(arrows)*. *(B)* Another patient with acute subdural hematoma appearing black on T_2-weighted MR sequence *(arrows)* because of deoxyhemoglobin.

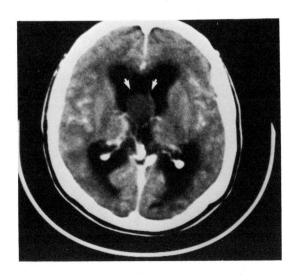

Figure 18–13. Colloid cyst in a 43-year-old female with headache and memory loss. CT scan shows a low-density midline lesion with associated hydrocephalus *(arrows)*. Surgery confirmed a colloid cyst arising from a cavum septum pellucidum with obstruction bilaterally of the foramina of Monro.

OBSTRUCTIVE HYDROCEPHALUS

Headache may follow ventricular obstruction, especially if the obstruction is acute. The diagnosis of hydrocephalus is obvious on either CT or MR. Intravenous contrast material is important in MR and CT for excluding possible causes of obstruction, especially tumors. In addition to malignant neoplasms, many strategically located benign lesions, such as colloid cysts, choroid plexus papillomas, craniopharyngiomas, and paraventricular meningiomas, can produce ventricular obstruction. Headache in these cases may be chronic or positional and unassociated with other neurologic findings. Discovering these lesions is particularly important, because a complete surgical cure is often possible (Figures 18–13, through 18–15). Stenosis of the aqueduct of Sylvius or foramen of Monro can be partial and intermittent, often presenting in adult life with intermittent headaches. Relative ventricular size can aid in pinpointing the site of ventricular obstruction. MR affords the advantage of direct sagittal and coronal imaging, which reproducibly demonstrates the foramina of Monro, the aqueduct of Sylvius, and the inferior fourth ventricle, all common sites of obstruction not easily seen on CT (El Gammal et al., 1987) (Figure 18–16).

INFLAMMATORY DISEASE

Until very recently, meningitis and encephalitis could not be reliably imaged. Diagnosis could only be made by lumbar puncture and clinical examination. This changed dramatically with the advent of intravenous MR contrast agents. Because injected chelated gadolinium will localize to any hyperemic tissue, early inflammation of dura, arachnoid, or pial membranes can be discriminated

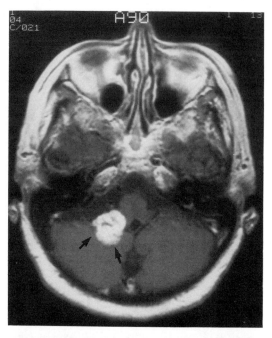

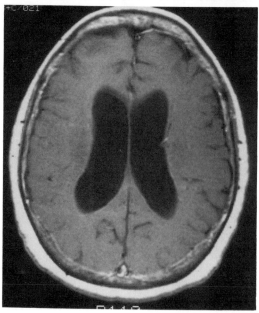

Figure 18–14. Choroid plexus papilloma in a 66-year-old female with frontal headache and loss of balance. *(A)* MR image with intravenous contrast shows a 2-cm enhancing mass in foramen of Luschka *(arrows)*. *(B)* Higher section demonstrates hydrocephalus, thought to be the result of overproduction of cerebrospinal fluid by neoplasm. A choroid plexus papilloma was found at surgery.

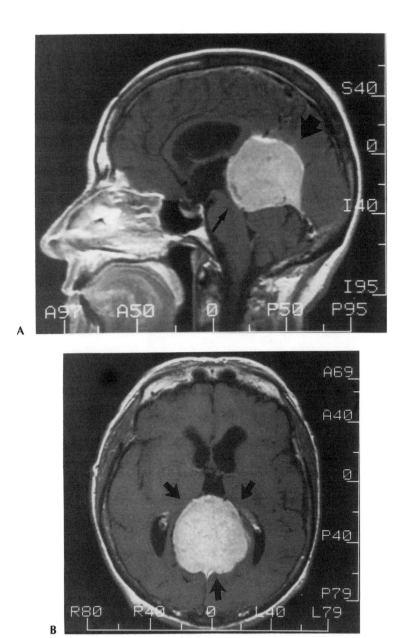

Figure 18–15. Tentorial meningioma in a 67-year-old female with occipital head pain and recent gait disturbance. Sagittal *(A)* and coronal *(B)* MR images with intravenous contrast show a 5-cm mass arising from the tentorium and posterior falx *(large arrows)*. Hydrocephalus is present secondary to aqueductal obstruction *(small arrow)*. A meningioma was successfully removed at surgery.

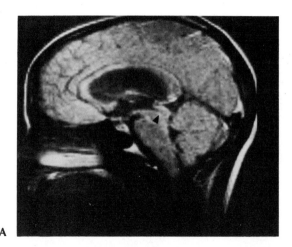

A

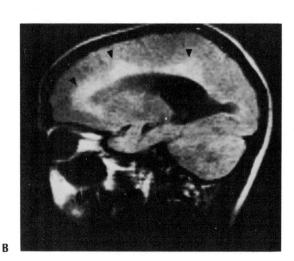

B

Figure 18–16. Aqueductal stenosis in a middle-aged female with a long-standing history of intermittent headaches. *(A)* Sagittal MR image best demonstrates narrowing of the aqueduct of Sylvius *(arrowhead)* with enlargement of the third and lateral ventricles. *(B)* A more lateral MR image shows periventricular high signal areas, suspicious for transependymal CSF migration *(arrowheads).*

from surrounding tissue (Figure 18–17). Granulomatous meningitides are particularly noteworthy because they tend to be localized, rather than disseminated, thereby posing difficult clinical diagnostic dilemmas. Recently, however, the diagnoses of fungal and tuberculous meningitides have been made when compelling MR findings warranted surgical biopsy, even in the presence of unimpressive or nondiagnostic cerebrospinal fluid findings. Early intervention should reduce the high mortality of these diseases (Desai et al., 1991).

Encephalitis is far more sensitively imaged by MR than by CT. Herpes simplex encephalitis is virtually always positive on MR scans within the first 48 hours of infection (Schroth et al., 1987) (Figure 18–18). The numerous infectious encephalitides seen as a complication of AIDS have all been demonstrated by MR, with the single exception of HIV encephalitis (Balakrishnan et al., 1990) (Figure 18–19). The secondary complications of central nervous system infections include venous sinus thrombosis, vasculitis, mycotic aneurysms, infarc-

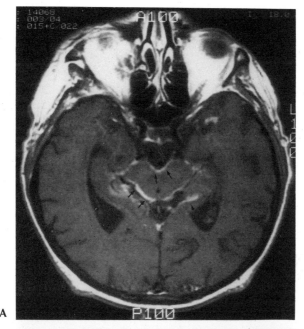

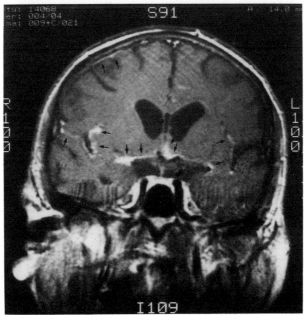

Figure 18–17. Coccidioidomycosis meningitis. Axial *(A)* and coronal *(B)* MR images with intravenous contrast show enhancement of the pia–arachnoid in the basal cisterns, Sylvian fissure, and convexity *(arrows)*, suggesting meningeal inflammation. The diagnosis of coccidioidomycosis was established by cerebrospinal fluid studies.

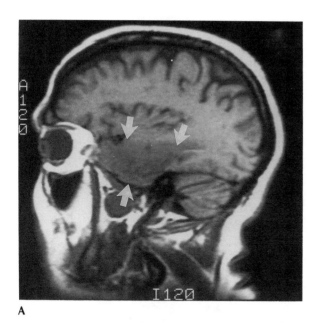

A

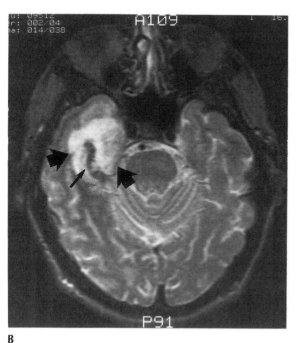

Figure 18–18. Herpes
encephalitis in a 61-year-old
male with headache, fever,
and obtundation. *(A)* Sagittal
MR image shows swelling of
the temporal lobe and low
signal changes suggesting
edema *(arrows)*. *(B)* Axial
T₂-weighted sequence
confirms edema *(large black
arrows)* and also demonstrates
a darker region, suggestive of
hemorrhage *(small black
arrow)*. Open brain biopsy
established the diagnosis of
herpes encephalitis. The rapid
diagnosis and initiation of
therapy resulted in a favorable
outcome.

B

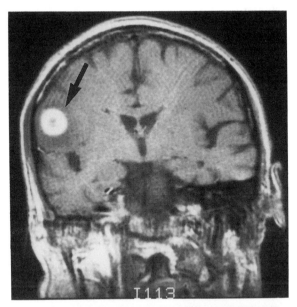

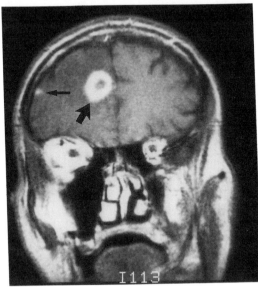

Figure 18–19. Toxoplasmosis in a 49-year-old HIV-positive male with fever and headaches. Coronal MR images with intravenous contrast show multiple enhancing "donut lesions" (*arrows*), typical of toxoplasmosis.

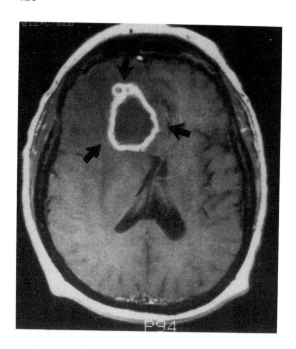

Figure 18–20. Frontal abscess in a 71-year-old female on immunosuppressive chemotherapy for leukemia, presenting with headache and slurred speech. Axial MR image with intravenous contrast shows 3-cm necrotic mass in left frontal lobe *(arrows)* surrounded by edema. A pyogenic abscess secondary to staphylococcus was surgically removed.

tion, and hydrocephalus. MR is important in determining or establishing the suspicion of these sequelae. Often arteriography or MRA will be necessary for definitive diagnosis.

Cerebral abscesses have been diagnosed earlier since the advent of CT and MR, and are now frequently seen during the cerebritis phase. Their response to antibiotic therapy can be easily followed. The appearance of abscesses in different phases of evolution can be characterized to provide greater precision in the timing of surgical intervention (Figure 18–20).

MISCELLANEOUS HEAD AND FACE PAIN

Because headache is such a nonspecific symptom, the yield of radiologic investigation in patients with headache alone is expectedly low in the absence of neurologic symptoms (Morrill et al., 1990). Studies have found a less than 1% incidence of abnormal CT scans in patients with chronic headache in the absence of other neurologic findings (Baker, 1983). The presence of an abnormal electroencephalogram increases the yield significantly. In one study, the surgical removal of lesions considered to be the probable cause for "chronic recurrent headache" produced no relief following surgery. This led investigators to conclude that the lesions were probably unrelated to the patients' headaches and evidently represented incidental findings (Weisberg, 1982). Routine necropsy studies have shown a high incidence of asymptomatic pituitary adenomas and meningiomas (Weisberg, 1975; Wood et al., 1957) (Figure 18–21).

Benign intracranial hypertension, also known as pseudotumor cerebri, presents with headache and papilledema. Scan findings in these patients are usually nonspecific but occasionally demonstrate small ventricles, cisterns, and sulci. Because of anatomic variability, the significance of these findings is made more apparent when sequential scans demonstrate a change. The primary purpose of radiographic investigation in these patients is to exclude a mass lesion (Silbergleit et al., 1989).

Patients with uncomplicated migraine are rarely investigated radiologically. Of 200 patients with the clinical diagnosis of migraine who underwent CT, only two clinically unsuspected lesions were detected in the occipital lobe—a glioma and an angioma; four other patients showed evidence of ischemia in the occipital cortex (Weisberg et al., 1984). Recent MR studies have demonstrated multifocal white matter lesions in between 25 and 50% of migraine patients, a nonspecific finding usually ascribed to axonal demyelination from microangiopathic ischemia (Kuhn and Shekar, 1990). Arteriography performed during acute migraine attacks has shown arterial spasm (Figures 18–22 and

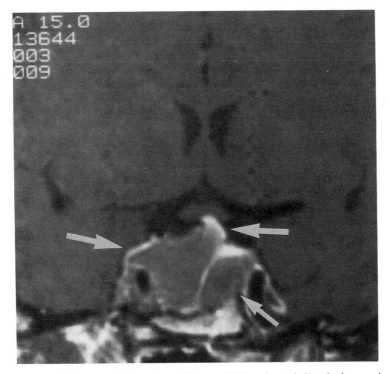

Figure 18–21. Pituitary adenoma in a 42-year-old female with headaches and normal endocrine function. Coronal MR image with intravenous contrast shows large pituitary adenoma with suprasellar extension, chiasm encroachment, and cavernous sinus invasion (arrows).

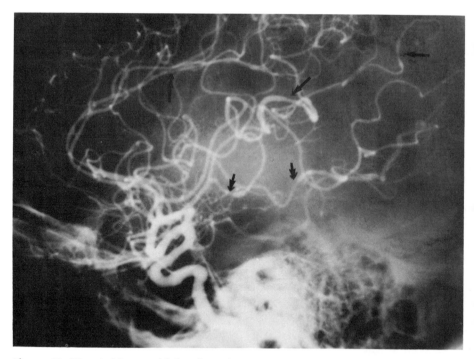

Figure 18–22. A 35-year-old female with migrainous headaches. Arteriogram during acute attack of migraine shows multiple areas of segmental arterial narrowing, compatible with vasospasm *(arrows)*. A similar appearance can be seen with vasculitis. The patient was not restudied to document reversibility.

18–23). Cerebral blood flow studies performed on migraineurs using xenon or SPECT have confirmed localized perfusion aberrations during and between attacks (Strickland, 1990). Infarcts and hemorrhages have been reported as a rare complication of migraine, documented by both CT and MR. When migraine is associated with neurologic deficits, MR is most sensitive in excluding unsuspected surgical lesions such as aneurysms or vascular malformations.

Patients with cluster headaches, temporal arteritis, or trigeminal neuralgia do not merit radiologic investigation unless atypical neurologic features are present. Atypical trigeminal neuralgia has been reported with posterior fossa and middle fossa tumors, aneurysms, and vascular malformations (Dandy, 1934) (Figures 18–24 and 18–25). MR imaging has also demonstrated multiple sclerosis plaques at the trigeminal root entry zone (Hutchins et al., 1990). Because only MR is capable of demonstrating both vascular and cranial nerve detail simultaneously, recent studies have been able to depict fifth nerve compression by ectatic and redundant arteries in the cerebellopontine angle. This encouraging anatomic information should be helpful to surgeons planning posterior fossa decompression procedures for trigeminal neuralgia or other cranial neuropathies (Tash et al., 1989).

Diseases of the paranasal sinuses, skull base, temporomandibular joints,

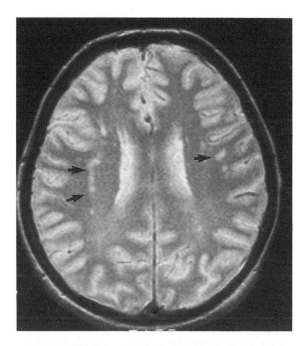

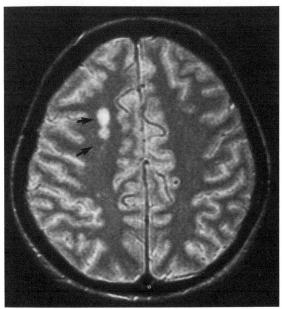

Figure 18–23. Migraine with aura in a 48-year-old female. Axial T$_2$-weighted images show multiple "bright" foci in the white matter, a nonspecific finding described in some migraine patients.

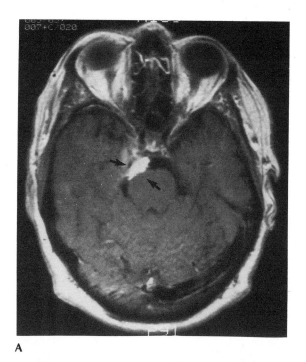

A

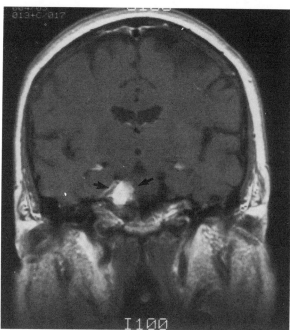

B

Figure 18–24. Petroclival meningioma in a 61-year-old female with atypical trigeminal neuralgia on the right. Axial *(A)* and coronal *(B)* MR images with intravenous contrast show an enhancing mass in the right prepontine and trigeminal cisterns *(arrows)*. The trigeminal nerve and ganglion were found to be compressed by a meningioma at surgery.

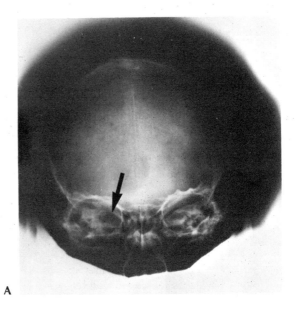

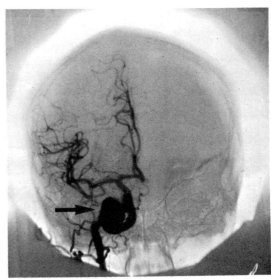

Figure 18–25. Aneurysm of the petrous carotid artery in a 73-year-old female with a 4-year history of facial pain. *(A)* Skull radiograph (anteroposterior view) shows erosion of the right petrous apex *(arrow)*. *(B)* Angiogram shows a large aneurysm arising from the petrous segment of the right internal carotid artery *(arrow)*.

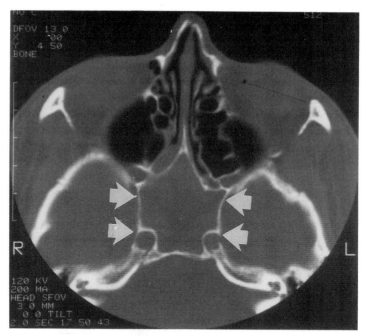

Figure 18–26. Sphenoid sinusitis in a 27-year-old female with head and eye pain. CT scan shows opacification of the sphenoid sinus compatible with sinusitis *(arrows)*. The other sinuses were clear. Plain sinus radiographs were normal. Treatment for sinusitis resulted in complete relief of symptoms.

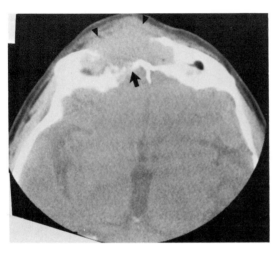

Figure 18–27. Carcinoma of the frontal sinus in an 83-year-old male with frontal head pain and a history of chronic polypoid sinusitis. CT scan best demonstrated a mass in the frontal sinus with destruction of the sinus walls *(arrow, arrowheads)*. The histologic diagnosis was squamous cell carcinoma.

and cervical spine occasionally present with headache or facial pain. Although conventional sinus radiographs are often used to screen for sinus disease, CT is far more accurate in visualization of sphenoid and ethmoid disease, which may cause occult headache (Figure 18–26). Limited sinus CT can currently be performed quickly and inexpensively and is increasingly preferred as a screening tool (Kennedy and Loury, 1988) (Figures 18–27 and 18–28). MR imaging in the sagittal plane is the best method for evaluating the upper cervical spine and temporomandibular joints, often sites of referred head pain (Figure 18–29). Both CT and MR have proven useful in discovering and staging tumors of the

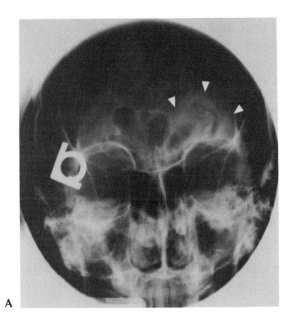

A

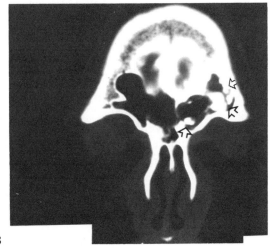

Figure 18–28. Frontal osteomyelitis. *(A)* Sinus radiograph (Caldwell view) shows sclerosis and poor delineation of the frontal sinus wall *(arrowheads).* A bony density is identified within the sinus. *(B)* CT scan in coronal view shows sinus wall erosion with multiple sequestered bony fragments within the sinus *(arrows),* compatible with chronic osteomyelitis.

B

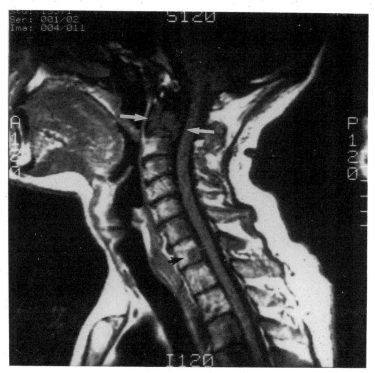

Figure 18–29. Cervical spine metastases in a 69-year-old male with severe occipital headaches. Sagittal MR of the cervical spine shows complete destruction and marrow replacement of the dens *(white arrows)*, with encroachment on the spinal cord. Additional lesions can also be seen in other cervical vertebrae *(black arrow)*. The diagnosis of metastatic prostate carcinoma was established.

nasopharynx and parapharyngeal spaces and in demonstrating bone destruction of the skull base (Schellhas, 1988) (Figures 18–30 and 18–31).

SUMMARY

Many organic causes of head pain can be diagnosed or excluded by radiographic procedures. MR imaging and CT have dramatically altered neurologic diagnosis, having largely replaced more invasive and less accurate procedures. With the few exceptions noted, all other radiographic procedures have been confirmatory or additive in diagnosing intracranial disease. CT and MR have also facilitated patient therapy and management, provided earlier diagnoses, and contributed to reduced hospital costs. Imaging technology continues to expand so rapidly that close cooperation between clinician and neuroradiologist is mandatory to ensure that each patient receives the proper procedures in the proper sequence.

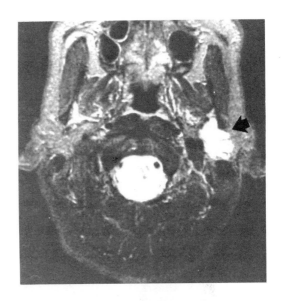

Figure 18–30. Parotid tumor in a 33-year-old male with atypical left facial and temporal pain. MR image shows an enlargement of the deep lobe of the parotid gland with increased signal intensity compatible with tumor *(arrow)*.

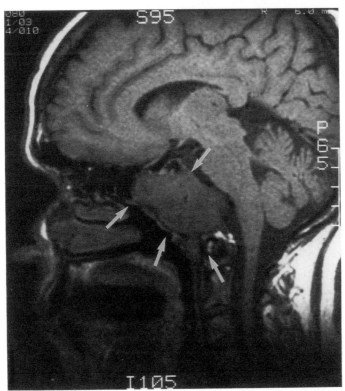

Figure 18–31. Metastasis to the skull base in a 64-year-old female with breast carcinoma and retro-orbital head pain. Sagittal MR image shows a 5-cm mass at the skull base, destroying the basisphenoid and clivus *(arrows)*. Biopsy confirmed a metastasis.

REFERENCES

Alavi, J.B., A. Alavi, J. Chambers et al. (1988). Predicting survival in glioma patients. *Cancer 62:*1074–1078.

Baker, H.L., Jr. (1983). Cranial CT in the investigation of headache: Cost-effectiveness for brain tumors. *J. Neuroradiol. 10:*112–116.

Balakrishnan, J., P.S. Becker, A.J. Kumar et al. (1990). Acquired immunodeficiency syndrome: Correlation of radiologic and pathologic findings in the brain. *Radiographics 10:*201–215.

Breger, R.K., R.A. Papke, K.W. Pojunas et al. (1987). Benign extraaxial tumors: Contrast enhancement with Gd-DTPA. *Radiology 163:*427–429.

Christie, J.H., M. Hirofumi, T.G. Raymundo et al. (1976). Computed tomography and radionuclide studies in the diagnosis of intracranial disease. *Am. J. Roentgenol. 127:*171–174.

Dandy, W.E. (1934). Concerning the cause of trigeminal neuralgia. *Am. J. Surg. 24:*447.

Davis, K.R., J.P. Kistler, R.C. Heros et al. (1982). Neuroradiologic approach to the patient with a diagnosis of subarachnoid hemorrhage. *Radiol. Clin. North Am. 20:*87.

Dean, B.L., B.P. Drayer, C.R. Bird et al. (1990). Gliomas: Classification with MR imaging. *Radiology 174:*411–415.

Desai, S.P., C. Bazan III, W. Hummell et al. (1991). Disseminated CNS histoplasmosis. *AJNR Am. J. Neuroradiol. 12:*290–292.

El Gammal, T.E., M.B. Allen, and B.S. Brooks (1987). MR evaluation of hydrocephalus. *AJNR Am. J. Neuroradiol. 8:*591–597.

Fobben, E.S., R.I. Grossman, S.W. Atlas et al. (1989). MR characteristics of subdural hematomas and hygromas at 1.5 T. *AJNR Am. J. Neuroradiol. 10:*687.

Glickson, J.D. (1989). Clinical NMR spectroscopy of tumors: Current status and future directions. *Invest. Radiol. 24:*1011–1016.

Gomori, J.M., R.I. Grossman, H.I. Goldberg et al. (1985). Intracranial hematomas: Imaging by high-field MR. *Radiology 157:*87–93.

Haughton, V.M., A.A. Rimm, L.F. Czervionke et al. (1988). Sensitivity of Gd-DTPA-enhanced MR imaging of benign extraaxial tumors. *Radiology 166:*829–833.

Healy, M.E., J.R. Hesselink, G.A. Press et al. (1987). Increased detection of intracranial metastases using intravenous gadolinium-DTPA. *Radiology 165:*619–624.

Heindel, W., J. Bunke, S. Glathe et al. (1988). Combined ^{1}H-MR imaging and localized ^{31}P-spectroscopy of intracranial tumors in 43 patients. *J. Comput. Assist. Tomogr. 12:*907–916.

Hesselink, J.R., C.F. Dowd, and M.E. Healy (1988). MR imaging of brain contusions: A comparative study with CT. *AJNR Am. J. Neuroradiol. 9:*269–278.

Heyk, H. (1968). Examination and differential diagnosis of headache. In *Handbook of Neurology,* Vol. 5 (P.J. Vinken and G.W. Bruyn, eds.), p. 2536. North-Holland Publishing, Amsterdam.

Hounsfield, G.N. (1973). Computerized transverse axial scanning (tomography); Part I. Description of system. *Br. J. Radiol. 46:*1016–1022.

Huckman, M.S., J.S. Fox, and R.G. Ramsey (1976). Computed tomography in the diagnosis of pseudotumor cerebri. *Radiology 119:*593.

Hutchins, L.G., H.R. Harnsberger, J.M. Jacobs et al. (1990). Trigeminal neuralgia (tic douloureux): MR imaging assessment. *Radiology 175:*837–841.

Johnson, P.C., S.J. Hunt, and B.P. Drayer (1989). Human cerebral gliomas: Correlation of post mortem MR imaging and neuropathologic findings. *Radiology 170:* 211–217.

Just, M. and M. Thelen (1988). Tissue characterization with T1, T2 and proton density values: Results in 160 patients with brain tumors. *Radiology 169:*779–785.

Kennedy, D.W. and M.C. Loury (1988). Nasal and sinus pain: Current diagnosis and treatment. *Semin. Neurol. 8:*303–314.

Komiyama, M., H. Yagura, M. Baba et al. (1987). MR imaging: The possibility of tissue characterization of brain tumors using T1 and T2 values. *AJNR Am. J. Neuroradiol. 8:*65–70.

Kuhn, M.J. and P.C. Shekar (1990). A comparative study of magnetic resonance imaging and computed tomography in the evaluation of migraine. *Comput. Med. Imaging Graph. 14:*149–152.

Masaryk, T.J., M.T. Modic, J.S. Russ et al. (1989). Intracranial circulation: Preliminary clinical results with three-dimensional (volume) MR angiography. *Radiology 17:* 793.

Morrill, B., E.B. Blanchard, K.D. Barron et al. (1990). Neurologic evaluation of chronic headache patients: Is laboratory testing always necessary? *Biofeedback Self Regul. 15:*27–35.

Patronas, N.J., G. DiChiro, C. Kuft et al. (1985). Predictions of survival in glioma patients by means of positron emission tomography. *J. Neurosurg. 62:*816.

Rodesch, G., P. VanBogaert, N. Mavroudakis et al. (1990). Neuroradiologic findings in leptomeningeal carcinomatosis: The value interest of gadolinium-enhanced MRI. *Neuroradiology 32:*26–32.

Salazar, O.M., P. Van Houtte, W.M. Plassche, Jr. et al. (1981). The role of computed tomography in the diagnosis and management of brain tumors. *Comput. Tomogr. 5:*256–267.

Schellhas, K.P. (1988). Medical imaging in the evaluation of facial pain. *Semin. Neurol. 8:*265–271.

Schroth, G., K. Kretzschmer, J. Gawehn et al. (1987). Advantages of magnetic resonance imaging in the diagnosis of cerebral infections. *Neuroradiology 29:*120–126.

Silbergleit, R., L. Junck, S. Gebarsky et al. (1989). Idiopathic intracranial hypertension (pseudotumor cerebri): MR imaging. *Radiology 170:*207–209.

Stack, J.P., R.T. Ramsden, N.M. Antoun et al. (1988). Magnetic resonance imaging of acoustic neuromas: The role of gadolinium-DTPA. *Br. J. Radiol. 61:*800–805.

Strickland, N.H. (1990). Mechanisms of classical migraine: New insights from radiology. *Br. J. Hosp. Med. 43:*282–286.

Sze, G., J. Shin, G. Krol et al. (1988). Intraparenchymal brain metastases: MR imaging versus contrast-enhanced CT. *Radiology 168:*187–194.

Tash, R.R., G. Sze, and D.R. Leslie (1989). Trigeminal neuralgia: MR imaging features. *Radiology 172:*767–770.

Vinuela, F., J. Dion, P. Lylyk et al. (1989). Update on interventional neuroradiology. *Am. J. Roentgenol. 153:*23–33.

Weisberg, L.A. (1975). Asymptomatic enlargement of the sella turcica. *Arch. Neurol. 33:*483.

Weisberg, L.A. (1982). Incidental CT findings. *J. Neurol. Neurosurg. Psychiatry 45:* 715.

Weisberg, L.L., C. Nice, and M. Katz (1984). Head and face pain. In *Cerebral Computed Tomography: A Text-Atlas,* 2nd ed., p. 279. W.B. Saunders, Philadelphia.

Wood, M.W., R.J. White, and J.W. Kernchan (1957). One hundred intracranial meningiomas found incidentally at necropsy. *Neuropathol. Exp. Neurol. 16:*337.

19

Headache Associated with Abnormalities in Intracranial Structure or Pressure

STEPHEN D. SILBERSTEIN
JOHN MARCELIS

Headache is the most common clinical manifestation of altered intracranial pressure. However, most headaches are not caused by an abnormality of intracranial structure or pressure. Clinical syndromes associated with these disorders include post–lumbar puncture headache, spontaneous intracranial hypotension, brain tumor, idiopathic intracranial hypertension, hydrocephalus, intracranial hemorrhage, and subdural hematoma. Disruption of cerebrospinal fluid (CSF) production, flow, or absorption may lead to alterations in intracranial pressure and thus to headache. Mass lesions can produce traction on pain-sensitive intracranial structures, impede CSF flow, or directly increase pressure by mass effect, all of which can produce headache. Each disorder may produce unique symptoms that have diagnostic value. Intracranial hypotension is characterized by orthostatic headache. Intracranial hypertension frequently has an associated headache whose characteristics depend on both the pressure elevation and local activation of pain-sensitive structures.

The Headache Classification Committee of the International Headache Society (IHS) (1988) classifies these disorders as "Headache associated with non-vascular intracranial disorder [7.0]." Patients may experience worsening of a pre-existing headache or may develop a new form of headache (including migraine, tension-type headache, or cluster headache) in close temporal relationship to a nonvascular intracranial disorder. Causality is *not* necessarily implied. The diagnostic criteria are:

1. Symptoms and/or signs of intracranial disorder
2. Confirmation by appropriate investigation
3. Headache as a new symptom or of a new type occurs temporally related to intracranial disorder

Included in this category are benign (idiopathic) intracranial hypertension, low-CSF-pressure headache, intracranial neoplasm, and "headache associated with other intracranial disorders," which are described in detail in this chapter.

Intracranial hematoma, subdural hematoma, and subarachnoid hemorrhage are classified as "Headache associated with vascular disorders [6.0]." They are described briefly in this chapter and in more detail in Chapter 12.

CEREBROSPINAL FLUID

Production, Flow, and Absorption

The major source of CSF is the choroid plexus, a series of invaginations of the ependyma into the roofs and walls of the ventricles by the blood vessels of the pia mater. Some CSF is also formed in extrachoroidal sites. The choroid plexus of each lateral ventricle is continuous with the choroid plexus of the third but separate from that of the fourth ventricle. The choroid epithelium, continuous with the ependymal lining of the ventricles, is composed of a single row of epithelial cells folded into villi around a core of blood vessels and connective tissue (Fishman, 1992). The choroid plexus epithelium and perivascular basement membranes are permeable to large molecules, such as horseradish peroxidase (HRP). However, there is a barrier to the movement of HRP back and forth between blood and the ventricular cavity in the form of tight junctions between choroidal and perivascular cells (Fishman, 1992; Milhorat, 1972).

It was believed that the CSF was an ultrafiltrate of blood until Flexner (1934) measured the components of CSF and blood and found higher concentrations of magnesium and chloride and lower concentrations of glucose, proteins, amino acids, uric acid, calcium, phosphate, and potassium in the CSF. Both active transport and serum dialysis are involved in CSF production (Milhorat, 1972).

Whereas hydrostatic pressure initiates the transfer of water and ions to the choroidal epithelium, active transport of sodium, potassium, and chloride, coupled to an adenosine triphosphatase (ATPase), plays a key role in CSF secretion. Choroid carbonic anhydrase, which catalyzes the formation of carbonic acid from water and carbon dioxide, plays an important role in CSF production. Inhibition of choroid carbonic anhydrase by acetazolamide decreases CSF production. Specific transport systems exist in the choroid plexus for organic acids and bases, monosaccharides, purines, amino acids, and vitamins (Carpenter, 1978; Fishman, 1992; Milhorat, 1972). Most proteins are excluded from the CSF by the blood–brain barrier.

The estimated rate of CSF formation in humans is 0.37 ± 0.1 ml/minute (500 ml/day) and is unaffected by changes in intracranial pressures from -10 to 240 mm H_2O (Milhorat, 1972). The total CSF volume is renewed every 6 to 8 hours.

The CSF flows from the lateral and third ventricles through the cerebral aqueduct into the fourth ventricle. CSF can enter the cisterna magna through the single midline foramen of Magendie or the cerebellomedullary cistern by the paired lateral foramina of Luschka. CSF then circulates into the subarachnoid space surrounding the brain and spinal cord, moving toward the cerebral convexities and points of absorption (Milhorat, 1972). Some CSF may pass into the central canal of the spinal cord.

CSF may be propelled through the subarachnoid space by postural effects, the ciliary action of ventricular ependymal cells, the bulk flow from newly formed CSF, and ventricular transmitted arterial pulsations emanating from the choroid plexus. Because no single mechanism can satisfactorily explain all aspects of CSF flow, more than one mechanism may be working.

CSF is passively absorbed by the arachnoid villi, fingerlike extensions of arachnoid cells that project from the subarachnoid space into the vascular spaces (Milhorat, 1972). These are grouped, like protruding cauliflower clumps, into parasagittal venous lakes parallel to the superior sagittal sinus, as well as at the proximal root sleeves. The arachnoid villi function as one-way valves with a critical opening pressure between 20 and 50 mm H_2O. Hydrostatic pressure differences between the CSF and venous sinuses produce large CSF blebs that migrate from the CSF to the luminal surface of the villi and produce bulk movement of CSF into the bloodstream. Because the capacity for absorption is two to four times greater than the production rate, there is a sizable absorption reserve (Wald, 1989).

CSF Pressure

The pressure level in the right atrium is the zero reference level for measuring the lumbar CSF pressure. In humans, in the lateral recumbent position the average CSF pressure is 150 mm H_2O, with a range from 50 to 200 (Fishman, 1992; Gamache et al., 1987; Milhorat, 1972). Recently Corbett and Mehta (1983) measured CSF pressures between 200 and 250 mm H_2O in normal, nonobese controls, suggesting that the upper limit of normal may be 250 mm H_2O. If simultaneous pressures are taken from the cerebral ventricles, cisterna magna, and lumbar sac during a change from the recumbent to the erect posture, there is a significant change in pressure throughout the system. The pressure rises to 375 to 565 mm H_2O in the lumbar sac, becomes 0 at the level of the cisterna magna, and can fall to -85 mm H_2O in the ventricles (Freemont-Smith and Kubie, 1929; Loman, 1934; Loman et al., 1935; Milhorat, 1972; Von Storch et al., 1937). The height of the hydrostatic column is not the only factor determining pressure, because the increase in lumbar pressure in the erect position is only one half to two thirds that due to hydrostatic pressure. The elasticity of the dura and volumetric change in the cerebral veins may be of critical importance in determining pressure (Milhorat, 1972).

Seven factors determine the CSF pressure: CSF secretion pressure, CSF absorption rate, intracranial arterial pressure, intracranial venous pressure, brain bulk, hydrostatic pressure, and presence of intact surrounding coverings. Normally transmitted venous pressure is the most important determinant of CSF pressure (Milhorat, 1972). Intracranial pressure can be elevated by: increased CSF formation, decreased CSF absorption, increased intracranial venous pressure, interruption of normal CSF flow, increase in brain bulk, in-

Table 19-1 Mechanisms for elevated intracranial pressure

Increased CSF production or secretion pressure
Decreased CSF absorption
Increased venous pressure
Obstruction of normal CSF flow
Increase in brain bulk
    Mass lesion/cerebral edema
Increased bulk or pressure in dura
Combination of above

creased bulk or pressure of the dura, or a combination of these factors (Table 19-1).

Elevated intracranial pressure can be produced when a mass lesion reaches a critical size, obstructs the intracranial venous system, or obstructs the CSF pathways. According to the Monro-Kellie doctrine, any increase in intracranial volume leads to increased intracranial pressure; because an adult's skull has rigid walls, it forms a closed chamber with a small exit, the foramen magnum, that alone provides an outlet for CSF into the vertebral canal. The contents of the skull (the blood, the brain, and the CSF) are virtually incompressible, and any addition to the contents, as with a tumor, bleed, or acute hydrocephalus, can only occur by expelling blood, CSF, or brain matter from the cranial cavity. This provides a small, relatively unforgiving, compensatory mechanism for raised pressure. When all local and general compensatory mechanisms are exhausted, intracranial hypertension will develop (Zulch et al., 1974).

In normal subjects, minor CSF pressure pulsations are seen that are synchronous with respiration between 2 and 5 mm and synchronous with systole between 1 and 2 mm. Patients with intracranial hypertension monitored continuously with isovolumetric pressure transducers show frequent rapid pressure fluctuations. The first two are related to respiration and systole. The third type, now called plateau waves (Figure 19-1), is an acute elevation of pressure, lasting 5 to 20 minutes, that can reach levels as high as 600 to 1,300 mm H_2O. Increased headache associated with restlessness, impaired consciousness, rigidity, nausea, and vomiting may occur with the pressure wave. At times there may be no change in the patient's condition despite extreme elevations of intracranial pressure (Fishman, 1992).

INTRACRANIAL HYPOTENSION

Normal intracranial pressure is 70 to 200 mm H_2O. Symptoms of intracranial hypotension occur with pressures below 50 to 90 mm H_2O. At times the CSF pressure is not measurable and CSF can only be obtained by aspiration (Fishman, 1992). Intracranial hypotension (Table 19-2) can be either spontaneous, with no evidence of CSF leak or systemic illness, or symptomatic, which may be associated with a CSF leak (Marcelis and Silberstein, 1990).

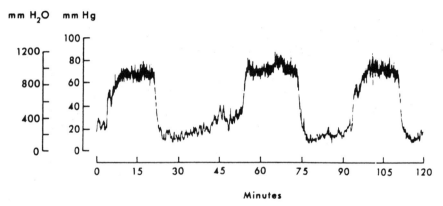

Figure 19–1. Plateau waves as visualized with an intracranial pressure transducer in a patient with a malignant brain tumor. During the waves, a rapid increase in signs of cerebral dysfunction was noted. (Reproduced with permission from Fishman, R. A. (1992). *Cerebrospinal Fluid in Diseases of the Nervous System*, 2nd ed. W. B. Saunders, Philadelphia.)

The most common cause of intracranial hypotension is lumbar puncture, whether done diagnostically, for myelography, or for anesthesia. Head or back trauma, craniotomy, and spinal surgery can produce CSF hypotension as a result of a dural tear or a traumatic avulsion of a nerve route, resulting in a CSF leak (Front and Penning, 1973; Kieffer et al., 1971; Sharrock, 1980). In addition, craniotomy or trauma can produce intracranial hypotension not associated with a CSF leak as a result of decreased CSF formation, decreased cerebral blood flow, or both (Bell et al., 1960). CSF rhinorrhea (spontaneous, post-traumatic, or secondary to a pituitary tumor) and spontaneous dural tears can produce intracranial hypotension. Systemic medical illness, including severe dehydration, hyperpnea, meningoencephalitis, uremia, severe systemic infection, and infusion of hypertonic solution, can cause intracranial hypotension.

Headache, the most common clinical symptom of intracranial hypotension

Table 19–2 Causes of low-pressure headache syndrome

Spontaneous intracranial hypotension
Symptomatic
  Lumbar puncture: diagnostic, myelographic and spinal anesthesia
  Traumatic: head or back trauma
    with CSF leak (dural tear, traumatic nerve root avulsion)
    without CSF leak
  Postoperative: craniotomy, spinal surgery, postpneumonectomy (thoracoarachnoid fistula)
    with CSF leak
    without CSF leak
  Spontaneous CSF leak: CSF rhinorrhea, occult pituitary tumor, dural tear
  Systemic illnesses: dehydration, diabetic coma, hyperpnea, meningoencephalitis, uremia, severe
    systemic infection

Table 19–3 Features of low-CSF-pressure headache

Pain: Aggravated by upright position, relieved with recumbency; aggravated by head shaking and jugular compression

Associated symptoms: Nausea, vomiting, dizziness, tinnitus, photophobia, anorexia, and generalized malaise

Physical exam: Within normal limits (rare neck stiffness, slow pulse rate ["vagus pulse"])

Lumbar puncture: Opening pressure from 0 to 30 mm H_2O CSF in the lateral decubitus position

(Table 19–3), is dramatically positional. It begins on assuming the erect position and is relieved with recumbency (orthostatic headache). Headache occurs in almost all patients with intracranial hypotension. The headache may be frontal, occipital, or diffuse and may vary in intensity from dull to severe and throbbing. The pain is aggravated by head shaking and jugular compression and is not usually relieved with analgesics. Other symptoms include anorexia, nausea, vomiting, vertigo, and tinnitus. The physical examination is usually normal, but may show mild neck stiffness and a slow pulse rate (vagus pulse). Spinal fluid pressure usually ranges from 0 to 30 mm H_2O (Von Storch et al., 1937). The CSF composition is usually normal, but there may be a slight protein elevation and a few red blood cells.

Headache Mechanism

In the presence of intracranial hypotension, intracranial pressure falls more on assuming the upright position than when intracranial pressure is normal. This may produce more traction on the brain's supporting structures. Traction on these pain-sensitive structures (blood vessels and dural sinuses) may cause headache in the upright position. A more important mechanism for the production of headache may be secondary compensatory venous dilation (Cass and Edelist, 1974; Dalessio, 1972). Magnetic resonance imaging (MRI) has shown intracranial CSF volume loss following lumbar puncture, which is seen mainly in the cortical sulci. The volume loss correlates to the presence of a post–lumbar puncture low-CSF-pressure headache (Grant et al., 1991). No change in position of the intracranial structures is demonstrated, suggesting that traction or displacement of the intracranial structures is not the cause of post–lumbar puncture headache. The loss of CSF volume is compensated by venodilation. Jugular compression, which increases both venous dilation and intracranial pressure, aggravates low-pressure headache. This suggests that the mechanism of post–lumbar puncture headache is *not* decreased intracranial pressure itself but decreased CSF volume and secondary painful venous dilation (Grant et al., 1991).

The diagnosis of low-CSF-pressure headache is easily made in the presence of orthostatic headache, particularly if there is an obvious cause, such as a recent lumbar puncture, head or back trauma, craniotomy, or one of the associated medical illnesses (Table 19–2). If no etiology is apparent or the diagnosis is uncertain, lumbar puncture (perhaps at the time of cisternography) is indicated, following a neuroimaging procedure (computerized tomography [CT] or MRI).

Subdural hematomas due to tears in bridging veins have been associated with intracranial hypotension (Sipe et al., 1981). Slitlike ventricles have also been reported (Murros and Fogelholm, 1983).

If the cause of the syndrome is known, one should proceed with the appropriate treatment modalities. If the cause is not known, one should proceed with cisternography or ionic myelography to search for a CSF leak. Occult CSF rhinorrhea can be ruled out by the lack of radioisotope collection in the nose. Nonionic (Pantopaque) myelography may reveal dural tears even when cisternography and ionic myelography are normal (K. Campbell, unpublished observations, 1991).

Lumbar Puncture Headache

Headache is the most common complication of lumbar puncture, occurring in 15 to 30% of patients (Dripps and Vandam, 1954; Tourtellote et al., 1964). The clinical picture is that of intracranial hypotension (Table 19–3). The onset of postural headache varies from 15 minutes to 4 days, but can be delayed up to 12 days (Dripps and Vandam, 1954; Raskin, 1988). The longer the patient is upright the longer it takes the headache to subside with recumbency (Raskin, 1988, 1990). Untreated, the headache can last 2 to 14 days (most commonly 4 to 8 days) or even months (Tourtellote et al., 1964). The more severe the headache, the more frequently it is associated with dizziness, nausea, vomiting, and tinnitus (Vilming et al., 1989).

Post–lumbar puncture headache is more common in younger patients and in women, who are affected twice as often as men (Dripps and Vandam, 1954; Raskin, 1990, 1988; Tourtellote et al., 1964; Vilming et al., 1989). This sex difference is most marked in younger women in most, but not all, studies (Lee et al., 1991; Raskin, 1988). A lower incidence of post–lumbar puncture headache in patients with higher opening pressures has been reported (Vilming et al., 1989). Torrey (1979) observed that post–lumbar puncture headache was rare among schizophrenic patients, perhaps because of their insensitivity to pain. This finding was not confirmed in another study (Daniels and Sallie, 1981). There is no evidence that post–lumbar puncture headache is prevented by keeping the patient supine after the procedure, keeping the patient prone after the procedure, removing the needle with the patient prone and head down, or maintaining adequate hydration (Fishman, 1992; Raskin, 1988; Tourtellote et al., 1964). Evidence suggests that using a small-gauge needle (smaller than 22 gauge) may decrease the incidence of post–lumbar puncture headache (Geurts et al., 1990; Raskin, 1990; Rasmussen et al., 1989); however, these needles are very difficult to use. Recently, a nontraumatic lumbar puncture needle has been developed, that reportedly is associated with a lower incidence of post–lumbar puncture headache (Engelhardt et al., 1991).

Vilming et al. (1989) have reported a 7% incidence of short-duration, non-postural, post–lumbar puncture headache. This has not been included in past series such headaches, and it is uncertain whether this is a low-grade post–lumbar puncture headache or is totally unrelated.

It is believed that post–lumbar puncture headache is due to low CSF pressure secondary to CSF leakage. In fact, dural holes and subdural collections of CSF have been observed at laminectomy or autopsy performed after lumbar puncture (Fishman, 1992; Tourtellote et al., 1964). Kunkle (as reported by Engelhardt et al., 1991) induced post–lumbar puncture headache in normal subjects by draining CSF. Headache appeared when pressure was reduced by removing 20 ml of CSF. The estimated intracranial pressure fell to between -220 and -290 mm H_2O from a normal -100 mm H_2O in the sitting position. Spinal drainage performed on a patient who had a prior section of the fifth and ninth cranial nerves and upper left cervical nerves did not produce left-sided headache (Fishman, 1992). No direct correlation exists between the degree of low pressure on a subsequent lumbar puncture and the presence of headache (Raskin, 1990), but a correlation exists between CSF volume loss and headache (Grant et al., 1991). Jugular compression increases the severity of headache despite increasing intracranial pressure, suggesting that headache is not caused solely by intracranial hypotension (Raskin, 1990).

As the post–lumbar puncture headache improves, the associated tinnitus and feeling of ear blockage disappear. An anatomic connection between the subarachnoid space and the cochlea would allow development of labyrinthine hypotension and cochlear symptoms (Fishman, 1992).

Spontaneous Intracranial Hypotension

If no secondary cause of intracranial hypotension is present and no dural leak can be demonstrated, spontaneous intracranial hypotension should be considered (Huber, 1970; Lasater, 1970; Lindquist and Moberg, 1949; Marcelis and Silberstein, 1990; Schaltenbrand, 1938). Recent studies suggest that CSF hyperabsorption, first described by Schaltenbrand (1938) as "spontaneous aliquorrhea," may be the cause of this unique syndrome. Schaltenbrand described three possible mechanisms to explain the pathophysiology of the syndrome: decreased CSF production, CSF hyperabsorption, and CSF leakage from small occult dural tears. The symptoms of spontaneous intracranial hypotension are the same as the symptoms of CSF hypotension produced by other causes. By definition, there is no evidence of CNS trauma or prior lumbar puncture.

Marcelis and Silberstein (1990), Labadie et al. (1976), Kraemer et al. (1987), and Molins et al. (1990) have reported cases of spontaneous intracranial hypotension in which the radionuclide cisternogram showed rapid uptake in the bladder and kidneys and rapid transport of isotope with no evidence of CSF leak. DiChiro et al. (1976) believe that this is abnormal and consistent with CSF hyperabsorption. Some cases do show slowing of isotope flow and an associated Arnold–Chiari malformation, suggesting that more than one mechanism may be operative (S. D. Silberstein, unpublished observations, 1992). Rando and Fishman (1992) reported two cases of spontaneous intracranial hypotension secondary to CSF spinal leaks that were demonstrated by radionuclide cisternography. These cases with chronic leaks are different than the cases without leaks reported above.

Sable and Ramadan (1991) found meningeal enhancement on gadolinium-enhanced cranial MRI in a 34-year-old woman with severe post-traumatic positional headache. Pannullo et al. (1992) found meningeal enhancement in four cases of intracranial hypotension (two spontaneous, two post–lumbar puncture) on evaluation several weeks after headache onset. One spontaneous case had a negative meningeal biopsy. After the patient recovered, the meningeal enhancement disappeared. Meningeal enhancement could account for the low CSF pressure by enhancing arachnoid villi CSF transport. Meningeal inflammation could, in addition, produce pain in dilated venous sinuses.

Treatment of Intracranial Hypotension

Many types of treatment for intracranial hypotension have been proposed, including bed rest, peripheral intravascular volume expansion, steroids (Kraemer et al., 1987; Murros and Fogelholm, 1983), caffeine (Sechzer and Abel, 1978), blood patch (Baker, 1983; Gaukroger and Brownridge, 1987; Gormley, 1960; Parris, 1987), abdominal binder, and continuous intrathecal saline infusion (Peterson et al., 1987) (Table 19–4). Treatment should be based on etiology (Table 19–2). Any associated illness should be treated and, if a CSF leak exists, it should be treated appropriately and repaired if identified and accessible. The treatment of post–lumbar puncture headache and spontaneous intracranial hypotension are similar. Postcraniotomy hypotension is not discussed.

Treatment of low-CSF-pressure headache begins with the noninvasive therapeutic modalities (Table 19–4) of bed rest and an abdominal binder; however, these modalities, if prolonged, are not cost-effective. If there is no improvement, intravenous or oral caffeine may provide significant relief.

Caffeine produces intracerebral arterial constriction, probably through blockade of brain adenosine receptors (Raskin, 1988). In a controlled double-blind prospective study, Sechzer and Abel (1978) showed that intravenous caffeine sodium benzoate (500 mg given by intravenous slow push) was dramatically effective in 75% of patients with low CSF pressure who had undergone previous lumbar puncture. This can be repeated in 12 to 24 hours.

A brief trial of steroids in combination with bed rest, abdominal binder, or caffeine may prove to be beneficial. If no relief is obtained in 24 hours, a quick steroid taper is recommended because of potential side effects. If the patient continues to be symptomatic after a noninvasive medical approach, a blood patch is indicated.

With a 96.8% success rate (Cass and Edelist, 1974) the blood patch, originally described by Gormley (1960), is the most successful treatment for low-CSF-pressure headache (Bart and Wheeler, 1978; Gormley, 1960; Millette et al,

---

Table 19–4   Treatment of low-CSF headache

Bed rest
Abdominal binder
Caffeine
Steroids
Epidural blood patch
Continuous epidural saline infusion

1982). It is performed by infusing 10 to 20 ml of autologous blood into the epidural space under sterile conditions. Many investigators have recently performed blood patches for the newly recognized spontaneous intracranial hypotension syndrome and have described similar results.

The presumed mechanism of action of the blood patch is an immediate gelatinous tamponade of a dural leak followed by fibrin deposition and fibroblastic activity. Collagen deposition and scar formation are complete within 3 weeks. However, this mechanism has recently been challenged by several investigators who have noted recurrence of orthostatic headache 4 to 6 months after successful blood patch (Raskin, 1988). They propose that compression of the dural sac with an increment in CSF pressure may serve as a signal that deactivates the low-CSF-pressure headache, possibly by antagonizing adenosine receptors (Raskin, 1988).

If the headache of intracranial hypotension recurs, repeat blood patch should be performed, or a continuous intrathecal saline infusion (Bart and Wheeler, 1978; Peterson et al., 1987) may be attempted. In this procedure, an epidural catheter is placed at the L_{2-3} level and a saline infusion begun at a rate of 20 ml/hour and continued up to 72 hours.

INTRACRANIAL HYPERTENSION

Many disorders are associated with the syndrome of increased intracranial pressure (Table 19–5). It may be difficult to correlate the features associated with intracranial mass displacement with the underlying pathologic process. Some have tried to categorize a syndrome of "general intracranial hypertension" consisting of headaches, vomiting, and papilledema (Zulch et al., 1974). However, the presence of increased intracranial pressure is not always associated with either headache or papilledema, and no direct correlation exists between the degree of pressure elevation and the presence of headache. Although it has been stated that headache does not always occur with mild to moderate eleva-

Table 19–5 Syndromes of increased intracranial pressure

Primary
  Idiopathic intracranial hypertension with papilledema
  Idiopathic intracranial hypertension without papilledema
Secondary
  Hydrocephalus
  Mass lesion
    neoplasm
    stroke—hematoma
  Meningitis/encephalitis
  Trauma
  Major intracranial and extracranial venous obstruction
  Drugs: vitamin A, nalidixic acid, anabolic steroids, steroid withdrawal
  Systemic diseases: renal disease, hypoparathyroidism, systemic lupus erythematosus

tions of intracranial pressure because there is no associated traction or distortion of pain-sensitive structures, at least two conditions in which this is not the case (acute hydrocephalus and idiopathic intracranial hypertension) must be recognized. The mechanisms underlying the cause of head pain in these situations are not understood and may not involve traction on pain-sensitive structures only.

Intracranial Neoplasms

Headache occurs at presentation in approximately 36 to 50% of patients with brain tumors and develops in the course of the disease in 60%. Headache is a rare initial symptom in patients with pituitary tumors, craniopharyngiomas, or cerebellopontine angle tumors (Jaeckle, 1991; Lavyne and Patterson, 1987). Headache is a very common initial symptom with infratentorial tumors (other than cerebellopontine angle tumors), occurring in 80 to 85% of patients (Kunkle et al., 1942; Northfield, 1938). Elevation of intracranial pressure is not necessary for its production. In one series of 72 patients with brain tumor from the New York Hospital, headache occurred in those patients without elevated intracranial pressure (19 of 23) as often as it did in those with increased intracranial pressure (46 of 49) (Lavyne and Patterson, 1987). The headache is usually generalized, but in 30 to 80% of patients it overlies the tumor (Jaeckle, 1991; Lavyne and Patterson, 1987). Supratentorial tumors that impinge on structures innervated by the ophthalmic division of the fifth cranial nerve may produce frontotemporal headache, whereas posterior fossa tumors may compress the ninth and 10th cranial nerves and typically produce occipitonuchal pain.

Traction on pain-sensitive intracerebral vessels, transient herniation of hippocampal gyri, traction on cranial or cervical nerves, or elevation of intracranial pressure are postulated mechanisms of headache development.

> Fay (1937) and shortly later Ray and Wolff (1940) stimulated the tentorium, the meninges, the major intracranial vessels at the skull base, and the cranial nerves of patients undergoing cranial surgery under local anesthesia. They found that stretching or distorting these structures produced headache. Stimulation of the supratentorial compartment caused the sensation of pain in the forehead, which suggested that these structures were innervated by the trigeminal nerve. Pain brought on by stimulating structures in the posterior fossa was probably transmitted by the 9th and 10th cranial nerves and the upper three cervical nerves because the pain was referred to the posterior half of the head.
>
> These observations formed an early basis for the understanding that one cause of headache is traction of major intracranial structures such as the large arteries and veins. . . . Studies performed on volunteers in the 1940s and 1950s documented the fact that the infusion of mock spinal fluid at pressures as high as 850 mm of water did not usually produce headache. This suggests that elevation of intracranial pressure by itself does not produce headache (Ray and Wolff, 1940).

Although increased CSF pressure is not necessary for headache development, it clearly plays a role in a group of patients with central nervous system neoplasms, acute obstructive hydrocephalus, and idiopathic intracranial hypertension. The rate of the change in pressure may be critical. Sudden increases in intracranial CSF pressure by tumors obstructing the foramen of Monro or the cerebral aqueduct may cause abrupt, severe headache associated with gait disturbance, syncope, incontinence, or visual obscurations. Why a significant number of patients with brain tumors do not have headache is not clear. Perhaps the tumor spares pain-sensitive structures or occurs in patients with high headache thresholds. In a study conducted at the Mayo Clinic, Rushton and Rooke (1962) looked at the characteristic headache features of 221 patients with brain tumors. Only 60% of the patients had headache. The location of the tumor had no significant bearing on the presence or absence of headache. However, 17 of the 59 patients with posterior fossa tumors had neurolemmomas, which have a lower incidence of headache. In this series, brain tumor headache severity was mild to moderate in 63% of patients and severe in 37%. The headaches were intermittent in 85% and throbbing in 15%. Five of the patients had exertional headache. The headache lateralized to the side of the tumor in 40 of 132 patients (30%). The headaches were aggravated by changing position in 20%, and by coughing or exertion in 25%. Fifty percent of the patients had nausea or vomiting. Twenty-five percent of the patients had headache during sleep, on arising, or both. Increased intracranial pressure was observed in 56 of 132 patients with headache and in 5 of 89 patients without headache.

Heyck (1968) surveyed 778 patients with cerebral tumor. In 422 (54%), headache was the earliest or principal symptom. In general, no difference in headache frequency was noted between rapidly growing and slow-growing tumors. Patients with rapidly growing posterior fossa tumors have a 90.4% incidence of headache as an early symptom. The headache can occur intermittently and mimic migraine. Pepin (1991) reported a 44-year-old woman with metastatic adenocarcinoma who met the IHS criteria for migraine with aura. Within 5 months there was an increase in headache frequency and the development of papilledema.

Headaches are a more common symptom of brain tumor in children (over 90%) than in adults (approximately 60%) (Zulch et al., 1974). Konig and Charney (1982) reported on 72 children with brain tumor headache. The following characteristics were found to occur frequently: headache awakening the child from sleep or present on awakening, severe or prolonged headache, increased severity or frequency of headache, and increased frequency of vomiting. A total of 68 children (94%) with headache had neurologic signs. In 96%, diagnostic clues appeared within 4 months of the onset of headache. Rossi and Vassella (1989) compared 600 children with migraine to 67 children with brain tumors. Characteristic features in the brain tumor group included nocturnal headache or headache present on arising, both associated with vomiting and increased frequency of headache. These symptoms were present in 32% of the brain tumor group and 10% of the childhood migraine group. Nocturnal headache or headache present on arising associated with vomiting or progressive neurologic symptoms or signs occurred in 65 of 67 children with brain tumor within 2 months of the onset of their headaches. Zammarano et al. (1989) found 5 of 2,416 children with tumor who presented with migraine-like headache without signs of tumor. Because changes in cognition may be the first sign of tumor, children with headache must be observed long enough to establish that they have normal growth and intellectual and motor development.

In conclusion, there is a significant overlap between the headache of brain tumor and migraine and tension-type headache. Any neurologic sign or symptom occurring with a headache, any headache of recent onset, or a headache that has changed in character requires a thorough evaluation. A careful search for papilledema and focal neurologic signs must be done. Morning or nocturnal headache associated with vomiting and increased headache frequency can be seen with both migraine and brain tumor. Neuroimaging with CT (with contrast) or MRI should be done in suspected cases.

Generalizations concerning headache and brain tumor localization include the following:

1. The headache of brain tumor may be referred from a distant intracranial source. It overlies the tumor in about one third of patients.
2. Supratentorial tumor pain is frequently vertex or frontal in location.
3. Infratentorial tumor pain is frequently occipital, and cervical muscle spasm may be present.
4. Posterior fossa tumors almost always have an associated headache.
5. Posterior fossa or cervicomedullary junction tumors (or structural abnormalities) may be associated with cough or exertional headache.
6. Hemispheric tumor pain is usually appreciated on the same side of the head as the tumor.
7. Chiasmal or sellar tumor pain may be referred to the vertex.

Pseudotumor Cerebri (Idiopathic Intracranial Hypertension)

The syndrome of idiopathic intracranial hypertension (IIH), also known as pseudotumor cerebri or benign intracranial hypertension, is a condition of increased intracranial pressure of unknown cause that occurs predominantly in obese women of child-bearing age. Definitive diagnosis cannot be made without excluding brain tumors and other intracranial mass lesions, infections, hypertensive encephalopathy, pulmonary encephalopathy (related to chronic carbon dioxide toxicity), and obstruction of the cerebral ventricles from whatever cause. The adjective "benign" is no longer employed because, although spontaneous recovery usually occurs, this is not invariable and, indeed, permanent visual loss may occur. In fact, visual loss occurs in 80% of patients and blindness occurs in 10% (Giuseffi et al., 1991; Wall and George, 1991). The symptoms of IIH are those of generalized increased intracranial pressure, with headache occurring in most, but not all, patients. Transient visual obscuration (Sadun et al., 1984), an episode of visual clouding in one or both eyes usually lasting seconds, occurs with all forms of increased intracranial pressure with papilledema but is not a specific symptom. Transient visual obscurations can occur in patients *without* increased intracranial pressure who have elevated optic disks from other causes (disk edema, nerve sheath tumors, drusen, and coloboma). Other common symptoms include pulsatile tinnitus, diplopia, and visual loss. Some patients report shoulder and arm pain (perhaps secondary to nerve

Table 19–6 Features of IIH

Headache: Chronic tension-type headache with migrainous features, may be present on awakening; can be intermittent or absent

Associated features: Pulsatile tinnitus, transient visual obscurations, diplopia, visual loss, shoulder and arm pain

Patients: Predominantly obese women aged 20 to 50

Physical and neurologic exam: Within normal limits, except for papilledema, visual loss, obesity, and a sixth nerve palsy

Neuroradiology: CT or MRI shows no evidence of intracranial mass, hydrocephalus, or venous sinus thrombosis (empty sella may be present)

Lumbar puncture: Demonstrates increased CSF pressure with a normal composition (may show decreased protein)

No other causes of increased CSF pressure present

---

root dilation) and retro-orbital pain (Giuseffi et al., 1991). Signs include papilledema and sixth nerve palsy.

IIH occurs with a frequency of about 1 case per 100,000 per year in the general population, and 19.3 cases per 100,000 per year in obese women ages 20 to 44 (Durcan et al., 1988). The patient with IIH is commonly a young, obese woman with chronic daily headache, normal laboratory studies, normal neurologic examination (except for papilledema), and an empty sella (Table 19–6).

The pathophysiology of IIH is unknown. Postulated mechanisms include increased rate of CSF formation, increased intracranial venous pressure, decreased rate of CSF absorption, and increase in brain interstitial fluid (edema). Recent studies suggest that decreased rate of absorption at the arachnoid villi and interstitial brain edema are the major contributors (Bjerre et al., 1982; Borgeson and Gjerris, 1987; Donaldson, 1981; Fishman, 1979, 1984; Gjerris et al., 1985; Janny et al., 1981; Johnston, 1973; Johnston and Paterson, 1974; Van Alphen, 1986). Malm et al. (1992) have found that the disturbances of CSF hydrodynamics in IIH persist for years. They believe that the mechanism for the development of increased CSF pressure is a result of a rise in venous sagittal sinus pressure (secondary to extracellular edema causing venous obstruction), or a low conductance for CSF reabsorption producing a compensatory increase in CSF pressure.

The headache profile of patients with IIH has been recently elucidated. In one study, 93% of patients described their headache as the most severe ever (Wall, 1990). Chronic daily headache present on awakening and pulsating in character, retro-ocular pain with eye movement, and associated symptoms of nausea, vomiting, and pulsatile tinnitus are common features.

Ninety-three percent of the patients were women, and 93% were obese. The mean age was 31 years. Headache was reported by 92%. Of those having headache, 73% had chronic daily headache, 93% said it was the most severe ever, and 83% said it was pulsatile. Nausea occurred in 57%, vomiting in 38%, and orbital pain in 43%. Transient visual obscuration was present in 71%, diplopia in 38%, and visual loss in 31% (Wall, 1990). Others have commented about the nonspecificity of the headache and its lack of severity. This may be the result of a nonsystematic analysis of headache symptoms (Corbett, 1989; Foley, 1955).

Occasionally patients with IIH are incidentally found to have papilledema while being examined for another purpose. Five to 10% of patients are essentially asymptomatic (Corbett, 1989). Loss of visual field and visual acuity are the only significant complications of IIH with papilledema. Visual loss occurs as: (1) transient visual obscuration, consisting of grayouts or blackouts in the vision in one or both eyes lasting seconds and commonly provoked by posture; (2) loss of visual acuity, either gradual or abrupt, as a result of enlargement of the blind spot, macular edema, subretinal hemorrhage, ischemic optic neuropathy, or venous status retinopathy; or (3) gradual loss of visual field, similar to the loss in glaucoma (rarely appreciated by the patient until it is severe) (Corbett, 1989). Ophthalmologic examination should include intraocular pressure, visual fields (Goldmann or Humphrey), optic disk photos, visual acuity, and search for a relative afferent pupil (Corbett, 1989).

Intracranial hypertension may be either *idiopathic,* with no clear identifiable cause, or *symptomatic,* a result of venous sinus occlusion, radical neck dissection, hypoparathyroidism, vitamin A intoxication, systemic lupus erythematosus, renal disease, or drug side effects (nalidixic acid, danocrine, steroid withdrawal) (Table 19–5) (Corbett, 1989). There is no evidence to associate IIH with pregnancy, hypertension, diabetes, thyroid disease, iron-deficiency anemia, or the use of tetracyclines or oral contraceptives. Arterial hypertension may be overreported in patients with IIH if a large blood pressure cuff is not used for obese patients (Giuseffi et al., 1991).

Symptomatic intracranial hypertension can be secondary to changes in cranial venous outflow, which may influence intracranial pressure by increasing cerebral blood volume, producing brain edema, and impairing CSF absorption. Intracranial venous outflow obstruction can be caused by chronic otitis, head trauma, tumors, hypercoagulable states, and cerebral edema (Malm et al., 1992). Extracranial venous outflow obstruction occurs with surgical ligation and further compression of venous outflow. Cranial venous outflow hypertension can also occur without obstruction in patients with arteriovenous malformations, cardiac failure, and pulmonary failure (Johnston et al., 1991).

IIH without Papilledema

A small subgroup of patients with intracranial hypertension without papilledema has been described (Lipton and Michelson, 1972; Marcelis and Silberstein, 1991; Scanari et al., 1979; Spence et al., 1980). Patients, particularly obese women, with chronic daily headache and symptoms of increased intracranial pressure (i.e., pulsatile tinnitus, history of head trauma or meningitis, an empty sella on neuroimaging studies, or a headache that is unrelieved by standard therapy) should have a diagnostic lumbar puncture. The clinical, historic, radiographic, and demographic characteristics are identical to those of patients with papilledema except for: (1) possible association with prior head trauma or meningitis; (2) extended delay in diagnosis, which requires lumbar puncture in the absence of papilledema; and (3) no evidence of visual loss as seen in patients with IIH with papilledema.

Why there is no papilledema in these cases of intracranial hypertension is not known. Congenital or acquired optic nerve sheath defects, "chronic IIH" with resolution of papilledema, or early IIH are alternative explanations.

Other Causes of Elevated Intracranial Pressure

Hydrocephalus

Obstructive hydrocephalus is the result of interference with normal CSF flow. Clinical presentation depends on the site and cause of obstruction and the patient's age. In infants, before the sutures are closed, the skull enlarges and increased intracranial pressure and headache are not features. In adults, hydrocephalus can produce elevated intracranial pressure and headache that occurs on awakening, is typically occipital, and is associated with neck stiffness, vomiting, and transient visual obscurations (Milhorat, 1972).

The acute increase in intracranial pressure that occurs with ventricular obstruction or shunt malformation in a treated hydrocephalic patient usually causes severe headache followed by visual disturbances. Because vascular perfusion of the brain is reduced as intracranial pressure approaches mean systemic arterial pressure, permanent neurologic deficit or death can result if emergency ventricular drainage is not instituted. Lumbar puncture is contraindicated if this situation is suspected, and papilledema may not occur. Although descriptions of headache with hydrocephalus vary, usually the pain is intense, bilateral, and exacerbated by moving or straining.

Headache is not a characteristic feature of normal-pressure hydrocephalus. The clinical picture includes disturbances of gait, mentation, and micturition. Almost all patients with this problem have a gait disturbance, varying from a slight apraxia to a total inability to walk. When these patients are tested, almost all of them will demonstrate significant memory impairment, distractibility, inability to maintain attention, and decreased concentration span. Later, sphincter incontinence may occur. Concern for incontinence is lacking or reduced and micturition may be performed in front of others, much in the manner of children. Bowel incontinence is less common, although flatus is often expelled without concern for social niceties. Sphincter incontinence is a late sign, rarely seen early in the course of this disease.

Other symptoms include dizziness, light-headedness, faintness or weakness, falling spells, and brief episodes of unconsciousness. Headache, which is often the primary symptom of acute obstructive hydrocephalus, is absent. However, patients with idiopathic intracranial hypertension have now been shown to develop symptomatic hydrocephalus and continue to have headache. These are cases of high-pressure hydrocephalus that resemble the normal-pressure syndrome (Malm et al., 1992).

Central Nervous System Disorders

Central nervous system trauma, hemorrhage, infarct, abscess, and infection may produce acute or chronic intracranial hypertension. The diagnosis is usually obvious, but atypical subacute presentations of subdural hematomas, arteriovenous malformations, and chronic meningitis can be difficult to diagnose. These are discussed in more detail in Chapter 12.

The rupture of an intracranial aneurysm is usually associated with an acute, severe, incapacitating headache that may radiate down the neck. The presence of meningismus, briefly altered consciousness, and vomiting are common and, with a positive CT scan, clinch the diagnosis. Headache may result from tearing pain-sensitive vessels, blood-induced chemical arachnoiditis, or acute hydrocephalus (Edmeads, 1986). The warning leaks of subarachnoid hemorrhage do not produce acute intracranial hypertension and are discussed in Chapter 1 and 12.

Headache is present in 36 to 68% of patients with intracerebral parenchymal hemorrhages (Kase et al., 1982; Mohr et al., 1978). Thalamic hemorrhages can cause a severe, bilateral, diffuse headache secondary to intraventricular rupture. Lobar hemorrhage can produce less severe, ipsilateral, frontal headache. Cerebellar hemorrhage can produce an increasingly severe, diffuse headache if there is rupture into the fourth ventricle, with development of acute hydrocephalus and intracranial hypertension.

Headache is one of the most common manifestations of a chronic subdural hematoma. Severe bitemporal pain, insidious in onset and fluctuating in intensity, can occur, accompanied by changes in cognition (leading to dementia), personality changes, focal weakness, and seizures. Because less than half the patients may give a prior history of head trauma, a high index of suspicion is necessary to make a diagnosis. Percussion tenderness over the subdural hematoma is a characteristic sign (Campbell and Caselli, 1989).

Treatment Modalities

The treatment of elevated intraspinal pressure syndromes is varied and depends on the underlying cause (Table 19–7). In many cases, the history, clinical examination, and neuroradiographic studies may define the syndrome, with distinctive therapy preceding any further diagnostic studies. Thus, cerebral neoplasm, abscess, acute meningitis, subarachnoid hemorrhage, subdural hematoma, acute obstructive hydrocephalus, cerebral infarct, and arteriovenous malformation may be treated with appropriate surgical (drainage, shunt) or medical (antibiotics, hyperventilation, steroids, hypertonic osmotic diuretics) intervention.

In patients with IIH (with or without papilledema), chronic meningitis, and subarachnoid hemorrhage, diagnosis is based on lumbar puncture following

Table 19–7 Treatment of IIH

Eliminate symptomatic causes
Weight loss if obese
Standard headache treatment
Carbonic anhydrase inhibitors and loop diuretics
Short course of high-dose corticosteroids
Serial lumbar punctures
Lumboperitoneal or ventriculoperitoneal shunt
Optic nerve sheath fenestration

neuroimaging. If lumbar puncture is unremarkable and intracranial pressure is elevated to greater than 200 mm H_2O (in nonobese subjects), IIH is the likely diagnosis (Corbett and Mehta, 1983). Routine blood chemistries (prothrombin time, partial thromboplastin time, antinuclear antibodies, VDRL, fluorescence immunoassay for antibodies, SMA-12, SMA-6, thyroxine, and thyroid-stimulating hormone) and serologies are helpful.

Once the diagnosis of IIH is made, secondary causes should be sought and eliminated. Over 50 diseases, conditions, toxins, or pharmaceuticals have been associated with IIH (Corbett, 1989). The obese patient should be encouraged to lose weight. If the patient is asymptomatic and has no visual loss, then no treatment is indicated. Careful ophthalmologic follow-up is needed. If there is no papilledema, or papilledema with no visual loss, and the only complaint is headache, it should be treated aggressively.

The headache of patients with IIH and papilledema has been reported to respond frequently to standard headache treatment, including β-adrenergic blockers, calcium channel antagonists, antidepressants, monoamine oxidase inhibitors, anticonvulsants, analgesics, and ergotamine preparations. Surgical treatment of IIH has been directed toward preventing visual loss secondary to papilledema (Table 19–7). Improvement in headache is a felicitous side benefit in many patients with optic nerve sheath fenestration.

If rigorous headache therapy is unsuccessful, or if there is visual loss, then a 4- to 6-week trial of furosemide or a potent carbonic anhydrase inhibitor (acetazolamide) should be made. These drugs have been shown to decrease the frequency and severity of elevated intracranial pressure headache (Corbett and Thompson, 1989; Weisberg, 1975).

The use of high-dose steroids (prednisone or dexamethasone) is controversial, but may be effective in IIH (Corbett, 1989; Weisberg, 1975). Rebound headache is common when steroids are withdrawn, and prolonged steroid use produces many adverse side effects. If steroid therapy is initiated, a brief, 2- to 6-week course is recommended.

Lumbar puncture typically relieves headache in IIH (Lipton and Michelson, 1972; Paterson et al., 1961; Weisberg, 1975). Because CSF is rapidly replaced, prolonged symptomatic relief may reflect a persistent CSF leak. Alternately, transient reduction of CSF pressure may allow decompression of the arachnoid villi, allowing for prolonged enhanced CSF absorption. Repeated lumbar puncture is effective in temporarily controlling the headache of increased intracranial pressure; its long-term usefulness is controversial.

In patients with IIH who have visual loss or severe incapacitating headache that does not respond to medical therapy or repeated lumbar puncture, surgical management may be needed. Subtemporal decompression, lumboperitoneal shunt, ventriculoperitoneal shunt, and optic nerve sheath fenestration have been used to treat patients with IIH and papilledema (Corbett and Thompson, 1989; Corbett et al., 1988; Digre and Corbett, 1988; Donaldson, 1986; Donaldson and Binstock, 1981; Foley, 1977; Foley and Posner, 1975; Greer, 1965; Maxner et al., 1987; Paterson et al., 1961; Sismanis, 1987; Spence et al., 1980; Wall, 1990). Subtemporal decompression is effective, but because it is cosmetically unattractive and is occasionally complicated by seizures or stroke, it has largely been replaced with shunting procedures.

Spence et al. (1980) successfully treated six patients who had IIH without papilledema with a lumboperitoneal shunt. This procedure, however, has a high reoperation rate, the potential for development of herniation and a new hindbrain herniation headache, and multiple serious complications. A ventriculoperitoneal shunt may now be the preferred shunting procedure.

Optic nerve sheath fenestration (ONSF) entails surgical incision of the dura covering the intraorbital optic nerve. The proposed mechanism in patients with IIH involves improved axoplasmic flow in the optic nerve and continuous intraorbital CSF drainage and absorption. In patients with papilledema and headache treated with ONSF, Corbett et al. (1988) have shown 65% efficacy in relieving medically uncontrolled headache. Using a modified optic nerve sheath decompression procedure, headache was relieved in 13 of 17 patients with IIH (Sergott et al., 1988). Although ONSF has been performed on patients with unilateral papilledema, to our knowledge it is untried in patients with IIH without papilledema. Without threatened vision loss, the small risk of visual loss due to the surgery in patients with IIH and absence of papilledema probably outweighs potential benefits.

Patients with IIH should have periodic neurologic follow-up. The neurologist is involved in lowering the intracranial pressure, controlling the headache, documenting changes in the neurologic examination, and encouraging weight loss. Persistently elevated CSF pressure may predispose these patients to visual loss, and papilledema should be looked for at every visit.

CONCLUSION

Disturbances of CSF production, flow, and absorption produce intracranial hypotension and hypertension. Although the etiology of each disease process is unique, headache is common to most, and each condition demonstrates certain characteristic headache profile features. Further understanding of the CSF and headache pathogenesis may help to provide new and improved therapeutic measures.

REFERENCES

Baker, C.C. (1983). Headache due to spontaneous low spinal fluid pressure. *Minn. Med.* 66:325–328.

Bart, A.J. and A.S. Wheeler (1978). Comparison of epidural saline infusion and epidural blood placement in the treatment of post lumbar puncture headache. *Anesthesiology* 48:221–223.

Bell, W.B., R.J. Joynt, and A.L. Sahs (1960). Low spinal fluid pressure syndromes. *Neurology* 10:512–521.

Bjerre, P., J. Lindholm, and C. Gyldensted (1982). Pseudotumor cerebri: A theory on etiology and pathogenesis. *Acta Neurol. Scand.* 66:472–481.

Borgesen, S.E. and F. Gjerris (1987). Relationships between intracranial pressure, ventricular size, and resistance to CSF outflow. *J. Neurosurg.* 67:535–539.

Campbell, J.K. and R.J. Caselli (1989). Headache and other craniofacial pain. In *Neurology in Clinical Practice—the Neurological Disorders*, (W.G. Bradley, R.B. Daroff, G.M. Fenichel, and C.D. Marsden, eds.), p. 1514. Butterworth-Heineman, Boston.

Carpenter, M.B. (1978). Meninges and cerebrospinal fluid. In *Core Text of Neuroanatomy*, 2nd ed., pp. 8–10. Williams & Wilkins, Baltimore.

Cass, W. and G. Edelist (1974). Post spinal headache. *JAMA* 227:786–787.

Corbett, J.J. (1989). Diagnosis and management of idiopathic intracranial hypertension (pseudotumor cerebri). *Focal Points 1989: Clinical Modules for Ophthalmologists,* American Academy of Ophthalmology, Vol. 7, Module 3, pp. 1–12.

Corbett, J.J. and M.P. Mehta (1983). Cerebrospinal fluid pressure in normal obese subjects and patients with pseudotumor cerebri. *Neurology* 33:1386–1388.

Corbett, J.J., J.A. Nerad, D.T. Tse, and R.L. Anderson (1988). Results of optic nerve sheath fenestration for pseudotumor cerebri: The lateral orbitotomy approach. *Arch. Ophthalmol.* 106:1391–1397.

Corbett, J.J. and H.S. Thompson (1989). The rational management of idiopathic intracranial hypertension. *Arch. Neurol.* 46:1049–1051.

Dalessio, D. (ed.) (1972). *Wolff's Headache and Other Head Pain,* 3rd ed. Oxford University Press, New York.

Daniels, A.M. and R. Sallie (1981). Headache, lumbar puncture, and expectation. *Lancet* 1:1003.

DiChiro, G., M.K. Hammock, and W.A. Bleyer (1976). Spinal descent of cerebrospinal fluid in man. *Neurology* 26:1–8.

Digre, K.B. and J.J. Corbett (1988). Pseudotumor cerebri in men. *Arch. Neurol.* 45:866–872.

Donaldson, J.O. (1981). Pathogenesis of pseudotumor cerebri syndromes. *Neurology* 31:877–880.

Donaldson, J.O. (1986). Endocrinology of pseudotumor cerebri. *Neurol. Clin.* 4:919–927.

Donaldson, J.O. and M.L. Binstock (1981). Pseudotumor cerebri in an obese woman with Turner syndrome. *Neurology* 31:758–760.

Dripps, R.D. and L.D. Vandam (1954). Long term followup of patients who received 10,098 spinal anesthetics. *JAMA* 156:1486–1491.

Durcan, F.J., J.J. Corbett, and M. Wall (1988). The incidence of pseudotumor cerebri: Population studies in Iowa and Louisiana. *Arch. Neurol.* 45:875–877.

Edmeads, J. (1986). Headache in cerebrovascular disease. In *Handbook of Clinical Neurology,* Vol. 4 (F.C. Rose, ed.), p. 278. Elsevier, Amsterdam.

Engelhardt, A., S. Oheim, and B. Neundorrfer (1991). Post lumbar puncture headache: Experiences with an "atraumatic" needle. *Cephalalgia* 11(Suppl. 11):356–357.

Fay, T. (1937). Mechanism of headache. *Arch. Neurol. Psychiatry* 37:471–473.

Fishman, R.A. (1979). Pathophysiology of pseudotumor. *Ann. Neurol.* 5:496.

Fishman, R.A. (1984). The pathophysiology of pseudotumor cerebri. An unsolved puzzle [editorial]. *Neurology* 41:257–258.

Fishman, R.A. (1992). *Cerebrospinal Fluid in Diseases of the Nervous System,* 2nd ed. W.B. Saunders, Philadelphia.

Flexner, L.B. (1934). The chemistry and nature of the cerebrospinal fluid. *Physiol. Rev.* 14:161–187.

Foley, J. (1955). Benign forms of intracranial hypertension—"toxic" and "otitic" hydrocephalus. *Brain* 78:1–41.

Foley, K.M. (1977). Is benign intracranial hypertension a chronic disease? *Neurology* 27:388.

Foley, K.M. and J.B. Posner (1975). Does pseudotumor cerebri cause the empty sella syndrome? *Neurology* 25:565–569.

Freemont-Smith, F. and L. Kubie (1929). Relation of vascular hydrostatic pressure and osmotic pressure to cerebrospinal fluid pressure. *Proc. Assoc. Res. Nerv. Ment. Dis.* 8:154.

Front, D. and L. Penning (1973). Subcutaneous extravasation of CSF demonstration by scinticisternography. *J. Nucl. Med.* 15:200–201.

Gamache, F.W., R.H. Patterson, and J.F. Alksne (1987). Headache associated with changes in intracranial pressure. In *Wolff's Headache and Other Head Pain*, 5th ed. (D.J. Dalessio, ed.), pp. 352–355. Oxford University Press, New York.

Gaukroger, P.B. and P. Brownridge (1987). Epidural blood patch in treatment of spontaneous low CSF pressure headache. *Pain* 29:119–122.

Geurts, J.W., M.C. Haanschoten, R.M. Van Wijk et al. (1990). Post-dural headache in young patients. *Acta Anaesthesiol. Scand.* 34:350–353.

Giuseffi, V., M. Wall, P.Z. Siegal, and P.B. Rojas (1991). Symptoms and disease associations in idiopathic intracranial hypertension (pseudotumor cerebri): A case control study. *Neurology* 41:239–244.

Gjerris, F., S. Sorenson, S. Vorstrup, and O.B. Paulson (1985). Intracranial pressure, conductance to cerebrospinal fluid outflow, and cerebral blood flow in patients with benign intracranial hypertension (pseudotumor cerebri). *Ann. Neurol.* 17: 158–162.

Gormley, J.B. (1960). Treatment of post-spinal headache. *Anesthesiology* 21:565–566.

Grant, R., B. Condon, I. Hart, and G.M. Teasdale (1991). Changes in intracranial CSF volume after lumbar puncture and their relationship to post-LP headache. *J. Neurol. Neurosurg. Psychiatry* 54:440–442.

Greer, M. (1965). Benign intracranial hypertension: VI obesity. *Neurology* 15:382–388.

Headache Classification Committee of the International Headache Society (1988). Classification and diagnostic criteria for headache disorders, cranial neuralgia, and facial pain. *Cephalalgia* 8(Suppl. 7):1–96.

Heyck, H. (1968). Examination and differential diagnosis of headache. In *Handbook of Clinical Neurology*, Vol. 5 (P.J. Vinken and G.W. Bruyn, eds.), pp. 25–36. Elsevier, Amsterdam.

Huber, M. (1970). Spontaneous hypoliquorrhea: Seven observations. *Schweiz. Arch. Neurol. Neurochir. Psychiatry* 106:9–23.

Jaeckle, K.A. (1991). Clinical presentation and therapy of nervous system tumors. In *Neurology in Clinical Practice* (W.G. Bradley, R.B. Daroff, G.M. Fenichel, and C.D. Marsden, eds.), pp. 1008–1030. Butterworth-Heinemann, Boston.

Janny, P., J. Chazal, G. Colnet et al. (1981). Benign intracranial hypertension and disorders of CSF absorption. *Surg. Neurol.* 15:168–174.

Johnston, I. (1973). Reduced CSF absorption syndrome. Reappraisal of benign intracranial hypertension and related conditions. *Lancet* 2:2418–2421.

Johnston, I., S. Hawke, M. Kalmagyi, and C. Antyeo (1991). The pseudotumor syndrome. *Arch. Neurol.* 48:740–747.

Johnston, I. and A. Paterson (1974). Benign intracranial hypertension: II. CSF pressure and circulation. *Brain* 97:301–312.

Kase, E.S., J.P. Williams, D.A. Wyatt, and J.P. Mohr (1982). Lobar intracerebral hematomas: A clinical and CT analysis of 22 cases. *Neurology* 32:1146–1150.

Kieffer, S.A., J.M. Wolff, W.B. Prentice, and M.K. Loken (1971). Scinticisternography in individuals without known neurological disease. *Am. J. Roentgenol.* 112: 225–236.

Konig, P.J. and E.B. Charney (1982). Children with brain tumor headaches. *Am. J. Dis. Child. 136*:121-124.

Kraemer, G., H.C. Hanns, and D. Eissner (1987). CSF hyperabsorption: A cause of spontaneous low CSF pressure headache [abstract]. *Neurology 37*(Suppl. 1):238.

Kunkle, E.C., B.S. Ray, and H.G. Wolff (1942). Studies on headache: The mechanisms and significance of headache associated with brain tumor. *Bull. N.Y. Acad. Med. 18*:400.

Labadie, E.L., J.V. Antwerp, and C.R. Bamford (1976). Abnormal lumbar isotope cisternography in an unusual case of spontaneous hypoliquorrheic headache. *Neurology 26*:135-139.

Lasater, G.M. (1970). Primary intracranial hypotension. *Headache 10*:63-66.

Lavyne, M.H. and R.H. Patterson (1987). Headache and brain tumor. In *Wolff's Headache and Other Head Pain*, 5th ed., (D.J. Dalessio, ed.), pp. 343-349. Oxford University Press, New York.

Lee, T., N. Maynard, P. Anslow et al. (1991). Post-myelogram headache—physiological or psychological? *Neuroradiology 33*:155-158.

Lindquist, T. and E. Moberg (1949). Spontaneous hypoliquorrhea. *Acta Med. Scand. 132*:556-561.

Lipton, H.L. and P.E. Michelson (1972). Pseudotumor cerebri syndrome without papilledema. *JAMA 220*:1591-1592.

Loman, J. (1934). Components of cerebrospinal fluid pressure as affected by changes in posture. *Arch. Neurol. Psychiatry 31*:679-681.

Loman, J., A. Myerson, and D. Goldman (1935). Effects of alteration of posture on cerebrospinal fluid pressure. *Arch. Neurol. Psychiatry 33*:1279-1284.

Malm, J., B. Kristensen, P. Markgren, and J. Ekstedt (1992). CSF hydrodynamics in idiopathic intracranial hypertension: A long-term study. *Neurology 42*:851-858.

Marcelis, J. and S.D. Silberstein (1990). Spontaneous low cerebrospinal fluid pressure headache. *Headache 30*:192-196.

Marcelis, J. and S.D. Silberstein (1991). Idiopathic intracranial hypertension without papilledema. *Arch. Neurol. 48*:392-399.

Maxner, C.E., M.I. Freedman, and J.J. Corbett (1987). Asymmetric papilledema and visual loss in pseudotumor cerebri. *Can. J. Neurol. Sci. 14*:593-596.

Milhorat, T.H. (1972). *Hydrocephalus and the Cerebrospinal Fluid*. Williams & Wilkins, Baltimore.

Millette, P.C., A. Paqacz, and C. Charest (1982). Epidural blood patch for the treatment of chronic headache after myelography. *J. Assoc. Can. Radiol. 33*:236-238.

Mohr, J.P., L.R. Caplan, J.W. Melski et al. (1978). The Harvard Cooperative Stroke Registry: A prospective register. *Neurology 2*:754-762.

Molins, A., J. Alvarez, J. Somalla et al. (1990). Cisternographic pattern of spontaneous liquoral hypotension. *Cephalalgia 10*:59-65.

Murros, K. and R. Fogelholm (1983). Spontaneous intracranial hypotension with slit ventricles. *J. Neurol. Neurosurg. Psychiatry 46*:1149-1151.

Northfield, D.W.C. (1938). Some observations on headache. *Brain 61*:133.

Pannullo, S., J. Reich, and J. Posner (1992). Meningeal enhancement associated with low intracranial pressure. *Neurology 42*(Suppl. 3):430.

Parris, W.C.V. (1987). Use of epidural blood patch in treating chronic headache: Report of six cases. *Can. J. Anaesth. 34*:403-406.

Paterson, R., N. Depasquale, and S. Mann (1961). Pseudotumor cerebri. *Medicine (Baltimore) 40*:85-99.

Pepin, E.P. (1991). Symptomatic headache of recent onset posing as migraine with aura. *Headache Q. 2*:23-27.

Peterson, R.C., D.P. Freeman, C.A. Knox, and B.E. Gibson (1987). Successful treatment of spontaneous low cerebrospinal fluid pressure headache. [abstract]. *Ann. Neurol. 22:*148.

Rando, T.A. and R.A. Fishman (1992). Spontaneous intracranial hypotension: Report of two cases and review of the literature. *Neurology 42:*481–487.

Raskin, N.H. (1988). Headaches caused by alterations of structure or homeostasis. In *Headache,* 2nd ed., pp. 283–316. Churchill Livingstone, New York.

Raskin, N.H. (1990). Lumbar puncture headache: A review. *Headache 30:*197–200.

Rasmussen, B.S., L. Blom, P. Hansen, and S.J. Mikkelsen (1989). Postspinal headache in young and elderly patients. *Anesthesia 44:*571–573.

Ray, B.S. and H.G. Wolff (1940). Experimental studies on headache. Pain sensitive structures of the head and their significance in headache. *Arch. Surg. 41:*813–853.

Rossi, L.N. and F. Vassella (1989). Headache in children with brain tumor. *Childs Nerv. Syst. 5:*307–309.

Rushton, J.G. and E.D. Rooke (1962). Brain tumor headache. *Headache 2:*147–152.

Sable, S.G. and N.M. Ramadan (1991). Meningeal enhancement and low CSF pressure headache. An MRI study. *Cephalalgia 11:*275–276.

Sadun, A.A., J.N. Currie, and S. Lessell (1984). Transient visual obscurations with elevated optic discs. *Ann. Neurol. 16:*489–494.

Scanari, M., S. Mingrino, D. d'Avella, and V. DellaCort (1979). Benign intracranial hypertension without papilledema: A case report. *Neurosurgery 5:*376–377.

Schaltenbrand, G. (1938). Neure Anschauen zor Pathophysiologie der Liquorzirkulation. *Zentralb. Neurochir. 3:*290–300.

Sechzer, P.H. and L. Abel (1978). Post-spinal anesthesia headache treated with caffeine. Evaluation with demand method. Part 1. *Curr. Ther. Res. 24:*307–312.

Sergott, R.C., P.J. Savino, and T.M. Bosley (1988). Modified optic nerve sheath decompression provides long-term visual improvement for pseudotumor cerebri. *Arch. Ophthalmol. 106:*1384–1390.

Sharrock, N.E. (1980). Postural headache following thoracic somatic paranvertebral nerve block. *Anesthesiology 52:*360–362.

Sipe, J.C., J. Zyroff, and T.A. Waltz (1981). Primary intracranial hypotension and bilateral isodense subdural hematomas. *Neurology 31:*334–337.

Sismanis, A. (1987). Otologic manifestations of benign intracranial hypertension syndrome: Diagnosis and management. *Laryngoscope 97:*1–17.

Spence, J.D., A.L. Amacher, and N.R. Willis (1980). Benign intracranial hypertension without papilledema: Role of 24 hour cerebrospinal fluid pressure monitoring in diagnosis and management. *Neurosurgery 7:*326–336.

Torrey, E.F. (1979). Headaches after lumbar puncture and insensitivity to pain in psychiatric patients. *N. Engl. J. Med. 301:*111.

Tourtellote, W.W., A.F. Haerer, G.L. Heller et al. (1964). *Post-Lumbar Puncture Headaches.* Charles C Thomas, Springfield, IL.

Van Alphen, H.A.M. (1986). Migraine, a result of increased CSF pressure: A new pathophysiologic concept (preliminary report). *Neurosurg. Rev. 9:*121–124.

Vilming, S.T., H. Schrader, and I. Monstad (1989). The significance of age, sex, and cerebrospinal fluid pressure in post lumbar puncture headache. *Cephalalgia 9:*99–106.

Von Storch, T., A. Carmichael, and T. Banks (1937). Factors producing lumbar cerebrospinal fluid pressure in man in the erect position. *Arch. Neurol. Psychiatry 38:*1158.

Wald, S.L. (1989). Disorders of cerebrospinal fluid circulation and brain edema. In *Neurology in Clinical Practice* (W.G. Bradley, R.B. Daroff, G.M. Fenichel, and C.D. Marsden, eds.) pp. 1212–1213. Butterworth-Heineman, Boston.

Wall, M. (1990). The headache profile of idiopathic intracranial hypertension. *Cephalalgia 10*:331–335.

Wall, M. and D. George (1991). Idiopathic intracranial hypertension: A prospective study of 50 patients. *Brain 114*:155–180.

Weisberg, L.A. (1975). Benign intracranial hypertension. *Medicine 54*:197–207.

Zammarano, C.B., M.L. D'Ancona, and M.C. Miceli (1989). Headache and cerebral neoplasm in childhood. In *Headache in Children and Adolescents* (G. Lanzi, U. Balottin, and A. Cernibori, eds.), pp. 177–178. Elsevier, Amsterdam.

Zulch, K.J., H.D. Mennel, and V. Zimmerman (1974). Intracranial hypertension. In *Handbook of Clinical Neurology* (P.J. Vinken and G.W. Bruyn, eds.), Vol. 16 pp. 89–149. Elsevier, Amsterdam.

20

Life Stress, Personality Factors, and Reactions to Headache

RUSSELL C. PACKARD

Headache is a disorder of diverse etiology occurring in a variety of contexts. Life stress, personality factors, and the patient's own reactions to pain influence all headache sufferers. Each individual reacts to life stresses differently, and his or her unique personality influences the headache pattern. The same person may react to a headache differently at different times, at one time being able to take two aspirin and ignore the headache, and at another time fearing the worst and becoming totally incapacitated. The headache complaint always involves a dynamic balance between cause, sensation, and reaction for each individual (Packard, 1979a).

Living is a constant, dynamic process of responding to internal and external stimuli, pressures, and demands. An accurate evaluation of stress or personality factors in a headache patient is complicated by the changing susceptibility to these stimuli as patients grow and adapt to life's circumstances. Thus, these factors may exert an inconsistent and variable influence on headache attacks. At age 20, a perfectionistic patient might suppress feelings of anger that might trigger periodic migraine (and/or tension-type headache), but at age 30 that patient may be less perfectionistic and better able to express his or her feelings. Such adaptive changes could result in headache improvement (Saper, 1983). This variability makes it difficult to isolate the numerous emotional and biologic headache stressors. Most specialists agree, however, that careful attention to these influences is important in the evaluation and management of patients with headache. This chapter reviews these areas in detail.

LIFE STRESS AND HEADACHE

Physicians have long been aware that emotionally stressful factors could trigger headaches. In the late 1880s, Breuer and Freud (1955) noticed that complaints of headache often disappeared after patients reached an improved emotional equilibrium. Harold Wolff (1963), in his investigations on psychiatric factors in headache, wrote: "Since the human animal prides himself on 'using his head,' it is perhaps not without meaning that his head should be the source of so much discomfort . . . or that the vast majority of discomforts and pains of the head . . . are accompaniments of resentments and dissatisfactions" (preface).

The first five classification groups of the American Medical Association's Ad Hoc Committee on Classification of Headache (1962) encompassed those headaches that, in the committee's words, "may be the principle manifestation of temporary or sustained difficulties in life adjustment." These groups were vascular headaches of migraine type, muscle contraction headache, combined headache (vascular and muscle contraction), headache of nasal vasomotor reaction, and headaches of delusional, conversion, or hypochondriacal states. "Temporary or sustained difficulties in life adjustment" could easily be termed "life stress."

The primary purpose of the new international classification developed by the Headache Classification Committee of the International Headache Society (IHS) (1988) was research, so operational diagnostic criteria were made as specific and sensitive as possible. The IHS committee acknowledged the difficulty involved in classifying an entity that has no objective laboratory tests or physical findings. Consequently, even tension-type headache is classified by descriptive criteria (quality of pain, tenderness of pericranial muscles, etc.) and diagnostic criteria (number of episodes, duration of attacks, etc.). Mechanisms of this type of headache were for the most part considered unknown, but in many cases "psychogenic etiologies are suspected." Previously used terms for the tension-type headache classification were tension headache, muscle contraction headache, stress headache, and psychogenic headache, among others. Aggravating factors such as stress generally were not discussed for individual headache types, including migraine. Headaches occurring as "temporary or sustained difficulties in life adjustment" were simply not addressed. Searching the new classification for the role of "psychosocial stress" or "anxiety" in headache, the reader is referred to the Definition of Terms section of the *Diagnostic and Statistical Manual of Mental Disorders* (3rd ed., revised) (American Psychiatric Association, 1987).

Stress has been variously defined. Rose and Gawel (1979) have commented, "Stress is one of the most misused words in the English language and its precise meaning is often forgotten." They define it from the Oxford Dictionary as simply "a demand upon energy." They believe this is a difficult concept to apply to the human body and not a factor that can easily be measured. Selye (1976) defined stress as "the non-specific response of the body to any demand made upon it." Schafer (1983) modified this definition slightly by defining stress as "an arousal of mind and body in response to demands made upon it."

A common thread in these definitions seems to be the word "demand." It seems clear that one cannot go through life without certain demands being placed on energy, body, and/or mind. Stress is an ever-present, universal part of life. We constantly think, feel, and act with some degree of arousal. It cannot be avoided. Response to stress involves virtually every set of organs and tissues in the body, and thoughts and feelings are clearly intertwined with physiologic processes. Behavior such as being short tempered, fast talking, or accident prone may also be an outward expression of stress.

The concept of stress often carries a negative connotation of "something harmful that should be avoided." This is not always the case, however, because arousal of heart rate, blood pressure, muscle tension, and perception is intrinsically neither helpful nor harmful but simply a fact of life. The effects of stress, however, can become either positive or negative. Positive stress can be useful in a wide range of circumstances, from helping us respond with strength and quickness to avoid a car accident to helping us meet a deadline or take an examination. The challenge, then, is not to "avoid stress" but to learn the danger signals and symptoms so that it can be more effectively managed.

When the level of arousal becomes too high (or too low), either temporarily or chronically, then positive stress can give way to distress (Schafer, 1983). This type of situation may lead to stress-related symptoms such as trembling hands, churning stomach, tight shoulders, edginess, or poor concentration. If a person ignores or "doesn't listen to" these early warning symptoms, they may become chronic and trigger several stress-related illnesses, such as migraine, tension-type headache, peptic ulcer disease, irritable colon, or high blood pressure. It is important to bear in mind that reactions to stress are a function of perception, experiences, social support systems, and one's capacity to respond adequately or adapt (Christensen, 1981). One's reaction to both stress and headache may be biologically determined (see Chapter 3).

The psychophysiologic mechanisms whereby migraine and tension-type headaches may develop are more fully discussed in the chapters dealing with these specific headache types. The manner in which stress provokes migraine is still unclear, as is the reason some attacks occur after a period of prolonged stress and not during the period of stress (Saper, 1983). Simply stated, stress can contribute to headache development in three ways: (1) intense reaction to stress may be a biologic marker for headache; (2) stress may produce long-term "wear and tear," producing changes in neurotransmitter function and receptor density; or (3) stress may alter central nociception (stress can produce either hypo- or hyperalgesia). This effect may account for aggravation of a pre-existing headache.

In a longitudinal study of 114 tension and migraine headache subjects (Jones, 1989), the relationship between the stressors of everyday life and headaches was evaluated. The results suggested that stressful events of everyday life may be causally related to headache onset and to increases in headache intensity; appraising stressful events as amenable to change and engaging in a broad range of coping responses may reduce the occurrence of headache in the face of those events; and failure to recognize the personal significance of a stressful event and the absence of a strong emotional response may render the individual vulnerable to a subsequent headache attack. These results were considered to strengthen the rationale for the continued application of stress management techniques to the control of recurrent headache.

The line between psychological distress symptoms and psychiatric illness often is not distinct. Symptoms tend to shade gradually into more serious states of anxiety or depression. Psychological distress symptoms frequently accompany physical illness or headache because of the intricate interplay of mind and body. This topic is discussed further in the last section of the chapter.

Evaluation of Stress

Emotionally stressful factors may trigger headache, and the intensity of reaction to stress may be a comorbid condition associated with headache. Unfortunately, stressful issues are often clouded over, presented in a vague manner, or concealed by patients. Although at times the patient is truly unaware of stressful events, often he or she is aware of stress but believes the physician will not be interested or does not have time. Patients also may perceive such complaints as a sign of weakness (Brodsky, 1984). Some physicians may, in fact, want to avoid this type of evaluation because it does take time, involvement with the patient, and some awareness of life stress factors and issues (Packard, 1983). Lance (1981) believes that careful attention must be given to the patient as a person and to his or her environment at work and at home in an attempt to prevent unnecessary fluctuations in stress or emotional tone. The physician must be aware of some common and high risk stressors, because patients frequently are unaware of these factors and their role in symptom formation.

Change
One of the major factors to consider is unpredictability and change (Brett, 1980). This may involve social change, referring to the environment in which the patient lives and works, or personal change in an individual's life, such as moving, changing jobs, getting older, retiring, or becoming more assertive (Schafer, 1983). Toffler (1971), in *Future Shock,* discussed the accelerating pace of social change in our current age with increased population growth and crowding, rapid technologic growth, and new knowledge. In such a rapidly changing world, more frequent and faster adjustments are needed and more stress can set in.

Even though human beings have an excellent capacity to adjust and adapt to change, this varies depending on the individual (Schafer, 1978). We also can easily delude ourselves into believing that we are adapting simply because we feel "comfortable" with a highly demanding job, the fast pace of our life, or a bad marriage. This apparent adjustment is really not successful adaptation. In time our bodies give way in one form or another. Selye (1976) maintained that our deep adaptive reserves are limited and can be used up. It is important to note how frequent a "change" in one's headache pattern may reflect a change in one's circumstances or life situation.

Life Pace
It is important to get some concept of the patient's pace of life. Patients are frequently overloaded, always trying to cram more into each hour, day, or week. A good example is the so-called Type A personality, who is driven to accomplish as much as possible in the shortest possible time (Dembrosky et al., 1978). He or she is often chronically impatient with "wasted time" and the slow pace of others. Friedman and Rosenman (1974) pointed out that American

culture places a high value on speed, numbers, and accomplishments. It is not unusual for these patients to outwardly present as "free of stress" because they have deluded themselves into believing they are race horses. However, a fast pace of life without pause for rest can be a significant source of tension, stress, and distress that may lead to headache symptoms or a change in headache pattern. Some headache patients will report two jobs, a divorce, family responsibilities, church duties, community activities, and no awareness of stress. Interestingly, although these patients are seeking explanations for and relief from headache, they frequently will not have time for doctor appointments, biofeedback, or biofeedback practice.

Transitions

Another type of experience that frequently causes distress is transition from one set of habits to another. This is similar to and actually represents a form of change, but every change requires a transition, and transition requires an adjustment. These factors even have been quantitated to some extent by the Holmes-Rahe social readjustment rating scale (1967). For instance, a geographic move, even to a better job or a nicer neighborhood, still represents a change from the familiar to the unfamiliar. A promotion involves a role transition. Marriage, divorce, and remarriage are common transitional stressful factors. Also, becoming a parent or a student can bring about major life-style changes. A serious loss can be a very traumatic occurrence, especially the loss of a spouse or home. Even retirement may represent a type of loss. Whatever the loss, people pass through remarkably similar steps of mourning (Horowitz, 1976).

Many studies have documented the contribution of individual life changes to physical and psychological distress (Rahe, 1979). Another common pattern among highly stressed patients, however, involves too much change in too short a time. A growing number of studies have shown that the greater the clustering of life events, the greater the chance of developing symptoms or becoming ill (Garrity et al., 1977; Rahe, 1968). Again, patients with headaches will often present with a "laundry list" of recent changes, transitions, and events all clustered together with little awareness of the role these may be playing in their headache symptom formation.

Work Stress, Role Conflicts, and Expectations

A recent comprehensive review by Brodsky (1984) of 2,000 patients over an 18-year period discussed work stress and its role as a stressor. Exploring a patient's feelings about his or her job situation and role in life is very important. A role is the cluster of expectations associated with a social or work position, such as teacher, student, husband, or neighbor. When someone's desires conflict with the expectations of others, a role conflict may result. Probably the most common example of this is a job problem in which a person is unable or unwilling to do what others expect because he or she may want something different or his or her skills do not fit the situation. Conflicting expectations almost always create stress.

The expectations of a patient with headache are equally important to clarify, especially if the patient is expecting or hoping for "total relief." This expectation is rarely expressed verbally but frequently expressed on a patient history form (Packard, 1987). Patients with headache may also be expecting or wanting something from the doctor other than what the doctor expects, such as an explanation of the cause of headache rather than pain relief (Packard, 1979b). These are important issues to clarify.

The physical environment is often taken for granted, but noise has been noted to be perhaps the most troublesome and common of all stressors in the physical environment. Girdano and Everly (1979) pointed out that noise can produce a stress response in three ways: by causing physiologic reactions from stimulation of the sympathetic nervous system, by being annoying and subjectively displeasing, and by disrupting ongoing activities. Another distressing stressor in the physical environment may be improper lighting (Ivancevich and Matteson, 1980). The increased amount of time spent by many individuals in front of a computer screen can also be quite irritating, and can aggravate or even precipitate some headaches. Temperature at either extreme also can have direct and indirect effects on stress.

Other Stressors

Other important areas of stress include understimulation (Schafer, 1983), social isolation or loneliness (Berkman and Syne, 1976), financial uncertainty or unemployment, and a number of minor but irritating "daily hassles." These "daily hassles," according to Lazarus (1981), may do the most damage of all. They frequently involve concern about weight, health of a family member, rising prices, home maintenance, and overwork. Neurotic lifestyles can also lead to chronic or intermittent stressful situations, such as when patients' fear of failure, fear of success, or perception of what they think they should be is in conflict with what they actually are. Patients who are rigid and perfectionistic have their own problems and difficulties. These are discussed in the section on Personality Factors in Headache.

When Patients Deny Stress

Many patients who present with headache initially deny having any emotional difficulties or any stress in their lives. This should not discourage the examiner from a careful evaluation of the patient's situation preceding or accompanying the onset of headache. The factors noted above should be listened for carefully. The coincidence of a major change or an acute emotional state and the appearance of headache is quite suggestive, even if the connection between the psychological event and the symptom is unrecognized by the patient (Packard, 1980). Does a headache "always" occur on weekends? A situation like this should be explored in detail (Nattero et al., 1989). At times a relative or close friend may clarify many confusing areas, whereas further direct questioning of the patient will probably be of little benefit. Patients must essentially be allowed to tell their own stories at their own rates. It is often helpful to have the patient begin keeping a headache diary, so that he or she may report events before and during a headache and grade the headache's intensity. This may enable him or her to develop an awareness of feelings or situations that were previously ignored or denied. It also can be useful for evaluating treatment. Another simple but effective technique to learn about the headache patient as a person is to ask the patient to "write about himself [herself]" (Bana et al., 1988).

The examiner should be alert for clues concerning psychological stresses that may be related to the patient's difficulties. An angry rejection or denial of possible psychologic factors is in itself evidence of underlying emotional conflict. Some people simply are not in touch with their inner needs and feelings, however, and find it difficult to verbalize them. Sometimes even a colloquial phrase used by a patient may be helpful in discovering areas of conflict or difficulty. The author recently explored in detail a remark by several headache patients that they had "a really good one [headache]" (Packard et al., 1989). The headache often turned out to be "good" in a relative sense, in that it had somehow served to help the patient avoid a more unpleasant emotional situation.

Indirect questioning may help bring the psychological factors to light. Ask the patient what he or she does for fun. It is surprising how many patients who describe a wonderful and problem free life cannot think of a single thing that is fun. This realization will often open an important doorway to emotional issues. Ask whether the patient has ever known anyone with a similar type of headache problem. The answer may reveal unconscious attitudes about the patient's own situation and clues concerning the origin. Ask what the headache keeps the patient from doing. This may provide material concerning the psychodynamic significance of the symptoms as well as the secondary gain. It is equally important to find out how the spouse reacts to the patient's headache. One of two patterns may emerge: a spouse who is an understanding and sympathetic caretaker, or just the opposite, one who totally lacks sympathy and understanding. It may be helpful to ask if the patient is concerned about a brain tumor, a common fear that is seldom expressed spontaneously.

PERSONALITY FACTORS IN HEADACHE

Personality factors have been intensively studied in migraine because it is a fairly well-defined syndrome. The thinking about personality factors in migraine has gone through an interesting evolutionary process over the years. Early studies in the 1930s and 1940s were heavily psychoanalytic; then, as the varied and interesting vascular and biochemical discoveries came to light, migraine became "psychosomatic" (Pearce, 1977) and the physiologic aspects seemed to become more central. In the past 10 years there has been a tendency to split into two camps. One group paid scant attention to personality factors, as was evidenced in *Advances in Migraine Research and Therapy* (Rose, 1982), which did not contain a single paragraph on personality factors. Others in the "organic" camp considered headache to be "perturbed serotonergic neurotransmission" (Raskin, 1988). The other camp would quietly try to remind their colleagues that headaches occur in people for many different reasons (Adler et al., 1987). Recently there have been signs that the camps are beginning to blend together again. In an elegant article comparing and contrasting the neural and vascular theories of migraine, Blau (1990) reported how many symptoms during the premonitory phase, such as yawning, food craving, tiredness, and mood change, may reflect a hypothalamic dysfunction. In the end, "drugs provide only one aspect of treating some patients; other patients need . . . reassurance, or the opportunity to confide in or share feelings with another human being" (Blau, 1990).

It is clear that personality factors are important to consider in all headache sufferers. As noted elsewhere in this chapter, every headache is a multifactorial symptom occurring in a person with a unique personality. The headache is not an abstraction with an existence in a pool of chemicals or blood vessels. Even if headaches are caused primarily by hereditary and/or physiologic factors, treatment must still be directed for the most part to the person suffering from the headache (Lance, 1981; Packard, 1979a). This section reviews personality factors and their role in headache.

Personality Factors and Migraine

Early Studies
In 1743, Junkerius wrote that the primary cause of migraine is anger, especially when it is tacit and suppressed (Jonckheere, 1971). This theme echoes regularly through the early case studies of migraine patients. In an early study, Touraine and Draper (1934) suggested that it may be possible to identify a "constitutional" personality susceptible to migraine, with retarded emotional development but superior intelligence, frequent exaggerated dependence on the mother, and rather unsatisfactory sexual adjustment.

Knopf (1935), in a detailed study of 30 cases of migraine, described migraineurs as being "dignified," very ambitious, reserved, repressed, sensitive, domineering, resentful of authority, and, perhaps the most serious defect, possessing very little sense of humor. Fromm-Reichman (1937), in describing a series of eight patients treated by psychoanalysis, related the etiology of migraine to envious hostile impulses, often followed by guilt and turned back against the self.

Wolff (1937), in a paper on personality features and reactions of subjects with migraine, described these persons as compulsive, perfectionistic, rigid, ambitious, competitive, unable to delegate responsibility, and chronically resentful. Selinsky (1939) described migraine as particularly frequent in women with intellectual abilities and inhibited behavior, commonly the harried housewife. Trowbridge et al. (1943) believed the patient with migraine was deliberate, often to the point of displaying hesitation that rendered decisions difficult. It was difficult for these patients to face new situations, and frequently they had an exaggerated feeling of personal insecurity. Marcussen (1949) and Alexander (1950) related the occurrence of migraine to suppressed resentment and anger or a state of repressed rage.

In the 1950s, although several studies continued to stress the inflexible, perfectionistic, rigid, resentful, and ambitious personality pattern of migraineurs (Weiss and English, 1957), Friedman and Brenner (1950) commented that the relationship to suppressed anger was not entirely specific and that other conflicts might occasionally precipitate a migraine attack. Friedman (1958) went on to state that he believed that personality manifestations were extremely variable in migraine patients and may include a variety of emotional factors, most of which are unconscious. They may be hostility, identification with a family figure, the wish to remain in a position of dependency, or a means to gain love, affection, or attention. The most frequent conflicts concerned hostile impulses associated with feelings of guilt. There was little evidence of specificity of the precipitating or psychodynamic factors. Friedman concluded that not all patients with migraine were compulsive, perfectionistic, or rigid.

Kolb (1963) believed that the majority of migraine patients seen by psychiatrists showed a rigid form of behavior in which they denied the expression of direct or verbal aggression. These patients often came from families who took great pride in attainment. In a dynamic formulation, the consequence of the arousal of conflict, with associated anxiety over inevitably emerging hostility (while trying to maintain the family standards as a means of continuing the desired relationships), formed the interpersonal matrix that triggered the headache. Boag (1968) reviewed these early studies in detail and summarized a wide range of personality characteristics that could be described in patients suffering from migraine. There seemed to be general agreement that repressed anger was a major common factor. However, Boag believed there was considerable evidence that this is not always true and that other emotional states, particularly anxiety or depression, may be equally important in some cases. Many of these conclusions are subject to selection bias (i.e., patients with headache who consult with psychiatrists) and the lack of adequate control groups.

Recent Studies

Jonckheere (1971) noted that 11 of 16 "typical" patients with migraine headaches were obsessional, aggressive, or both, and that their aggression, along with their headaches, had a tendency to disappear when psychotherapy permitted the expression of underlying emotional states. Using detailed histories and psychometric tests in a controlled study of 100 patients with migraine, Henryk-Gutt and Rees (1973) found that emotional stress was important, because over half of their subjects suffered their first migraine attacks during a period of emotional stress. However, there was no objective evidence that the subjects experienced greater stress than the controls. They concluded that migraine subjects were predisposed by constitutional factors (and not by environmental factors) to experience a greater than average reaction to a given quantity of stress. They were unable to confirm that migraine subjects were especially obsessional or ambitious and suggested that previous studies were insufficiently comprehensive because the groups studied were self-selected and not fully representative of migraine subjects in general.

In a review study, Phillips (1976) concluded that there was only minimal support for the view that migraine sufferers were more neurotic than age-matched normal subjects. In a random sample of 1,500 patients in a general practice, he found 39 migraine patients, 24 tension-type headache patients, and

5 with migraine and tension-type headaches. No significant group differences were found in neuroticism, extroversion, or psychotic behavior. These cases, collected without reference to a headache complaint, cannot be distinguished from normal subjects.

In a review of four studies using the Minnesota Multiphasic Personality Inventory (MMPI) (Martin, 1972; Martin et al., 1967; Rogado et al., 1974; Steinhilber et al., 1960), 325 subjects with various types of headache complaints showed a common profile characterized by a "conversion V." This suggested that the patients' anxiety was being held in check by compulsive defenses and expressed by somatic complaints. Although psychological factors may be a cause of or provide a predisposition to headache, it has been suggested that neuroticism observed in headache patients may be a consequence of the risks of sudden intense pain or of adaptation to being a patient.

One recent MMPI study (Invernizzi et al., 1989) explored the correlation of headache duration and neurotic personality traits. The results from 418 patients with migraine, tension-type, and mixed headaches showed no correlation between any of the MMPI scale scores and duration of illness. Patients with mixed headaches did show significantly elevated scores on the MMPI scales, and the authors hypothesized that the role of personality characteristics in this group of subjects could play a significant role in the transition from a simple to a mixed headache pattern.

The role of psychopathology and/or personality variables in the etiology of chronic headaches has been discussed for many years. It has consistently been found that chronic headache patients show significant elevations on a variety of parameters for psychopathology in comparison to nonheadache populations (Andrasik et al., 1982; Blanchard et al., 1984; Kudrow, 1979; Sternbach et al., 1980). The question has been whether these personality disturbances predispose a patient to or somehow "cause" chronic headaches to develop or are they the consequence of living with chronic head pain for years. Blanchard et al. (1989) analyzed psychological test results of 492 chronic headache patients and found no support for the hypothesis that headache "causes" psychopathology. There was modest support for the hypothesis that psychopathology "causes" headache.

Recent studies indicate the absence of a discreet border between migraine and tension-type headache (Cohen, 1978). In a controlled study of personality in headache types by Passchier et al. (1984), there was very little difference in personality factors among migraine and tension-type headache patients. Achievement motivation was found to be elevated in both headache groups. The tension-type headache patients also exhibited greater rigidity in comparison to the migraine headache group and to the controls, a finding not reported in earlier studies. Both headache groups showed higher achievement motivation, rigidity, and fear of failure than controls. (Recent epidemiologic evidence does not support these conclusions [see Chapter 3] and suggests that Passchier et al.'s conclusion may be a selection artifact.) No evidence was found for higher prevalence of neuroticism or obsessive-compulsive behavior in the headache groups.

An interesting study to be mindful of when soliciting subjects for headache research (especially in regard to exploring personality factors) through media advertisements is that of McAnulty et al. (1986). Their MMPI findings provide strong evidence that research subjects who are prompt to respond to limited media coverage requesting headache research participants exhibit significantly higher levels of psychopathology than later volunteers. The elevated MMPI scores could not simply be attributed to a more severe headache experience. Questions also have been raised about whether private headache clinics might attract a "different psychological crowd" than a university research setting. In a comparison of just such a situation, no differences were observed between settings (Blanchard et al., 1990).

In summary, it is difficult to derive a concise statement regarding personality factors in migraine. In broad terms, migraine seems to represent a neurovascular mechanism for coping with stressful life situations. It is probable that many stresses—social, economic, and psychological—may activate this unique neurovascular response. Some of the factors described may be very important in some patients and of lesser importance in others. If these personality factors are identified, they can be useful in the evaluation and management of these patients. As an example, a structured individual who has migraine attacks only on Saturday mornings may be helped by having him arise a bit earlier or plan his weekend activity in advance. Other patients may be able to deal with accumulating tension and repressed or suppressed hostility up to a certain point, but beyond this they cannot continue, and a headache may ensue that forces the patient to a halt.

It is clear that awareness of personality characteristics and the stresses that provoke or aggravate the migraine response is essential to effective treatment. The physician has a unique opportunity to assist the patient in modifying his or her responses to the external factors he or she considers stressful, and also, more importantly, to change the patient's reaction to any unrealistically rigid internal demands that may be present.

Personality Factors and Other Headache Types

Tension-Type Headache

Chronic tension-type headaches are associated with tension, anxiety, depression, repressed hostility, unresolved dependency needs, or psychosexual conflicts (Saper, 1983). One can see that many of the personality factors discussed in the previous sections also are associated with tension-type headache development, although the actual mechanisms are still unclear (Lance, 1981). These may be the most common headaches seen in medical practice and are often demonstrably associated with or occur with emotional stress or tension (Packard, 1979a, 1983). Friedman (1958) found emotional factors to be present in 100% of his patients with tension-type headaches.

One of the difficulties in delineating personality factors in cases of tension-type headache has been the vague and ambiguous terminology applied prior to the new IHS criteria. Terms such as "psychogenic," "nervous," and "tension" have been used in different senses by different authors (Blumenthal, 1968). The term "psychogenic headache" has been shown by at least one study to be variously defined and neither precise nor diagnostic (Packard, 1976). There always seems to be some doubt as to whether tension implies emotional or muscle tension.

Graham (1964) believed that a deep-seated reflex, apparently little altered by evolution, underlies tension-type headache. He compared the turtle shrugging back its head and the ape pulling its head down between its shoulders in the face of fear or danger to what people now do before the "slings and arrows of outrageous fortune." This may occur in occupational settings, attempts to reduce the pain of a migraine headache, or painful disorders of the neck, but occurs most often as part of a total reaction against psychological pressures. Although it seems clear that these headaches often are related to environmental stress, anxiety, or strongly repressed or suppressed anger, there does not seem to be any clear personality type or profile associated with them. Adler et al. (1987) have done a thorough review.

Patients with chronic tension-type headache frequently overuse medication and revert to episodic headache when the overuse is eliminated. With reduction of drug overuse, not only headache but depression frequently improves, suggesting a common causation for both conditions.

Cluster Headache

Cluster headaches seem to occur more often in men who drink and smoke more than the average male (Kudrow, 1979). Psychological tests and MMPI studies on a series of cluster headache patients demonstrated high scores on traits such as conscientiousness, perseverence, responsibility, self-sufficiency, precision, and resourcefulness; the patients were also found to be tense, frustrated, driven, and overwrought (Kudrow, 1979). MMPI results from patients with migraine and cluster headaches are almost indistinguishable (Kudrow, 1983).

A more detailed study of a small number of cluster headache patients demonstrated obsessive-compulsive behavior traits in aggressive, hard-driving, goal-oriented men. These men seemed to push themselves until they faltered because of the symptoms or until they reached their set goals, at which time they often collapsed with a seige of headache. Many times it was noted that a cluster seemed to begin during or just after stressful events in the person's life (Graham, 1968). Graham also described facial characteristics shared by many cluster headache patients and identified the leonine facial appearance. Observations have also suggested the presence of sustained stress and/or rage that may provoke a bout of episodic cluster, and a disturbance of sleep and mood may also occur prior to the onset of the headaches (Kudrow, 1980).

Some believe that the cluster headache patient may display the most deep-seated emotional difficulties of all (Adler et al., 1987). Cluster patients will not acknowledge these difficulties and will invariably deny them. The typical cluster patient is often an "iron-clad man." There are frequently severe and overwhelming early losses, often of a parent. According to Graham (1990), some of these patients give histories of strenuous attempts to please parents or other authorities in their childhood years, only to be rewarded with disfavor or even physical violence. It is remarkable that, in describing these occurrences, cluster headache patients show little feeling. They seem to have shut off the most upsetting emotional experiences of their lives behind a steel door. They do not betray intense emotion because they do not consciously feel intense emotion, but when the cluster headache begins! . . . then there is tearing, thrashing, overwhelming agitation, depression, aggression, and sometimes even suicide. These problems are so well repressed and the affect is so isolated from awareness that they may be undetectable on the MMPI. These patients are often extremely resistant to traditional forms of psychotherapy but may be helped with a less confrontive type of treatment, along with medical treatment.

REACTIONS TO HEADACHE

Illness has the capacity to initiate strong regressive tendencies in an individual (MacKinnon and Michels, 1971). Whereas one patient may submit to these tendencies by lapsing into a helpless and dependent state, another may deny and/or try to hide his or her symptoms and insist on maintaining usual activity. If headaches become long lasting, chronic, or severely disabling, they may provoke a variety of psychological reactions in the patient and his or her family. This section considers some common patterns of reaction among patients with headache. An awareness by the physician of these patterns can lead to improved treatment planning and management of patients with headache problems.

Personality and Emotional Reactions to Headache

Any major change in an individual's body functioning and way of living requires adaptation. Headache often represents a change that is unplanned, unscheduled, and unwanted, as well as producing pain and possibly other symptoms that may make adaptation difficult. The individual's reaction to this type of problem often depends on several factors, but especially important is his or her own basic personality and the degree to which he or she has responded successfully to previous life stresses. Basic personality structure has become an important element in the psychological management of any patient who is physically ill, even when the patient is psychologically a normal, well-functioning person (Kahana and Bibring, 1964). Naturally, if there is a marked accentuation of character traits, neurotic or psychotic symptoms, limited capacity for work, or impaired ability for social relationships, treatment becomes more difficult.

The basic nature and severity of the headache is also important, including its actual meaning and symbolic significance to the patient. Many laymen still look at the head and brain as synonymous (Kolb, 1959). The family dynamics for coping play an important role, as do situational demands from the patient's environment, such as level of responsibility and work. Expectations of both the patient and the physician are also important, especially if the patient is hoping for or expecting total relief (Packard, 1987). In addition, even a well-designed treatment regimen will fail without patient compliance. In one of the few studies to investigate adherence by patients treated for recurrent headache disorders,

Packard and O'Connell (1986) found that over 50% of headache sufferers failed to adhere to drug treatment regimens. Reasons for noncompliance are many, but some reflect patients' reactions to and attitudes about their headache problem. Sometimes a brief educational intervention designed to address the problem of patient adherence may yield significant improvements in standard therapies (Holyroyd et al., 1989).

Fortunately, most headaches are minor, short-lived, and self-limited symptoms that impose little or no actual disability, and anxiety is self-limited; however, headache can become disabling, both physically and emotionally. It can drain an individual's energy, cause lost time at work, disrupt the family, and lead to medication overuse or abuse (Mathew, 1987). Anxiety generalized by more significant headache or poor coping ability may even interfere sufficiently with the patient's adaptive capacity that he or she will be unable to participate in the management of his or her own care or headache problem (Horenstein, 1983). Simple anxiety in headache patients usually responds well to reassurance, a good physician–patient relationship, and a period of well-being or stability of the underlying headache symptom (Graham, 1987). The more a patient's life has changed, however, the more overwhelming the emotional response is likely to be, and certain types of reaction can often be defined. The most common of these are denial, depression, hostility, anger, and dependency (Horenstein, 1983).

Denial

Denial is not uncommon as a reaction to illness (Weinstein and Kahn, 1955). Denying the extent of one's symptoms by withdrawal may temporarily relieve the attendant anxiety. Denial may also protect the patient from painful reality by delaying necessary steps in diagnosis and treatment. For instance, many headache patients continue to work while feeling ill with a headache, continue a hectic pace that may aggravate their symptoms, or may not have time to see their doctor or take their medication. This type of reaction may actually be part of the underlying process that causes or precipitates some headaches. In a sense, it is "easier" for the patient to get a headache or have one get worse than to deal with underlying fears, concerns, guilt, or harsh expectations. A patient may also delay treatment by seeking other medical advice, trying fads, or rejecting advice or medication.

Denial may also be coupled with projection, and the patient may externalize the cause for his or her discomfort by blaming family members or even the physician. By this mechanism, the patient may deny his or her own role as causative in an auto or industrial accident that produced a post-traumatic headache. It may serve as a barrier to the patient's acceptance of his or her diagnosis, assumption of responsibility for participation in his or her own care, and involvement in long-term planning. These difficulties frequently arise with headache patients who are searching for a cure or total relief, despite explanations and the definition of realistic goals. Patients may even nod in understanding, only to call back in 2 days, reporting, "the headache isn't gone." Another common difficulty is the patient who is continually searching for "the cause," despite adequate evaluation, testing, and reassurance.

For the most part, denial tends to disappear with time and requires little special treatment other than careful explanation and understanding on the part of the physician. When one is confronted with a patient who is actively in a period of denial, it is often fruitless and frustrating to demand the patient's involvement in planning or participation in headache management. Prolonged or severe degrees of explicit denial may require psychotherapeutic intervention, which the patient may reject. These situations may occur if there is hypochondriasis, in which the patient has a poor sense of self-worth and turns to the physician to obtain what is not solidly established by the spouse or family (Adler, 1981). These patients will often be demanding, searching, complaining, and unresponsive to explanations and treatment measures.

A patient presenting with a continuous or chronic headache and denial of any emotional and interpersonal difficulties, idealization of family relationships, excessive activity prior to the onset of the headache, and excessive passivity after the onset of headache would fit a profile of "pain-prone disorder," as described by Blumer and Heilbronn (1981). These pain-prone patients are often not candidates for psychotherapy and are best managed in a pain or headache clinic, where a treatment team consistently de-emphasizes pain from headache, encourages activity, and slowly eliminates treatment with analgesics (Blumer, 1986). Denial also represents a key feature in conversion headache, in which the patient may complain bitterly about headache but seem affectually indifferent (Packard, 1980).

Depression

Depression is a common reaction to chronic headache, but depression and headache are prevalent clinical problems that often coincide (Diamond, 1985). One may antedate the other or they may appear simultaneously. Depression may occur in a "realistic sense" when the patient is aware of his or her limitations with headache and its direct effect on his or her life, or it may be enhanced by the many symbolic meanings that the patient may attach to his or her problem. These reactions may vary considerably from one patient to another and vary with each individual's situation. For instance, a migraine headache with a 5-minute visual aura may provoke considerable anxiety and depression in an airline pilot, who anticipates occupational disability and dependency. This type of situation in a laborer would most likely be of trivial meaning. The symbolic meaning of headache invariably plays some part in the patient's reaction to illness.

The under-recognition of pain and depression has been highlighted by the effectiveness of antidepressants in treating pain with or without accompanying depression. It is an increasing practice of pain centers or headache clinics to focus on the diagnosis of depression and to treat the condition with antidepressant medication. It is not clear whether depression is simply a psychological consequence of the pain or headache experience, or represents part of a reverberating circuit between pain and depression, or is an aspect of a fundamental psychobiologic disorder (Lindsay and Wyckoff, 1981).

Recent epidemiologic evidence suggests that migraine, anxiety, depression, and panic disorder are comorbid conditions. Subjects with anxiety in early life may later develop migraine and then depression and may have an increased risk of panic disorder and suicide (see Chapter 3). Whatever the precise mechanisms involved, mounting evidence suggests that headache and depression are best viewed as a single entity rather than a condition in which each aspect is merely a symptom of the other. Further aspects of depression in headache and the biochemistry of affective disorders in headache can be found elsewhere in this book.

Hostility, Anger, and Dependency

Hostility and anger may dominate one's reaction to headache. Many patients with headache have difficulty expressing angry or hostile feelings. Frequently these feelings emerge as a reaction to a headache (i.e., the patient is angry because he or she has a headache or because there is no cure). In this situation the patient's family and/or physician may be the object of this displaced anger. If patients have difficulty expressing their feelings, their behavior may become passive–aggressive, they may become depressed, and/or their headache may become worse.

An underlying quality of anger is common when the headache is post-traumatic in nature (Massey and Scherokman, 1983). The patient may blame others entirely for his or her difficulty and deny his or her own responsibility or negligence. He or she may try to punish those responsible for the difficulty through lawsuits. Gain or search for compensation may become a predominant element in the patient's reaction to post-traumatic headache, although this is not a problem in all post-traumatic headache patients (Speed, 1985). As long as these issues of anger and denial remain unresolved, the patient is likely to remain symptomatic, respond poorly to management, and develop new symptoms, especially in response to treatment.

Dealing with a patient's anger requires more patience and thoughtfulness than many physicians can muster (Groves, 1978). In treatment, the psychological issues should be defined as clearly as possible, appropriate investigations should be conducted, and a therapeutic contract established with the patient in which therapeutic goals are mutually defined and pursued.

The development of dependency and the abandonment of efforts at independence frequently complicate long-term headache problems. Dependency reactions can often be anticipated when patients have a past history of passivity and immaturity. Once established, these reactions are difficult to manage. The patient who reacted initially with depression may also evolve into one who is quite dependent.

A hostile patient will often elicit a reciprocal feeling of anger in the physician that may lead to distancing from or rejection of the patient (Gorlin and Zucker, 1983). Such behavior only intensifies the patient's reaction. A coping strategy would be to simply acknowledge and analyze the patient's anger, use behavioral approaches, and not attempt to like the unlikable patient. If the situation is intolerable, the patient is best transferred to another physician.

Comments

The management of emotional reactions to headache is based on a good patient–physician relationship. It may be helpful for the physician to realize that the patient's emotional reaction is not conscious or voluntary. Also, to some degree the family and others in the environment participate in the development and management of the emotional disorder. As effective treatment is instituted and physical improvement ensues, the emotional reactions tend to become less severe. In patients with persistent denial, depression, hostility, or dependency, a psychiatric evaluation or psychotherapy should be considered.

SUMMARY

The intertwining factors of life stress, personality factors, and reaction to headache affect all headache sufferers. An accurate evaluation of these factors is often difficult because most patients experience a changing susceptibility to these stimuli as they grow and adapt, resulting in an inconsistent and variable influence on headache attacks. Despite this, careful attention to these factors is important for effective evaluation and management of headache patients.

Emotionally stressful factors are often clouded over or denied by headache patients. Life stresses such as change, life pace, transitions, work stress, role conflict, and differing expectations of patients and physicians and their role in symptom formation must be evaluated.

Personality factors in migraine have been studied intensively for many years. Earlier studies of preselected patients seeing psychiatrists focused on psychodynamic aspects of repressed anger, compulsiveness, rigidity, and perfectionism as causative factors in migraine. Recent studies have shown less specificity for these personality factors in migraine. Awareness of personality features and characteristics in patients with headache can be useful in both diagnosis and treatment. Migraineurs have an increased incidence of the comorbid conditions of anxiety, depression, and panic disorder, suggesting that these disorders and migraine may have a common biologic basis.

Headaches, unplanned, unscheduled, and unwanted, may provoke a variety of reactions depending on the patient's basic personality. The most common reactions—denial, depression, hostility, anger, and the development of dependency—are usually not conscious or voluntary, and will improve with a good patient–physician relationship and/or resolution of symptoms. If they persist, a psychiatric evaluation or psychotherapy may be required.

REFERENCES

Ad Hoc Committee on Classification of Headache (1962). Special report. *JAMA 179:* 717–718.

Adler, C.L., S.M. Adler, and R.C. Packard (1987). *Psychiatric Aspects of Headache.* Williams & Wilkins, Baltimore.

Adler, G. (1981). The physician and the hypochondriacal patient. *N. Engl. J. Med. 304:* 1394–1396.

Alexander, F. (1950). *Psychosomatic Medicine.* W.W. Norton & Co., New York.

American Psychiatric Association (1987). *Diagnostic and Statistical Manual of Mental Disorders,* 3rd ed., rev. American Psychiatric Press, Inc., Washington, DC.

Andrasik, F., E.B. Blanchard, J.G. Arena et al. (1982). Psychological functioning in headache sufferers. *Psychosom. Med. 44:*171–182.

Bana, D.S., J.R. Graham, and E. Spierings (1988). Headache patients as they see themselves. *Headache 28:*403–408.

Berkman, L.F. and S.L. Syne (1976). Social class, susceptibility and sickness. *Am. J. Epidemiology 104:*1–8.

Blanchard, E.B., F. Andrasik, and J.G. Arena (1984). Personality and chronic headache. In *Progress in Experimental Personality,* Vol. 13, (B.A. Maher, ed.). Academic Press, New York.

Blanchard, E.B., S.M. Baskin, K.A. Appelbaum et al. (1990). Similarities and differences in MMPI profiles of headache patients at a headache clinic and university setting. *Headache Q. Curr. Treat. Res. 1:*51–53.

Blanchard, E.B., C.A. Kirsch, K.A. Appelbaum et al. (1989). The role of psychopathology in chronic headache: Cause or effect? *Headache 29:*295–301.

Blau, J.N. (1990). Migraine theory and therapy: Their relationship. *Headache Q. Curr. Treat. Res. 1:*15–22.

Blumenthal, L.S. (1968). Tension headache. In *Handbook of Clinical Neurology,* Vol. 5 (P.J. Vinken and G.W. Bruyn, eds.), pp. 157–171. North-Holland Publishing, Amsterdam.

Blumer, D. (1986). Chronic muscle contraction headache and the pain prone disorder. In *Psychiatric Aspects of Headache* (C.L. Adler, S.M. Adler, and R.C. Packard, eds.), pp. 124–130. Williams & Wilkins, Baltimore.

Blumer, D. and M. Heilbronn (1981). The pain prone disorder: A clinical and psychological profile. *Psychosomatics 22:*395–402.

Boag, T.F. (1968). Psychogenic headache. In *Handbook of Clinical Neurology,* Vol. 5 (P.J. Vinken and G.W. Bruyn, eds.), pp. 247–257. North-Holland Publishing, Amsterdam.

Brett, J.M. (1980). The effect of job transfer on employees and their families. In *Current Concepts in Occupational Stress* (C.L. Cooper and R. Payne, eds.), pp. 99–136. John Wiley & Sons, New York.

Breuer, J. and S. Freud (1955). Case histories. In *The Complete Psychological Works of Sigmund Freud, Vol. 2, Studies on Hysteria* (J. Strachey, ed. and transl.), p. 23. The Hogarth Press, London.

Brodsky, C.M. (1984). Long-term work stress. *Psychosomatics 25:*361–368.

Christensen, J.F. (1981). Assessments of stress: Environmental, intrapersonal, and outcome issues. In *Advances in Psychological Assessment,* Vol. 5 (P. McReynolds, ed.), pp. 62–123. Jossey-Bass, San Francisco.

Cohen, M.J. (1978). Psychophysiological studies of headache: Is there similarity between migraine and muscle contraction headaches? *Headache 18:*189–196.

Dembrosky, T.M., M. Feinleib, S.E. Haynes et al. (1978). *Coronary Prone Behavior.* Springer-Verlag, New York.

Diamond, S. (1987). Depression and headache. In *Psychiatric Aspects of Headache* (C.L. Adler, S.M. Adler, and R.C. Packard, eds.), pp. 259–274. Williams & Wilkins, Baltimore.

Friedman, A.P. (1958). The mechanism and treatment of migraine and tension headache. *Mississippi Valley Med. J. 80:*141–146.

Friedman, A.P. and C. Brenner (1950). Psychological mechanisms in chronic headache. *Proc. Assoc. Res. Nerv. Ment. Dis. 29:*605–608.

Friedman, A.P., J.C. VonStorch, and H.H. Merritt (1954). Migraine and tension headache; a clinical study of two thousand cases. *Neurology 4:*773–774.

Friedman, M. and R.H. Rosenman (1974). *Type A Behavior and Your Heart,* Chap. 13. Fawcett Crest, New York.

Fromm-Reichmann, F. (1937). Contribution to the psychogenesis of migraine. *Psychoanal. Rev. 24:*26–33.

Garrity, T.F., M.D. Marx, and G. Somes (1977). Personality factors in resistance to illness after recent life changes. *J. Psychosom. Res. 21:*23–32.

Girdano, D.A. and G.S. Everly (1979). *Controlling Stress and Tension,* pp. 100–101. Prentice-Hall, Englewood Cliffs, NJ.

Gorlin, R. and H.D. Zucker (1983). Physician's reactions to patients. *N. Engl. J. Med. 308:*1059–1063.

Graham, J.R. (1964). Treatment of muscle contraction headache. In *Modern Treatment,* Vol. 1, pp. 1399–1403. Harper & Row, New York.

Graham, J.R. (1968). Cluster headache. *Proceedings of the International Symposium on Headache,* Chicago, October, pp. 21–23.

Graham, J.R. (1987). The headache patient and the doctor. In *Psychiatric Aspects of Headache* (C.S. Adler, S.M. Adler, and R.C. Packard, eds.), pp. 34–40. Williams & Wilkins, Baltimore.

Graham, J.R. (1990). Cluster headache: The relation to arousal, relaxation, and autonomic tone. *Headache 30:*145–151.

Groves, J.E. (1978). Taking care of the hateful patient. *N. Engl. J. Med. 298:*883–887.

Headache Classification Committee of the International Headache Society (1988). Classification and diagnostic criteria for headache disorders, cranial neuralgias, and facial pain. *Cephalalgia* 8(Suppl. 7):1–96.

Henryk-Gutt, R., and W.L. Rees (1973). Psychological aspects of migraine. *J. Psychosom. Res. 17:*141–153.

Holmes, T.H. and R.N. Rahe (1967). The social readjustment rating scale. *J. Psychosom. Res. 11:*213–218.

Holyroyd, K.A., G.E. Coringley, J.D. Pingel et al. (1989). Enhancing the effectiveness of abortive therapy: A controlled evaluation of self-management training. *Headache 29:*148–153.

Horenstein, S. (1983). Emotional aspects of neurologic disease. In *Clinical Neurology* Vol. 4 (A.B. Baker and L.H. Baker, eds.), Chap. 64, pp. 1–3. Harper & Row, New York.

Horowitz, M.J. (1976). *Stress Response Syndrome,* p. 56. Jason Aronson, Inc., New York.

Invernizzi, G., C. Gala, M. Buono et al. (1989). Neurotic traits and disease duration in headache patients. *Cephalalgia 9:*173–178.

Ivancevich, J.M. and M.T. Matteson (1980). *Stress and Work,* p. 113. Scott, Foreman and Company, Illinois.

Jonckheere, P. (1971). The chronic headache patient. *Psychother. Psychosom. 19:*53–61.

Jones, N.F. (1989). Cognitive, behavioral and emotional responses to stressful events: A study of their relationships to headache activity. *Cephalalgia* 9(Suppl. 10): 248–249.

Kahana, R.J. and G.L. Bibring (1964). Personality types in medical management. In *Psychiatry and Medical Practice in the General Hospital* (N.E. Zinberg, ed.), pp. 108–123. International University Press, New York.

Knopf, O. (1935). Preliminary report on personality studies in thirty migraine patients. *J. Nerv. Ment. Dis. 82:*270–285.

Kolb, L.C. (1959). Psychiatric and psychogenic factors in headache. In *Headache, Diagnosis and Treatment* (A.P. Friedman and H.H. Merritt, eds.). F.A. Davis, Philadelphia.

Kolb, L.C. (1963). Psychiatric aspects of the treatment of headache. *Neurology 13:* 34–37.

Kudrow, L. (1979). MMPI pattern specificity in primary headache disorders. *Headache 19:*18–24.

Kudrow, L. (1980). *Cluster Headache: Mechanisms and Management.* Oxford University Press, London.

Kudrow, L. (1983). Cluster headache: new concepts. In *Neurologic Clinics: Symposium on Headache*, Vol. 1. (R.C. Packard, ed.), pp. 369–383. W.B. Saunders, Philadelphia.

Lance, J.W. (1981). Headache. *Ann. Neurol. 10:*1–10.

Lazarus, R.S. (1981). Little hassles can be dangerous to health. *Psychol. Today 58:*62.

Lindsay, P.G. and M. Wyckoff (1981). The depression-pain syndrome and its response to antidepressants. *Psychosomatics 2:*571–577.

MacKinnon, R.A. and R. Michels (1971). The psychosomatic patient. In *The Psychiatric Interview in Clinical Practice,* p. 365. W.B. Saunders, Philadelphia.

Marcussen, R.M. (1949). Vascular headache experimentally induced by presentation of pertinent life experiences: Modification of course of vascular headache by alternations of situations and reactions. *Proc. Assoc. Res. Nerv. Ment. Dis. 29:* 609–614.

Martin, M.J. (1972). Muscle contraction headache. *Psychosomatics 13:*16–19.

Martin, M.J., H.P. Rome, and W.M. Swenson (1967). Muscle contraction headache: a psychiatric review. *Res. Clin. Stud. Headache 1:*184–204.

Massey, W. and B. Scherokman (1983). Post-traumatic headaches. In *Neurologic Clinics: Symposium on Headache* Vol. 1, (R.C. Packard, ed.), pp. 457–464. W.B. Saunders, Philadelphia.

Mathew, N. (1987). Headache patients and drug abuse. In *Psychiatric Aspects of Headache* (C.L. Adler, S.W. Adler, and R.C. Packard, eds.), pp. 289–297. Williams & Wilkins, Baltimore.

McAnulty, D.P., M.A. Rappaport, P.J. Brantley et al. (1986). Psychopathology in volunteers for headache research: Initial versus later respondents. *Headache 26:*37–38.

Nattero, G., C. DeLorenzo, L. Biale et al. (1989). Psychological aspects of weekend headache sufferers in comparison with migraine patients. *Headache 29:*93–99.

Packard, R.C. (1976). What is psychogenic headache? *Headache 16:*20–23.

Packard, R.C. (1979a). Psychiatric aspects of headache. *Headache 19:*168–172.

Packard, R.C. (1979b). What does the headache patient want? *Headache 19:*370–374.

Packard, R.C. (1980). Conversion headache. *Headache 20:*266–268.

Packard, R.C. (1983). Emotional aspects of headache. In *Neurologic Clinics: Symposium on Headache* Vol. 1 (R.C. Packard, ed.), pp. 445–456. W.B. Saunders, Philadelphia.

Packard, R.C. (1987). Expectations: Of patients with headache and their physicians. In *Psychiatric Aspects of Headache,* (C.S. Adler, S.M. Adler, and R.C. Packard, eds.), pp. 29–33. Williams & Wilkins, Baltimore.

Packard, R.C., F. Andrasik, and R. Weaver (1989). When headaches are good. *Headache 29:*100–102.

Packard, R.C. and P. O'Connell (1986). Medication compliance among headache patients. *Headache 26:*416–419.

Passchier, J., H. VanderHelm-Hylkema, and J.F. Orlebeke (1984). Personality and headache type: A controlled study. *Headache 24:*140–146.

Pearce, J. (1977). Migraine: A psychosomatic disorder. *Headache* 17:125–128.

Phillips, C. (1976). Headache and personality. *J. Psychosom. Res.* 20:535–542.

Rahe, R.A. (1968). Life change measurement as a predictor of illness. *Proc. R. Soc. Med.* 61:1124–1126.

Rahe, R.A. (1979). Life change events and mental illness: An overview. *J. Human Stress* 5:2–10.

Raskin, N. (1988). On the origin of head pain. *Headache* 28:254–257.

Rogado, A.Z., R.H. Harrison, and J.R. Graham (1974). Personality profiles in cluster headache, migraine, and normal controls. *Arch. Neurobiol.* 37(Suppl.):227–241.

Rose, C.L. (ed.) (1982). *Advances in Migraine Research and Therapy.* Raven Press, New York.

Rose, C.L. and M. Gawel (1979). What brings on a migraine attack? In *Migraine: The Facts,* p. 42. Oxford University Press, London.

Saper, J.R. (1983). Migraine: Precipitating factors. In *Headache Disorders: Current Concepts and Treatment Strategies,* p. 34. Wright-PSG Publishers, Littleton, MA.

Schafer, W. (1978). *Stress, Distress and Growth.* International Dialogue Press, Davis, CA.

Schafer, W. (1983). *Wellness through Stress Management,* pp. 24–26. International Dialogue Press, Davis, CA.

Selinsky, H. (1939). Psychologic study of the migrainous syndrome. *Bull. N. Y. Acad. Med.* 15:757–763.

Selye, H. (1976). *The Stress of Life,* p. 412. McGraw-Hill, New York.

Speed, W.G. (1987). Psychiatric aspects of post-traumatic headache. In *Psychiatric Aspects of Headache* (C.S. Adler, S.M. Adler, and R.C. Packard, eds.), pp. 201–206. Williams & Wilkins, Baltimore.

Steinhilber, R.M., J.S. Pearson, and J.G. Rushton (1960). Some psychological considerations of histamic neuralgia. *Proc. Staff Meetings Mayo Clin.* 35:691–699.

Sternbach, R.A., D.J. Dalessio, M. Kunzel et al. (1980). MMPI patterns in common headache disorders. *Headache* 20:311–315.

Toffler, A. (1971). *Future Shock.* Bantam Books, New York.

Touraine, G.A. and G. Draper (1934). The migrainous patient; a constitutional study. *J. Nerv. Ment. Dis.* 80:1–23.

Trowbridge, L.S., O. Cushman, et al. (1943). Notes on the personality of patients with migraine. *J. Nerv. Ment. Dis.* 97:509–517.

Weatherhead, D.L. and R.C. Packard (1987). Conversion headache. In *Psychiatric Aspects of Headache* (C.S. Adler, S.M. Adler, and R.C. Packard, eds.), pp. 194–200. Williams & Wilkins, Baltimore.

Weinstein, E.A. and R.L. Kahn (1955). *Denial of Illness.* Charles C Thomas, Springfield, IL.

Weiss, F. and I.S. English (1957). *Psychosomatic Medicine.* W.B. Saunders, Philadelphia.

Wolff, H.G. (1937). Personality features and reactions of subjects with migraine. *Arch. Neurol. Psychiatry* 37:895–921.

Wolff, H.G. (1963). Cranial pain sensitive structures. In *Headache and Other Head Pain,* 2nd ed. (H.G. Wolff, ed.), pp. 59–97. Oxford University Press, New York.

21

Behavioral Management of Headache

ALAN H. ROBERTS

Headache is one of the most frequently encountered pain complaints. It is estimated that approximately 80% of people experience a headache in any given year (Waters, 1975). Most of these people will not consult a physician. When they do, it is ordinarily because the headaches are unusual, because the pain has become a source of concern, or because it is interfering with the patient's ability to function. Of patients seeking treatment for headaches, the vast majority are diagnosed as having migraine, tension-type, or a combination of both. Most often a diagnostic evaluation, a prescription, and reassurance are sufficient to resolve the problem satisfactorily. For a subgroup of patients with otherwise benign headache, however, the problem may become chronic. It is this group of headache patients that presents the greatest challenge to clinicians.

It is well recognized that there is a relationship between illness and behavior (Fordyce, 1976; Mechanic, 1962). Succinctly put, *illness* is what a person has, whereas *illness behavior* is what a person does. The simplicity of this statement belies the complexity of the relationship between the two.

The physiologic definition of pain includes a psychological component. This psychological component has a profound impact on both the evaluation and treatment of pain. The complex relationships among the physiologic components, the psychological components, and the manifestations of pain through behavior are most clearly evident in the management of chronic headaches. For the clinician to focus only on the physiologic aspects of pain (as in diagnosis) or the sensory aspects of pain (as in treatment) is to ignore what is often the most critical integrant of the problem: the social, motivational, and affective properties that, in turn, become apparent in behavior.

These complex components of the experience of pain generally are not a major problem for the acute pain associated with an injury that persists only until healing occurs. When pain becomes chronic, however, as so often happens with headaches, psychological and socioenvironmental factors play an increasing role in the experience of pain, the expression of pain through behavior, and the patient's response to treatment. Pain is neither psychogenic nor somatic (Fordyce, 1991). It is an interaction among psychological, social, and environmental factors that modulate nociceptive stimulation and the response to treatment (Turk and Holzman, 1986).

Pain has been defined as "an unpleasant sensory and emotional *experience* associated with actual or potential tissue damage, or described in terms of such damage" (IASP Subcommittee on Taxonomy, 1979). As an experience, one person's pain cannot be known directly by another. For that reason, it must be judged by observing the patient's vocalizations, facial expressions, posture, or peripheral autonomic responses. The patient may be asked to describe, rate, or categorize his or her pain; all of these are behaviors.

Until the 1960s, there were few legitimate forms of treatment available to chronic headache sufferers other than pharmacologic and related medical procedures. Around that time, three psychological approaches to pain management emerged, all of which have application to the management of chronic headache. These consist of operant techniques intended to alter the behaviors of patients, biofeedback and relaxation techniques aimed at altering the physiology of the patient, and cognitive techniques designed to change the patient's thinking (McGrath and Craig, 1989).

The first of these is represented by Wilbert E. Fordyce's application of operant behavioral conditioning techniques to the management of chronic pain and illness (Fordyce, 1976, 1986). The second approach is represented by the application of biofeedback techniques to the treatment of headaches (Sargeant et al., 1972). The third is the use of cognitive techniques to treat chronic pain (Meichenbaum and Turk, 1976; Turk et al., 1983). Each of these approaches can be considered separately, but in clinical practice they may be used simultaneously.

OPERANT BEHAVIORAL TECHNIQUES

Following Fordyce's publication of the operant behavioral methods he developed for treating chronic pain and illness (Fordyce, 1976), their use has become almost universal in legitimate pain treatment programs and clinics in the United States (Fordyce et al., 1985). Instead of assuming either a medical or a psychological cause for disability associated with pain, the behavioral methods focus directly on the actions or behaviors of patients and their families. Behavior modification techniques are used to help patients change selected behaviors in order to improve function. They are not used to treat pain directly.

Some Basic Concepts

The rationale and methods of operant behavioral applications are best understood in terms of some basic concepts. *Behavior* refers to the overt or observable actions of a patient. Focusing on behavior does not deny the reality of inner, covert, or cognitive events. Isolating behavior as a focus for treatment simply recognizes that the clinician cannot observe directly or modify the subjective experiences of a patient. Only the external expressions of the patient's experience are accessible. The term "pain behaviors" refers to observable expressions of pain by the patient.

An *operant* is an expressed behavior that may be governed by a *reinforcer* or reward that follows the behavior. Although pain behaviors are usually, although not invariably, initiated by some actual or potential tissue damage, they may persist beyond healing for many reasons. Among these reasons is the possibility that they may have been reinforced (rewarded) by powerful consequences in the patient's environment. These consequences are sometimes referred to as *contingencies*, because the occurrence of the reinforcers is contingent on the occurrence of the pain behaviors. In the behavioral analysis of pain, attention is focused on the relationship between the occurrence of a pain behavior and the consequent occurrence of a reinforcing contingency.

Operant pain behaviors such as crying, moaning, or holding the head usually begin as a direct response to a noxious stimulant. In addition, these operants may result in contingencies that are rewarding to the patient. When this happens, the reinforced behavior is strengthened and is more likely to occur again. Similarly, when healthy (well) behaviors are not reinforced, they are likely to diminish in strength and frequency. In managing the illness behavior of a chronic headache patient, an attempt is made to reverse this chain of events. If illness behaviors are not reinforced they are less likely to occur. Healthy behaviors are strengthened when they are consistently reinforced.

Potential reinforcers for the *excess disability* (Roberts, 1986a,b) associated with chronic headaches may include medications for pain, sleep, or tension; solicitousness from family members or others; attention from physicians or other health care professionals; financial incentives for disability; relief from situations in which the patient has difficulties coping, such as employment outside the home, responsibilities, or sexual demands; or a variety of other family, social, medical, or work-related factors. For each patient, the determination of applicable reinforcers must be assessed and managed separately.

It follows that the *goals* of behavioral treatment for chronic headaches (chronic pain behaviors) are different from the goals of traditional medical treatment. Operant behavioral methods are not intended to treat headache "pain." Rather, they are intended to treat excess disability (Roberts, 1986a,b) and expressions of suffering. The treatment goal is to render the chronic headache patient functional again and as normal in behavior as possible. This is done by changing the relationships between the disabling illness behaviors and their reinforcing contingencies.

Behavioral Assessment

Candidates for contingency management are patients with chronic headaches of greater than 3 months' duration who have not responded to appropriate medical treatment and who are functionally disabled by their headaches. When medications, biofeedback training, or relaxation training have failed, the most difficult patients often respond to contingency management techniques.

Consider a patient with migraine headaches that have been managed medically for several years. The headaches wax and wane, but when they have worsened, they have responded to changes in medication. Follow-up visits have averaged two to three times a year. Then, gradually, the headaches seem to worsen. There are more frequent office visits. The intensity of the headaches increases and they last longer. Medications are changed or increased and the patient is using more prescription analgesics. The physician receives more and more phone calls from the patient and occasionally from a desperate spouse.

The patient is spending more time in bed and losing more work time. There begin rare and then more frequent emergency room visits, and injectable medications are administered perhaps once or twice a month. The physician recognizes that medications may be exacerbating the headaches but cannot justify withholding them in light of the patient's expressions of suffering. Current stresses in the patient's life have been discussed (Feuerstein et al., 1983; Headache Classification Committee of the International Headache Society, 1988; Levor et al., 1986), and the patient insists that the headache is his or her chief source of stress. This patient clearly has analgesic rebound headache and requires a multidimensional treatment plan (see Chapter 5).

Such patients have been described by several researchers and clinicians (Blanchard et al., 1989a; Burg, 1987; Vanast, 1987a,b) and are candidates for operant behavioral management. Blanchard et al. (1989a) have defined a group of patients like this who are refractory to biofeedback and relaxation therapies and suggest that these kinds of headache patients are candidates for contingency management.

The behavioral treatment of these patients begins with a behavioral assessment. In this assessment the clinician does not focus on the medical problem responsible for the symptoms and complaints. Instead, the focus is on the behavioral consequences of headaches. Helpful questions to ask in a behavioral assessment include the following:

What makes the headache worse (going to work, stress, arguing, heat, cold, etc.)?

What makes the headache better (heat, cold, dark room, massage, peace and quiet, medications, etc.)?

What does the spouse or other family members do to help (assume home chores, leave the patient alone, provide emotional support, etc.)?

Is the patient receiving any disability payments or anticipating doing so?

Is litigation pending? If so, how large a settlement is anticipated?

If the headaches could be "cured," what would the patient do that is not being done now (return to work outside the home, assume more homemaking tasks, participate in family recreation and other activities, exercise, sex, etc.)?

What does the spouse say or do when the patient has a headache? Is the headache a source of conversation at home or at work? Does the spouse or others know when the patient has a headache without being told? If so, what is the response? What could the respondent do instead?

The responses to questions like these provide the clinician with data concerning pain behaviors and potential reinforcers for alternative well behaviors. They define the extent of disability and assist in constructing behavioral treatment goals. These goals should be defined to help the patient return to normal levels of function for age and sex.

Components of Treatment

The usual operant program includes several components, but these vary from patient to patient depending on the outcome of the behavioral analysis. The individualized programs are designed to decrease all controllable reinforcers for pain behaviors and disability while increasing reinforcers for healthy behaviors.

A critical component in operant programs is withdrawal of the patient from all medications with addiction potential. Although there is still some controversy about medication rebound headaches, there is increasing evidence of the profoundly reinforcing consequences of medications that initially reduce headaches at the time they are taken (Anderson, 1975; Baumgartner et al., 1989; Göbel et al., 1992; Michultka et al., 1989; Rowsell et al., 1973).

Caffeine is a frequent and particularly pernicious source of reinforcement for headache pain. Found in both over-the-counter and prescription medications as well as common beverages, it is often overlooked because of the frequency of its use, its general social acceptance, and the common perception that it is benign. Caffeine, however, improves mood (Lieberman et al., 1987) and rapidly reduces some vascular headaches (Greden et al., 1980). Withdrawal from caffeine may be negatively reinforcing by stimulating rebound headaches (Greden et al., 1980). Finally, caffeine has additional reinforcing properties because of its independent analgesic effects (Ward et al., 1991).

Yet another destructive form of medication for chronic headaches is analgesics administered by injection. This too is often overlooked as a potential reinforcer for headaches because the patient may be receiving the injections only once or twice a month. Because of the infrequency of use, the patient is considered not to be dependent on the injected drugs. Milligan and Atkinson (1991) have recently demonstrated, however, that 85% of patients receiving injections for chronic pain have a return-of-pain interval that coincides with the proximity of their next clinic appointment. They term this phenomenon "the two week syndrome."

Some recent studies have shown that medications and behavioral treatments can be equally effective (Holroyd and Penzien, 1990). Fordyce (1976) has demonstrated how headache pain may be reinforced by medications prescribed for pain. The reinforcing qualities of these medications are strengthened further when they are prescribed prn ("as needed") because the taking of medication is associated with feeling better. When the medication wears off, the headache rebounds. The mechanism for this can be either physiologic or psychological but probably is both.

In operant treatment, patients are slowly withdrawn from all medications that may be reinforcing the headache pain. Any patient who overuses medication is likely to have an operant component to the pain. Put another way, if the patient is overusing medication, the medication is, by definition, reinforcing and must be withdrawn. Multiple drugs should be reduced to a minimum. Nonaddicting (i.e., nonreinforcing) medications should be prescribed on a time-contingent rather than a pain-contingent basis so as to reduce the relationship between pain reduction and the medication.

A major goal of operant treatment is to increase physical activity. This is often accomplished in a physical therapy exercise program, which will reinforce slowly increasing activity and withdraw reinforcement for time spent being inactive. A number of operant techniques to accomplish this have been described by Fordyce (1976), Roberts (1986a,b), and others.

A final and often necessary treatment strategy is to teach family members to stop reinforcing pain behaviors and pain complaints and instead to reinforce normal activities. It is also very useful to work with the patient's health care support system to accomplish these same ends.

The most recent critical evaluation of these methods is the analysis by Fordyce et al. (1985). More recent reviews of behavioral treatment methods (Holroyd and Penzien, 1986, 1990; Iezzi et al., 1989) have tended to focus more on biofeedback and related techniques.

In summary, operant behavioral management is an effective treatment for the most difficult of chronic headache patients. For those who have failed medical management and alternative behavioral techniques, it may be the only feasible approach. The majority of chronic headache patients can be treated on an outpatient basis unless they are severely addicted to their medications. It is important to keep in mind that these methods do not imply a psychoneurotic etiology for the headache; they are valid for any person excessively disabled by headache. The purpose of treatment is to manage the disability and not an underlying psychogenic cause for the problem (see also Chapter 5).

BIOFEEDBACK AND RELATED TECHNIQUES

Biofeedback is a technique used to display some aspect of a patient's physiologic functioning to the patient with the expectation that he or she will be able to use that information to attain increased voluntary control over the physiologic function being displayed. The physiologic function must be detected, transduced, amplified, and then displayed. Typical functions include heart rate, skin temperature, skin conductance, peripheral blood flow, muscle tension, and blood pressure. It is generally understood that the measured functions must be displayed (fed back) to the patient immediately and continuously.

Theoretically, a person who is well motivated and rewarded can learn to increase or decrease voluntarily the rate or amplitude of the function being measured so as to control that function. For example, Roberts and his colleagues (Roberts et al., 1973, 1975) demonstrated that human subjects could learn to control the skin temperature of their hands reliably so as to make one hand warmer or colder than the other and then reverse the sequence on demand.

The study and development of biofeedback emerged from two contrasting movements (Roberts, 1985). The first was stimulated by the scientific fields of learning theory, psychophysiology, and the experimental analysis of behavior. The question of most interest to those disciplines at the time was the issue of whether or not the autonomic nervous system could be taught to respond to instrumental operant conditioning or whether autonomous nervous system responses could be shaped only by classic conditioning—a theoretical rather than a clinical issue.

The second movement developed from the work of Jacobson on progressive relaxation (1938), Schultz on autogenic training (Schultz and Luthe, 1969), and interest in altered states of consciousness, transcendental meditation, Yoga, Zen Buddhism, the relaxation response, and similar "self-control" procedures. Roberts (1985) and Yates (1980) provided brief accounts of these historic antecedents to biofeedback treatment. Despite 20 or more years of research, the relationship between the scientific study of these two areas (altered states and operant learning of autonomic responses) and the clinical application of biofeedback is still highly controversial (Duckro, 1990, 1991; Roberts, 1985; Shellenberger and Green, 1986).

Biofeedback Methods

The two most frequent applications of biofeedback to headaches are the training of patients to warm their hands and to reduce muscle tension. In the former, temperature measuring devices are attached to the patient's fingers. Information about increases or decreases in temperature are fed back to the patient immediately and continuously through visual display or by means of an increasing or decreasing auditory tone. Muscle tension is recorded using electromyographic (EMG) measuring devices that are strategically placed to record muscle activity of the head, face, neck, shoulders or upper back. This information is also fed back to the patient visually or by means of an auditory signal.

Although peripheral skin temperature is usually associated with the treatment of migraine headaches and muscle tension with the treatment of tension-type headaches, in practice both are generally used with both kinds of headaches. Only one study comparing patients with migraine with or without aura has shown differential effectiveness using biofeedback (Gauthier et al., 1988).

Relaxation training is also taught to patients by biofeedback therapists. Often the patients are provided with tape recordings of progressive relaxation, guided imagery, or autogenic instructions. The patient is expected to listen to these recordings at home, thus practicing relaxation techniques. Sometimes these tapes are confused with the concept of biofeedback and patients are simply provided with tapes and sent home to practice on their own. It is very unlikely that this practice by itself will have much positive effect on the outcome of headaches of any variety.

Efficacy

Biofeedback and relaxation techniques increasingly are becoming a part of standard practice in the comprehensive treatment of tension-type and migraine headaches. Recent reviews and meta-analytic studies of the efficacy of biofeedback in treating chronic migraine and tension-type headaches (Andrasik, 1989, 1990; Andrasik and Blanchard, 1987; Blanchard and Andrasik, 1987; Jessup, 1989; Turk and Rudy, 1991) concluded that biofeedback, relaxation training, or combinations of the two improve headaches when compared to no treatment, some other psychological treatments, and even pharmacologic treatments. Between 35 and 50% of treated patients report at least 50% reduction in headache activity. One third to one half of treated patients do not improve. Although clinically impressive, these figures are well within the range of effectiveness that can be attributed solely to nonspecific effects (Roberts et al., in press).

When biofeedback and relaxation training are compared, there is little evidence that one is any better than the other (Jessup, 1989). Reich (1989) compared biofeedback, relaxation training, and electrical stimulation in a longitudinal study. Patients were randomly assigned to short-term (less than 15 sessions) or long-term (more than 15 sessions) treatment. All treatments reduced the intensity and frequency of headaches. Reich also reported that certain combinations of variables (biofeedback, relatively short chronicity, and longer term treatment) were the best predictors of success.

Mechanisms of Treatment Effects

The mechanisms by which biofeedback and relaxation treatments reduce headache activity are not understood. Most hypothesize that headaches are at least partly associated with stress and that the treatments somehow reduce the effects of tension. The 1962 Ad Hoc Committee on Classification of Headache specifically stated that tension-type headaches occur as part of the individual's reaction to life stress. The more recent revision (Headache Classification Committee of the International Headache Society, 1988) is less explicit but still instructs clinicians to evaluate psychosocial stressors. Bakal (1982) and others have speculated that tension-type and migraine headaches may have a common etiology. Although biofeedback and relaxation training may reduce peripheral autonomic activity, the relationship of this to "stress" in general and to the etiology of tension-type and migraine headaches remains caliginous at best.

Despite the demonstrated efficacy of biofeedback and relaxation training in reducing the frequency and intensity of headache activity, there is as yet no convincing evidence that these techniques are either necessary or sufficient methods of treatment (Roberts, 1985). Biofeedback, as used in clinical practice, includes many components in addition to physiologic feedback information. Examples are education to acquire relaxation skills, stress management training, counseling by the therapist, and medication changes. A universal component is a variety of nonspecific and placebo effects that may be very powerful when compared to alternative therapies (Roberts et al., in press). Any of these may account for the inability of researchers to demonstrate specific effects or the superiority of biofeedback to other modalities such as relaxation training. For example, Kewman and Roberts (1980), in a double-blind study of biofeedback and migraine headaches, found no evidence of specific effects. Temperature training to cool the hands was just as effective as hand-warming training.

Recently Blanchard et al. (1991) compared the use of home practice of biofeedback with no home practice in a study using hand-temperature training to manage migraine headaches. Although both treatment groups improved compared to a no-treatment control group, there was no advantage for the group practicing at home between sessions. This is an important finding because regular home practice has been considered to be a major, perhaps necessary, component for the successful application of biofeedback in clinical settings. This study raises additional questions about what is being learned and how it exerts treatment effects.

Some studies (Blanchard et al., 1983) find a dose–response relationship between target biofeedback responses and headache response. Other studies (Morrill and Blanchard, 1989; Werbach and Sandweiss, 1978) do not. Blanchard and his colleagues recently provided hand temperature norms for 221 headache patients, 105 hypertensive patients, 45 patients with irritable bowel syndrome, and 56 normal controls (Blanchard et al., 1989b). Across five conditions of measurement, they found that their migraine headache groups had significantly lower hand temperatures than did the other groups.

Maintenance of Improvement

Most studies of biofeedback efficacy have reported only short-term treatment effects. More recently, a few studies have attempted long-term follow-up of patients treated with biofeedback and relaxation training (Andrasik and Holroyd, 1983; Blanchard et al., 1987a,b, 1988; Ford et al., 1983). These studies have reported effectiveness maintained for as long as 5 years. One study, for example, followed 9 tension-type and 12 migraine headache patients prospectively for 5 years (Blanchard et al., 1987a). They reported that 78% of tension-type headache and 91% of migraine headache patients were still improved. Another study by the same group (Blanchard et al., 1988) compared home-based, minimal therapist contact treatment of chronic tension-type headaches with a clinic-based treatment protocol. With up to 2 years of follow-up, they found the minimal treatment protocol to be at least as effective as treatment in the clinic.

Holroyd's group (Holroyd et al., 1989) compared biofeedback and relaxation training treatment with medical pharmacologic treatment prospectively for 3 years. Nineteen of 21 successfully treated patients in both groups continued to show lower headache activity than before treatment. The medication-treated patients were more likely to have required further medical treatment and they were also more likely to still be using prophylactic or narcotic medications. Although the number of patients followed was small and there was no untreated control group, Holroyd et al. concluded that improvements with behavioral treatment may be more likely to be maintained without additional treatment than similar improvements with medications. They acknowledge the preliminary nature of their conclusions.

In another study (Sovac et al., 1981), biofeedback combined with relaxation was found to be similar in effectiveness to propranolol and analgesics. Mathew (1981) compared biofeedback to a variety of drugs and combination of drugs to treat migraine and mixed migraine–tension-type headache patients. Biofeedback was found to be more effective than abortive and analgesic treatment. Although prophylactic medication exceeded biofeedback effectiveness, the addition of biofeedback to prophylactic medication increased effectiveness by about 10 to 20% and the greatest improvement occurred with the combination of prophylactic medication and biofeedback.

Two studies have compared EMG biofeedback and medical treatment for tension-type headaches. In the first (Bruhn et al., 1979), biofeedback outcomes were superior to those achieved using "the most suitable" medical treatment. The second study (Paiva et al., 1982) compared EMG biofeedback to diazepam and placebo treatments. Diazepam was superior to biofeedback initially. At follow-up, however, the patients treated with medication deteriorated while those treated with biofeedback showed treatment gains.

Although a number of procedures have been proposed for enhancing long-term maintenance (Lynn and Freedman, 1979), few, if any, have so far been shown to be effective. Overall, studies of the relationship between effectiveness, maintenance, and such variables as amount of practice are mixed (Turk and Rudy, 1991). Some studies do, but most studies do not provide evidence of a relationship between practice and maintaining improvement (Turk and Rudy, 1991). When a relationship has been shown between practice and effectiveness or maintenance, it may be because those who do not improve simply stop practicing. Those who improve for any reason, whether or not related to specific or nonspecific effects, may be reinforced to continue practice (superstitious response learning). The recent study by Blanchard et al. (1991) further questions the utility of practice.

Cost-Effectiveness

Some studies raise questions about the potential cost-effectiveness of biofeedback and relaxation training. This is particularly true of studies exploring minimal therapist interventions (Blanchard et al., 1988; Richardson and McGrath, 1989) and comparing behavioral with pharmacologic treatments (Holroyd et al., 1989; Sovac et al., 1981). Two reports have specifically addressed the issue of cost-effectiveness in a preliminary way. Blanchard et al. (1985a) reported that comparable headache reduction can be obtained from mainly self-administered home treatment when compared to therapist-administered clinic treatment. They then concluded that home treatment is more cost-effective. Amar et al. (1989) reviewed some preliminary data that led her to speculate that behavioral medicine treatments can be cost-effective.

COGNITIVE–BEHAVIORAL THERAPY

The cognitive–behavioral approach to treating headaches is different from both biofeedback, which is intended to alter the patient's physiologic status, and operant behavioral treatment, which is intended to reduce a patient's maladaptive illness behaviors. The goal of cognitive therapy techniques is to provide patients with a set of problem-solving and coping skills that they can use to manage stressors and situations that are thought to be associated with pain (Meichenbaum and Turk, 1976; Turk et al., 1983). Broader and more diverse than either operant behavioral pain management or biofeedback techniques, cognitive–behavioral therapies include treatment approaches described as rational–emotive therapy, coping skills therapy, self-instructional training, problem-solving therapy, and self-control approaches (Turk et al., 1983). These treatment methods are typically active, time limited, and structured. The goal of therapy is to help the patient correct maladaptive and distorted ideas and dysfunctional beliefs. Patients are helped to become aware of the role that negative thoughts and images play in maintaining the maladaptive behaviors. Specific examples of applications of these methods are provided by Holzman et al. (1986) and Turk et al. (1983).

In the case of headaches, cognitive–behavioral therapy focuses on the relationships among cognitions, feelings, and behaviors and how these variables contribute to the maintenance of both psychological and physical problems. The treatment concentrates on helping patients manage their pain before it becomes severe. In particular, cognitive stress coping training provides patients with a set of flexible problem-solving skills that they can use to manage situations or stressors that are associated with headaches.

Most often, these techniques have been studied in combination with other methods. Andrasik (1990) called attention to the fact that cognitive techniques play a role in all psychological treatments for headache in that patients must be educated to accept and understand the treatment, must be motivated to practice learned skills to achieve therapeutic proficiency levels, and must be willing to apply what is learned to their daily lives. It goes without saying that similar cognitive factors also apply to medical treatment. Andrasik (1990), Turk et al. (1983), and McCarran and Andrasik (1987) have all reviewed the relatively few empirical studies of cognitive therapy for headaches. In general, cognitive treatments seem to improve migraine and tension-type headaches at levels comparable to biofeedback.

Richardson and McGrath (1989) compared cognitive–behavioral therapy in the clinic, the same therapy with only minimal therapist contact, and waiting-list control patients in a randomized control trial. At 6 months' follow-up, both treatment groups had reduced headache frequency, intensity, and peak intensity when compared to the control patients. As would be expected, the minimal therapist contact treatment was considered to be more cost-effective.

Richter et al. (1986) compared relaxation training, cognitive coping training, and placebo treatments for migraine headaches in a pediatric population. They found both active treatments to be superior to placebo but not different from each other. The active treatments reduced headache activity and frequency but not duration or intensity. Those patients with more severe headaches responded better than those with milder headaches. Unless the activity and frequency of headaches before and after treatment are perfectly correlated, however, this is an inevitable consequence of regression toward the mean (Dawes, 1988).

The Blanchard research group has recently reported on two studies using cognitive therapy treatments for migraine headaches (Blanchard et al., 1990a,b) and two for tension-type headaches (Appelbaum et al., 1990; Blanchard et al., 1990c). In a comparison of thermal biofeedback combined with relaxation training, thermal biofeedback combined with cognitive therapy, an attention placebo treatment, and headache monitoring for patients with migraine headaches (Blanchard et al., 1990b), all three treatment groups (including the attention placebo group) improved compared to headache monitoring. There were no differences among the three treatment groups, however.

In the other study of migraine headaches (Blanchard et al., 1990a), two home-based treatment groups were compared. The first used thermal biofeedback and relaxation and the second received cognitive stress coping instructions. A control group monitored their headaches. Both treatment groups reduced headache activity and medication use compared to controls. They did not, however, differ from each other.

The two studies of these treatments applied to tension-type headaches appear to contradict each other. The first (Appelbaum et al., 1990) evaluated the effects of adding cognitive therapies to a home-based relaxation treatment. They concluded that both treatment groups improved when compared to a control group but did not differ from each other. The second (Blanchard et al., 1990c) showed some advantage to adding a cognitive therapy component to progressive muscle relaxation.

Summarizing, relatively few studies of the effectiveness of cognitive therapy strategies applied to headaches are available. The preliminary findings suggest that further research is justified, as is often the case in early research on psychological treatment, but the efficacy and power of these approaches is yet to be determined. Adding these techniques to other behavioral methods may or may not increase efficacy but, if it does, the added effects appear not to be very impressive so far. Still, these methods do no harm when compared, for example, to some of the potential effects of medications, especially for children and pregnant women. Thus continued work in this area seems reasonable, especially for special groups.

SPECIAL GROUPS

Two special groups stand out with respect to behavioral management: the elderly and children. Some studies have reported a negative correlation between aging and response to biofeedback and related treatments (Blanchard et al., 1985b; Diamond and Montrose, 1984; Holroyd and Penzien, 1986). Arena and Hightower (1988), in a study of relaxation therapy for tension-type headache in the elderly, pointed out that, despite the decline of effectiveness for the elderly, some do learn with more extended treatment.

Kabela et al. (1989) tried various combinations of relaxation, cognitive coping, and biofeedback in an uncontrolled series of headache patients ages 60 to 77. At 1 month's follow-up they found clinically significant reductions in both headache activity and medication use. They found their results to be encouraging and recommended prospective controlled evaluations of the elderly with long-term follow-up. These kinds of studies of the elderly are mostly conspicuous in their absence.

There seems to be somewhat greater interest in the application of behavioral methods to children and adolescents. Lascelles et al. (1989) have described therapeutic techniques that can be used with adolescents who have migraine headaches. Reviews of studies of behavioral applications to pediatric headaches (Andrasik, 1989; Andrasik et al., 1986; Duckro and Cantwell-Simmons, 1989; Larsson, 1989) have been published and support the use of these techniques with this special group. In particular, Larsson's review (1989) supports the efficacy of relaxation as a viable first approach to treating both migraine and tension-type headaches in adolescents. His recent follow-up with Melin of 108 adolescents treated with behavioral methods (1989) showed 80 to 85% of patients improved at 5 to 6 months and 3 to 4 years. The treatments were administered in a school-based treatment program (Larsson et al., 1987). Guibert et al. (1990) have evaluated variables associated with compliance with behavioral treatments of headaches in both children and adolescents. Children with fewer headaches were more likely to adhere to treatment, as were older children.

Two studies of relaxation (McGrath et al., 1988) and biofeedback (Burke and Andrasik, 1989) support the effectiveness of these techniques with children and adolescents through 1 year's follow-up. Andrasik (1990) pointed out that children and adolescents appear to be more enthusiastic about psychological interventions and may respond at a level superior to adults. Nonpharmacologic treatments, if effective, would be particularly attractive for this special group. There is no reason to believe that these techniques are any less effective for pediatric headaches than for adult headaches (Andrasik, 1989).

SUMMARY

Behavioral management approaches for headaches are of three types: those that attempt to change the patient's behavioral responses to pain, those that attempt to alter the patient's thinking and coping responses, and those that are intended to alter the patient's physiologic responses. There is some overlap among them in application. All are, to some degree, effective in managing chronic headaches. Because, by definition, chronic headaches are those that have not responded to medical treatment, it is clear that these methods can contribute in important ways to the management of distressing and disabling headaches. All of these methods address complex biobehavioral and social components of headaches in ways that are often neglected in standard medical care, and this may account for their effectiveness when medical treatments are ineffective.

Operant behavioral management techniques are comprehensive and are most likely to be effective when other treatments have failed. They are generally reserved for more functionally disabled patients. Biofeedback methods are more often used but generally are more controversial. A large number of clinicians in psychology seem to believe that the clinical issues contributing to this controversy cannot be addressed by research (Newman and Howard, 1991). Some have pointed out that the clinical research is sometimes poorly conceived or executed and that is undoubtedly true. Others have argued (e.g., Duckro, 1990, 1991) that such research is not possible at this time. Still others (e.g., Roberts, 1985) have taken the position that competent and applicable research is available and is simply being misunderstood or ignored by clinicians. The ways in which biofeedback and relaxation techniques improve headaches is unknown, thus contributing to the continuing controversy. They may be effective because of a variety of nonspecific and specific effects that are poorly understood (Roberts et al., in press). Because between one third and one half of patients with migraine, tension-type headache, or both appear to benefit from these treatments, however, they are appropriate for use in comprehensive management programs for chronic headaches. Younger patients seem to benefit most and older patients least, but all patients are eligible candidates.

The research relating to cognitive management techniques for chronic headaches is sparse. There is no evidence suggesting that they are less effective than biofeedback and relaxation techniques. Adding cognitive therapy to other behavioral therapies probably does not increase efficacy to a clinically significant degree, but this needs to be further evaluated.

For all of these behavioral methods, questions remain unanswered concerning mechanisms, efficacy, and matching treatments to patients. Refinements of these various strategies are sorely needed. Questions concerning cost-effectiveness are only recently beginning to be addressed. Overall, however, all of these methods are benign, more so than some medical treatments, and all have been shown to be effective for some patients when selectively and appropriately applied. It follows that they deserve to be considered when deciding on treatment for chronic headaches.

REFERENCES

Ad Hoc Committee on Classification of Headache (1962). Classification of headache. *JAMA 179:*717–718.
Amar, P., R. Shellenberger, C. Schneider, and R. Steward (1989). *Cost-effectiveness and Clinical Efficacy of Biofeedback Therapy: Guidelines for Third Party Reimbursement.* Association for Applied Psychophysiology and Biofeedback, Wheat Ridge, CO.
Anderson, P.G. (1975). Ergotamine headache. *Headache 15:*118–121.
Andrasik, F. (1989). Biofeedback applications for headaches. In *Clinical Perspectives on Headaches and Low Back Pain* (C. Bischoff, H.C. Traue, and H. Zenz, eds.), pp. 181–200. Hogrefe Publishing, Lewiston, ME.
Andrasik, F. (1990). Psychological and behavioral aspects of chronic headache. *Neurol. Clin. 8:*961–976.
Andrasik, F., D.D. Blake, and M.S. McCarran (1986). A biobehavioral analysis of pediatric headache. In *Child Health Behavior: A Behavioral Pediatrics Perspective* (N.A. Krasnegor, J.D. Arasteh, and M.F. Cataldo, eds.), pp. 394–434. John Wiley & Sons, New York.
Andrasik, F. and E.B. Blanchard (1987). The biofeedback treatment of tension head-

ache. In *Biofeedback: Studies in Clinical Efficacy* (J.P. Hatch, J.G. Fisher, and J.D. Rugh, eds.), pp. 281–321. Plenum, New York.

Andrasik, F. and K.A. Holroyd (1983). Specific and nonspecific effects in the biofeedback treatment of tension headaches: 3-year follow-up. *J. Consult. Clin. Psychol. 51:*634–636.

Appelbaum, K.A., E.B. Blanchard, N.L. Nicholson et al. (1990). Controlled evaluation of the addition of cognitive strategies to a home-based relaxation protocol for tension headache. *Behav. Ther. 21:*293–304.

Arena, J.G. and N.E. Hightower (1988). Relaxation therapy for tension headache in the elderly: A prospective study. *Psychol. Aging 3:*96–98.

Bakal, D.A. (1982). *The Psychology of Chronic Headache*. Springer-Verlag, New York.

Baumgartner, C., P. Wessely, C. Bingöl et al. (1989). Long-term prognosis of analgesic withdrawal in patients with drug-induced headaches. *Headache 29:*510–514.

Blanchard, E.B. and F. Andrasik (1987). Biofeedback treatment of vascular headache. In *Biofeedback: Studies in Clinical Efficacy* (J.P. Hatch, J.G. Fisher, and J.D. Rugh, eds.), pp. 1–79. Plenum, New York.

Blanchard, E.B., F. Andrasik, K.A. Appelbaum et al. (1985a). The efficacy and cost-effectiveness of minimal-therapist-contact, non-drug treatment of chronic migraine and tension headache. *Headache 25:*214–220.

Blanchard, E.B., F. Andrasik, D.D. Evans et al. (1985b). Behavioral treatment of 250 chronic headache patients: A clinical replication series. *Behav. Ther. 16:*308–327.

Blanchard, E.B., F. Andrasik, D.E. Neff et al. (1983). Four process studies in the behavioral treatment of chronic headache. *Behav. Res. Ther. 21:*209–220.

Blanchard, E.B., K.A. Appelbaum, P. Guarnieri et al. (1987a). Five-year prospective follow-up on the treatment of chronic headache with biofeedback and/or relaxation. *Headache 27:*580–583.

Blanchard, E.B., K.A. Appelbaum, P. Guarnieri et al. (1988). Two studies of the long-term follow-up of minimal-therapist contact treatments of vascular and tension headache. *J. Consult. Clin. Psychol. 56:*427–432.

Blanchard, E.B., K.A. Appelbaum, N.L. Nicholson et al. (1990a). A controlled evaluation of the addition of cognitive therapy to a home-based biofeedback and relaxation treatment of vascular headache. *Headache 30:*371–376.

Blanchard, E.B., K.A. Appelbaum, C.L. Radnitz et al. (1989a). The refractory headache patient. I. Chronic, daily, high-intensity headache. *Behav. Res. Ther. 27:*403–410.

Blanchard, E.B., K.A. Appelbaum, C.L. Radnitz et al. (1990b). A controlled evaluation of thermal biofeedback combined with cognitive therapy in the treatment of vascular headache. *J. Consult. Clin. Psychol. 58:*216–224.

Blanchard, E.B., K.A. Appelbaum, C.L. Radnitz et al. (1990c). A placebo-controlled evaluation of abbreviated progressive muscle relaxation and relaxation combined with cognitive therapy in the treatment of tension headache. *J. Consult. Clin. Psychol. 58:*210–215.

Blanchard, E.B., P. Guarnieri, F. Andrasik et al. (1987b). Two-, three-, and four-year prospective follow-up on the behavioral treatment of chronic headache. *J. Consult. Clin. Psychol. 55:*257–259.

Blanchard, E.B., B. Merrill, D.A. Wittrock et al. (1989b). Hand temperature norms for headache, hypertension and irritable bowel syndrome. *Biofeedback Self Regul. 14:*319–331.

Blanchard, E.B., N.L. Nicholson, C.L. Radnitz et al. (1991). The role of home practice in thermal biofeedbacks. *J. Consult. Clin. Psychol. 59:*507–512.

Bruhn, P., J. Olesen, and B. Melgaard (1979). Controlled trial of EMG feedback in muscle contraction headache. *Ann. Neurol. 6:*34–36.

Burg, H.E. (1987). Variable somataform disorder presenting as intractable chronic headache. *Headache 27:293.*

Burke, E.J. and F. Andrasik (1989). Home- vs. clinic-based biofeedback treatment for pediatric migraine: Results of treatment through one-year follow-up. *Headache 29:434–440.*

Dawes, R.M. (1988). *Rational Choice in an Uncertain World.* Harcourt Brace Jovanovich, San Diego.

Demjen, S. and D. Bakal (1986). Subjective distress accompanying headache attacks: Evidence for a cognitive shift. *Pain 25:187–194.*

Diamond, S. and D. Montrose (1984). The value of biofeedback in the treatment of chronic headache: A four-year retrospective study. *Headache 24:5–18.*

Duckro, P.N. (1990). Biofeedback in the management of headache—Part 1. *Headache Q. 1:290–298.*

Duckro, P.N. (1991). Biofeedback in the management of headache—Part 2. *Headache Q. 2:17–22.*

Duckro, P.N. and E. Cantwell-Simmons (1989). A review of studies evaluating biofeedback and relaxation training in the management of pediatric headache. *Headache 29:428–433.*

Feuerstein, M., L. Bortolussi, M. Houle, and E. Labbé (1983). Stress, temporal artery activity, and pain in migraine headache: A prospective analysis. *Headache 23: 296–304.*

Fitzpatrick, R.M., A.P. Hopkins, and O. Harvard-Watts (1983). Social dimensions of healing: A longitudinal study of outcomes of medical management of headaches. *Soc. Sci. Med. 17:501–510.*

Ford, M.R., C.F. Stroebel, P. Strong, and B.L. Szarek (1983). Quieting response training: Long-term evaluation of a clinical biofeedback practice. *Biofeedback Self Regul. 8:265–278.*

Fordyce, W.E. (1976). *Behavioral Methods for Chronic Pain and Illness.* C.V. Mosby, St. Louis.

Fordyce, W.E. (1986). Learning processes in pain. In *The Psychology of Pain,* 2nd ed. (R.A. Sternbach ed.), pp. 49–65. Raven Press, New York.

Fordyce, W.E. (1991). On opioids and treatment targets. *Am. Pain Soc. Bull. 1:1–4.*

Fordyce, W.E., A.H. Roberts, and R.A. Sternbach (1985). The behavioral management of chronic pain: A response to critics. *Pain 22:113–125.*

Gannon, L.R., S.N. Haynes, J. Cuevas, and R. Chavez (1987). Psychophysiological correlates of induced headaches. *J. Behav. Med. 10:411–427.*

Gauthier, J., C. Fradet, and C. Roberge (1988). The differential effects of biofeedback in the treatment of classical and common migraine. *Headache 28:39–46.*

Göbel, H., M. Ernst, J. Jeschke et al. (1992). Acetylsalicylic acid activates antinociceptive brainstem reflex activity in headache patients and in healthy subjects. *Pain 48:187–195.*

Greden, J.F., B.S. Victor, P. Fontaine, and M. Lubetsky (1980). Caffeine-withdrawal headache: A clinical profile. *Psychosomatics 21:411–418.*

Guibert, M.B., P. Firestone, P. McGrath et al. (1990). Compliance factors in the behavioral treatment of headache in children and adolescents. *Can. J. Behav. Sci. 22:* 37–44.

Headache Classification Committee of the International Headache Society (1988). Classification and diagnostic criteria for headache disorders, cranial neuralgias and facial pain. *Cephalalgia 8*(Suppl. 7):1–96.

Holroyd, K.A., J.F. Holm, D.B. Penzien et al. (1989). Long-term maintenance of improvements achieved with (abortive) pharmacological and nonpharmacological treatments for migraine: Preliminary findings. *Biofeedback Self Regul. 14:* 301–308.

Holroyd, K.A. and D.B. Penzien (1986). Client variables and the behavioral treatment of recurrent tension headache: A meta-analytic review. *J. Behav. Med. 9:*515–536.

Holroyd, K.A. and D.B. Penzien (1990). Pharmacological versus non-pharmacological prophylaxis of recurrent migraine headache: A meta-analytic review of clinical trials. *Pain 42:*1–13.

Holzman, A.D., D.C. Turk, and R.D. Kerns (1986). The cognitive-behavioral approach to the management of chronic pain. In *Pain Management: A Handbook of Psychological Treatment Approaches* (A.D. Holzman and D.C. Turk, eds.), pp. 31–50. Pergamon Press, New York.

IASP Subcommittee on Taxonomy (1979). Pain terms: A list with definitions and notes on usage. *Pain 6:*249–252.

Iezzi, A., H.E. Adams, R.N. Pilou, and S.S. Averitt (1989). Psychological management of headache pain. In *Handbook of Chronic Pain Management* (C.D. Tollison, ed.), pp. 264–274. Williams & Wilkins, Baltimore.

Jacobson, E. (1938). *Progressive Relaxation.* University of Chicago Press, Chicago.

Jessup, B. (1989). Relaxation and biofeedback. In *Textbook of Pain,* 2nd ed. (P.D. Wall and R. Melzack, eds.), pp. 989–1000. Churchill Livingston, New York.

Kabela, E., E.B. Blanchard, K.A. Appelbaum, and N. Nicholson (1989). Self-regulatory treatment of headache in the elderly. *Biofeedback Self Regul. 14:*219–228.

Kewman, D. and A.H. Roberts (1980). Skin temperature biofeedback and migraine headaches: A double-blind study. *Biofeedback Self Regul. 5:*327–345.

Larsson, B. (1989). Psychological treatment of recurrent headache in adolescents. In *Headache in Children and Adolescents* (G. Lanzi, U. Balottin, and A. Cernibori, eds.), pp. 325–332. Excerpta Medica, Amsterdam.

Larsson, B. and L. Melin (1989). Follow-up on behavioral treatment of recurrent headache in adolescents. *Headache 29:*249–253.

Larsson, B., L. Melin, M. Lamminen, and F. Ullstedt (1987). A school-based treatment of chronic headaches in adolescents. *J. Pediatr. Psychol. 12:*553–566.

Lascelles, M.A., S.J. Cunningham, P. McGrath, and M.J.L. Sullivan (1989). Teaching coping strategies to adolescents with migraine. *J. Pain Symptom Management* 4(3):135–145.

Levor, R.M., M.J. Cohen, B.D. Naliboff et al. (1986). Psychosocial precursors and correlates of migraine headache. *J. Consult. Clin. Psychol. 54:*347–353.

Lieberman, H.R., R.J. Wurtman, G.G. Emde, and I.L. Coviella (1987). The effects of caffeine and aspirin on mood and performance. *J. Clin. Psychopharmacol. 7:* 315–319.

Lynn, S.J. and R.R. Freedman (1979). Transfer and evaluation of biofeedback treatment. In *Maximizing Treatment Gains: Transfer Enhancement in Psychotherapy* (A. Goldstein and F. Kahfer, eds.), pp. 445–485. Academic Press, New York.

Mathew, N.T. (1981). Prophylaxis of migraine and mixed headache: A randomized control study. *Headache 21:*105–109.

McCarran, M.S. and F. Andrasik (1987). Migraine and tension headaches. In *Anxiety and Stress Disorders: Cognitive Behavior Assessment and Treatment* (L. Michelson and M. Ascher, eds.), pp. 465–483. Guilford Press, New York.

McGrath, P.J. (1990a). Paediatric pain: A good start. *Pain 41:*253–254.

McGrath, P.A. (1990b). *Pain in Children: Nature, Assessment, Treatment.* Guilford Press, New York.

McGrath, P.J. and K.D. Craig (1989). Developmental and psychological factors in children's pain. *Pediatr. Clin. North Am. 36:*823–836.

McGrath, P.J., P. Humphreys, J.T. Goodman et al. (1988). Relaxation prophylaxis for childhood migraine: A randomized placebo-controlled trial. *Dev. Med. Child Neurol. 30:*626–631.

Mechanic, D. (1962). The concept of illness and behavior. *J. Chronic Dis. 15:*189–194.

Meichenbaum, D.H. and D.C. Turk (1976). The cognitive-behavioral management of anxiety, anger, and pain. In *The Behavioral Management of Anxiety, Depression, and Pain* (P.O. Davidson, ed.), pp. 1–33. Brunner/Maze, New York.

Melzack, R. (1986). Neurophysiological foundations of pain. In *The Psychology of Pain,* 2nd ed. (R.A. Sternbach, ed.), pp. 1–24. Raven Press, New York.

Michultka, D.M., E.B. Blanchard, K.A. Appelbaum et al. (1989). The refractory headache Patient-II: High medication consumption (analgesic rebound) headache. *Behav. Res. Ther. 27:*411–420.

Milligan, K.A. and R.E. Atkinson (1991). The "two-week syndrome" associated with injection treatment for chronic pain—fact or fiction? *Pain 44:*165–166.

Morrill, B. and E.B. Blanchard (1989). Two studies of the potential mechanisms of action in the thermal biofeedback treatment of vascular headache. *Headache 29:* 169–176.

Newman, F.L. and K.I. Howard (1991). Introduction to the special section on seeking new clinical research methods. *J. Consult. Clin. Psychol. 59*(2):8–11.

Paiva, T., J.S. Nunes, A. Moreira et al. (1982). Effects of frontalis EMG biofeedback and diazepam in the treatment of tension headache. *Headache 22:*216–220.

Reich, B.A. (1989). Non-invasive treatment of vascular and muscle contraction headache: A comparative longitudinal clinical study. *Headache 29:*34–44.

Richardson, M. and P.J. McGrath (1989). Cognitive-behavioral therapy for migraine headaches: A minimal-therapist-contact approach versus a clinic-based. *Headache 29:*352–357.

Richter, I.L., P.J. McGrath, P.J. Humphreys et al. (1986). Cognitive and relaxation treatment of paediatric migraine. *Pain 25:*195–203.

Roberts, A.H. (1985). Biofeedback: Research, training, and clinical roles. *Am. Psychol. 40:*938–941.

Roberts, A.H. (1986a). Excess disability in the elderly: Exercise management. In *Geropsychological Assessment and Treatment* (L. Teri and P.M. Lewinsohn, eds.), pp. 87–119. Springer-Verlag, New York.

Roberts, A.H. (1986b). The operant approach to the management of pain and excess disability. In *Pain Management: A Handbook of Physicological Treatment Approaches* (A.D. Holzman and D.C. Turk, eds.), pp. 10–30. Pergamon Press, New York.

Roberts, A.H., D.G. Kewman, and H. MacDonald (1973). Voluntary control of skin temperature: Unilateral changes using hypnosis and feedback. *J. Abnorm. Psychol. 8a:*163–168.

Roberts, A.H., D.G. Kewman, L. Mercier, and M. Hovell (in press). The power of nonspecific effects in healing: Implications for psychosocial and biological treatments. *Clin. Psychol. Rev.*

Roberts, A.H., J. Schuler, J. Bacon et al. (1975). Individual differences and autonomic control: Absorption, hypnotic susceptibility, and the unilateral control of skin temperature. *J. Abnorm. Psychol. 84:*272–279.

Rowsell, A.R., C. Neylan, and M. Wilkinson (1973). Ergotism-induced headache in migranous patients. *Headache 13:*65–67.

Sargeant, J.D., E.E. Green, and E.D. Walters (1972). The use of autonomic training in a pilot study of migraine headaches. *Headache 12:*120–124.

Schultz, J.H. and W. Luthe (1969). *Autogenic Therapy.* Grune & Stratton, New York.

Shellenberger, R. and J. Green (1986). *From the Ghost in the Box to Successful Biofeedback Training.* Health Psychology Publications, Greeley, CO.

Solomon, F. and K.G. Cappa (1987). Is chronic daily headache a form of tension headache? *Headache 27:*302–303.

Sovac, N., M. Kunzel, R. Sternbach, and D.J. Dalessio (1981). Mechanism of the biofeedback therapy of migraine: Volitional manipulation of the psychophysiological background. *Headache 21:*89–92.

Turk, D.C. and A.D. Holzman (1986). Chronic pain: Interfaces among physical, psychological, and social parameters. In *Pain Management: A Handbook of Psychological Treatment Approaches* (A.D. Holzman and D.C. Turk, eds.), pp. 1–9. Pergamon Press, New York.

Turk, D.C., D. Meichenbaum, and M. Genest (1983). *Pain and Behavioral Medicine: A Cognitive Behavioral Perspective.* Guildford Press, New York.

Turk, D.C. and T.E. Rudy (1991). Neglected topics in the treatment of chronic pain patients—relapse, noncompliance, and adherance enhancement. *Pain 44:*5–28.

Vanast, W.J. (1987a). Research strategies in benign, almost daily headache: I. The Edmonton criteria for patient inclusion. *Headache 27:*295–296.

Vanast, W.J. (1987b). Research strategies in benign, almost daily headache: II. District study groups based on age at consultation and age at onset. *Headache 27:*296.

Ward, N., C. Whitney, D. Avery, and D. Dunner (1991). The analgesic effects of caffeine on headache. *Pain 44:*151–155.

Waters, W.E. (1975). Epidemiology of migraine. In *Modern Topics in Migraine* (J. Pearce, ed.), pp. 8–21. William Heinemann, London.

Werbach, M.R. and M.A. Sandweiss (1978). Peripheral temperatures of migraineurs undergoing relaxation training. *Headache 18:*211–214.

Yates, A.J. (1980). *Biofeedback and the Modification of Behavior.* Plenum Press, New York.

22

Clinical Observations on Headache

DONALD J. DALESSIO
STEPHEN D. SILBERSTEIN

HEADACHE GAMES: DEALING WITH THE DIFFICULT HEADACHE PATIENT

In 1978 James E. Groves published his now-classic paper on "Taking Care of the Headache Patient." He described four classes of patients who might strike dread into a physician's heart, but was careful to note that a single patient might encompass more than one of these attributes. His four stereotypes were:

1. *Clingers:* patients whose demands escalate from mild and appropriate requests for reassurance to repeated cries for explanation, review, and critique of their multiple complaints. Often, repeated requests for drugs are made, especially analgesics and sedatives. These patients devise multiple ruses for gaining and securing attention.
2. *Entitled Demanders:* patients who use intimidation, threats, and induction of guilt (in their physician) to get what they want. They frequently threaten litigation, or at least allude to it. They may attempt to coerce the physician into playing along with their insurance ploys. Often they will seek disability status for dubious medical problems. If provoked, they may be dangerous.
3. *Manipulative Help-Rejecters:* patients for whom nothing works. No therapeutic regimen is ever successful. Often possessed of multiple complaints, they frequently describe allergies to multiple compounds. For example, "I'm allergic to all antibiotics." Despite the absence of therapeutic responses, they return again and again to the physician's office to report that, once again, the physician has failed. Many of these patients are depressed but refuse to recognize depression when it is suggested to them.
4. *Self-Destructive Deniers:* patients who often practice poor health habits but refuse to give them up. They request care, diagnosis, and treatment of all types but refuse to alter destructive life-styles. Some of this behavior could be considered suicidal over the long term.

To these four stereotypes, we have added a fifth called, for lack of a better name, the day-ruiner. The day-ruiner usually arrives on the office doorstep, notes in hand, prepared to settle in for a prolonged period of intense discussion. Many of these patients appear to have found special comfort in prepaid organizations such as health maintenance organizations, which allow them to visit the physician's office frequently without the pain of paying for the interaction. They are characterized by striking adaptiveness, and are capable of turning an ordinary 15-minute visit into an hour-long verbal wrestling match. Furthermore, they are often late but insist on being seen nonetheless, and they are frequently married to persons of similar personality. The day-ruiner is best described as demanding, manipulative, tangential, disorganized (or hyperorganized), frustrating, complaining, litigious, disputatious and cantankerous.

These stereotypes are familiar to most practicing physicians. Like other difficult patients, they sometimes engage in games with headache as the primary complaint, hence the term "headache games."

Headache Games

It is important at this point to provide a disclaimer. Headache patients are generally easily treated. Many do not require medical assistance, and those who do usually respond to standard treatments. They are anxious to return to their endeavors, and aggravated by the annoyance that headache invariably produces. Of course, there are exceptions—persons with migraine or cluster headache, or even tension-type headache, who need more careful management of their headache problems. Here again, most patients respond to appropriate therapies, and the vast majority can be helped by a knowledgeable physician.

A small group of headache patients remains. This is the chronic group, characterized by persisting complaints and resistance to treatment, and often very difficult to deal with professionally. It is this group that we have characterized, and separated, into the 10 headache games that follow.

Headache Game #1
This is the "You're my last hope, doctor" game:

> None of the other doctors I've seen have done me any good. Most of them shouldn't have licenses. All they're interested in is money. They order too many tests. But I know you'll be different, doctor.

Commentary. Do not fall into this trap. Often this game is played by the person who accompanies the headache patient. Both parties (husband and wife, or mother and child, for example) may contribute. It is unlikely that all previous physicians seen by the patient have been greedy and incompetent. You can be sure that you are next on the list for this form of doctor bashing.

Solution. Advise that you are not a magician, and no miracles are likely to occur. We tell patients that physicians all use the same medications. If you suspect your patient is litigious, be especially careful about criticizing your colleagues. Be helpful, assertive, and supportive, but maintain your distance from these patients.

Headache Game #2
This is the "It's my diet" game:

> I know it's some food I'm eating. Of course I've given up most foods and all I eat now are scallions and broccoli with garlic powder. I never touch sugar, and meat is so bad for you. But I keep having headaches. Could I have some allergy tests?

Commentary. We generally advise a healthy diet with regular meals and provide guidance regarding this matter. Although diet may be a provoking factor in migraine, it is important to point out that it is only one factor among many. Eating a rigidly restricted diet is unwise. It tends to reinforce obsessive habit patterns and the concept that some foods are "bad for you."

Solution. Send the patient for professional nutritional help, or have him or her purchase a cookbook for migraine patients. Or devise dietary guidelines of your own, and instruct the patient in their use. Eating should be one of life's great pleasures. Emphasize that to your patient.

Headache Game #3
This is the "It's my sinuses" game:

> I've had my nose fixed, and two Caldwell-Lucs, and turbinates removed, but I keep having sinus troubles. I can't breathe through my nose and the pain at the bridge of my nose is awful. It radiates through my ears and down the back out my tailbone. If only I could get my nose and sinuses straightened out, everything would be fine.

Commentary. This is an example of obsessive preoccupation with a single organ system. Although chronic sinusitis can produce chronic headache, the diagnosis is usually readily evident. Given today's modern methods of investigation, there should be no real problem of establishing the diagnosis or excluding it. The pain pattern described here is also bizarre, and does not fit anatomic guidelines.

Solution. Once a problem has been thoroughly investigated, one should move on to other etiologies. Discourage dwelling on a single organ system. Change the topic. Do not abet the situation by agreeing to another consultation, another study, or another operation.

Headache Game #4
This is the "It's my TMJ" game, "and my tongue burns, too."

> I've been to three dentists, had complete caps, my bite has been reworked, and I almost had both TM joints replaced, but at the last minute I decided against that procedure. My teeth and gums burn all the time and my mouth is so sore I just can't stand it. Do you think it could be my dental fillings? Should I have another gum biopsy?

Commentary. Unless you are doubly trained in dentistry, our advice is to deflect questions about temporomandibular joint (TMJ) disease to the dental profession. If patients come to us and advise their problem is with the TMJ, we tell them immediately that they have been referred incorrectly, and we try to steer them appropriately.

Solution. Our test for TMJ disease is to have the patient open and close the mouth repeatedly. If there's no pain and if the mouth capacity is adequate, we would look elsewhere for a headache etiology. Magnetic resonance imaging of the TMJ may show degenerative changes, but that is true of almost every joint in the body, as one ages. Conservative treatment of this problem is best. Try not to contribute to what may be an oral fixation, often a problem in these patients.

Headache Game #5
This is the "I need Demerol" game:

> Now look doctor, let's get one thing straight. I don't respond to anything but Demerol [or Percodan]. I'm allergic to everything else, or it doesn't work, so don't give me any NSAIDs, antidepressants, anxiolytics, et cetera, et cetera, and furthermore, I'm resistant to Demerol so I need big doses, like 200 mg, and maybe repeated once or twice. And I'm not an addict, I know my body.

Commentary. This patient is seeking drugs. Requests for a specific narcotic, with a specific dose, should always arouse suspicion. However, addiction implies daily use, with increasing doses to achieve the same effect. Appearing at an emergency room once every several months for an injection is not addiction.

Solution. Other drugs can be employed in this situation and are, in fact, more effective. Both sumatriptan and dihydroergotamine (DHE-45) can be used. If only Demerol or another narcotic relieves your patient, it can be employed provided such use does not become a habit. You can always just say no.

Headache Game #6
This is the "Everything is wonderful in my life" Game:

> I have such terrible headaches and I don't know why. My husband [wife] is so understanding, what a saint. My son is Phi Beta Kappa at Harvard and my daughter just won three gold medals at the Olympics. We live in a beautiful house with plenty of money and I love my Jaguar convertible. And of course we travel constantly, always first class, staying at the best hotels, in season. Do you suppose if something was wrong I'd feel better?

Commentary. This is the Pollyanna syndrome. Nobody has a perfect life, marriage, or relationship with a spouse and children. Patients like this need to learn that it is normal to have some problems that are difficult to resolve, and they may do well in self-help group sessions where they can learn to vocalize deficiencies and gain support from group dynamics.

Solution. These patients are generally more easily managed than some of the other game players. A behavioral consultation may be helpful. Often biofeedback is useful in this situation. Work with the patient with regular visits and reassurance.

Headache Game #7
This is the "I need alternative medicine" game:

> All the doctors keep giving me are tranquilizers and pills. I know it's a hidden infection. I had food allergy testing and turned up positive to *Candida.* I'm on an anti-*Candida* diet and it isn't easy but I'm sticking to it. I haven't seen any improvement yet but I know I'm on the right track. I'd like your opinion, doctor, about *Candida,* and do you believe in homeopathy, chelation, and acupressure?

Commentary. If patients wish to pursue alternatives to mainstream medicine, we do not raise objections. It is important, however, not to put your personal imprimatur on these projects, especially if they turn out to be expensive and unsuccessful. Be honest and give your opinion without becoming overbearing, angry, and dictatorial. Remember, you are not the patient's parent or caretaker, and you are not responsible for another's behavior.

Solution. Always guide your patient in the directions you believe are appropriate. Be specific in your recommendations, rather than providing alternatives and telling the patient that "It's your choice." That's the essence of a professional opinion. Try not to become offended if your advice is not followed. A little humility is helpful. None of us has all the answers.

Headache Game #8
This is the "I'm allergic to everything" game:

> I've been so weak and fatigued, and the headaches, my God, my head feels like it's splitting with water rushing out and my scalp is on fire and it hurts when I blink. But I found out I'm allergic to light, sound, smell, and touch and so I'm moving to a colony in the high desert where there's no smog or odors or perfumes, where the air and water are clean and pure, and I'm going to grow everything organically and live like people are supposed to live. I'll show organized medicine. I'll make it all the way back, then I'm going to write a book and be on the Oprah show.

Commentary. Make sure that patients such as this are worked up to rule out endocrine disease, myasthenia, and the like. If that has been done, advise the patient that no disease has been found, and that allergy is not a cause of chronic fatigue. If the patient persists and begins to quote from those who lead the clinical ecology movement, advise that chronic fatigue has been a problem for every generation, and was called "the vapors," or neurasthenia, or effort syndrome in past years.

Solution. Treat the patient's opinion with courtesy and respect, but do not agree with him or her, especially if you believe that the proposed solution is not correct professionally. Suggest that the patient transfer to the care of another physician with a different outlook. Be honest but firm, and do not argue with the patient.

Headache Game #9

This is the "I need another test" game:

> I'm sure there's something the matter, but the doctors can't find it. I've had three CAT scans, three MRI's, a TCD, an LP, and a bone scan, and it's all negative. Have you heard of the magnetoencephalograph? Should I have one of those? I'm going to keep going til I find an answer and I don't care how much it costs Medicare! They owe me—I worked hard 40 years and always paid my taxes. By the way, do you accept assignment?

Commentary. This patient is hypochondriacal and believes that a disease is present, despite overwhelming evidence to the contrary. If you follow the patient long enough, of course, the patient will be correct. We are all mortal, and, sooner or later, a discoverable disease will appear. Furthermore, if patients are covered by third-party insurance, or by government funding, the cost of studies is not felt by them, which compounds the problem.

Solution. With newer tests of neurologic function, you may be able to convince these patients that no serious disease is present, particularly by going over the films with them. If this fails, and further work-up is demanded, then stand your ground. Although there are no rewards for denying studies, it is still the honorable thing to do if you believe a study is not indicated.

Headache Game #10

This is the "impossible situation" game:

> Hey, man, it's 2:00 in the morning and I'm having a terrible headache. I've been barfing since supper. I need a shot but I don't have any medicine or syringes or needles. Could you call something in to a pharmacy? I don't want to go to an emergency room, either, it costs too much. And I don't know of any pharmacy that's open and I don't have their telephone number either. I'd sure like some help. Do you have any suggestions? And by the way, before you order anything I need to remind you, in case you have forgotten, that I'm allergic to most medications. What if what you are going to give me doesn't work?

Commentary. There are impossible situations in medicine, and this is one of them. The patient knows it full well. If, by some miracle, you could relieve him of all of his complaints, would he be happier? Probably not. It's especially disheartening when one hears the last sentence above, because the patient, or his enabler, begins to question your plan of treatment before it is even undertaken. Negative thinking of this type is always counterproductive.

Solution. Deferred.

On Prescription Renewals

A final note on problem patients concerns prescription renewals. For the most part, prescriptions are renewed because the patient finds the medication useful and needs more. However, prescription renewals are a legal act and extend the physician–patient contract. Hence, you need to see your patient at reasonable intervals, depending on the drug ordered. This requires a good deal of record keeping, secretarial and clerical help, and overhead for telephone expenses, among others. Thus, it is surprising that so few physicians charge for this service. We never have done so.

Here is a partial list of reasons for prescription renewals that we have found either amusing or irritating:

1. My purse (wallet) was stolen, with my medicines.
2. I've lost the prescription.
3. I've switched pharmacies ($\times 2$, $\times 3$, $\times 4$).
4. By mistake I flushed the medicine down the toilet.
5. My medications all got wet in the rain.
6. My dog (cat, pig) ate the medications.
7. I'm on vacation, I left my medications at home.
8. I couldn't reach my regular doctor during the week so I'm calling you on the weekend (or at 2:00 A.M.).
9. My medications were in my pants and I laundered them by mistake.
10. My grandmother has used all my medicines and I didn't even know it.
11. My suppositories have melted.
12. The triplicate prescription has expired.
13. I didn't have your prescription filled when you wrote it, but now I need it.

Discussion and Conclusions

Are there other guidelines to follow when dealing with difficult patients of these types? Four rules apply.

First, do not dump difficult patients on your colleagues, under the guise of consultation. It is perfectly acceptable to ask for a second opinion, especially regarding management, but this should be done with the expectation that the patient will be returning to you. If you do transfer the patient to a colleague, it is appropriate to call and advise about your problems with the patient. At least then your colleague is forewarned.

Second, do not argue with difficult patients, especially about billing, insurance coverage, and disability status. When possible, pass them along to an ombudsman who is, preferably, not a physician. Many times an ombudsman skilled in interpersonal relationships can resolve issues with courtesy and dispatch, and smooth over ruffled feelings, even if only temporarily.

Third, do not become involved physically. This also applies to any sort of sexual liaison. Physicians are assumed to be trustworthy by patients, and one simply cannot violate that trust. There is no excuse for placing hands on a patient in other than a professional manner for other than professional reasons.

Fourth, do not become disillusioned. Most patients are not in the above categories. Medicine remains a calling, a service profession, and a worthwhile life's pursuit. With attention to courtesy and tactful use of some of the suggestions outlined above, even difficult headache patients can be managed successfully.

SOME OLD CLINICAL SAWS THAT NEED COMMENT

Unilaterality

If headache is always on the same side, should one suspect an aneurysm? What does it mean to have a persistent focal headache? Should the patient be studied? Are angiograms indicated?

The patient's history must be taken seriously, but is the patient providing the diagnosis, or is the history confusing both patient and physician? Focal headaches imply focal disease. The clinician should be alert for local infection such as sinusitis or inflammation (cranial arteritis) or diseases of the facial organs, including the eyes and nose. He or she should also be concerned about endocrine and metabolic diseases, especially diabetes. However, if the headache is typically migrainous, or suggests cluster headache, then it should be accepted as such. Aneurysms are, by and large, nonpainful entities. Angiomas do not often produce pain. Angiomas may rupture, bleed, clot, calcify, provoke seizures, and eventually inhibit learning, but they do not usually hurt.

Many patients with migraine always have their headache on the same side, and there is no requirement that the headache must shift from side to side. This first maxim, then, has produced many unnecessary studies and evoked much needless worry among clinicians. If focal disease is not present, the clinician should accept the persistent repetition of unilateral throbbing head pain as compatible with headache of several types, including migraine and cluster headaches.

Association of Vascular Lesions and Migraine

Are aneurysms common in patients with migraine?

Migraine is a common disease. Aneurysms are infrequent, but it is reasonable to assume that the two entities may occasionally appear in the same patient. There is little evidence that the two syndromes are related. Asymptomatic aneurysms are asymptomatic. If an aneurysm begins to expand rapidly, it will produce a particularly severe localized pain that is not likely to be mistaken for recurrent vascular headache. Those aneurysms that do rupture evoke catastrophic headache, with associated neurologic signs and symptoms, and are related to a sterile inflammatory reaction produced by the presence of blood in the subarachnoid space.

Is migraine a common feature of cerebral arteriovenous anastomoses?

It is true that angiomas may leak briefly and repeatedly. Because the source of the bleeding is usually from anomalous, often venous, blood vessels and is not arterial in type, the headache is not so intense as in subarachnoid bleeding. If sufficient blood is liberated into the subarachnoid space, signs of meningeal irritation will also occur, indistinguishable from those associated with subarachnoid bleeding produced by the rupture of a typical berry aneurysm. Hemispheric angiomas may produce almost any neurologic sign or symptom related to bleeding, calcification, and the production of seizures. Large angiomas may also produce headache.

Is headache therapy straightforward and easy, once the diagnosis is made?

Successful treatment of a patient with headache may not be easily accomplished. The care and sympathy with which the physician relates to his or her patients is indispensable to effective management of each individual headache problem. Cures should not be promised. It is enough to advise the patient that attempts will be made to reduce the intensity and frequency of the headaches. The art of medical practice may be more important than scientific pharmacology. Patience and perseverance on the part of both physician and patient may be necessary. The physician may find that his or her therapeutic suggestions have not achieved the desired result. It is important, then, not to become angry at the patient. Sometimes simple structuring of the environment will help the patient modify some of his or her life goals. At times, the patient will demand a type of practical office psychotherapy, an informal program directed toward guidance and re-education of his or her emotional responses. With careful attention to the whole patient, some resolution of the problem can be achieved in the majority of headache complaints. If the physician suspects a serious thought disorder, psychiatric consultation is mandatory.

Allergy

Is migraine frequently caused by allergy?

It has not been possible to demonstrate that migraine results from any significant or specific antigen–antibody reaction, whether the antigen be an inhaled pollen, an injected material, or food. There is no specific correlation between positive skin tests for various allergens and the appearance of migraine. Dietary migraine may be related to the ingestion of vasoactive substances in a person predisposed to overactivity of vasomotor responses. Thus, long trials of hyposensitization to presumed allergens are not indicated in the chronic treatment of migraine. Hives, allergic rhinitis, ectopic eczema, bronchial asthma, and other manifestations of true allergic reactions cannot be equated with the migraine episode.

MIGRAINE EQUIVALENTS

Migraine may express itself in forms other than hemicranial pain, and these different modes of expression are known as migraine equivalents. The equivalents are paroxysmal, recurrent symptom complexes characterized by the following:

1. Lack of demonstrable organic lesion
2. Previous history of typical migraine headache
3. Replacement of headaches by the equivalent syndrome
4. Absence of symptoms between attacks
5. Family history of migraine
6. Relief from the equivalent syndrome using appropriate drugs

Migraine equivalents may take many forms, including abdominal, ophthalmic, and psychic.

Abdominal migraine is characterized by recurrent episodes of vomiting and/or abdominal pain in association with symptoms of the migraine attack. It is the most common visceral manifestation of migraine. Although it has been reported in patients from infancy to old age, it is most common between the ages of 2 and 11 years, and males are most often affected. Abdominal migraine is often characterized by a prodromal period of yawning, listlessness, drowsiness, or the typical aura of a migraine attack. The episode usually starts suddenly and is precipitated by a specific or stressful experience. The pain may be situated anywhere in the abdomen, but is usually epigastric or periumbilical. The individual bout of pain varies in severity, usually lasts 1 to 6 hours, and is frequently characterized by severe nausea and vomiting. There may also be a typical headache, constipation or diarrhea, lethargy, stuporous sleep, or irritability associated with the attack. Electroencephalography done during the attack may show a mild generalized dysrhythmia, with high-voltage slow waves, thought to be indicative of cerebral hypoxia.

Ophthalmic migraine is also a reasonably well-recognized syndrome, characterized by temporary scotomas, amblyopias, or hemianopsias that occur at the height of the migraine attack instead of acting as a prodrome to the unilateral headache. Many of these patients are men. Some may develop ophthalmic migraine without the subsequent headache.

"Psychic migraine" is probably more common than realized and is characterized by transient mood disorders or psychotic states that replace a typical unilateral headache. Often there is a short prodromal period of lethargy or vigor, followed by a mood disorder lasting from a few hours to days. Many patients experience similar symptoms prior to a typical migraine attack, but in psychic migraine no headache occurs.

Various autonomic dysfunctions are common in patients with migraine. These include Raynaud phenomenon, flushing, and even, on occasion, hemorrhage into the skin. Recurrent febrile episodes as a migraine equivalent have been reported. Recently three young women have been seen, with reasonably typical migraine, who have, in addition, a form of connective tissue disease not clearly defined, perhaps a mixed connective tissue disease or Sjögren syndrome.

HEADACHE AND METABOLIC DISEASE

Headache may be a nonspecific complaint of a number of metabolic disorders, particularly those that lead eventually to disordered cognitive states. These include, but are not limited to, hypernatremia, hyponatremia, acid–base abnormalities, and failure of the liver and kidneys. Generally, however, headache is a minor symptom in these conditions, which are marked by increasing irritability and weakness, confusion, disorientation, and, eventually, coma. As cerebral cortical functions deteriorate, headache is no longer a complaint. Exceptions to the above are:

1. *Hypercapnia:* Some individuals with chronic respiratory failure, primarily those with hypercapnia, will develop severe headache. Marked dilation of cerebral vasculature may occur, and at times papilledema may result. Not all patients with hypercapnia and respiratory failure develop headache, but there clearly is an increase in headache that is roughly proportional to the degree of hypercapnia.
2. *Acidosis:* Acidosis may be associated with headache. The cause is assumed to be the vasodilation that can occur as cerebral autoregulation is affected by the acidotic state.
3. *Hypoglycemia:* Hypoglycemia is associated with a headache that is usually holocranial and may be steady or throbbing.
4. *Thyroid disease:* Headache occurs particularly with hypothyroidism and generally disappears as the disturbance of metabolic function is corrected.
5. *Parathyroid disease:* A particularly intense form of chronic headache is seen in patients with hyperparathyroidism. Generally, the pain is bilateral, and muscular tenderness may be present. The headache is generally improved as the disease is corrected (usually by surgery), but this may take as long as six months to accomplish.

The diagnosis of headache related to metabolic disease has been enhanced by the development of automated multichannel laboratory devices, which measure multiple functions from a single aliquot of the patient's blood. It is prudent to obtain this study in all patients with chronic headache that is otherwise unexplained.

GENERAL REMARKS ON MIGRAINE THERAPY

Counseling

There are three basic approaches to migraine therapy: (1) the symptomatic approach, using medications to abort the acute attack; (2) a preventive approach, using methods of prophylaxis; and (3) prevention by encouraging adjustments in the patient's behavior to avoid situations or substances known to precipitate migraine. Once the diagnosis is established, it is good practice to educate the patient about his or her disorder with a detailed description of suspected mechanisms and common precipitating factors. Contributing psychological factors should also be noted, with encouragement for the patient to communicate personal feelings about what has been presented. Patients are often relieved to find out that their head pain is neither secondary to an organic disease nor "merely" psychogenic.

Abortive versus Prophylactic Therapies

The frequency and duration of migraine attacks are the principal criteria for deciding between the abortive and the prophylactic approach. If the migraine attacks occur two or more times a month, each lasting a day or more, then it is appropriate to consider prophylaxis.

It is important to provide the patient with treatment alternatives that cover all of the potential types of head pain identified in the history. Migraine patients often suffer from tension-type headaches. Also, some patients on prophylactic medications experience "breakthrough" migraine attacks. Abortive medications can be used in this contingency; one should also identify in what circumstances the patient should contact the physician during an attack for further treatment.

All medications in the proposed treatment regimen should be discussed in relation to latency periods, side effects, and complications. With patients on supplemental or replacement estrogen therapy, some adjustments in dose and scheduling may be desirable. Also, patients with a history of chronic head pain often develop a strong over-reliance on analgesics. It is always important to consider the possibility of an established pattern of drug abuse and to provide specific guidance about the use or avoidance of pain medications other than those prescribed.

SURGERY FOR CLUSTER HEADACHE

When should one operate for cluster headache? When medical therapy fails, is the obvious answer. How one constitutes failure is another question. However, if multiple medical therapies have been employed without success, and if the patient is becoming desperate, surgery should at least be considered.

Surprisingly, there is a large and venerable history of surgery for cluster headache, stretching back over five decades and longer. Multiple operations have been proposed, performed, and eventually abandoned. These have included, among others, resection of the ipsilateral greater superficial petrosal nerve, sphenopalatine ganglionectomy, section of the nervus intermedius, and cryosurgery of the facial arteries.

Attention is now focused on the trigeminal ganglion and, in effect, the operations proposed are those usually undertaken in the surgical treatment of trigeminal neuralgia. Cluster headache can be considered as a form of trigeminal vascular reflex response, involving the autonomic nervous system on one side of the face, and from this aspect the operations make sense. In effect, one must injure the ganglion to the extent that the reflex response, which we call cluster headache, is interrupted.

This can be done in several ways. Glycerol injections given into the trigeminal cistern produce the least hypesthesia, and these can be repeated more than once. Percutaneous radiofrequency gangliorhizolysis is preferred by some physicians. With this technique one can expect more facial sensory loss. Finally, posterior fossa sensory rhizotomy can be performed in truly intractable cases. Significant facial hypesthesia and corneal anesthesia may occur after this operation but, nonetheless, these problems can usually be managed. We generally suggest proceeding from one operation to another, depending on the intensity of the cluster headaches and the response to the surgery, moving from the procedure that does the least "damage" to those that produce more sensory loss.

To summarize, surgical therapy is rarely employed in cluster headache patients because medical therapy is almost always successful given the self-limited nature of this syndrome. In an occasional patient with chronic cluster headache who is unrelieved by variegated medical regimens, surgical therapy can at least be contemplated. In this situation, surgical procedures on the trigeminal ganglion/root are most effective.

REFERENCES

Groves, J.E. (1978). Taking care of the hateful patient. *N. Engl. J. Med. 298*:883–887.

Index